Nursing Management for the Elderly THIRD EDITION

Edited by

DORIS L. CARNEVALI, RN, MN

Associate Professor, Emeritus
Community Health Care Systems
School of Nursing, University of Washington, Seattle

MAXINE PATRICK, RN, DrPH

Professor, Physiological Nursing
School of Nursing, University of Washington, Seattle

With 27 contributors

 **J. B. Lippincott Company**
Philadelphia

Acquisitions Editor: Barbara Nelson Cullen
Coordinating Editorial Assistant: Jennifer E. Brogan
Production Manager: Lori J. Bainbridge
Production: P. M. Gordon Associates
Compositor: Pine Tree Composition, Inc.
Printer/Binder: Courier Book Company/Westford

6   5   4   3

Library of Congress Cataloging-in-Publication Data

Nursing management for the elderly / edited by Doris L. Carnevali,
    Maxine Patrick ; with 27 contributors. — 3rd ed.
        p.   cm.
    Includes bibliographical references and index.
    ISBN 0-397-54898-2
    1. Geriatric nursing.   I. Carnevali, Doris L.   II. Patrick,
Maxine.
    [DNLM: 1. Geriatric Nursing.   2. Nursing, Supervisory. 152 N9747]
RC954.N892   1993
610.73'65—dc20
DNLM/DLC
for Library of Congress   92-20793
                                                              CIP

Any procedure or practice described in this book should be applied by the health-care
practitioner under appropriate supervision in accordance with professional standards of
care used with regard to the unique circumstances that apply in each practice situation.
Care has been taken to confirm the accuracy of information presented and to describe
generally accepted practices. However, the authors, editors, and publisher cannot accept
any responsibility for errors or omissions or for consequences from application of the
information in this book and make no warranty, express or implied, with respect to the
contents of the book.

Every effort has been made to ensure drug selections and dosages are in accordance with
current recommendations and practice. Because of ongoing research, changes in government regulations, and the constant flow of information on drug therapy, reactions, and
interactions, the reader is cautioned to check the package insert for each drug for indications, dosages, warnings, and precautions, particularly if the drug is new or infrequently used.

To our parents
Hannah and Helmer Scholin
and
Signe and Ernest Lambrecht
Their skill and zest in living their
later years as fruitfully as their
younger ones, despite age-related
changes and eventual chronic disease, inspired us to try to contribute
professionally to the health and well-
being of other elderly people.

Contributors

James Bennett, DMD
Professor Emeritus (Hospital Dental
    Service)
Oregon Health Sciences University
Portland, Oregon

Lynn Berry, MN, ARNP
Gerontological Nurse Practitioner
Bethany of the Northwest
Everett, Washington

Carol A. Blainey, RN, MN, CDE
Associate Professor
Department of Physiological Nursing
University of Washington
Seattle, Washington

Marian Caudill, MN, ARNP, CS
Geriatric Clinical Specialist
Whitman Nursing Administration Consultant
Walla Walla, Washington

Lee-Ellen Copstead, EdD, NCC, ARNP
Associate Professor
Intercollegiate Center for Nursing
    Education
Spokane, Washington

Lynda Crandall, RN, C, GNP
Gerontological Nurse Practitioner
Oregon State Hospital
Geropsychiatric Treatment Program
Outreach and Consultation Service
Salem, Oregon

Ruth Craven, RN, EdD
Associate Professor, Department of
    Physiological Nursing
Assistant Dean, Continuing Nursing Education
University of Washington
Seattle, Washington

Howard Creamer, PhD (Deceased)
Formerly Associate Professor
Chairman, Oral Microbiology and
    Immunology
School of Dentistry
Oregon Health Sciences University
Portland, Oregon

Denise Renton Davignon, MN, ARNP,
    GNP
Clinical Instructor
Department of Physiological Nursing
University of Washington
Research Associate
General Internal Medicine
Seattle Veterans' Affair Medical Center
Seattle, Washington

Connie Davis, MN, CS
Research Associate
General Internal Medicine
Seattle Veterans' Affairs Medical Center
Seattle, Washington

Kris Dietsch, MN, ARNP
Gerontological Nurse Practitioner
Cascade Vista and Evergreen Vista
    Convalescent Centers
Redmond, Washington

Carolyn H. Enloe, MN, ARNP
Clinical Instructor
Department of Physiological Nursing
University of Washington
Institutional Nursing Consultant
Nursing Home Complaint and Resolution
    Unit
State of Washington
Seattle, Washington

Sharon Filipcic, MN, ARNP
Gerontological Nurse Practitioner
Bessie Burton Sullivan Skilled Nursing
    Residence
Instructor
School of Nursing
Seattle University
Seattle, Washington

Marsha D. Fretwell, MD
Clinical Associate Professor of Medicine
Brown University School of Medicine
Medical Director, The Aging 2000 Project
Providence, Rhode Island

Margaret Heitkemper, RN, PhD
Professor
Department of Physiological Nursing
University of Washington
Seattle, Washington

Nancy Hoffart, RN, PhD
Assistant Professor
School of Nursing
University of Kansas Medical Center
Kansas City, Kansas

Joan M. Karkeck, MS, RD, CD
Director of Clinical Dietetic Programs
Nutrition Sciences
University of Washington
Seattle, Washington

Suzanne C. Lareau, RN, MS
Pulmonary Clinical Nurse Specialist
Jerry L. Pettis VA Medical Center
Assistant Clinical Professor of Nursing
Loma Linda University
School of Nursing
Loma Linda, California

Maria Linde, RN
Nurse Coordinator
American Parkinson's Disease I&R Center
Clinical Associate
Department of Physiological Nursing
University of Washington
Seattle, Washington

Thomas R. McCormick, DMin
Senior Lecturer
Department of Medical History and Ethics
University of Washington
School of Medicine
Seattle, Washington

Susan A. Morgan, PhD, C, GNP
Private Practice/Consultant
Adjunct Associate Professor
Vanderbilt University
Nashville, Tennessee

Deanna Ritchie, RN, MN
Cardiac Clinical Specialist
Rehabilitation Medicine
Seattle Veterans' Administration Hospital
Seattle, Washington

Nancy Roben, RN, C, BSN
Clinical Associate
Department of Physiological Nursing
University of Washington
Nurse Practitioner, Ambulatory Care
Seattle Veterans Administration Hospital
Seattle, Washington

Vera S. Wheeler, MN, OCN
Clinical Nurse Specialist, Cancer Nursing
    Service
National Institutes of Health
Bethesda, Maryland

Cynthia P. White, RPh
Geriatric Pharmacist
Long-term Care Pharmacist Consultant
Kirkland, Washington

Robert Wills, MD
Geropsychiatrist, Private Practice
Bellevue, Washington

Bonnie Worthington-Roberts, PhD
Professor
Nutritional Sciences/Epidemiology
University of Washington
Seattle, Washington

Reviewers

Teresa A. Dolan, DDS, MPH
Assistant Professor
Department of Community Dentistry
University of Florida
College of Dentistry
Gainesville, Florida

Cathy S. Heriot, PhD, RN
Assistant Professor
Medical University of South Carolina
College of Nursing
Charleston, South Carolina

Kaye Ann Herth, PhD, RN
Associate Professor
Northern Illinois University
School of Nursing
DeKalb, Illinois

Barbara Liegel, MS, RN, C
Geriatric Nurse Practitioner
University of Wisconsin Hospital and Clinics
Madison, Wisconsin

Melody J. Marshall, PhD, RN
Associate Professor
University of Florida
College of Nursing
Gainesville, Florida

Donna Rane-Szostak, EdD, RN, C
Assistant Professor
Northern Illinois University
School of Nursing
DeKalb, Illinois

Georgia L. Stevens, PhD, RN, CS
Adjunct Assistant Professor
The Catholic University of America
School of Nursing
Washington, DC

Preface

The Third Edition of *Nursing Management for the Elderly* continues its strong emphasis on nursing and the underlying knowledge that enables nurses to make accurate nursing diagnoses and sound treatment decisions. It is written for nursing students, clinicians, and practitioners in all settings who give direct care to older patients and their families.

This edition has been extensively revised and updated. Fifteen new contributors, almost all of whom are directly involved in the care of older patients and their families, have written for this edition. Their practical experience, based on clinical care and current knowledge, provides a useful guide for management of nursing care of the elderly. A new section has been added on ethical and legal issues and governmental policies as they affect health care for elderly people in general and in nursing situations specifically. Part Four has been reorganized to include neurologic (stroke and Parkinson's disease) as well as behavioral problems.

There are seven new chapters, covering the following topics: ethical issues (Chapter 4), governmental policies (Chapter 5), cognitive changes of normal aging (Chapter 15), daily living with Alzheimer's disease (Chapter 18), Parkinson's disease (Chapter 20), genital problems (Chapter 26), and incontinence and urinary problems (Chapter 29).

We have tried to include much of the new information on the care of the elderly, such as minimum data set, nutritional assessment, and federal guidelines for urinary incontinence. A bibliography concerning circadian rhythm effects on the cardiovascular system is also included.

The Third Edition continues the pattern developed in the previous edition of separating nursing and medicine. Nurses are required to make clinical judgments in the medical field on a regular basis, based on their medical knowledge. Medical knowledge also is used in nursing diagnosis and treatment planning. Therefore, it has been included in this nursing text. The organizational structure of the content for both medicine and nursing is comparable. A generic approach has been used with terminology—i.e., signs and symptoms, diagnosis, or treatment apply to either medicine or nursing.

Daily Living ↔ Functional Health Status is the nursing model used in this edition. This model describes a nursing focus for diagnosis and treatment that addresses the balancing of specifically identified requirements in daily living with the functional capacities and external resources that can be mobilized to meet these requirements in health-related areas. The model is described in Chapter 1. Nursing diagnosis and treatment of older individuals and their families requires a knowledge base that includes information from a variety of areas including normal aging, factors affecting daily living with aging, and high-risk pathology and its medical treatment, all of which are addressed.

The content is divided into five parts.

Part 1: Nursing's Discipline-Specific Focus in Providing Health Care for the Elderly. In the three chapters in this section, readers will find:

An operational definition of nursing's discipline-specific focus for providing care for the elderly and a practical description of the way in which the nursing model is used in the book

An exploration of the impact of nurses' values and beliefs about aging and the aged on their practice

Assessment structure and approaches used with older individuals.

Part 2: Ethical and Governmental Issues Associated with Nursing Care of the Elderly. Two chapters address ethical, legal, and governmental policy issues that affect the elderly and their nursing care. In Chapter 5, acquired immunodeficiency syndrome is discussed in relation to governmental policies, rather than as a high-risk disease of the elderly.

Part 3: Normal Aging. Nine chapters describe normal aging in areas that form a foundation for nursing diagnosis and treatment. Each chapter contains enough information so that the reader does not need to consult specialty texts unless more in-depth information is required. References and selected readings offer guidance in seeking more information. These chapters address:

The characteristics of the aged population

Tasks in daily living, particularly associated with the later stages of life

Normal changes in aging structure and function

Laboratory values for the elderly

Responses to medications and problems associated with medication taking

Oral health and important aspects of nursing responsibility in helping to maintain oral health, particularly in dependent, frail elderly

Nutrition for health maintenance and deterrents that nurses may need to diagnose and treat

Characteristics of families and caretakers and some of their specific problems in providing support and care to older members of the family

The reality of diminishing resources and losses and how these can affect quality of life for the older person.

All chapters have been updated, and a change in format has been made in Chapter 9 on laboratory values. Written by a gerontological nurse practitioner, the content is presented in a table, alphabetically arranged by categories. These age-related values are important in making nursing judgments. The format increases the usability of content, and the most recent norms for adults and older adults are included.

Part 4: Neurologic and Behavioral Problems in the Elderly. Cognitive changes of normal aging and delirium and dementia have been separated into two chapters. Daily living with Alzheimer's disease is a separate chapter, and some of the material that was incorporated into the chapter on daily living with behavioral problems in the Second Edition is now found in the Alzheimer's chapter. In addition, a chapter has been added on Parkinsonism, and the chapter on stroke has been moved to this section.

Part 5: High-Risk Pathophysiology in the Elderly: Medical and Nursing Management. The 13 chapters in this section address selected high-risk conditions in the elderly and their medical and nursing management. The intent is to cover common problems and not to include every system or disease that affects elderly people. Arranged alphabetically, the chapters include discussion on cancer, cardiovascular problems, diabetes mellitus, gastrointestinal problems, genital problems, hearing loss, hypertension, incontinence and urinary tract infections, musculoskeletal problems, renal failure, respiratory problems, skin problems, and vision problems.

In this book, the age group described as elderly is over 70 years, and the person who seeks health care services is called a *patient*. This term is not intended to place the individual in a dependent relationship to the nurse. The pronoun "he" is used in a generic sense to mean both male and female patients, and "she" is used to refer to both male and female nurses. These pronouns are used to maintain the flow of the text.

D. L. C.
M. P.

Contents

PART FOUR
NEUROLOGIC AND BEHAVIORAL PROBLEMS IN THE ELDERLY

PART FIVE
HIGH-RISK PATHOPHYSIOLOGY IN THE ELDERLY: MEDICAL AND
NURSING MANAGEMENT

PART ONE

Nursing's Discipline-Specific Focus in Providing Health Care for the Elderly

Part One sets the perspective for the entire book. The opening chapter describes the Daily Living↔Functional Health Status nursing viewpoint. This model requires nurses to integrate the data on an individual's or family's functional capacities and external resources with data on the current and future daily living requirements these capacities and resources must meet. Nursing diagnosis then identifies any imbalance between specific requirements in daily living and the person's capacities to meet them in an effective and satisfying way. Nursing treatment is seen as complementing or supplementing any functional capacities of external resources that are needed to achieve optimum balance.

Chapter 2 examines the relationship between societal and personally held values associated with aging and the resultant nursing care. Finally, Chapter 3 addresses the physical assessment of older individuals. Written by a gerontological nurse practitioner with many years of experience, it is practical and specific. A Minimum Data Set, now a requirement for nursing homes, is included.

1
Health Care for the Elderly: Nursing's Area of Accountability

DORIS CARNEVALI

Providing nursing care for older people is a major area of responsibility in the caseloads of nurses in almost all health care settings, aside from those that are specifically oriented to geriatric care. There is also a growing awareness that the older person comes with different capacities and resources than people in younger age groups. Thus, a specialized gerontologic-geriatric body of knowledge is required to provide effective nursing care to the older person in both general and specialized clinical areas. At one time health care was considered synonymous with medical care. Now health-illness care is seen as an area that often benefits from multiple perspectives and management skills. This broader perspective is particularly appropriate for the aged person whose health problems tend to have multiple ramifications.

Nurses are accustomed to a multidisciplinary approach in giving care. They have a long history of being the most constant health care providers in many settings. Thus, nurses have been carrying out the *tasks* of other disciplines when others were either off duty or working elsewhere. Tasks, however, are only one dimension of the service these professionals have been prepared to provide.

In the field of geriatrics and gerontology, nurses will undoubtedly continue to assume multidisciplinary roles, particularly in home care and long-term care settings. Given this likelihood, it becomes important, if older persons are not to get second-class care, that nurses alter their vision of their surrogate roles from the *tasks* to focus on the *perspective*, the basic knowledge and basic skills of those disciplines. Nurses need to see themselves functioning in lieu of that other professional, seeing the patient and family through that discipline's eyes. They need to know how that discipline gathers information for its data base and what its orientation is to the management of patient problems that fall within their domain. Further, nurses need to be aware of *what they know* and *what they do not know* about these other disciplines and to use this awareness as a basis for making decisions about when to consult, when to refer, and when to retain management of a patient's care.

By the same token, the reverse is also important. Nurses need to hold persons in other disciplines accountable for the quality of nursing care that they deliver when they function in lieu of the nurse. Other disciplines need to know nursing's contribution to care, nursing's techniques of gathering information for the nursing data base, and the basic knowledge and approach used in management of a patient's and family's problems in the nursing domain. Professionals in other disciplines must be aware of what they know and do not know about nursing so that they too will make astute decisions and appropriately use nursing consultation and referral.

A model may help to clarify these territories and relationships. Figure 1–1 shows a petal-

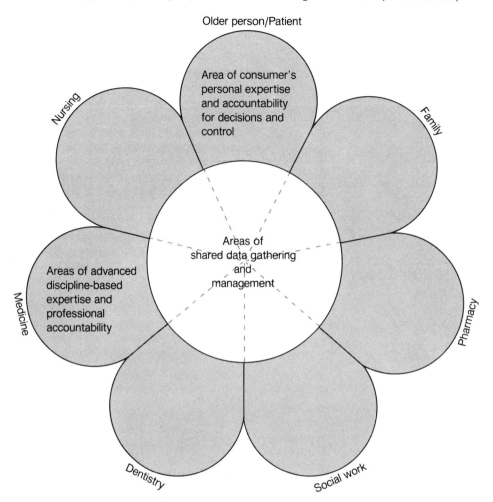

FIGURE 1-1   Model of patient and professional expertise and shared contributions on a treatment team.

type arrangement of patient and professional contributions on a treatment team. Solid lines and shaded areas are used to suggest areas of discipline expertise and accountability that cannot be easily shared or delegated to others, while intermittent lines denote blurring and sharing of responsibility, knowledge, perspective, and care. This particular prototype diagram has seven petals; however, it should be imagined as changeable, with fewer or greater numbers of components as the presenting treatment team requires. The comparable size of wedges is not meant to indicate area of responsibility in any one situation, only a designated territory of personal or discipline expertise and accountability.

Figure 1-1 suggests several general ideas and relationships:

1. The patient, family, and any disciplines involved in providing care bring a personal or discipline-based perspective and expertise as well as accountability to the situation.
2. At *basic* levels both data gathering and management are shared, usually being assumed by whatever professional (or layperson) the patient selects to encounter or is already encountering.
3. When involved in a health care situation, each one has an area of accountability for the quality of this care, whether the assessment and care is personally given or is performed by a person from another discipline territory.
4. The care provider or participant from each discipline has a degree of specialized knowledge and expertise that goes beyond that

normally expected of persons not so professionally trained. Therefore, consultation or referral is appropriate whenever patient problems require more than the basic knowledge and skills available from current care providers.*

5. The patient and family have expertise and skills that are significant and valuable. The consultation and referral process applies to them as validly as to the professionals.

This model has been presented initially in a very general approach. Petals have been labeled merely to demonstrate the disciplines commonly involved in health care for the elderly who might be involved in a presenting situation; other disciplines or groups could as easily be substituted. Quality of care for the geriatric patient is best achieved through this shared/collegial approach.

Clinical Nursing Practice and Care of the Elderly

In long-term care and assisted living care settings, the older age group predominates; however, in home care, ambulatory care, and acute care institutions older patients are a part of an age-mixed clientele. Thus, busy nurses in emergency rooms, critical care units, acute care units, and ambulatory care settings need to be able to adjust their thinking as they move from the older person to younger individuals and back again. This requires knowledge and expertise in the gerontologic-geriatrics field as it applies to the specific clinical area as well as the body of knowledge that is needed for the care of younger individuals.

This book assumes that nurses in all care settings function in two major health care domains. They traditionally and routinely provide care from a medical perspective as nurse practitioners or as nurses carrying out delegated medical functions (case finding, monitoring patient status from the medical perspective, and implementing medical treatment). Nurses also have primary accountability for diagnosing and treating patients from a nursing perspective. The nursing body of knowledge

*A problem here is that nurses have been trained to consult and refer, but not to expect to be consulted or receive referrals when nursing problems exist that require advanced nursing expertise.

has as one element knowledge from the medical domain. For this reason, knowledge in both medical and nursing domains is addressed in each clinical chapter of this book.

Knowledge Needed to Practice in the Medical Domain in the Care of the Elderly

Health care given to the older person from a medical perspective primarily uses knowledge in the fields of normal physiology and structure, normal age-related changes and their effects on pathology, pathophysiology, and psychopathology, medical treatment options, and response to medical treatment. Medical practice uses this knowledge in order to prevent, cure, stabilize, and palliate health conditions that usually involve pathology, pathophysiology, and psychopathology. Knowledge in the medical domain, used by physicians or nurses to provide medical care to older individuals, is shown in Figure 1–2.

The target for medical diagnosis and treatment is primarily the individual identified as the patient. Rarely are others in the patient's situation formally diagnosed and treated, unless they also enter the patient role. The exception may be psychotherapy or counseling where families are involved.

Nursing Diagnosis and Treatment of the Elderly

A nursing perspective in diagnosing and treating the elderly uses different approaches. The point of view for looking at the person's situation is different, the knowledge base is different, the diagnostic targets are more inclusive, the data base is different, the diagnoses are different in character and language, the prognostic variables are different, and so are the treatment modalities and the evaluation criteria. Unchanged are the treatment goals of: prevention, minimizing, or delay of health problems, cure or resolution, stabilization and palliation, or support when health problems in the nursing domain cannot be prevented or cured. The health problems involved are those in the nursing domain.

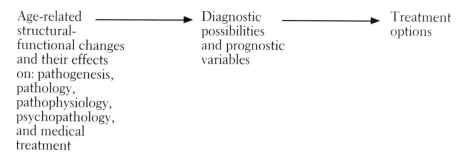

Age-related structural-functional changes and their effects on: pathogenesis, pathology, pathophysiology, psychopathology, and medical treatment ⟶ Diagnostic possibilities and prognostic variables ⟶ Treatment options

FIGURE 1–2   Knowledge in the medical domain for diagnosis and treatment of older individuals. (Adapted with permission from Carnevali D, Reiner A. The cancer experience: nursing diagnosis and management. Philadelphia: J.B. Lippincott, 1990.)

Targets for Nursing Diagnosis and Treatment

The patient is the primary target for nursing diagnosis and treatment just as in medicine. However, because of nursing's focus on daily living and functioning, patient well-being often depends on nursing diagnosis and appropriate treatment for other individuals involved in that person's daily living. For example, when the patient has pathology that creates increasing dependence on others, the diagnosis and treatment of the daily living and functional capacities of the spouse, other family members, or care givers can be as crucial as that of the patient. Throughout this book, patient situations are presented in which the diagnosis and treatment of individuals in the support system are critical to the well-being of the patient.

A Perspective for Nursing Diagnosis and Treatment

In this book, the nursing perspective for diagnosis and treatment of older individuals integrates their functional capacities and external resources with the daily living context within which that functioning takes place. In this model, Daily Living generates requirements that must be met, while Functional Capacities and External Resources provide the resources to meet those requirements. The relationships between the requirements of daily living and the resources to meet those requirements can be seen as a balance as shown in Figure 1–3.

Balances or imbalances between requirements and resources can be seen as a totality.

More often, nursing diagnosis and treatment deal with imbalances between specific requirements in daily living and the often compromised functional capacities and external resources for managing them.

A balance may be achieved at a variety of levels. A healthy older person may have many requirements in daily living and have the functional capacities and external resources to meet them, achieving a sense of well-being and satisfaction with the quality of life in the process. At the other extreme an older person may have greatly compromised functional capacities, but the requirements in daily living can be reduced commensurately and appropriate external resources can be added so that it is possible to achieve balance at a much lower level and yet maintain some satisfaction with quality of life.

Nursing diagnosis and treatment can address areas in all three components: daily living, functional capacities, and external resources. Any aspect of daily living can be modified to try to make its requirements fit with available resources. Specific functional capacities can be improved, modified, or supplemented. External resources can be located, recruited, maintained, discontinued, or adjusted to fit the needs of the situation.

Health (using this model) may be defined as the achievement of a balance between health-related requirements of daily living and the resources for meeting those requirements in such a way that well-being and a degree of satisfaction with quality of life is attained. This suggests that health, from a nursing perspective, can occur in daily living whether the older person is well and fully functional, living with chronic illness, acutely ill, terminally ill, or dying. In *any* clinical situation nursing can address aspects

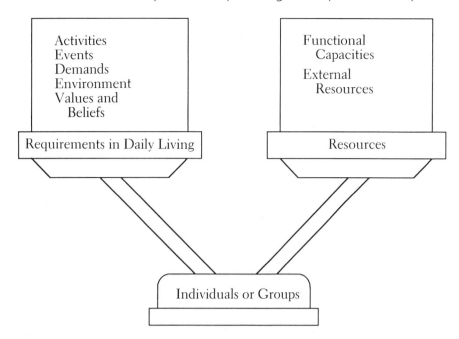

FIGURE 1-3   The relationships between the requirements of daily living and the resources to meet those requirements. (Adapted with permission from Carnevali D, Reiner A. The cancer experience: nursing diagnosis and management. Philadelphia: J.B. Lippincott, 1990.)

that promote a balance between health-related requirements and resources for daily living at an appropriate level and promote satisfaction with quality of life for the patient and those who share the daily living.

The relationship of this model to nursing diagnosis, prognosis, and treatment can be better understood if the major categories are divided into subcategories.

Nursing Phenomena and the Category of Daily Living

Daily living is seen to be made up of five subcategories. These include activities in daily living, events in daily living, demands of daily living, environment for daily living, and values and beliefs affecting daily living.

ACTIVITIES IN DAILY LIVING

The category of activities in daily living includes anything that the individual does as a part of daily living that is relevant to the presenting health situation. The activities may in-

volve those of the patient as well as others who share that daily living and thus affect the patient. This includes not only care givers and family members, but also health care workers.

USUAL OR UNUSUAL ACTIVITIES

Activities in daily living of concern in the older patient's situation may be *usual*, as in well-established patterns of daily living. Eating, sleeping, and eliminating are examples that come easily to mind. But the patient situation may also require the nurse to consider other activities such as driving a car, being sexually active, shopping for food, cooking, and caring for a pet. For example, if the husband had a stroke and has a wife who has been a nurse, her usual activities may include providing personal hygiene, giving medications, driving the car, engaging in rehabilitation activities, and interpreting stroke-related changes in behavior. On the other hand, the wife might be someone whose usual activities didn't include providing care to an adult. Nursing treatment often involves modifying activities of daily living that are usual. Since what is usual varies markedly from one individual or family to another, it becomes important to diagnose and treat those situations where modifying the usual activities creates difficulties.

Activities may be *unusual* for the patient or for those who share the daily living. Sometimes changes in functioning make usual activities unusual, e.g., the person who has had a stroke and has altered fields of vision, hemiplegia, or aphasia finds that usual tasks have become quite unusual. The person who receives a new diagnosis of diabetes finds eating and self-monitoring to be unusual activities. Individuals who have been diagnosed as having cancer find that relating to others becomes unusual (Carnevali and Reiner, 1990). Certainly activities related to participating in diagnostic and medical treatment tend to be unusual, and living in a health care institution creates a host of unusual activities both for the patient and the family. Diagnosis and treatment of activities that are unusual become an important aspect of helping patients and care givers to manage daily living in health-related areas.

With shortened hospital stays, older patients are returning home with medical treatments and technology involving activities in daily living that are unusual for the patient and care givers. These are important areas for nursing diagnosis and treatment if daily living is to be effectively managed.

On the other hand, there are times when activities are usual for the patient, but unusual for the nurse. Successful, experienced diabetics sometimes face this situation as do individuals who have become expert in managing specialized kinds of health technology.

PAST, PRESENT, AND FUTURE ACTIVITIES

Past, present, and future activities are a nursing consideration in data collection, diagnosis, and treatment. *Past activities* can influence the capacity and attitude of the individual in participating in present activities, making the person more or less skilled and responsive. *Present and future activities* need to be considered in terms of the functional capacities and external resources for carrying them out.

SIGNIFICANCE OF ACTIVITIES

The significance of an activity to those who are involved is also a nursing consideration. Nursing is often involved in modifying activities in daily living in health-related areas. For the el-

derly, the experience of many years has offered opportunities to develop both high and low priorities for particular activities in daily living, strong emotional attachments to some and less for others. The importance and meaning of activities to the older person or the family is a factor to be considered when changes are being contemplated or undertaken.

EVENTS IN DAILY LIVING

Events are special occasions in the daily living of the individual. These events may be personal or health related. It is important to look at events through the eyes of the individual, because what may be an activity in daily living to the nurse may well be an event to the patient.

TIME FACTORS

Past events can shape the participation of the patient or family member in current events. For example, past experience with radiation or chemotherapy can make the patient reluctant to undergo further treatment of this type. Or in a more positive vein, long-term memories of participation in earlier social or religious holidays may be used to help cognitively impaired older persons to take part in the current celebration. *Current and future events* need to be considered and modified to keep them within the functional capacities of the patient.

SIGNIFICANCE

Events, like activities in daily living, can vary in their significance for participants in the health situation. Data on the significance of an event can be used to determine the priority of attention and resources the older patient and the family are willing to allocate to a given event.

It is also possible that health care providers and patients may differ in the significance they assign to an event. This potential conflict can create major difficulties and misunderstandings and is therefore an important area for nursing diagnosis and treatment.

DEMANDS OF DAILY LIVING

Demands of daily living are *expectations* that influence behavior or emotional response. These demands can arise from three sources: self, others, and possessions.

SELF-EXPECTATIONS

One's expectations of oneself can shape both behavior and attitudes. Examples of this in the older person can include self-expectations about independence or dependence, control in daily living, response to symptoms, the role of the older person in relation to family and health personnel, body image, etc.

DEMANDS OF OTHERS

Demands of others can come from family members, others in the daily living situation (e.g., residents in a long-term care setting), health care providers, friends, religious or social groups, and bureaucracies. For example, the paper work associated with third-party payers creates demands that can be overwhelming to older people.

The demands that come from a variety of sources can be congruent with each other and with the older person's expectations. Often they are stressfully incongruent and disruptive to effective management of daily living. Nurses are frequently involved in the diagnosis and treatment of conflicting demands being made on the patient or family.

DEMANDS OF POSSESSIONS

Possessions can create major problems for the fragile and dependent older person. The care of pets, a car, and the immediate environment can become increasingly difficult if strength and endurance decrease, vision is impaired, and other functional capacities diminish.

ENVIRONMENT FOR DAILY LIVING

For diagnostic and treatment purposes, nursing's perspective on the environment involves the locale and milieu within which the person's daily living takes place, whether it is a home or institutional setting. It involves physical, microbial, and sensory dimensions. For diagnosis and treatment of the individual or family, the elements of the environment that have priority are those that are linked to the areas of compromised functioning or deficits in external resources. For example, where there is immunosuppression, the microbial environment is important; where mobility is compromised, distances, stairs, the height of chairs, and the placement of objects become important; for the visually impaired, lighting, railings, and the placement of carpets and furniture must be considered; for the individuals with urinary urgency or diarrhea, access to the bathroom becomes crucial.

For almost all older individuals the adequacy and appropriateness of the sensory environment is a critical environmental consideration. This is true in both home and institutional settings.

VALUES AND BELIEFS AFFECTING DAILY LIVING

Health care often involves choices and decisions in which the individual's and family's values and beliefs are strong influences. Data on values or beliefs that may be linked with particular health decisions can be valuable as plans are formulated for health care treatment in either the medical or nursing realm. Such data also may be used to understand responses to health care. Examples of obvious value and belief situations involve prolonging life or not, or acceptance versus rejection of treatment on the basis of religious beliefs. However, subtle values or beliefs may influence health care decisions, e.g., the woman's belief that the obligation to care for her husband has precedence over self-care (Gaynor, 1991); or the belief that medical science and technology can diagnose and treat all health problems, or conversely that medical science and technology have grave limitations.

In the elderly, values and beliefs may have become strongly established. They may or may not be congruent with those held by other family members or by health care providers. Where there is incongruence, consideration of difficulties in managing health-related daily living is an important area for nursing diagnosis and treatment.

Categories of Functional Capacities

Functional capacities involve all of the individual's or family's internal resources for meeting the requirements of daily living. Functional Capacities (see box on p. 10) includes some of the major areas. It can be seen that pathology, pathophysiology, psychopathology, and medical treatment can influence these functional capacities. A functional capacities conceptualization views body changes in terms

Functional Capacities

Strength	Capacity to handle physical or emotional work at a given point in time
Endurance	Capacity to continue with a physical, mental, or emotional workload over time
Cognition	Capacity to accurately process stimuli and information
Sensory abilities	Capacity of sense organs to take in external stimuli and transmit them to the central nervous system. The resources to control external stimuli to create a satisfying and effective sensory environment
Mood	Usual temperament (trait), e.g., optimism versus pessimism, usual anxiety level, etc., plus emotional response to the presenting health-related situation (state)
Knowledge	Status of acquired subject matter in areas relevant to managing daily living and level of ability to use that knowledge (recall, comprehension, application, synthesis, evaluation)
Desire	Will or motivation to participate in health-related activities and behavior
Courage	Capacity to take risks in health-related areas
Skills	Psychomotor and interpersonal competencies in health-related activities
Communication	Capacity to make oneself understood by others

of capacity to meet requirements in daily living rather than as a manifestation of aging, disease, or response to medical treatment.

External Resources

Some individuals and families experience major health problems and manage the stresses and adjustments remarkably well because they have adequate, appropriate resources and support systems. In contrast, other individuals and families fail to manage daily living with even minor health difficulties because there are major deficits in external resources or those that are available are not appropriate. Therefore, functional capacities to manage the requirements of daily living can be augmented or diminished by the nature of external resources that are available and used.

With many older individuals and families the external resources become more precarious and undependable even as their func-tional capacities become more fragile. Nursing diagnosis and treatment for the older individual or family must concern itself with the status of external resources. The box on p. 11 indicates some of the major areas of external resources.

Knowledge Needed to Practice in the Nursing Domain of the Care of the Elderly

Given this focus on the older person's daily living, functional capacities, and external resources, the knowledge needed to diagnose and treat elderly individuals and their families in the nursing domain differs from that of the medical domain shown in Figure 1–1. Both begin with normal age-related structure and functioning as each affects pathogenesis, pathology, pathophysiology, psychopathology, and response to medical activities. However, nursing knowledge then moves to focus on the

External Resources

Architecture	The arrangement of rooms, facilities, stairs, elevators, space, equipment in one's housing
Communication	Telephone, postal services
Financial resources	Income, securities, health insurance, monetary obligations, debts
Housing	The availability and security of preferred housing arrangements, furnishings, and amenities
Neighborhood	The character, safety, services, facilities, density of people, distances
People	Personal networks of nuclear and extended family, friends, and groups that are available to call on or those that can call on the person
Pets	Dogs, cats, birds, fish, and other animals available for contact or as a responsibility
Services	Availability and usability of health care, governmental, and social services from any source
Supplies and equipment	Availability of needed supplies and equipment
Technology	State of the art and the availability of technology associated with the presenting health situation
Transportation	Nature, availability, and usability of transportation facilities, either personal or municipal

effect of these changes on functional capacities, daily living, and external resources. The diagnostic areas focus on any difficulties in effective management of daily living, functioning, and management of external resources. Prognostic variables may include some associated with medical prognosis; however, there are others that deal with dimensions of daily living and external resources as well as functional capacities that are not dependent on the pathology and its treatment. Knowledge about treatment options focuses on modifications in the requirements of daily living, enhancing or supplementing functional capacities, and management of external resources to promote effective daily living and satisfaction with quality of life. These areas of knowledge and their relationships are shown in Figure 1–4.

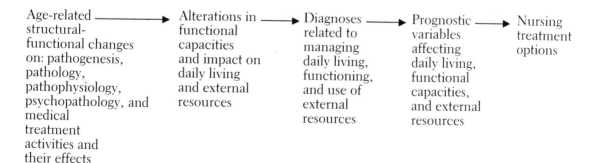

FIGURE 1–4   Knowledge in the nursing domain for diagnosis and treatment of older individuals. (Adapted with permission from Carnevali D, Reiner A. The cancer experience: nursing diagnosis and management. Philadelphia: J.B. Lippincott, 1990.)

The Nursing Domain and This Book

The Daily Living↔Functional Health Status approach to the domain of nursing can be used in terms of organizing and extending nursing's body of knowledge in research, taxonomic activities, and teaching as well as the topics and structure of writing. However, this book is directed to nurses who are caring for the elderly or students of nursing who wish to gain knowledge and expertise in giving nursing care to the elderly. Therefore, the concept is used with a practical, clinical orientation.

First the reader is offered knowledge about the normal responses to aging. Then the content moves on to the pathologic overlay to normal age-related status. In the sections involving pathology, an organizational system is used that structures both the biomedical and nursing knowledge in a *comparable* format to encourage organized storage of knowledge in long-term memory. This pattern of storage may, in turn, expedite effective retrieval as the nurse makes assessment, diagnostic, and prognostic judgments, as well as treatment (intervention) decisions.

With this purpose in mind the clinical chapters have been divided into two sections. The first section addresses the knowledge nurses need to have in order to understand the pathology and medical treatment of common psychological and physiologic problems of the elderly. Nursing's role requires its clinicians to

1. Make biomedical judgments when physicians are not present in both case-finding and ongoing contacts
2. Implement delegated medical care in an intelligent, expert manner
3. Monitor patient response to medical treatment and take appropriate action on the findings

All of these delegated nursing functions from the medical field require nurses to have a solid working knowledge of the biomedical domain.

Beyond these delegated medical functions, nurses need knowledge of pathology and its treatment as well as medical data on patient status and response to treatment for clinical judgments and treatment decisions in the nursing area. This knowledge base and the patient information are an integral part of nursing's

data bases, diagnoses, prognoses, and treatment (intervention) plans. This then is the rationale for its inclusion in the book and for addressing this content first in each chapter or section.

The structure and sequence of the subject matter in each of the clinical chapters is based on the use of knowledge in diagnostic reasoning and decision-making thought patterns (Carnevali and Reiner, 1990; Carnevali and Thomas, 1993). Knowledge of risk factors and signs and symptoms is needed as part of the assessment process of problem sensing, activating of diagnostic possibilities, and subsequent gathering of additional data to determine which of the diagnostic possibilities most accurately categorizes the presenting situation. Thus, in each topic, whether pathology or daily living, risk factors and manifestations (signs and symptoms) are addressed first. Then alternatives of closely related phenomena (differential diagnoses) are considered when this is appropriate, e.g., solitude— a comfortable, often chosen status of being by oneself—versus loneliness— a painful deficit in desired interpersonal relationships that may occur whether one is alone or with others and a condition requiring intervention and treatment. Prognosis is a factor influencing treatment. Therefore knowledge of prognostic variables and possibilities associated with particular diagnoses is considered prior to treatment decisions and content. Potential complications also are considered before treatment decisions are made; therefore this content is addressed prior to the subject of treatment options. The final sections of each topic will address the treatment (interventions) options and evaluation areas.

This book is based on five major assumptions about professional health care:

1. The disciplines of nursing and medicine have two distinct but closely related domains that shape their perspectives in viewing presenting clinical situations, approaches to collecting patient data, diagnosing and making prognoses, consideration of treatment options, and evaluation of patient response to treatment.
2. The health care of people, particularly the elderly, will be more effective if the discipline-specific differences in care are retained but integrated.
3. The nursing role requires nurses to make clinical judgments and engage in therapeu-

tic activities in both the nursing and medical fields.

4. The critical thinking—data collecting and processing patterns required for arriving at diagnostic and treatment decisions—is identical for all clinical disciplines; only the discipline-specific perspective and expertise vary.

5. The organization of knowledge used in storing clinical knowledge in long-term memory can be a factor in its retrieval for clinical judgments and decision making.

Based on these assumptions, you will find that a shared terminology has been chosen that highlights the *commonalities* of thinking and the organization of knowledge for storage, while emphasizing the *differences* in the disciplines' perspectives and knowledge base. Thus, in both the pathophysiologic and daily living areas the content for assessment is labeled *risk factors* and *signs and symptoms*, rather than use these labels for the biomedical portion and *assessment areas* for the nursing portion. Similarly the term *treatment* is used for both biomedical and nursing sections rather than shift to the currently popular term *intervention* in the nursing sections.

Health care for the elderly, particularly the frail or ill elderly, virtually cries out for nurses who confidently recognize their distinct discipline-specific contribution to health care and who have command of the special knowledge of gerontology and geriatrics to add to a solid foundation of nursing knowledge and basic clinical expertise. It is the intent of this book to contribute to that consciousness of the special nursing expertise and to the particular knowledge associated with expert nursing care for the elderly.

References and Other Readings

Carnevali D, Reiner A. The cancer experience: nursing diagnosis and management. Philadelphia: JB Lippincott, 1990.

Carnevali D, Thomas M. Diagnostic reasoning and treatment decision making in nursing. Philadelphia: JB Lippincott, 1993.

Gaynor SE. The long haul: the effects of home care on caregivers. Image 1991; 22:208.

2

The Nurse's Philosophy of Aging and the Aged: Its Impact on Nursing Practice

DORIS CARNEVALI

The individual nurse's practice is shaped by the focus of the diagnostic–management model or by the knowledge and skill used in applying the model to patient care. In a very basic way the care of the elderly also is influenced by the beliefs and values* the nurse holds about the elderly clientele for whom she provides health care services.

Beliefs and values are a strong influence on all aspects of nursing diagnosis and management—the data one notices, the words used to describe what is noticed, the priorities set, the decisions made, the formulation of diagnostic statements, the care prescribed, the way care is delivered, and the criteria set for evaluation. At times, values and beliefs form a conscious basis for behavior. For example, the belief that "Honesty is the best policy" may be a very conscious thought that precedes the return of change to a store clerk who has made an error in the shopper's favor. More often the values and beliefs are subtle, pervasive influences. In other words, beliefs and values shape the nurse's behavior whether or not she is aware of it. This is a particularly important insight for those who are in the helping professions. Here, the risk of inflicting one's own beliefs and values on those who are dependent becomes very

great. In the case of nurses involved in the care of the dependent elderly, often with ongoing day-to-day contact, one can see the opportunities and the risks of the situation. It becomes very easy and comfortable to incorporate one's own value and belief system unless purposeful thought is addressed to what is happening.

Given this risk of requiring others to comply with the care-provider's values, it becomes important for the nurse who is working with the elderly to know the *working* values and beliefs that are influencing the nursing care being given. (See the section on pp. 16–17 identifying values for techniques to determine one's working values.) It is important to see the relationship between these beliefs and values and the diagnosis and management evolving from them, including the style in which care is given.

Societal Factors and the Status of the Aged

Nurses are socialized first by their families and then by professionals, who are a part of a larger culture. It is reasonable to assume that the values a society or subculture holds regarding a group of its members will influence the attitudes, values, and beliefs its members are taught to hold toward that group. Subgroups within a society may be identified in a variety of ways. *Age* is one of them. So it is that differ-

---

Beliefs are ideas or opinions that a person or group holds to be true. Beliefs are not always rational. *Values* are preferences for or esteeming of certain activities, ideas, objects, kinds of persons, goals, and so forth.

ing cultures have varying values associated with identifiable age groups—children, adults, and the aged.

The status of the elderly within a society has been hypothesized to be related to several forces that are impinging on the entire society:

1. Extent of available resources in relationship to the needs of the population
2. Availability of written communication for transmission of knowledge, cultural patterns, and skills
3. Rate of change
4. Proportion of the society that falls within the group

SOCIETAL RESOURCES, PERSONAL PRODUCTIVITY, AND STATUS

It has been suggested that the status of the elderly is related to their productive capacity to carry their own weight and contribute to the society's product or, alternatively, to the resources available to the society to support nonproductive members. In more primitive societies, which were dependent on an environment with limited resources, the aged who survived their productive capability were left behind or sent out of the community. The group could not afford to value them as continuing members since they endangered the survival of the group. One reads of nomadic tribes who left behind members who could not keep up. In fact, for some tribes, the religious belief regarding life after death supported early death by holding that dead persons retained throughout eternity the body, age, beauty, and functional capacity they had at the time of death. Such beliefs made abandonment of a parent or cherished tribal member easier (Simmons, 1960).

In agrarian societies, including rural life in modern societies, the aged often have been able to contribute in ways that released younger stronger members to participate more actively in producing resources needed. Therefore, the aged were able to retain status and were valued as contributors to family and society.

Modern industrial society's decree of mandatory nonproductivity in the form of formal retirement from the work force places its elder members in a situation where loss of status is a high risk. They are less valued and therefore less wanted. The current concern those in the present work force have regarding funding pensions for an increasing number of members who no longer contribute, as well as concern for their own pensions later, is a manifestation of the risk to status faced by the elderly. Not only do the elderly not produce but also they place an increasing drain on others. This drain may take the form of money, as in pensions, but it may also involve time and physical and emotional energy (Callahan, 1987, 1990). In a personal sense, when family members not only cannot provide for themselves but also become a burden on others, they can be valued less and status decreases, even though love and affection for them may continue.

TRANSMISSION OF CULTURAL PATTERNS AND STATUS

Cultures that had no written language depended on the elders to teach succeeding generations the history, skills, and traditions of the society. Those with written and other advanced symbolic forms of communication seem to have less need of the wise and skilled elders.

The resurgence of interest and pride in cultural heritage has enhanced the status of many older persons who are the only sources of knowledge about the history, recipes, crafts, stories, arts, music, dances, and religion of the group. Once these are written, the songs recorded for posterity, the dances filmed and recorded, one wonders if again the elders will revert to a less valued status.

RATE OF CULTURAL CHANGE

The status of older persons has also been influenced by the rate of societal change. Slow rates of change have been associated with higher status for older members. The logic of this hypothesis is that when a culture is changing rapidly, the older generations lose their value as they become too out of tune with changing times to be useful to younger generations except as a baseline for measuring change. They are seen as knowing only how things were, not how they are.

We have to go no further than our own nursing profession to see the truth in the latter. How much value do currently competent young nurses place on a nurse who decides to return to the field after having been away from it for 5 years? The language is new, the technology has changed, the systems have been reorganized, the role and role relationships have been modified. Even currently practicing professionals struggle to keep up with change—witness the strong continuing education programs.

In a society afflicted with the condition of "future shock," the contributions of older people tend to lose value, and with it, unless other sources of value are seen, the people themselves are valued less.

PROPORTION OF ELDERLY AND STATUS

Another factor seen as leading to loss of status for older persons in a society is the size of the group in relation to the rest of the population. The rare rather than the commonplace is valued. In cultures in which most die young, survivors are revered. Where increasing numbers live long, being an elder member of the society becomes mundane, less valued. The elderly may even be viewed as depriving young people of jobs, housing, and resources.

An example of this may be seen in the changes occurring in the nursing profession. The career patterns of women in the nursing profession are changing from that of short careers with retirement to homemaking and family activities to long nursing careers combined with other activities. The result is that young nurses entering the field may have difficulty locating the job opportunities they prefer. How much value do eager, aspiring young graduates place on older nurses whose seniority deprives them of career opportunities?

If we look at just these factors and apply them to our current industrialized society (the older persons who consume more than they currently produce, who are becoming a growing proportion of the group to be supported by fewer young people) and if we add the widespread use of communication (the written word, other audiovisual media, computerization, and advanced technology) as well as the rate of societal change and rapid human technologic obsolescence, one sees that there is a great risk that older persons will be less valued. This societal attitude of decreased valuing can, in turn, subtly or overtly influence the values and beliefs that nurses, as products of this society, bring to bear as they provide health care services to the older age group.

On the other hand, the older age group is currently increasing in size. Many have adequate finances. As individuals remain healthy longer, they also represent a pool of available time and energy to contribute to society. Many are well educated, formally or informally. Businesses are recognizing their purchasing power. Politicians are recognizing their voting power. They are banding together in groups that enhance their self-esteem and promote issues concerned with their own and society's welfare.

Nurses need to be aware of the variety of societal values that have impact on the older person's self-image and the attitudes of health care providers.

IF YOU BELIEVE	YOU MAY TEND TO
Older people can't learn ("You can't teach an old dog new tricks")	Minimize teaching older adults about health, disease, coping behaviors (e.g., aged mastectomy patients received less teaching about arm exercises and coping with changed musculature than younger patients)
Intelligence decreases with age	Use simpler words and ideas than you do with younger people without checking to see if it is appropriate
Older people prefer to live in the past	Encourage reminiscing to the exclusion of including current ideas, future planning, and activities
	Negate the value of reminiscing

IF YOU BELIEVE *(Continued)*	YOU MAY TEND TO *(Continued)*
Older people tend to have "mental" problems	View behavior as reflecting age-related deviances with some skepticism
Kindness to older people means protecting them from being upset or stressed	Conceal information from them or modify the truth in terms of what you think is good for them
All older people end up in hospitals with illness	Emphasize illness care rather than prevention, maintenance, and self-care
Spunky patients are difficult patients	Avoid assertive patients
Interest in sex is inappropriate among the elderly, particularly among single elderly	Joke about sexual overtures or activities among older persons. Neglect to obtain data on interest in sexual activity and take this into account when prescribing and administering treatments
	Fail to consult them in the decision-making process when decisions will affect their sexual activity patterns
	Make no provision for protected privacy as a norm in the institutional setting
Older persons are not credible historians in reporting signs, symptoms, or health history data	Behave as if they don't really know what they are talking about when they report to you
	Patronize them, but don't take the reports seriously
	Check the data out with younger adults who are "more reliable"
Adult children should assume parenting or executor roles with aged parents	Talk over important decisions with the children rather than the parent
	Help the parent to make the decision already made by the children. Relate to the children as if they were in the parenting role and the parent as if he were in the child role
Body image is not important when one is older	Minimize the importance of grooming services and attractive clothing
	Fail to give information or budget for prosthetic devices and rehabilitative teaching
	Fail to help make the older person feel attractive
Competence decreases with old age, and therefore the elderly must be protected from risk	Require people to prove competence before trusting them to perform (e.g., not allow them control of their own money)
Older persons want to be with their own kind (i.e., other older persons)	Structure activities with age mates rather than other generations
The daily bath is more important than grooming habits of a lifetime	Equate personal cleanliness and neatness with good nursing care

IF YOU BELIEVE OLDER PERSONS HAVE A RIGHT TO	YOU WOULD TEND TO
Make decisions about their own lives	Include them in decision making in order to maintain this expectation for both care providers and consumers of health care services
Adequate data on which to make informed decisions	Provide information and help the person to explore options
Have their decisions accepted	Accept their decisions and assist in interpreting them to and implementing them with the system and family members
Time and attention of care providers and family	Schedule time to be with them
	Genuinely attend to them in any encounter rather than engaging in distancing maneuvers, professional business, or superficiality
Access to health care	Locate care where it is convenient to clusters of elderly
	Facilitate transportation
	Engage in architectural planning and furnishing to give access and provide appropriate support during waiting periods for those with limited mobility or endurance
Therapy including prevention, maintenance, and restoration	Chronologic age would not automatically rule out certain forms of care
Make decisions regarding health care with their finances in mind	Know their resources and attitude toward health expenditures
	Act in accordance with their wishes where possible
Live alone if they so choose and maintain their preferred style of living as long as possible	Seek services that would enable the person to remain in a preferred environment
Participate in decisions regarding change of lifestyle if and when this becomes necessary	Explore pros and cons of each option and predict and discuss transition problems
	Acknowledge the difficulty of changing one's lifestyle
	Support coping patterns of dealing with change
	Allow time for transition when this is possible
	Explain signs and symptoms of stress in making a change to the family and staff
Maintain independence in all areas as long as possible	Seek ways to foster and support independence on a daily basis in little as well as larger areas, rather than doing tasks for them

IF YOU BELIEVE OLDER PERSONS HAVE A RIGHT TO (Continued)	YOU WOULD TEND TO (Continued)
Maintain a personal environment with the person's own cherished belongings	Sacrifice neatness and uniformity if needed to provide a home environment
Maintain privacy	Where privacy must be violated, help them to understand rationale
Feel cared about	Seek ways to communicate personal interest in the individual
Talk about or avoid talking about dying	Take time to listen when the person indicates an interest and need to discuss dying
	Listen without judgment or engaging in distancing maneuvers
Be assertive in coping with the environment	Develop patterns of interaction that value and understand assertive responses rather than dampen them

Specific Beliefs and Implications for Nursing Care

Nurses maturing within any society undoubtedly assimilate the general societal attitudes and those of their more immediate families (Cunningham and Hutchinson, 1991). These attitudes, plus the process of professional socialization through training and clinical role models in practice, lead to the adoption of specific beliefs and values that affect the nursing care given to older adults. Some of these beliefs, commonly heard among nurses, are listed in the accompanying displayed material. Potential nursing behaviors that could result from these beliefs are also noted.

The stereotypes and beliefs in the first box (pp. 16–17) are of a negative nature. Although some of these beliefs would hold true for selected older adults, the beliefs are inappropriate if applied without validation across the board to all aged persons. Ideas for a bill of rights that might be created for the older clientele are given in a second box on pp. 18–19. Examine the ideas and discover the beliefs you hold. Explore the ways in which you currently implement them through the way in which you nurse your older patients.

The boxed material is a sample and is not to be considered as a full exploration. The reader no doubt will think of a variety of other values and stereotypes that influence the health care given to the elderly.

Strategies for Identifying Values Impinging on Health Care

When nurses are working with an older age population, whether to maintain wellness and independence or to provide high levels of care to dependent ailing persons, the question of an awareness of the values and beliefs involved becomes highly important—not just the platitudes that sometimes pass as the influencing values, but those that are genuinely affecting the responses of both the patient and the nurse. It is not easy to discover the real values that are inherent in a given presenting situation, yet it is important to ascertain them.

There are two strategies by which nurses can discover their personal *working values*. In the first, known values are stated explicitly, e.g., "I value the right of the older person to make decisions based on adequate information." After having selected a specific value, the nurse then proceeds to observe his or her practice and that of others to analyze how that value influences nursing behavior. If there are occasions when the older person is not given enough information to make an informed choice, or is not given the opportunity to make decisions about his or her own life, the extenuating circumstances are noted. Eventually a working value emerges that is a variant of the ideal value first cited. It may be something like, "I value the right of the older person to make decisions based on adequate information, except when

1. Pathology or response to treatment deprives him of cognitive ability.
2. The patient does not have sufficient energy for decision making.
3. The patient does not make decisions that I or the family believe are in his best interests.
4. I, the doctor, or the family believe that the patient should not have particular information about himself for the patient's own good."

This latter version of the working value makes the nurse aware of the circumstances under which she may not hold fully to the value of informed decision making. It is equally possible that the working value will emerge as having a strong component of always giving the patient all of the information needed to make informed decisions and pushing for decision making by the patient even under marginal conditions. These two variants will result in differing priorities and behavior on the part of the nurse. As a starting point the reader may select sample beliefs (values) from the displayed material and then derive the variations that are the working values actually held and actually modifying nursing practice.

The second strategy for discovering one's working values is to observe one's actual behavior on the clinical unit, e.g., the characteristics of patients who are valued and of those who are avoided, the priorities of activities, the language that is used, the way in which activities are carried out, and so on. One then can infer the values that are the genesis for the preferences, choices, style, and language. Some of these values may not be ones we would put on a nursing philosophy to be hung in a gilt frame on the wall. Some nurses have discovered that they value control and devalue people or circumstances that threaten their control. Others have found that they do not value as greatly those patients whose pathology has been generated by deliberate exposure to causative agents such as alcohol, drugs, smoking, promiscuity, and so on. An honest acceptance of one's working values has the merit of allowing one to recognize the nature of one's behavior and responses in the clinical situation.

A realistic appraisal of working values (not platitudes) can be a very useful personal exercise or staff development activity; it can pay off in greater self-awareness and more effective care.

References and Other Readings

Callahan D. Setting limits: medical goals in an aging society. New York: Simon & Schuster, 1987.

Callahan D. What kind of life: the limits of medical progress. New York: Simon & Schuster, 1990.

Cunningham N, Hutchinson S. Myths in health care ethics. Image 1991; 22:235.

Simmons LW. Aging in preindustrial societies (1945). In: Tibbitts C, ed. Handbook of social gerontology, societal aspects of aging. Chicago: University of Chicago Press, 1960:62.

3
Assessment in the Elderly

CAROLYN ENLOE

An adequate data base is the cornerstone for diagnosis and treatment of the elderly. Nurses use data from both the medical and nursing domains for nursing diagnosis and treatment. Further, given the positions they hold in the provision of health care for the elderly, they are often involved in collecting a medical data base as well as the nursing data base. For these reasons, collection of data from the elderly is covered from both nursing and biomedical perspectives.

The basic skills of history taking and the physical examination are not dealt with in this chapter. Instead, the emphasis is placed on the adaptations in both focus and strategies or techniques that are needed to assemble a valid data base with a clientele over age 70. (For basic level content, see the references at the end of this chapter.)

Over 90% of people classified as elderly are managing their daily living and their own health care at some level in noninstitutional settings. This means that the elderly or their families are themselves monitoring their own health status and implementing any prescribed medical or nursing regimens. Dysfunctions are being managed (or not managed) and are shaping daily living within the older person's particular situation. The older person is either integrating the treatment regimens into daily living with some level of desire, knowledge, and skill or choosing not to do so.

Thus, despite the fact that the majority of practicing nurses are employed in health care institutions, the health status and treatment regimen of the elderly must be viewed from the perspective of some level of self-care integrated into an established pattern of daily living in a particular living environment.

Compliance versus Participation Model

This self-monitoring and self-care orientation together with the long-term nature of many health problems in the elderly suggests that a compliance model in which the power or control is seen to rest with the health care provider is probably ineffective. In reality, it is the older person who chooses and engages in the level of integration of health monitoring and treatment in his life. Older persons have the basic day-to-day power and control, even though others may control some important resources. A participation model in which the older person's control is acknowledged and the nurse engages with him as coparticipant is more realistic and productive. Here each party brings knowledge, background, expertise, and some level of motivation and sense of responsibility to the relationship.

The participation model requires nurses to have a solid data base that identifies all of the facets of daily living as they are relevant to the presenting health problem—activities, events, demands, environment, values, and beliefs. Accurate data are also needed on available and usable internal and external resources. Only then can nurses work effectively with the elderly if help is needed, so as to determine the most effective, economic, and satisfying ways of incorporating health care and management of dysfunction into their lives and those of their families or companions.

Adaptations of the Assessment Process to the Elderly

Although many older persons can tolerate an assessment encounter taken in one sitting, some cannot. The content and timing need to be planned with care. Particular attention should be paid to the energy and endurance of the older person because fatigue will dramatically reduce the amount of information given.

ENVIRONMENT FOR THE ASSESSMENT

The environment or setting in which the assessment takes place also affects the success of the interaction. The room should provide privacy (often roommates have been found to become very involved in another person's interview with the nurse). The room should be well lighted and warm, with bathroom facilities nearby. Every effort should be made to eliminate as many potential distractions as possible, e.g., telephone calls and coming and going of personnel.

ASSESSMENT STRATEGIES

The introduction is important. It gives the older person information about the nurse who is doing the assessment. It explains the nurse's role in the system and the potential for a future relationship. It identifies the reason why sharing personal information is important. It also structures the focus for the interaction, whether it is pathology, functional status, daily living, or all of them.

Elderly people can be reticent to give information because many were not raised in a verbal tradition. For this reason and the fact that they may accept the myth of ageism, underreporting of symptoms often occurs. Making the older patient's data important and valuable is a crucial early strategy. Permission should be obtained to take notes during the assessment, since this may be misinterpreted by some older people who have had negative experiences with officials and bureaucracies in the past. They also need to know that they have the right to talk to the nurse "off the record." It is also normal for the older person not to share all of the information that nurses may think they need in the first interview. The older person will tend to share more as trust is built over several contacts. To pursue any other approach may cause the nurse to question her interviewing skills or communicate reproach to the patient, and either of these responses would be inappropriate.

Early on in the interview, evaluate the respondent for vision and hearing deficits. When a deficit is recognized, modify the technique and environment appropriately. For example, in the presence of hearing loss, position yourself with the light on your face to promote lipreading. Keep a magic slate on hand for the person with severe deafness. In extreme cases, you may have to resort to a self-report questionnaire, such as the Self-Evaluation of Life Function Scale (Linn, 1984).

Allow time for the older person to respond to questions. Data are lost when the interviewer fails to listen or does not allow adequate time for the person to process the question or make a request for information. When adequate time for the interview has not been allowed there is a tendency to try to rush the older person to get to the "important" data, i.e., data that the health care provider thinks are important. There is also a tendency to interrupt and redirect the conversation. In a study of physician and elderly patients history-taking interactions, it was found that only 23% of the elderly respondents were allowed to complete their opening statements. The mean time allowed the patients before physician interruption was 18 seconds. Most often it occurred after only a single concern had begun to be identified. The interviewer interrupted with direct questions. As a result the patients became inhibited in expressing their additional problems and concerns (Beckman and Frankel, 1984). Older persons take more time to process sensory input and their thoughts; therefore, nurses must incorporate this phenomenon into the planning and execution of the interview. Otherwise inadequate, skewed data will contribute to invalid, imprecise diagnoses in both the biomedical and nursing domain.

Many times the older person will be accompanied by a spouse or family member. Frequently this other person will attempt to answer the questions directed to the patient. Early on in the interaction, even if the older person is a poor historian, he should be interviewed alone. At this time, inquire as to patient's preference for giving data or having a family member do so, and then complete the arrangements as indicated by that preference. Family members can be interviewed separately for their perceptions and related problems in daily living.

It is also important to evaluate the older person's mental status early in the interaction. If doubt is present, testing of recent and remote memory can be validated by a family member or by testing. It is important to give a mental examination to establish a baseline. The test most often used is the Mini-Mental Status Examination given in Chapter 16 (Folstein, 1975).

Occasionally the older person will ramble from one subject to another or will cite multiple complaints. With rambling it becomes necessary to bring the person back on track. Refocusing strategies are detailed in Carnevali's text *Nursing Care Planning* (1983). With multiple complaints, it is helpful to restate all the problems presented and then to inquire about which one is most troublesome. Gather data on the primary problem, then return to the other complaints during the course of the interview. Some older persons avoid discussion of a specific content area. Note these areas of omission; they are frequently problematic. Return to them later in the interview rather than trying to force the issue at the time because this often stops information flow because of psychogenic discomfort.

On completion of the data gathering it is important to synthesize and organize the data into clusters of information and the problem areas they represent, e.g., the person who is seen after a fall, antecedent events revealing dizziness, imbalance, fear, or other specific etiology. The nurse summarizes the patient's strengths, the areas being managed well, and the problem areas that have emerged during the interaction. These are then validated with the person. It is wise then to ask a final question: "Is there anything else I should know in order to be of help to you?" Frequently the respondent will, at this time, tell you things that had been withheld or that were thought of during the interview. The question should be repeated until no more new information is given.

When the nurse–elderly person relationship is one that will continue, it is wise to negotiate the mutual expectations regarding continued diagnostic and planning activities. Since these expectations vary among clinicians and settings, it is not a component of the relationship that should be left to chance or taken for granted.

Focus of Nursing Assessment

The focus of the nursing assessment is on data from both sides of the balance—on the one side the requirements of daily living and on the other the internal and external resources for managing the daily living requirements, given the realities of aging either with health or illness. The interview should begin where the older person's current concerns and interests lie and go on from there. However, by the time the assessment is completed in one or more contacts the nurse should have subjective and objective data relevant to the presenting situation in the following five areas:

1. The person's perception of his health status
2. Usual or preferred patterns in daily living
3. Activities, events, demands, values, and beliefs in daily living that affect health status or are affected by functional status or the treatment regimen
4. Functional status
5. Status of external resources and environment for daily living

These areas are woven into the nursing assessment in whatever way is appropriate. For example, activities and demands of daily living may be addressed in relationship to areas of functional status that impact on them or they may be addressed as a separate initial section that is then used as functional capacities are discussed. Both objective and subjective data are collected (Carnevali, 1983).

FUNCTIONAL STATUS

The physician tends to collect data on organs, systems, and their functions in order to determine the pathology. The nurse uses some of the same data in order to determine the effect of functional status on daily living. Thus, where a functional deficit is noted, the nurse should collect data on the areas of living affected in the presenting situation.

These data are essential to the development of a usable nursing plan; however, asking questions in the same way and same order each time a problem is reported or noted will make for a monotonous interview. Often the person will indicate or give data without being asked. Listen first and then direct conversation or ask as needed to keep the interaction during the assessment natural and interesting for the person as well as efficient for the care provider.

CONTENT AREAS

Some functional areas are critical for collecting specific data to determine the balance between the requirements of daily living and the resources for managing those requirements (see the box on p. 25). When the nurse has access to the physician's findings on normal or pathologic status, these data become a foundation for the nursing assessment. However, when the nurse encounters the person before the physician, the nurse's assessment serves as the initial screening examination.

In the boxed material, the categories of functional health status are listed in alphabetical order, not necessarily the sequence the nurse would use. Most practicing clinicians or advanced students will have been taught or have developed a particular system or sequence that works for them. The presenting situation determines what problems should be addressed first in terms of urgency. What is important is that ultimately data are collected and recorded in each appropriate area so as to (1) discover or rule out health-related problems in daily living, (2) define them specifically enough to generate effective plans for nursing management, and (3) note if information is missing, negative or neutral to ensure that all questions are asked.

The introduction of a *problem area* may be done either by the patient or the nurse. The person may report on signs and symptoms, or the nurse may note objective data indicating some dysfunction. For example, the nurse may see that the person has swollen joints and the restricted movement associated with degenerative joint disease, yet the patient may not mention this as a problem. The nurse can approach the problem area with a question such as, "I noticed that you have some swollen joints. Do they give you any trouble?" If the person fails to bring up management areas such as discomfort, analgesia, and impaired activities, the nurse can express an interest in the kinds of ad-

---

Areas for Data Collection on Daily Living Associated with Presenting Functional Health Status

High risk areas of daily living being affected by current functional health status (includes consideration of activities, demands, events, and environmental features)

Activities, demands, events, and environmental features that trigger the condition, make it worse, or make it harder to live with

Activities or circumstances that are seen to alleviate symptoms or conditions

Alterations in daily living either made or contemplated in order to accommodate to the presenting functional health status

---

justment actually being made. The nurse's interest should be explained as interest in the nature of adjustments the person is making and the attitude toward the situation so that the usual management style can be more effectively used by the health care providers. In the nursing data base it is as important to know health situations in which persons feel they are managing well or are able to ignore deficits as it is to have data on less well-managed problems. Both can be significant in subsequent nursing management.

When the nurse has data about health problems already under medical treatment, such as diabetes, cancer, chronic obstructive pulmonary disease, alcoholism, and cerebrovascular accident, the person's skill and satisfaction in participating in the regimens and managing the disabilities should also be explored. (See specific chapters for guides.)

Although much of the data suggested here addresses a lifestyle characterized by self-care and some independence, these data are also important to the nurse assisting the older person to make a transition from self-care to greater dependency in an institutional setting, or the reverse. With older persons it is extremely important to identify and *use the resources and*

Categories of Functional Health Status

Breathing	Shortness of breath, pain on coughing, wheezing, bloody sputum
Circulation	*Heart:* Pain—nature, heaviness, episodes of rapid heartbeat, skipped beats, dizziness, blackouts
	Vessels: Varicose veins, cold hands or feet, "charley horses," leg pains—walking/at rest
Communication	Any problems making oneself understood by others (specify)
Eating	Appetite, enjoyment of food, diet or dieting, weight, chewing problems
	Cooking: Skill, enjoyment, resources
	Shopping: Transportation, skill, frequency, finances
	Eating patterns: Meals per day, typical foods
	Locale: Home or restaurant, alone or with others
Elimination	*Bowels:* Frequency, time, concerns, associated problems, medications
	Urine: Frequency, urgency, pain, leaking, up at night
Grooming	Importance to person, capabilities, frustrations
Mobility/safety	Patterns and location of activities, gait, accidents, balance, weakness, dizziness, stiffness, pain, status of feet and shoes, appropriate clothing available
Senses	Vision, hearing, use of glasses or hearing aid; tactile; sensory stimulation—desired or available
Sleep/rest	Sleep patterns—night/naps, number of pillows, medications, times up at night
Social/emotional/ cognitive	Memory problems, difficulties in comprehending, slowed response and processing time; satisfaction with social life, barriers, use of time, difficult times (see Chapter 16 for additional guides)

When a functional deficit is reported or observed, follow the guidelines mentioned earlier in the areas for data collection on daily living to determine a deficit's impact on the elderly person's daily living and the strategies used to cope with it.

strengths they have as soon as possible so that losses do not occur. The expression "What you don't use you lose" is particularly significant for the elderly. It is also important for the nurse to document not only the kind of assistance needed but also that which is acceptable to the individual. The two may be quite different.

EXTERNAL RESOURCES

The other component of the nursing data base as suggested by the models in Chapter 1 is that of the nature and status of the external resources. For the over-70 age group, both subjective and objective data are crucial. The categories of external resources (see boxed material on p. 26) have been found to be useful in the nursing care of the elderly. These areas seem to address again the problems of the older person living independently; however, many of them are applicable to care in an institution and discharge planning.

These, then, are the major areas of nursing assessment and the priorities associated with dealing with an older population. The emphasis is on how patients see the situation as well as the objective reality, how they have been managing to this point, how satisfied or frustrated they are with their adjustments, and what they see their needs to be.

Categories of External Resources or Barriers

Housing	*Type:* Single or multiple family dwelling, yard, apartment, hotel room, transient housing, no housing, retirement apartment
	Institutional: Intensive care unit, acute care unit, long-term care—single or multiple bed settings
	Features: Stairs, location of bathroom and tub, shower, lighting, cooking facilities, risk factors (e.g., wires, small rugs, etc.), heating and cooling
Personal network	Living alone; living with spouse, children, friend(s), other patients; pets; relationship with and distance from family members, friends, neighbors, professional health care givers; primary care giver status
Communication devices	Phone, emergency contacts, intercom systems
	In institutions: level of staffing on each shift
Transportation	Public transportation availability and convenience, personal rides, senior citizen passes, volunteer transportation for health care; barriers to use of vehicles; own car, status of driver's license, money for fuel and upkeep
Finances	Perceived adequacy, problem areas, resources, concerns
Need for support	Nature of desired support services; support that would not be acceptable; available support services; ability to maintain support systems, both mechanical and personal

The presenting situation with the patient and the style of the nurse will determine which of these areas are initially addressed and what will constitute the total nursing data base for a patient. These areas are suggested as having relevance to the plan of nursing management.

For more details on issues related to nursing assessment, see Carnevali (1983).

Medication History in the Nursing Assessment

There is an additional area that, in the older person, is wisely handled as a separate component of the assessment. That is the medication history. Nurses have found that with the myriad drugs that are used by many older persons—prescribed, over-the-counter, and home remedies—it becomes important to address their drug-taking patterns, systems, and attitudes as a separate, not integrated, part of the assessment. It is also an assessment that is repeated at intervals appropriate to the drug-taking patterns and skills of the elderly person as well as changes in status that affect the taking of medications.

Medication-taking behavior, previous patterns of drug* use, and associated beliefs about medications are an important component of the data base in particular with the older population. Although it is true that in some situations the clinical pharmacists will collect a portion of the data in a drug history, the nursing perspective is different from that of the pharmacist.[†]

The pharmacist focuses on the names and kinds of drugs being taken. The nurse adds some different dimensions that include the following:

1. Previous patterns of medication use
2. Attitudes toward medications and their effects

*The terms *drugs, medicines,* and *medications* are used interchangeably in this chapter. However, because of the negative connotation the word *drug* has for some older persons, it is suggested that the terms *medication* or *medicine* be used in talking with older people.

[†]Read this section in conjunction with Chapter 10.

3. Side effects experienced and allergies
4. Ethnic or religious influences on the treatment of illness and health maintenance

The nurse is also interested in any physical or environmental barriers to the safe and effective use of medications or treatments. So, although it is wise to check the pharmacist's data to avoid duplication, it usually is necessary for the nurse to gather additional data in order to develop effective nursing management plans for any older person.

BRINGING IN THE MEDICATIONS

Nurses who have worked with ambulatory elderly often ask the older person periodically to put all the medications he is using into a paper bag and bring them to the clinic or office. The person should be told that this request refers to all medicines prescribed by all doctors as well as products he has gotten over the counter in drug stores, supermarkets, natural food stores, ethnic shops, and so forth. Give examples of aspirin, vitamins, laxatives, antacids, and medicinal teas. The person should bring those medicines taken regularly as well as those used only occasionally, including those in the medicine cabinet for some time and those shared by friends, relatives, or neighbors.

The explanation is made to the person that information gained from seeing the medications, their labels, and dates as well as from talking to him about them will enable the nurse to be more effective in working with the patient in managing his health care and daily living. Indicate to the person that many patients require pretty large bags, since medications are so widely used.

The medication containers and labels offer a concrete point of departure for gaining an understanding of the person's knowledge about medications and patterns of medication taking. It may also disclose the use of multiple physicians and pharmacists, making for the increased risk of drug interactions, because no one pharmacist will have a complete drug file for discovering drug interaction risks.

SEQUENCE IN THE MEDICATION ASSESSMENT

There is a preferred sequence of topics in assessing the individual's medication-taking behavior. It begins with current prescription drugs and moves on to over-the-counter remedies and finally to home remedies. The rationale is that in sharing information one discusses areas requiring the least risk—drugs prescribed by the health care provider. Here the only risk probably is that of reporting the adjustment of doses, schedules, or noncompliance. The next increment in risk is with the use of over-the-counter products; these are sold by pharmacists or major firms and, therefore, could be seen by the person as having some modicum of health system or societal approval. The area that may seem riskiest of all for the elderly person is an honest discussion of the use of home remedies and ethnic practices used in the treatment of illness or in health maintenance. The attitude of the health care provider seeking this information can greatly reduce the difficulty in discussing ethnic practices.

DATA ON CURRENT DRUG-TAKING PRACTICES

KNOWLEDGE OF DRUGS

If the person brings in medications, each bottle can be talked about to determine his working knowledge of the following:

- The name of the drug
- The dosage (milligram per gram and number of tablets or amount)
- Timing of medication
- Purpose of the drug and any effects being noted
- Side effects—those the person monitors and those being experienced

For the new patient who does not bring in the drugs and cannot remember drug names, the nurse may ask such questions as:

Do you take any medicines for your heart? For your blood pressure? For your breathing?
Do you take any water pills? Vitamins? Tranquilizers? Specific types of medicines?

BARRIERS TO SAFE MEDICATION TAKING

Much of the medication assessment is a subjective approach—viewed from the elderly person's perspective. However, the person may have some blind spots with regard to some aspects of his capability to follow the medical regimen safely. Therefore, it becomes important for the nurse to gather objective data on these areas—from the medical data base and from observations of patient behavior during interactions. Some areas of high risk that predict decreased ability to participate safely and effectively in drug regimens include

- Vision deficits
- Hearing deficits (taking in instructions)
- Intellectual or memory deficits
- Strong aversion to taking any medication
- Patterns of drug abuse or addiction
- Financial constraints

Perhaps further afield but still relevant on occasion is the attitude of family or significant others toward the regimen.

In these and other areas, the nurse needs to note as specifically and precisely as possible the observations made and the inferences drawn regarding the risks to safe medication-taking activities. Nursing management of medication taking will be built on these data.

It is important to know that the risk of errors increases directly and significantly with increases in numbers of medications (Schwartz et al, 1964).

SYSTEM FOR DRUG TAKING

Another area of data gathering that is particularly important with the elderly is that of learning what system the individual uses to remember and take the right drugs in the right amount at the right time. Herein lies the risk of precarious or ineffective drug taking. The nurse should learn the following:

Does the person put a day's supply in separated containers so that in the evening there is a check on what has been taken?

For those with vision problems:

How does the person know what pill is in which bottle?

One elderly patient indicated that he recognized pills by the sound as he shook the bottles. Pharmacists suggest that different-sized, -colored, or -shaped bottles or raised strips of tape on the sides of bottles are safer techniques.

Schwartz and associates (1964) found in the study of medication errors of the elderly that persons who had a system for remembering to take their medicines made fewer errors than those without a system. Almost any predictable daily event can be used as a reminder. One respondent remembered his pills by taking them every time he ate oatmeal. This worked for him because he had once-a-day pills and ate oatmeal once every day.

TIMING IN RELATIONSHIP TO ACTIVITIES OF DAILY LIVING

Timing of drugs in relationship to the activities of daily living, particularly in relation to meals and sleep and in relationship to other drugs, can be important. Three times a day or even 9 AM–1 PM–6 PM can have quite different relationships to meals and sleep for a person who eats two meals a day at 11 AM and 7 PM and retires at midnight as compared with one who eats 7 AM–12 PM–5 PM and retires at 9 PM. Further, the way drugs are given in the hospital or nursing home may not be the time they should be taken at home. If something is to be taken "before breakfast," be certain that the person (1) eats breakfast and (2) eats breakfast before noon. Blood levels of certain medications, such as antibiotics, need to be maintained for the drug to be effective. This means taking the drug regularly over the 24-hour period; others do not require such regular round-the-clock intervals. Be certain that a round-the-clock regimen is actually required on a medication before subjecting the patient to setting an alarm and being awakened to take a pill at 2 AM. Also know the person's usual sleep patterns. Often it is possible to schedule the drugs so that they coincide with times the person is normally awake or falls back to sleep readily.

MODIFYING THE DRUG REGIMEN

Knowing whether or not older persons adjust their medications in relationship to their signs and symptoms, and how they do it, it also significant. One patient reported to the doctor that his heartbeat was "hard as a hammer" on digoxin, 0.25 mg daily, but was fine on half that amount. This same patient has chronic obstructive pulmonary disease and keeps a supply of tetracycline prescribed by the physician, which he takes when a respiratory infection threatens. He has a known history of being responsible and knowledgeable about recognizing his symptoms and taking drugs. Physicians, however, appreciate a telephone call when a patient begins such a self-controlled regimen because then a check can be maintained on the patient. Occasionally a drug change or an office call can prevent the development of a more serious problem.

A less knowledgeable patient was found from a drug history to be taking nitroglycerin and digoxin interchangeably for chest pain. Some people discontinue antibiotics as soon as symptoms disappear instead of taking the full course prescribed, and then they have a relapse. Others staunchly continue to take medications despite side effects.

Some people are born "savers" and, when money is scarce, many older persons find the expense of medications an almost unsupportable burden. For whatever reason, there are those persons who save medications to use should a condition recur. Others exchange medications with someone who has a "similar condition." These are difficult behaviors to deal with, but they certainly should be delineated and addressed as sensitively and positively as possible since they affect the therapy the older person achieves.

OBSERVING FOR RESPONSE TO MEDICATIONS AND GIVING FEEDBACK

Because of the increased risk of side effects of drugs in the elderly, another area of data that is important to the nurse is the patient's pattern of observing drug effects:

What is the person aware of that should be noted? Will the person remember better with written guidelines?

How does the person check on his responses? Does he have the capacity to notice signs and symptoms?

Does the person have the vocabulary to give usable data to the health care provider?

What is the person's attitude about giving feedback? For example, does he tend not to want to bother the doctor or nurse? Does he tend to ignore symptoms? Does he worry about every twinge?

Does the person know the best time to call? Does he have access to a telephone?

Does the person know when it is important to report symptoms promptly—regardless of the day or hour—and what can wait for office hours?

Flow sheets on which the person can record data on critical variables may be useful. This technique will control the person who tends to want to report unending minutiae as well as the one who does not know what to report. It also fosters the person's active participation in his own treatment. An example is given in Figure 3–1.

Members of the health team need to be aware of what behaviors they are fostering by their response to patients as they teach them or respond to their calls. Failure to answer simple questions, failure to return calls, and condescending attitudes toward data not seen as important to the professional all can contribute to patterns of inadequate patient feedback.

OVER-THE-COUNTER PRODUCTS

Patterns in the use of over-the-counter products are also important. If the nurse has sensed a reluctance to share information, this section of the assessment can be prefaced by a remark such as, "There are a lot of products available to us in the drug store and supermarkets that help with our health. Do you use any of them?" If the person's memory seems to require jogging, the nurse can ask about specific types of medicines such as antacids, antidiarrheals, cough and cold remedies, laxatives, vitamins, and ointments.

Another approach is to ask the person if he has a particular complaint and what he does to relieve it (e.g., Do you have headaches? What do you do for them?). Include other complaints such as heartburn, gas, indigestion, nausea, diarrhea, constipation, head colds, chest colds, aching joints, and skin problems.

Bertha Johnson	1/16	1/17	1/18	1/19
Weight	200	201	204	
Episodes of shortness of breath	2	2	4	
Swelling of ankles a.m./p.m.	0/+	+/++	++/+++	
Lasix 1 tab/day	9am	forgot	8:30	

FIGURE 3–1   Medication flow sheet example.

HOME REMEDIES

There is a greater likelihood that the older person has learned family ways of dealing with health problems and complaints. The person also may feel, or know from past experience, that health professionals will ridicule these folkways. A means of approaching this subject is to say something like, "My family had some ways of treating colds and aches and pains that worked pretty well. I still use some of them. Did you grow up with some of these too?" If the response is affirmative, the nurse may continue with, "Are there any that you still find useful?"

One form of home remedy is adjustment in diet for particular complaints. For example, in some cultures persons who feel that they have "high blood" (too much blood volume) will restrict red meats and other red foods, whereas if the condition is felt to be "low blood," they will increase their consumption of red foods (red meats, beets, red fruits). There are many dietary remedies suggested to prevent or treat arthritis or rheumatism; some people drink lemon juice first thing in the morning.

Home remedies are as effective in some aspects of care as more expensive medications (e.g., gargles of salt and hot water, cough medicine of honey and hot tea, steam for sinusitis, and rice water for diarrhea). If the health care provider suggests these home remedies and they resolve the problem, the elderly person will feel the provider's concern for him.

BELIEF IN MEDICATIONS

Another critical area that may emerge overtly is the credibility that drugs have for the person. Aside from religious groups that overtly disavow reliance on medications, individuals vary markedly in their beliefs about the efficacy of drugs. Some want a pill for any complaint—the more the better. Others endure major physical dysfunction and discomfort rather than take medications. Most persons fall somewhere between these two extremes but tend to lean toward one or the other. It is important for the nurse to specifically seek data on the preference the person has regarding medications. Even highly educated and sophisticated persons (often health professionals) who do understand the rationale for the medication may not take prescribed medications.

Current items in the media—television, radio, newspapers, magazines, and books—can strongly influence attitudes and drug-taking behavior. Therefore, it is important for the nurse to know what is currently in vogue or under attack. The nurse can check whether this input has influenced patients and their attitudes or behavior in relationship to these drugs.

The data in the medication assessment is critical to working realistically with an elderly person in effectively incorporating drug therapy into his life. The data should affect prescription; the way in which drugs and their effects, monitoring, and feedback are introduced and supervised; the assistance needed in developing a system for safe and accurate drug taking; and the risks of drug interactions. Understanding home remedies and patterns allows for better articulation of prescriptions with the person's and family's usual way of doing things.

The data collected by the nurse should be located in the patient's record in such a way that others who are involved in planning for medications can be aware of the patient's lifestyle in medication taking.

Recording the Nursing Data Base

Regardless of the record system being used—traditional, problem-oriented format, or a computerized data record—the nursing data base, including the medication history, needs to be easily located in the permanent legal record. The overall nursing assessment should be recorded on a special form located near the physical examination and medical history forms, so that an integrated composite, interdisciplinary view of the data is easily available. In addition, data collated to "SOAP" (subjective, objective, analysis, plan) current presenting problems would reappear on the progress page or on nursing notes, depending on the system.

As the older person moves from one nursing system to another, it seems only fair and cost-effective that the nursing data base be carried with him. In some ambulatory care clinics, for instance, patients regularly carry communication to and from nursing homes or home health-care nurses and the physician–nurse teams in the office or clinic.

The Medical History and the Elderly Patient

The purposes of taking a medical history are to:

Evaluate health in terms of existent and potential problems

Give focus to the physical examination by establishing which body systems need to be examined in detail

Gather data that will assist in construction of differential diagnostic and prognostic statements

A standard form for the medical history contains the following elements (Bates, 1991; Judge et al, 1989).

Identifying data
Chief complaint
Present illness
Past medical history
Family history
Personal history
Review of systems

Each element of the medical history seeks specific data about the patient. The use to which this information is applied will differ with the age group being evaluated.

IDENTIFYING DATA

A review of the introductory data section gives demographic information about the person. In this section a key element is found in the source reliability statement. Implicit in this notation is the mental status of the individual. Inferences made about the person's ability to give information then sets the tone for all of the remaining information presented. When patients are reliable historians, details of symptoms and concerns from their own perspectives will follow. When an older person cannot give a history, then the majority of information contained in the history will come from a secondary source, e.g., medical records or a family member.

CHIEF COMPLAINT

The chief complaint is a statement of the problem in the patient's word. It documents the reason for the physician–patient contact. Usually this is illness related and will be symptomatol-ogy that is problematic to the patient. If the patient has sought out the physician, nurse practitioner, or physician assistant for a routine health evaluation, then this section may state "routine health examination."

PRESENT ILLNESS

In the history of present illness, the elderly person's perceptions of all major problems are recorded. Both the onset and chronology of the problems are documented. Careful symptom analysis is noted. Time frame, progression, self-treatment, and past history pertinent to the major concerns are often included. The data reflects elements of information used to determine the differential diagnoses to be pursued (Carnevali and Thomas, 1993).

PAST MEDICAL HISTORY

Illnesses, injuries, operations, hospitalizations, and health practices are identified in the section called past history. In the elderly, careful analysis of these data often demonstrate the progression of chronic conditions. Sometimes information presented here may give a clue to a diagnosis of subtle problems. For example, a series of fractures over a 3-year period might lead the examiner to institute more detailed questioning regarding dizziness, vision, or balance problems. In the absence of these symptoms, one might wonder about possible osteoporosis or neurologic deficits.

FAMILY HISTORY

Under the category of family history, information is elicited on the health status of three generations of the immediate family. In the old who are the survivors, this type of data is of value in evaluating expectations of disease outcomes as well as the nature of family support systems.

PERSONAL HISTORY

The personal history section deals with environmental information in terms of places of residence and description of occupation. It documents relationships, activities of daily living, and the lifestyle of the person. It can give clues to ways to individualize approaches to preventative health strategies.

REVIEW OF SYSTEMS

The section called review of systems is a screening tool. It is organized under body systems. The information sought is the presence or absence of symptoms and disease states. Symptoms of each body system are pursued individually in order to pick up any major problem missed in the initial exploration of patient concerns. The review of systems data are usually limited to occurrence in the past year but also include documentation of ongoing health problems.

STRATEGIES IN TAKING THE MEDICAL HISTORY

Familiarize yourself with the medical history form before seeing the patient. Translate your questions into terminology that has meaning to a layperson. Phrase questions to seek one piece of information at a time. Pause, to allow the person time to process your request and formulate a response, but beware of lengthy silences (over a minute) because these can increase the stress on the respondent.

Moving from open-ended requests for information to more specific ones is an effective approach. Begin with statements such as "Tell me about . . ." and allow the person to complete the response. For every symptom presented gather information on these factors:

Location
Character and quality
Quantity—intensity or severity
Timing and setting (continuous, intermittent, etc.)
Factors that increase (e.g., position, activity)
Factors that decrease (e.g., self-treatment and results)
Presence of additional but associated symptoms

Listen carefully to the replies on open-ended questions, then narrow the focus by asking forced-choice questions, e.g., "Do you sleep through the night or do you wake frequently?" Specific closed questions are introduced after the patient has given all voluntary information. If one starts with the specific questions too early, the elderly patient tends to stop offering new information and simply replies to questions.

The Physical Examination

When the medical history has been completed, the focus of the physical examination is established. The decision is made to perform either a baseline total examination or a limited but detailed examination of body systems related to the specific complaints.

GENERAL GUIDELINES

With the elderly, who are often cold and may be at risk for hypothermia, it is necessary to limit exposure of body parts to a minimum. This is accomplished by careful draping to expose only the area to be examined.

Some older people need additional time to process information. Attention to the quality of instructions for performing maneuvers during the physical examination is critical. Some elderly persons with deficits in processing capacity will require that requests be made in one-level commands (e.g., raise your eyebrows) and this may need to be accompanied by the examiner's cuing (i.e., the examiner demonstrates the behavior by, in this instance, raising her own eyebrows). In a person who has severe cognitive deficits, some segments of the examination will have to be omitted. For example, if the person has an attention span of less than 30 seconds, neurologic sensory testing or other maneuvers requiring complicated instructions are impossible.

A major concern in working with the old–old is mobility and balance. Some physical examination techniques are not appropriate for this group (e.g., deep knee bends). Other techniques need modification, such as range of motion of the hip in an elderly person who has had a total hip replacement, or prosthesis. Care must be taken in performing any test that has the potential to result in injury or falls.

Some individuals have physical deformities that require modifications of positioning. For example, the person with severe kyphosis may have difficulty in maintaining the supine position. The person with contractures of the hip will require modifications in the lithotomy position. Wheelchair-bound patients and those who require walkers for balance cannot perform Romberg's test.

Psychomotor skills and rationale for testing are found in basic textbooks of physical examination (see the references at the end of the chapter). To organize the examination and to minimize examiner omissions and patient fatigue, three factors are considered:

1. Minimize patient change of position
2. Organize the body into units for examination—head to toe
3. Integrate the information sought by body systems

It is especially important in working with the elderly to prevent fatigue of the patient (and the examiner) during physical examinations. The entire body can be examined by placing the patient in a sequence of positions—standing, then sitting, supine, sitting again, and the lithotomy or sidelying position. If, in addition to following a set pattern of patient positioning, the examiner establishes the habit of standing at the *right side* of the patient, it will assist in recalling the results of the examination when writing a report.

Establishment of a systematic examination routine reduces missing data. The units can be organized in a head-to-toe sequence or, in the peripheral extremity, in a head-to-foot approach. To recognize subtle findings, a comparison is made of side-to-side findings (right side to left side in extremities, or symmetry in area examinations of the head, neck, and trunk). Using this technique, the patient becomes his or her own control.

To evaluate findings, the examiner must keep in mind the normal age changes universal to this population and identify the range of normal for this group. The latter is established only with the experience of multiple examinations and a solid knowledge base of what to see.

When nurses are learning physical examination techniques, it is important that they focus on and learn one body system at a time. As each body system is mastered, another is added. Over time, organization and mastery of the content of each body system permits the examiner to integrate all systems into anatomic units, resulting in a comprehensive integrated physical examination.

To identify the different results on physical examination between a younger adult and the elderly person, the reader is referred to the references at the end of the chapter. The focus of the physical examination performed by the nurse is primarily that of identification of functional strengths and deficits. The following areas of physical examination data are pertinent to this objective:

Mobility	Postural blood pressures (see Chapter 28)
	Gait analysis
	Visual acuity and peripheral fields
	Active range of motion
	Lower extremity pulses (femoral, dorsal pedalis, and posterior tibial)
	Light touch, vibration, and position sense
	Foot examination (toenails, calluses, corns)
Eating	Swallowing evaluation (cranial nerves IX and X)
	Coordination of upper extremities
	Dentition
	Height and weight
Elimination	Bowel sound evaluation
	Rectal sphincter tone
	Percussion of bladder size
	Pelvic floor relaxation (women)
Energy	Apical pulse rate and rhythm
	Neck vein evaluation
	Cardiac auscultation
	Respiratory rate and character
	Chest auscultation
	Inspection of lower extremities for edema
Cognition	Carotid artery palpation and auscultation
	Hearing screening tests
	Mental status testing if deficit present

In geriatric nursing, the objective of all assessments is to identify the strengths and resources, as well as the deficits and the problem areas—whether they are pathology related or concerned with managing daily living—as a basis for maintaining the maximum functioning of the elderly person and an optimum quality of life. An accurate and appropriate data base permits accurate and precise diagnosis and prognostic statements as a basis for planning effective treatment. Please see the information presented in Appendices 3–1, 3–2, and 3–3 for more information. The minimum data set required by federal law for patients admitted to nursing homes is shown in Display 3–1.

References and Other Readings

Andres R, Bierman E, Hazzard W. Principles of geriatric medicine. New York: McGraw-Hill, 1985.

Baker M. A selective review of client assessment tools in long-term care of people. Unpublished. Waltham, MA: Levinson Policy Institute, The Florence Heller Graduate School of Advanced Studies in Social Welfare, Brandeis University, October 1980.

Bates. A guide to physical examination. 5th ed. Philadelphia: JB Lippincott, 1991.

Beckman HB, Frankel RM. The effect of physician

behavior on the collection of data. Ann Intern Med 1984; 101:692.

Brammer L. The helping relationship: process and skills. 2nd ed. Englewood Cliffs, NJ: Prentice-Hall, 1984.

Brockelhurst JC, ed. Textbook of geriatric medicine and gerontology. 3rd ed. Edinburgh: Churchill-Livingstone, 1985.

Caird RI, Judge TG. Assessment of the elderly patient. 2nd ed. Philadelphia: JB Lippincott, 1978.

Calkins E, Ford AB, Katz PR. Practice of geriatrics. 2nd ed. WB Saunders, 1992.

Carnevali D: Nursing care planning: diagnosis and management. 3rd ed. Philadelphia: JB Lippincott, 1983.

Carnevali D, et al. Diagnostic reasoning in nursing. Philadelphia: JB Lippincott, 1984.

Carnevali D, Thomas M. Diagnostic reasoning and decision making in nursing. Philadelphia: JB Lippincott, 1993.

Cassel CK, Riensenberg DE, Sorenson LB, Walsh JR. Geriatric medicine. 2nd ed. New York: Springer-Verlag, 1990.

Cormier LS, Cormier WH, Weisser RJ. Interviewing and helping skills for health professionals. Monterey, CA: Wadsworth Health Sciences Division, 1984.

Covington TR, Walker JI. Current geriatric therapy. Philadelphia: WB Saunders, 1984.

DeBettignies BH, Mahurin RK. Assessment of independent living skills in geriatric populations. Clin Geriatr Med 1989; 5:461.

DeGowin E, DeGowin R. Bedside diagnostic examination. 5th ed. New York: Macmillan, 1987.

Ebaugh FG, ed. Management of common problems in geriatric medicine. Menlo Park, CA: Addison-Wesley, 1981.

Folstein MF, Folstein SE, Hugh PR. Mini-mental state: a practical method for grading the cognitive state of patients for the clinician. J. Psychiatr Res 1975; 12:189.

Grimes J, Iannopollo E. Health assessment in nursing. Monterey, CA: Wadsworth Health Sciences Division, 1982.

Hamdy C. Geriatric medicine: a problem-oriented approach. London: Bailliere Tindall, 1984.

Hillman RS. Clinical skills: interviewing, history taking and physical diagnosis. New York: McGraw-Hill, 1981.

Judge R, Zuidema G, Fitzgerald F. Clinical diagnosis: a physiologic approach. 5th ed. Boston: Little, Brown, 1989.

Linn MW, Linn BS. Self-evaluation of life function (self) scale: a short comprehensive self-report of health for elderly adults. J Gerontol 1984; 39:603.

Ouslander JG, Osterwell D, Morley J. Medical care in the nursing home. New York: McGraw-Hill, 1991.

Reichel W. Clinical aspects of aging. 3rd ed. Baltimore, MD: Williams & Wilkins, 1989.

Schrock M. Holistic assessment of the healthy aged. New York: John Wiley & Sons, 1980.

Schwartz D, Henley B, Zutz L. The elderly ambulatory patient. New York: Macmillan, 1964.

Strub RL, Black FW. The mental status examination in neurology. 2nd ed. Philadelphia: FA Davis, 1985.

Wasson JH, et al. Continuity of outpatient medical care in elderly men. JAMA 1984; 252:2413.

APPENDIX 3–1
Medical History Adaptation to the Elderly

Chief Complaint

Relate to FUNCTION in comparison to a STRICT PATHOLOGIC approach.

Review of Systems

General: anorexia, fatigue, thirst, weight loss.

Head: headaches, particularly new symptoms and any related to visual difficulties.

Eyes: Loss of peripheral fields or central vision. Pain. Difficulty with glare at night or movement between bright and dark environments. Recent (6 months) change in vision status.

Ears: Loss of hearing other than high frequency. Tinnitus. Recent (6 months) change.

Mouth: Denture fit. Dentition status. Changes in taste perception. Dry mouth.

Throat: Voice change or dysphagia.

Endocrine: Changes in behavior with cardiovascular or nervous system. Chronic constipation, confusion, lethargy. History of thyroidectomy. Fainting, dizziness, chest pains, urinary frequency, fungus infection. Weight loss with satisfactory appetite.

Cardiovascular: Mental confusion, swollen ankles bilaterally, difficulty sleeping or eating.

Developed by Bruno P, Enloe C, Fretwell M, et al. Gerontological Nurse Practitioner Program, Physiological Nursing Department, University of Washington, Seattle, Washington, 1981.

Rheumatic fever, hypertension. Medication (salt retaining steroids or anti-inflammatory drugs). History of emotional (anxiety) turmoil in past 3 days. Hypotension with change in position. History of stroke. Cough, chest pain, dyspnea, falls.

Gastrointestinal: Epigastric and retrosternal distress. Nocturnal discomfort. General malaise, confusion. Bowel pattern—use of medication for length of time and/or lack of bowel movement over 3 days. Change in bowel habits. Hard stool, leaking, incontinence. Diarrhea, vomiting, abdominal pain. Change in nutritional patterns over past few years (intake or content).

Genitourinary: Frequency, nocturia, dysuria, urgency. Difficulty starting and stopping stream. Incontinence. History of pelvic surgery, parturition, vaginal pruritis. Postmenopausal bleeding, breast mass. History of urinary tract infection, fever, confusion.

Musculoskeletal: Proximal muscle weakness, polymyalgia, early morning stiffness. History of recent fractures (nontraumatic), pain in limbs, back or joints. Security in ambulation/ mobility. Change in gait.

Neurologic: Dizziness, falls, loss of consciousness, transient dysphagia, confusion withdrawal, headache, fits, or disorder of speech. Memory changes. Changes in sexual activity.

Integumentary: Lesions: change in size, color bleeding, no healing. Lower extremity edema, discoloration, pruritis, or pain.

Personal and Past History Summary Data

Change in normal daily activity
Stress level or changes therein (anxiety, fear, anger, rejection)

Allergies
Immunizations
Current medications including over-the-counter medications
Hospitalizations/ surgical procedures.

APPENDIX 3-2
Checkpoints and Terminology for Physical Examination of Selected Body Parts

(Samples of guides used in teaching physical examination to gerontological nurse practitioner students)

Head and Neck

STRUCTURES

Hair, scalp, skull, face, eyes, ears, nose, mouth and neck

INSPECTION

Symmetry

PALPATION

External structures

SEQUENCE OF EXAMINATION

HEAD

General: Face
Ears: External structures (+ hx or pe: cover, alternate cover test)
Nose: External structures
Mouth: Remove dentures

External: Lips
Internal: Mucous membrane, gums, teeth, Stenson's ducts, Wharton's ducts, tongue, pharynx

These are samples of guides used in teaching gerontologic nurse practitioner students physical examination skills. They were developed for the Gerontological Nurse Practitioner Program in the Physiological Nursing Department, Seattle, WA, University of Washington, 1984.

NECK

1. Lymph nodes (start with preauricular, postauricular, occipital, submaxillary, submandibular, anterior chain, posterior chain, and end with supreclavicular.
2. (Go to back) Thyroid
3. Position of trachea

TERMINOLOGY

Eye: Amblyopia, anisocoria, arcus senilis, astheopia, AV notching (nicking), cataract, conjunctivitis, diplopia, ectropion, entropion, epiphora, exophthalmos, funduscopy, glaucoma, hyphema, hypopyon, iritis, miosis, mydriasis, nystagmus, OD/OS, optic atrophy, papilledema, phoria, photophobia, presbyopia, proptosis, ptosis, tropia, visual field, yoked muscles
Head: Aphonia, deglutition, dysphagia, dysphonia, epiphora, epistaxsis, laryngopharynx, nares, nasopharynx, odynophagia, oropharynx, otalgia, otitis, otorrhea, rhinorrhea, stridor, vallecula, vestibule

Respiratory System

STRUCTURES

Nails, nares, neck muscles, trachea, thorax: skin, bones, lung fields, abdominal muscles

INSPECTION

1. Symmetry
2. Interspaces for bulging and retraction, use of accessory breathing muscles
3. Curve of spine
4. AP ratio
5. Bony thorax

PALPATION

1. Excursion (free and easy, equal)
2. Measure inspiration versus expiration
3. Tactile fremitus
4. Costal angle and spine

PERCUSSION

1. All lung fields
2. Diaphragm excursion
3. (+ hx: check tenderness and for rib fracture)

AUSCULTATION

1. All lung fields (listen to full respiratory cycle and all sites in pattern)
2. (+ hx or findings: vocal fremitus through egophony, whispered pectorilogy, and egophony)

SEQUENCE OF EXAMINATION

SITTING POSITION

Hands: Check angle of nail bed and bogginess
Head: Observe nares
Neck: Observe for use of accessory muscles
Count rate and observe characteristics of respiration
Walk to Back: 1. Check trachea 2. Examine posterior chest: I, Pa, Pe, A*
Go to Front: 1. Examine anterior chest: I, Pa, Pe, A

TERMINOLOGY

Asthma, atelectasis, breathlessness, breath sounds (vesicular, bronchovesicular and bronchial)
Adventitious sounds: crackles (rales), gurgles, wheezes (rhonchi), and friction rub
Bronchiectasis, bronchitis, COPD, clubbing, collapse, compression, consolidation, crackle, crepitation, cyanosis, dyspnea, emphysema, empyeme, FET, FVC, FEV_1, fremitus, hemoptysis, kyphosis, pleural effusion, pleurisy, pneumonia, pneumothorax, respiration terms (CheyneStokes respiration, Biot's breathing, hyperpnea, eupnea, orthopnea, tachypnea, *etc.*), scoliosis, stridor, Valsalva maneuver

Cardiac and Blood Vessels

STRUCTURES

Nails, pulses, blood pressure, funduscopic examination of vessels, carotids, jugular veins, precordium, and heart

INSPECTION

1. Pulsations
2. Heaves

PALPATION

1. Pulsations
2. Characteristics of vessels
3. Thrills
4. Apical pulse
5. Carotid pulse wave

PERCUSSION

1. Optional
2. Size of heart

AUSCULTATION

1. All valve sites
2. Start at base and work to apex
3. Inching technique

SEQUENCE OF EXAMINATION

SITTING POSITION

Hands: Check circulation time
Upper extremities: Check radial, brachial (axillary) pulses
Head: Visualization of vessels
Neck: Observe neck veins
       Palpate carotid pulses
       Check for bruits

*I = inspection, Pa = palpation, Pe = percussion, A = auscultation

ANTERIOR THORAX

1. Inspect for heaves and pulsations
2. Palpate each valve area for pulsations or thrills
3. Auscultate from base to apex listening for: Rate and rhythm (1x) (If irregular, take radial pulse concurrently to check for pulse deficit)
4. S1, S2 (Normal? Split?)
5. Systole and diastole
6. Extra sounds
7. If murmur present, what location in cardiac cycle, and where radiates

SUPINE POSITION

Neck: Check neck veins (if + history, check for engorgement by lifting patient to 45 degree angle)

Anterior Thorax
1. Inspect
2. Palpate
3. Auscultate, as above

Abdomen
1. Inspect for pulsations
2. Auscultate aorta and femorals for bruits
3. Palpate femoral pulses (if bruits present, auscultate renals)

Lower Extremities
1. Inspect for trophic changes
2. Palpate popliteal, posterior tibial, and dorsal pedalis pulses

TERMINOLOGY

Aneurysm, angina pectoris, apex, arrhythmia, atrial fibrillation, atrial flutter, atrial tachycardia, AV block, base, bradycardia, bruit, cor pulmonale, cyanosis, diastole, dyspnea, edema (brawny and pitting), embolism, friction rub, gallop rhythm, hypertension, infarction, murmur, orthopnea, palpitation, paroxysmal, presystolic, protodiastolic, pulse, Raynaud's phenomena, shock, syncope, systole, tachycardia, thrill, varicose

Agranulocytosis, anemia, epistaxis, erythrocytosis, hematopoiesis, hemolysis, leukemia, leukocytosis, leukopenia, lymphadenopathy, lymphoma, polycythemia, purpura, splenomegaly, thrombocytopenia, thrombocytosis

Musculoskeletal System

STRUCTURES

Bones, muscles, and joints

INSPECTION

1. Symmetry, deformity (redness, swelling)
2. Active range of motion
3. Passive range of motion

PALPATION (EACH JOINT)

1. Tenderness
2. Crepitation, heat
3. Strength (performed in conjunction with active range of motion)
4. Tone (entire extremity)

SEQUENCE OF EXAMINATION

STANDING POSITION

Station: Romberg with and without eyes open
Gait: Walking, start, stop, and turning

SITTING POSITION

1. *Hands* (PIP, DIP, MCP)
   a. Shake hands
   b. Squeeze fingers
   c. Make a fist, check thumb
   d. Claw: individual finger
   e. Abduction (adduction only if deficit or positive history)
2. *Forearm* (wrist)
   a. Flexion
   b. Hyperextension
   c. Radial and ulnar deviation (circular movement)
   d. Pronation/supination
3. *Upper arm* (shoulder)
   a. Adduction, abduction, external rotation, internal rotation, extension, flexion
   b. Strength (3)
   c. Entire upper extremity (UE): tone
4. *Head* (cranium)
5. *Neck* (flexion, extension, rotation, lateral bending)
   a. Spinal curve
6. *Posterior thorax* (spine: flexion, extension, rotation, lateral bending *with pelvis fixed*)
7. *Anterior thorax* (bony configuration)
   a. Supine
8. *Abdomen* (symmetry, muscle tone)
9. *Thighs* (hip: flexion, extension, internal and external rotation)
   a. Strength (3)
10. *Lower leg* (knee: flexion, extension)

11. *Foot* (dorsiflexion, plantar flexion, inversion, eversion)
    a. Inspect sole of foot
12. Entire lower extremity (LE): tone

TERMINOLOGY

Abduction, active range of motion, adduction, ankylosis, bursa, calcific tendinitis, capsule, carpal tunnel, cavus foot, club foot, contracture, contralateral, crepitation, eversion, inversion, joint effusion, kyphosis, paresthesia, passive range of motion, pronation, rotator cuff of shoulder scoliosis, spondylolisthesis, subluxation, supination, supine, synovitis, tendinitis, thoracic outlet, valgus, varus

Nervous System

STRUCTURES

Mental status, cranial, sensory, motor nerves, and reflexes

INSPECTION

1. Atrophy, tremor (involuntary movement), fasciculation
2. If sensory defect, *map* location

PALPATION

(Strength: tested in multiple sclerosis [MS])

SEQUENCE OF EXAMINATION

History: Assess mental status

STANDING POSITION

Snellen test (distant vision acuity)
Station: Romberg with and without eyes open, drift
Gait: Walking, start, stop, and turning

SITTING POSITION

1. *Hands*
2. *Upper extremity coordination:* Rapid alternating movements (Pronation/supination) or finger-to-nose test
3. (*Upper arm*) shoulder shrug (XI)
4. *Head:*

General: Face (V and VII)
Eyes: Visual acuity Jaeger (II)
        Central vision (II)
        Peripheral fields (II)
        EOM (III, IV, VI)
        PERRLA (III) + chamber depth
        Fundoscopy
        Corneal reflex
Ears: 1. Rinne
        2. (Behavioral)
Nose: Olfactory (I) tested only with positive history
Mouth: Pharynx and gag reflex (IX and X)
        Tongue (XII)
5. *Neck:* Head/neck strength (XI)
6. *Posterior thorax*
7. *Anterior thorax*

SUPINE POSITION

8. *Abdomen:* (Sensory) regional testing all body dermatomes for
   a. Light touch
   b. Pain (temperature)
   c. Vibration (position)
   d. Stereognosis (graphesthesia, two-point discrimination)
   e. Abdominal reflexes
9. *Thighs*
10. *Lower leg*
11. *Foot*
    a. Coordination: rapid alternating movement (toe tapping) or heel-to-shin test
    b. Babinski
12. Reflexes (sitting position)
    a. Triceps
    b. Biceps
    c. Brachioradialis
    d. Knee
    e. Ankle

TERMINOLOGY

Anarthria, asphasia, ataxia, atrophy, bulbar palsy, dysarthria, dysmetria, dysphagia, dysphasia, dysneuria, extinction (suppression), fasciculation, graphesthesia, homonymous hemianopia, lower motor neurons, nystagmus, optic atrophy, optic neuritis, papilledema, paresis, plegia, proprioception, ptosis, sensory "level," scotoma, stereognosis, upper motor neurons

APPENDIX 3–3
Sequence and Guide for Integrated Physical Examination

Area	Patient Position	Technique	Skin	Musculoskeletal	Neurologic	Head and Neck	Cardiovascular and Lymphatics	Respiratory	Abdomen	Genitalia/Rectum	Misc. Data/Equipment
General inspection	Standing and walking (entering office)	I	Color, texture, exposed areas (face, arms)	Posture, gross skeletal deformities, muscle mass symmetry, gross joint ROM	Balance, gait, start-stop ability, handshake	(Expression eye contact)		Posture ± use of accessory muscles			Height, weight, temperature
	Sitting (during history) or removing coat	I		Gross ROM, shoulder, hip, knees, elbows	Gross coordination, balance, facial expression, mood		B/P both arms, pulse	Ability to speak and breath respiratory rate			
	Sign form	I		Fine motor	Coordination						
	Changes to examining gown	I	Color, texture	Spine AP curvature				Thorax configuration			
	Standing (at examiner's request)	PA	Turgor ± lesions on posterior surface	Spinal tenderness, alignment, ROM	Rhomberg position sense	Position of trachea, size of thyroid		Symmetry of expansion thorax			
		PE								CV tenderness	
Upper extremity	Sitting	I	Color, texture, integrity, fingernails	Muscle size and symmetry, ROM	Finger-nose coordination or pronation-supination, hand		Palm of hand, Circulation time	± Clubbing			
		PA	Temperature	Joint spaces, muscle strength, against examiner	Strength-grasp, position sense		Radial pulses, Epitrochlear nodes				
Head and neck	Sitting	I and PA	Hair color, skin integrity	II	Cranial nerves visual acuity, visual fields (confrontation)	Eye structures, position, ophthalmoscopic 1) red reflex 2) eye grounds	Jugular venous filling				Snellen test, flashlight, ophthalmoscope, otoscope, tuning fork, cotton ball

(Continued)

41

Area	Patient Position	Technique	Skin	Musculoskeletal	Neurologic	Head and Neck	Cardiovascular and Lymphatics	Respiratory	Abdomen	Genitalia/ Rectum	Misc. Data/ Equipment
				III, IV, VI	Perrla eom						
				V	Temporal (PA) Masseter Corneal reflex	Ear structures (PA) Lymph node otoscopic a) eardrum					
				VII	Facial movements, puff cheeks, eyelid strength (PA)						
				VIII	Weber test Rinne test	Nasal structures (PE) sinuses					
				IX X	Elevation soft palate and uvula, gag reflex	Oral structures, (PA) Cervical lymph chain (PA)	(PA) Carotid pulses				
				XI	Shoulder shrug, turn head against resistance	Salivary glands a) Parotid b) Submaxillary					
				XII	Protrude tongue, tongue against cheek	(PA) Submental and submandibular lymph nodes					
Thorax	Sitting	I	Color, texture	Symmetry & size			± Heaves, pulsations	Rate, character, resp. Costal angle			
Note	Begin on posterior chest and progress to anterior chest.	PA	Breast examination (3 positions) Turgor				Axillary lymphatic nodes, ± thrills, pulsations, apical impulse	Symmetry of expansion, fremitus.			
		PE						Patterning screen. Diaphragm excursion			

Area	Patient Position	Technique	Skin	Musculoskeletal	Neurologic	Head and Neck	Cardiovascular and Lymphatics	Respiratory	Abdomen	Genitalia/Rectum	Misc. Data/Equipment
		A+				± Bruits 1) Carotids	Rate, rhythm, S1, S2, ± Bruits over subclavian areas. ± murmurs identify (valve area, placement in cycle)	Normal breath sounds			Stethoscope
	Supine		Breast exam (PA)				Repeat cardiac assessment				Stethoscope
Abdomen	Supine	A					± Bruits 1) Aorta 2) Renal A 3) Femoral		Bowel sounds		Stethoscope
		I	± Scars striae, hair distribution pattern	Symmetry					Umbilicus movement: vascular, peristaltic, edema		
		PA	Temperature	Muscle tone integrity	Abdominal reflexes		Femoral pulses, inguinal nodes		Light abd wall; Deep: tenderness, or masses; position		
		PE							Organ size/location 1) liver 2) spleen 3) stomach		
Lower extremities	Supine	I	Color, texture, ± trophic change, ± edema	ROM	Muscle symmetry, Heel to knee-shin-angle or toe tapping						
		PA		Muscle group strength against examiner	Plantar response		DP pulses PT pulses ± edema		Brudzinski's sign Kernig's sign (optional)		
Total body (head to toe)	Supine				Touch Pain Vibration						Cotton ball Safety pin Tuning fork
											(Continued)

APPENDIX 3–3 (Continued)

Area	Patient Position	Technique	Skin	Musculoskeletal	Neurologic	Head and Neck	Cardiovascular and Lymphatics	Respiratory	Abdomen	Genitalia/ Rectum	Misc. Data/ Equipment
	Sitting				DTRs 1) triceps 2) biceps 3) Bradio-radialus 4) knee 5) ankle						Percussion hammer
Genitalia/ rectum	Standing	I								Structure of penis and scro-tum ± bulging-femoral, inguinal area	
Male:		PA								Shaft of penis, scrotal sac contents, inguinal ring	Flashlight Examina-tion gloves
	On left side or bending over exami-nation table	I PA								Rectal sphincter Prostate Rectal shelf	
Female:	Lithotomy	I PA								External struc-tures, va-gina and cervix, Pap smears Perform bimanual	Speculum; Gloves

Teaching tool developed by C. Enloe for the students in the Gerontological Nurse Practitioner Program, Physiological Nursing Department. Seattle, WA, University of Washington, 1984.

Abbreviations: I, inspection; PA, palpation; PE, percussion; A, auscultation.

Display 3–1 Minimum data set for nursing facility resident.

MINIMUM DATA SET
FOR NURSING FACILITY RESIDENT ASSESSMENT AND CARE SCREENING (MDS)
(Status in last 7 days, unless other time frame indicated)

Code "NA" or ⊝ = Information unavailable or untrustworthy

▨ = Write in the appropriate alpha or numeric response

☐ = Check (✓) if response is applicable

UPON COMPLETION OF THIS FORM, GO TO RAP TRIGGER LEGEND.

SECTION A. IDENTIFICATION AND BACKGROUND INFORMATION

1. **ASSESSMENT DATE**   ☐☐ — ☐☐ — ☐☐☐☐
   Month   Day   Year

2. **RESIDENT NAME**   (First)   (Middle Initial)   (Last)

3. **SOCIAL SECURITY NO.**   ☐☐☐ — ☐☐ — ☐☐☐☐

4. **MEDICAID NO. (If applicable)**

5. **MEDICAL RECORD NO.**

6. **REASON FOR ASSESSMENT**
   1. Initial admission assess.   4. Annual assessment
   2. Hosp/Medicare reassess.   5. Significant change in status
   3. Readmission assessment   6. Other (e.g., UR)

7. **CURRENT PAYMENT SOURCE(S) FOR N.H. STAY**   (Billing Office to indicate; check all that apply)
   a. Medicaid   a.
   b. Medicare   b.
   c. CHAMPUS   c.
   d. VA   d.
   e. Self pay/Private insurance   e.
   f. Other   f.

8. **RESPONSIBILITY/ LEGAL GUARDIAN**   (Check all that apply)
   a. Legal guardian   a.
   b. Other legal oversight   b.
   c. Durable power attrny./ health care proxy   c.
   d. Family member responsible   d.
   e. Resident responsible   e.
   f. NONE OF ABOVE   f.

9. **ADVANCED DIRECTIVES**   (For those items with supporting documentation in the medical record, check all that apply)
   a. Living will   a.
   b. Do not resuscitate   b.
   c. Do not hospitalize   c.
   d. Organ donation   d.
   e. Autopsy request   e.
   f. Feeding restrictions   f.
   g. Medication restrictions   g.
   h. Other treatment restrictions   h.
   i. NONE OF ABOVE   i.

10. **DISCHARGE PLANNED WITHIN 3 MOS.**   (Does not include discharge due to death)
    0. No   1. Yes   2. Unknown/uncertain

11. **PARTICIPATE IN ASSESSMENT**
    a. Resident   0. No   1. Yes   a.
    b. Family   0. No   1. Yes   2. No family   b.

12. **SIGNATURES** (Indicate section(s) completed next to name)
    Signature & Date of RN Assessment Coordinator
    _____
    Signatures, Titles & Dates of Others Who Completed Part of the Assessment
    _____
    _____
    _____
    _____

SECTION B. COGNITIVE PATTERNS

1. **COMATOSE**   (Persistent vegetative state/no discernible consciousness)
   0. No   1. Yes (Skip to SECTION E)

2. **MEMORY**   (Recall of what was learned or known)
   a. Short-term memory OK—seems/appears to recall after 5 minutes
   0. Memory OK   1. Memory problem ▲²   a.
   b. Long-term memory OK—seems/appears to recall long past
   0. Memory OK   1. Memory problem ▲²   b.

3. **MEMORY/ RECALL ABILITY**   (Check all that resident normally able to recall during last 7 days) Fewer than 3 ✓ = ▲²
   a. Current season   a.
   b. Location of own room   b.
   c. Staff names/faces   c.
   d. That he/she is in a nursing home   d.
   e. NONE OF ABOVE are recalled   e.

4. **COGNITIVE SKILLS FOR DAILY DECISION-MAKING**   (Made decisions regarding tasks of daily life)
   0. Independent—decisions consistent/reasonable ▲⁴
   1. Modified independence—some difficulty in new situations only ▲⁴ ▲²
   2. Moderately impaired—decisions poor; cues/supervision required ▲⁴ ▲²
   3. Severely impaired—never/rarely made decisions ▲²

5. **INDICATORS OF DELIRIUM —PERIODIC DISORDERED THINKING/ AWARENESS**   (Check if condition over last 7 days appears different from usual functioning)
   a. Less alert, easily distracted ●¹   a.
   b. Changing awareness of environment ●¹   b.
   c. Episodes of incoherent speech ●¹   c.
   d. Periods of motor restlessness or lethargy ●¹   d.
   e. Cognitive ability varies over course of day ●¹   e.
   f. NONE OF ABOVE   f.

6. **CHANGE IN COGNITIVE STATUS**   Change in resident's cognitive status, skills, or abilities in last 90 days
   0. No change   1. Improved   2. Deteriorated ●¹ ▲¹⁴

SECTION C. COMMUNICATION/HEARING PATTERNS

1. **HEARING**   (With hearing appliance, if used)
   0. Hears adequately—normal talk, TV, phone
   1. Minimal difficulty when not in quiet setting
   2. Hears in special situation only—speaker has to adjust tonal quality and speak distinctly
   3. Highly impaired/absence of useful hearing

2. **COMMUNICATION DEVICES/ TECHNIQUES**   (Check all that apply during last 7 days)
   a. Hearing aid, present and used   a.
   b. Hearing aid, present and not used   b.
   c. Other receptive comm. technique used (e.g., lip read)   c.
   d. NONE OF ABOVE   d.

3. **MODES OF EXPRESSION**   (Check all used by resident to make needs known)
   a. Speech   a.
   b. Writing messages to express or clarify needs   b.
   c. Signs/gestures/sounds   c.
   d. Communication board   d.
   e. Other   e.
   f. NONE OF ABOVE   f.

4. **MAKING SELF UNDERSTOOD**   (Express information content—however able)
   0. Understood
   1. Usually Understood-difficulty finding words or finishing thoughts
   2. Sometimes Understood-ability is limited to making concrete requests ▲⁴
   3. Rarely/Never Understood ▲⁴

5. **ABILITY TO UNDERSTAND OTHERS**   (Understanding verbal information content-however able)
   0. Understands
   1. Usually Understands-may miss some part/intent of message ▲²
   2. Sometimes Understands-responds adequately to simple, direct communication ▲² ▲⁴ ▲⁵
   3. Rarely/Never Understands ▲² ▲⁴ ▲⁵

6. **CHANGE IN COMMUNICATION/ HEARING**   Resident's ability to express, understand and hear information has changed over last 90 days
   0. No change   1. Improved   2. Deteriorated ●¹

SECTION D. VISION PATTERNS

1. **VISION**   (Ability to see in adequate light and with glasses if used)
   0. Adequate—sees fine detail, including regular print in newspapers/books
   1. Impaired—sees large print, but not regular print in newspapers/books ●³
   2. Highly Impaired—limited vision, not able to see newspaper headlines, appears to follow objects with eyes ●³
   3. Severely Impaired—no vision or appears to see only light, colors, or shapes ●³

● = Automatic Trigger   ▲ = Potential Trigger

1 - Delirium	5 - ADL Functional/Rehabilitation Potential	9 - Behavior Problems 13 - Feeding Tubes 17 - Psychotropic Drug Use
2 - Cognitive Loss/Dementia	6 - Urinary Incontinence and Indwelling Catheter	10 - Activities 14 - Dehydration/Fluid Maintenance 18 - Physical Restraints
3 - Visual Function	7 - Psychosocial Well-Being	11 - Falls 15 - Dental Care
4 - Communication	8 - Mood State	12 - Nutritional Status 16 - Pressure Ulcers

Form 1828HF   BRIGGS, Des Moines, IA 50306 (800) 247-2343   PRINTED IN U.S.A.   1 of 4   Rev. 3/91

(Continued)

Resident Name _____   I.D. Number _____

2.	VISUAL LIMITATIONS/ DIFFICULTIES	a. Side vision problems—decreased peripheral vision; (e.g., leaves food on one side of tray, difficulty traveling, bumps into people and objects, misjudges placement of chair when seating self) ●[3]	a.
		b. Experiences any of the following: sees halos or rings around lights, sees flashes of light; sees "curtains" over eyes	b.
		c. *NONE OF ABOVE*	c.
3.	VISUAL APPLIANCES	Glasses; contact lenses; lens implant; magnifying glass 0. No 1. Yes	

SECTION E. PHYSICAL FUNCTIONING AND STRUCTURAL PROBLEMS

1. ADL SELF-PERFORMANCE *(Code for resident's PERFORMANCE OVER ALL SHIFTS during last 7 days—Not including setup)*
- **0. INDEPENDENT**—No help or oversight—OR—Help/oversight provided only 1 or 2 times during last 7 days.
- **1. SUPERVISION**—Oversight encouragement or cueing provided 3+ times during last 7 days—OR—Supervision plus physical assistance provided only 1 or 2 times during last 7 days.
- **2. LIMITED ASSISTANCE**—Resident highly involved in activity, received physical help in guided maneuvering of limbs, or other nonweight bearing assistance 3+ times—OR—More help provided only 1 or 2 times during last 7 days.
- **3. EXTENSIVE ASSISTANCE**—While resident performed part of activity, over last 7-day period, help of following type(s) provided 3 or more times:
  - — Weight-bearing support
  - — Full staff performance during part (but not all) of last 7 days.
- **4. TOTAL DEPENDENCE**—Full staff performance of activity during entire 7 days.

2. ADL SUPPORT PROVIDED—*(Code for MOST SUPPORT PROVIDED OVER ALL SHIFTS during last 7 days; code regardless of resident's self-performance classification)*
- **0. No setup** or physical help from staff
- **1. Setup help only**
- **2. One-person physical assist**
- **3. Two+ person physical assist**

			1 SELF-PERFORMANCE	2 SUPPORT
a.	BED MOBILITY	How resident moves to and from lying position, turns side to side, and positions body while in bed for self-perf = ▲[5]		
b.	TRANSFER	How resident moves between surfaces—to/from: bed, chair, wheelchair, standing position (EXCLUDE to/from bath/toilet) 3 or 4 for self-perf = ▲[5]		
c.	LOCO-MOTION	How resident moves between locations in his/her room and adjacent corridor on same floor. If in wheelchair, self-sufficiency once in chair 3 or 4 for self-perf = ▲[5]		
d.	DRESSING	How resident puts on, fastens, and takes off all items of street clothing, including donning/removing prosthesis 3 or 4 for self-perf = ▲[5]		
e.	EATING	How resident eats and drinks (regardless of skill) 3 or 4 for self-perf = ▲[5]		
f.	TOILET USE	How resident uses the toilet room (or commode, bed-pan, urinal); transfers on/off toilet, cleanses, changes pad, manages ostomy or catheter, adjusts clothes 3 or 4 for self-perf = ▲[5]		
g.	PERSONAL HYGIENE	How resident maintains personal hygiene, including combing hair, brushing teeth, shaving, applying makeup, washing/drying face, hands, and perineum (EXCLUDE baths and showers)		

3.	BATHING	How resident takes full-body bath, sponge bath, and transfers in/out of tub/shower (EXCLUDE washing of back and hair. Code for most dependent in self-performance and support. Bathing Self-Performance codes appear below.) 3 or 4 for (a) = ▲[5] 0. Independent—No help provided 1. Supervision—Oversight help only 2. Physical help limited to transfer only 3. Physical help in part of bathing activity 4. Total dependence	a.	b.

4.	BODY CONTROL PROBLEMS	*(Check all that apply during last 7 days)*	
		a. Balance—partial or total loss of ability to balance self while standing ▲[11]	a.
		b. Bedfast all or most of the time ▲[11]	b.
		c. Contracture to arms, legs, shoulders, or hands	c.
		d. Hemiplegia/hemiparesis ▲[11]	d.
		e. Quadriplegia ▲[11]	e.
		f. Arm—partial or total loss of voluntary movement	f.
		g. Hand—lack of dexterity (e.g., problem using toothbrush or adjusting hearing aid)	g.
		h. Leg—partial or total loss of voluntary movement ▲[11]	h.
		i. Leg—unsteady gait	i.
		j. Trunk—partial or total loss of ability to position, balance, or turn body ▲[11]	j.
		k. Amputation	k.
		l. *NONE OF ABOVE*	l.

5.	MOBILITY APPLIANCES/ DEVICES	*(Check all that apply during last 7 days)*	
		a. Cane/walker	a.
		b. Brace/prosthesis	b.
		c. Wheeled self	c.
		d. Other person wheeled	d.
		e. Lifted (manually/ mechanically)	e.
		f. *NONE OF ABOVE*	f.
6.	TASK SEG-MENTATION	Resident requires that some or all of ADL activities be broken into a series of subtasks so that resident can perform them. 0. No 1. Yes	
7.	ADL FUNC-TIONAL REHAB. POTENTIAL	a. Resident believes he/she capable of increased independence in at least some ADLs ▲[5]	a.
		b. Direct care staff believe resident capable of increased independence in at least some ADLs ▲[5]	b.
		c. Resident able to perform tasks/activity but is very slow	c.
		d. Major difference in ADL Self-Performance or ADL Support in mornings and evenings (at least a one category change in Self-Performance or Support in any ADL)	d.
		e. *NONE OF ABOVE*	e.
8.	CHANGE IN ADL FUNCTION	Change in ADL self-performance in last 90 days 0. No change 1. Improved 2. Deteriorated ▲[14]	

SECTION F. CONTINENCE IN LAST 14 DAYS

1. CONTINENCE SELF-CONTROL CATEGORIES
(Code for resident performance over all shifts.)
- **0. CONTINENT**—Complete control
- **1. USUALLY CONTINENT**—BLADDER, incontinent episodes once a week or less; BOWEL, less than weekly
- **2. OCCASIONALLY INCONTINENT**—BLADDER, 2+ times a week but not daily; BOWEL, once a week
- **3. FREQUENTLY INCONTINENT**—BLADDER, tended to be incontinent daily, but some control present (e.g., on day shift); BOWEL, 2-3 times a week
- **4. INCONTINENT**—Had inadequate control. BLADDER, multiple daily episodes; BOWEL, all (or almost all) of the time.

a.	BOWEL CONTINENCE	Control of bowel movement, with appliance or bowel continence programs if employed	
b.	BLADDER CONTINENCE	Control of urinary bladder function (if dribbles, volume insufficient to soak through underpants), with appliances (e.g., foley) or continence programs, if employed 2, 3 or 4 = ▲[6]	
2.	INCONTINENCE RELATED TESTING	*(Skip if resident's bladder continence code equals 0 or 1 AND no catheter is used)*	
		a. Resident has been tested for a urinary tract infection	a.
		b. Resident has been checked for presence of a fecal impaction, or there is adequate bowel elimination	b.
		c. *NONE OF ABOVE*	c.
3.	APPLIANCES AND PROGRAMS	a. Any scheduled toileting plan	a.
		b. External (condom) catheter ▲[6]	b.
		c. Indwelling catheter ▲[6]	c.
		d. Intermittent catheter ▲[6]	d.
		e. Did not use toilet room/ commode/urinal	e.
		f. Pads/briefs used ▲[6]	f.
		g. Enemas/irrigation	g.
		h. Ostomy	h.
		i. *NONE OF ABOVE*	i.
4.	CHANGE IN URINARY CONTINENCE	Change in urinary continence or programs in last 90 days 0. No change 1. Improved 2. Deteriorated	

SKIP TO SECTION J IF COMATOSE

SECTION G. PSYCHOSOCIAL WELL-BEING

1.	SENSE OF INITIATIVE/ INVOLVE-MENT	a. At ease interacting with others	a.
		b. At ease doing planned or structured activities	b.
		c. At ease doing self-initiated activities	c.
		d. Establishes own goals	d.
		e. Pursues involvement in life of facility (i.e., makes/keeps friends; involved in group activities; responds positively to new activities; assists at religious services)	e.
		f. Accepts invitations into most group activities	f.
		g. *NONE OF ABOVE*	g.
2.	UNSETTLED RELATION-SHIPS	a. Covert/open conflict with and/or repeated criticism of staff ●[7]	a.
		b. Unhappy with roommate ●[7]	b.
		c. Unhappy with residents other than roommate ●[7]	c.
		d. Openly expresses conflict/anger with family or friends ●[7]	d.
		e. Absence of personal contact with family/friends	e.
		f. Recent loss of close family member/friend	f.
		g. *NONE OF ABOVE*	g.

● = Automatic Trigger   ▲ = Potential Trigger

1 - Delirium	5 - ADL Functional/Rehabilitation Potential	9 - Behavior Problems
2 - Cognitive Loss/Dementia	6 - Urinary Incontinence and Indwelling Catheter	10 - Activities
3 - Visual Function	7 - Psychosocial Well-Being	11 - Falls
4 - Communication	8 - Mood State	12 - Nutritional Status

13 - Feeding Tubes	17 - Psychotropic Drug Use
14 - Dehydration/Fluid Maintenance	18 - Physical Restraints
15 - Dental Care	
16 - Pressure Ulcers	

Resident Name _____   I.D. Number _____

3.	PAST ROLES	a. Strong identification with past roles and life status	a.
		b. Expresses sadness/anger/empty feeling over lost roles/status ●[7]	b.
		c. *NONE OF ABOVE*	c.

SECTION H. MOOD AND BEHAVIOR PATTERNS

1.	SAD OR ANXIOUS MOOD	*(Check all that apply during last 30 days)*	
		a. **VERBAL EXPRESSIONS of DISTRESS** by resident (sadness, sense that nothing matters, hopelessness, worthlessness, unrealistic fears, vocal expressions of anxiety or grief) ●[8]	a.
		DEMONSTRATED (OBSERVABLE) SIGNS of mental DISTRESS	
		b. Tearfulness, emotional groaning, sighing, breathlessness ●[8]	b.
		c. Motor agitation such as pacing, handwringing or picking ●[8]	c.
		d. Failure to eat or take medications, withdrawal from self-care or leisure activities ●[8] ▲[14]	d.
		e. Pervasive concern with health ●[8]	e.
		f. Recurrent thoughts of death—e.g., believes he/she is about to die, have a heart attack ●[8]	f.
		g. Suicidal thoughts/actions ●[8]	g.
		h. *NONE OF ABOVE*	h.
2.	MOOD PERSISTENCE	Sad or anxious mood intrudes on daily life over last 7 days—not easily altered, doesn't "cheer up" 0. No 1. Yes ●[8]	
3.	PROBLEM BEHAVIOR	*(Code for behavior in last 7 days)* 0. Behavior **not exhibited** in last 7 days 1. Behavior of this type occurred **less than daily** 2. Behavior of this type occurred **daily or more frequently**	
		a. **WANDERING** (moved with no rational purpose; seemingly oblivious to needs or safety) 1 or 2 = ●[9]	a.
		b. **VERBALLY ABUSIVE** (others were threatened, screamed at, cursed at) 1 or 2 = ●[9]	b.
		c. **PHYSICALLY ABUSIVE** (others were hit, shoved, scratched, sexually abused) 1 or 2 = ●[9]	c.
		d. **SOCIALLY INAPPROPRIATE/DISRUPTIVE BEHAVIOR** (made disrupting sounds, noisy, screams, self-abusive acts, sexual behavior or disrobing in public, smeared/threw food/feces, hoarding, rummaged through others' belongings) 1 or 2 = ●[9]	d.
4.	RESIDENT RESISTS CARE	*(Check all types of resistance that occurred in the last 7 days)*	
		a. Resisted taking medications/injection	a.
		b. Resisted ADL assistance	b.
		c. *NONE OF ABOVE*	c.
5.	BEHAVIOR MANAGEMENT PROGRAM	Behavior problem has been addressed by clinically developed behavior management program. (Note: Do not include programs that involve only physical restraints or psychotropic medications in this category.) 0. No behavior problem 1. Yes, addressed 2. No, not addressed	
6.	CHANGE IN MOOD	Change in mood in last 90 days 0. No change 1. Improved 2. Deteriorated ▲[1]	
7.	CHANGE IN PROBLEM BEHAVIOR	Change in problem behavioral signs in last 90 days 0. No change 1. Improved 2. Deteriorated ●[1]	

SECTION I. ACTIVITY PURSUIT PATTERNS

1.	TIME AWAKE	*(Check appropriate time periods—last 7 days)* Resident awake all or most of time (i.e., naps no more than one hour per time period) in the:	
		a. Morning 7a.m.–Noon (or when resident wakes up)	a.	c. Evening 5p.m.–10p.m. (or bedtime)	c.
		b. Afternoon Noon–5p.m.	b.	d. *NONE OF ABOVE*	d.
2.	AVERAGE TIME INVOLVED IN ACTIVITIES	0. Most—(more than 2/3 of time) ▲[10] 2. Little—(less than 1/3 of time) ▲[10] 1. Some—(1/3 to 2/3 time) 3. None ▲[10]	
3.	PREFERRED ACTIVITY SETTINGS	*(Check all settings in which activities are preferred)*	
		a. Own room	a.	d. Outside facility	d.
		b. Day/activity room	b.	e. *NONE OF ABOVE*	e.
		c. Inside NH/off unit	c.		

4.	GENERAL ACTIVITIES PREFERENCES (adapted to resident's current abilities)	*(Check all specific preferences whether or not activity is currently available to resident)*	
		a. Cards/other games	a.	f. Spiritual/religious activ.	f.
		b. Crafts/arts	b.	g. Trips/shopping	g.
		c. Exercise/sports	c.	h. Walking/wheeling outdoors	h.
		d. Music	d.	i. Watch TV	i.
		e. Read/write	e.	j. *NONE OF ABOVE*	j.
5.	PREFERS MORE OR DIFFERENT ACTIVITIES	Resident expresses/indicates preference for other activities/choices. 0. No 1. Yes ●[10]	

SECTION J. DISEASE DIAGNOSES

Check only those diseases present that have a relationship to current ADL status, cognitive status, behavior status, medical treatments, or risk of death. (Do not list old/inactive diagnoses.) (If none apply, check the NONE OF ABOVE box)

1.	DISEASES	**HEART/CIRCULATION**			r. Manic depressive (bipolar disease)	r.
		a. Arteriosclerotic heart disease (ASHD)	a.		**SENSORY**	
		b. Cardiac dysrhythmias	b.		s. Cataracts	s.
		c. Congestive heart failure	c.		t. Glaucoma	t.
		d. Hypertension	d.		**OTHER**	
		e. Hypotension	e.		u. Allergies	u.
		f. Peripheral vascular disease	f.		v. Anemia	v.
		g. Other cardiovascular disease	g.		w. Arthritis	w.
		NEUROLOGICAL			x. Cancer	x.
		h. Alzheimer's	h.		y. Diabetes mellitus	y.
		i. Dementia other than Alzheimer's	i.		z. Explicit terminal prognosis	z.
		j. Aphasia	j.		aa. Hypothyroidism	aa.
		k. Cerebrovascular accident (stroke)	k.		bb. Osteoporosis	bb.
		l. Multiple sclerosis	l.		cc. Seizure disorder	cc.
		m. Parkinson's disease	m.		dd. Septicemia	dd.
		PULMONARY			ee. Urinary tract infection—in last 30 days ▲[14]	ee.
		n. Emphysema/asthma/COPD	n.		ff. *NONE OF ABOVE*	ff.
		o. Pneumonia	o.			
		PSYCHIATRIC/MOOD				
		p. Anxiety disorder	p.			
		q. Depression	q.			
2.	OTHER CURRENT DIAGNOSES AND ICD-9 CODES	260–263.9 ●[12] 276.5 ▲[14] 291.0–293.1 ●[1]			
		a.			
		b.			
		c.			
		d.			
		e.			
		f.			

SECTION K. HEALTH CONDITIONS

1.	PROBLEM CONDITIONS	*(Check all problems that are present in last 7 days unless other time frame indicated)*	
		a. Constipation	a.	j. Pain—resident complains or shows evidence of pain daily or almost daily	j.
		b. Diarrhea ▲[14]	b.		
		c. Dizziness/vertigo ▲[14]	c.		
		d. Edema	d.	k. Recurrent lung aspirations in last 90 days	k.
		e. Fecal impaction	e.		
		f. Fever ▲[14]	f.	l. Shortness of breath	l.
		g. Hallucinations/delusions	g.	m. Syncope (fainting)	m.
		h. Internal bleeding ▲[14]	h.	n. Vomiting ▲[14]	n.
		i. Joint pain	i.	o. *NONE OF ABOVE*	o.
2.	ACCIDENTS	a. Fell—past 30 days ●[11]	a.	c. Hip fracture in last 180 days	c.
		b. Fell—past 31-180 days ●[11]	b.	d. *NONE OF ABOVE*	d.

(Continued)

Resident Name _____   I.D. Number _____

3.	STABILITY OF CONDITIONS	a. Conditions/diseases make resident's cognitive, ADL, or behavior status unstable—fluctuating, precarious, or deteriorating.	a.
		b. Resident experiencing an acute episode or a flare-up of a recurrent/chronic problem.	b.
		c. *NONE OF THE ABOVE*	c.

SECTION L. ORAL/NUTRITIONAL STATUS

1.	ORAL PROBLEMS	a. Chewing problem	a.	c. Mouth pain ●[15]	c.
		b. Swallowing problem		d. *NONE OF ABOVE*	d.

2.	HEIGHT AND WEIGHT	*Record height (a) in inches and weight (b) in pounds.* Weight based on most recent status in **last 30 days**; measure weight consistently **in accord with standard facility** practice—e.g., in a.m. after voiding, before meal, with shoes off, and in nightclothes. HT (in.) [a.] WT (lb.) [b.]	
		c. Weight loss (i.e., 5% + in **last 30 days**; or 10% in **last 180 days**) 0. No 1. Yes ●[12] ▲[14]	c.

3.	NUTRITIONAL PROBLEMS	a. Complains about the taste of many foods ●[12]	a.	d. Regular complaint of hunger ●[12]	d.
		b. Insufficient fluid; dehydrated ●[14]	b.	e. Leaves 25%+ food uneaten at most meals ●[12] ▲[14]	e.
		c. Did **NOT** consume all/almost all liquids provided during last 3 days ▲[14]	c.	f. *NONE OF ABOVE*	f.

4.	NUTRITIONAL APPROACHES	a. Parenteral/IV ▲[14] ●[12]	a.	e. Therapeutic diet ●[12]	e.
		b. Feeding tube ▲[14] ●[13]	b.	f. Dietary supplement between meals	f.
		c. Mechanically altered diet ●[12]	c.	g. Plate guard, stabilized built-up utensil, etc.	g.
		d. Syringe (oral feeding) ●[12]	d.	h. *NONE OF ABOVE*	h.

SECTION M. ORAL/DENTAL STATUS

1.	ORAL STATUS AND DISEASE PREVENTION	a. Debris (soft, easily movable substances) present in mouth prior to going to bed at night ●[15]	a.
		b. Has dentures or removable bridge	b.
		c. Some/all natural teeth lost—does not have or does not use dentures (or partial plates) ●[15]	c.
		d. Broken, loose, or carious teeth ●[15]	d.
		e. Inflamed gums (gingiva), oral abscesses, swollen or bleeding gums, ulcers, or rashes ●[15]	e.
		f. Daily cleaning of teeth/dentures If not checked = ●[15]	f.
		g. *NONE OF ABOVE*	g.

SECTION N. SKIN CONDITION

1.	STASIS ULCER	(i.e., open lesion caused by poor venous circulation to lower extremities) 0. No 1. Yes	
2.	PRESSURE ULCERS	*(Code for highest stage of pressure ulcer)*	
		0. No pressure ulcers	
		1. Stage 1 A persistent area of skin redness (without a break in the skin) that does not disappear when pressure is relieved ●[12] ●[16]	
		2. Stage 2 A partial thickness loss of skin layers that presents clinically as an abrasion, blister, or shallow crater ●[12] ●[16]	
		3. Stage 3 A full thickness of skin is lost, exposing the subcutaneous tissues—presents as a deep crater with or without undermining adjacent tissue ●[12] ●[16]	
		4. Stage 4 A full thickness of skin and subcutaneous tissue is lost, exposing muscle and/or bone ●[12] ●[16]	
3.	HISTORY OF RESOLVED/ CURED PRESSURE ULCERS	Resident has had a pressure ulcer that was resolved/cured in **last 90 days** 0. No 1. Yes	

4.	SKIN PROBLEMS/ CARE	a. Open lesions other than stasis or pressure ulcers (e.g., cuts)	a.
		b. Skin desensitized to pain/pressure/discomfort	b.
	If None Checked From C Thru G = ▲[11]	c. Protective/preventive skin care	c.
		d. Turning/repositioning program	d.
		e. Pressure-relieving beds, bed/chair pads (e.g., egg crate pads)	e.
		f. Wound care/treatment (e.g., pressure ulcer care, surgical wound)	f.
		g. Other skin care/treatment	g.
		h. *NONE OF ABOVE*	h.

SECTION O. MEDICATION USE

1.	NUMBER OF MEDI-CATIONS	(Record the number of *different medications used in* the last 7 days; enter "0" if none used.)	
2.	NEW MEDI-CATIONS	Resident has received new medications during the **last 90 days** 0. No 1. Yes	
3.	INJECTIONS	*(Record the number of days injections of any type received during the last 7 days.)*	
4.	DAYS RECEIVED THE FOLLOWING MEDICATION	(Record the number of days during last 7 days; *Enter "0" if not used; enter "1" if long-acting meds. used less than weekly.)*	
		a. Antipsychotics 1–7 = ▲[9] ▲[11] ▲[17]	a.
		b. Antianxiety/hypnotics 1–7 = ▲[9] ▲[11] ▲[17]	b.
		c. Antidepressants 1–7 = ▲[9] ▲[11] ▲[17]	c.
5.	PREVIOUS MEDICATION RESULTS	*(SKIP this question if resident currently receiving anti-psychotics, antidepressants, or antianxiety/hypnotics—otherwise* code correct response for last 90 days.) Resident has previously received psychoactive medications for a mood or behavior problem, and these medications were effective (without undue adverse consequences).	
		0. No, drugs not used 1. Drugs were effective 2. Drugs were not effective 3. Drug effectiveness unknown	

SECTION P. SPECIAL TREATMENTS AND PROCEDURES

1.	SPECIAL TREAT-MENTS AND PROCE-DURES	SPECIAL CARE—*Check treatments received during the last 14 days.*			
		a. Chemotherapy	a.	f. IV meds	f.
		b. Radiation	b.	g. Transfusions	g.
		c. Dialysis	c.	h. O₂	h.
		d. Suctioning	d.	i. Other _____	i.
		e. Trach. care	e.	j. *NONE OF ABOVE*	j.
		THERAPIES—*Record the number of days each of the following therapies was administered (for at least 10 minutes during a day) in the last 7 days:*			
		k. Speech—language pathology and audiology services			k.
		l. Occupational therapy			l.
		m. Physical therapy			m.
		n. Psychological therapy (any licensed professional)			n.
		o. Respiratory Therapy			o.
2.	ABNORMAL LAB VALUES	Has the resident had any **abnormal lab values** during the last 90-day period? 0. No 1. Yes 2. No tests performed	
3.	DEVICES AND RESTRAINTS	*Use the following code for last 7 days:* 0 Not used 1 Used less than daily 2 Used daily	
		a. Bed rails	a.
		b. Trunk restraint 1 or 2 = ▲[9] ●[18]	b.
		c. Limb restraint 1 or 2 = ▲[9] ●[18]	c.
		d. Chair prevents rising 1 or 2 = ▲[9] ●[18]	d.

● = Automatic Trigger   ▲ = Potential Trigger

1 - Delirium	5 - ADL Functional/Rehabilitation Potential	9 - Behavior Problems 13 - Feeding Tubes 17 - Psychotropic Drug Use
2 - Cognitive Loss/Dementia	6 - Urinary Incontinence and Indwelling Catheter	10 - Activities 14 - Dehydration/Fluid Maintenance 18 - Physical Restraints
3 - Visual Function	7 - Psychosocial Well-Being	11 - Falls 15 - Dental Care
4 - Communication	8 - Mood State	12 - Nutritional Status 16 - Pressure Ulcers

FACE SHEET FOR NURSING FACILITY RESIDENT ASSESSMENT AND CARE SCREENING (MDS)
BACKGROUND INFORMATION/INTAKE AT ADMISSION

I. IDENTIFICATION INFORMATION

1. RESIDENT NAME _____
   (First)   (Middle Initial)   (Last)
   ID# _____

2. DATE OF CURRENT ADMISSION
   Month — Day — Year

3. MEDICARE No. (SOC. SEC. or Comparable No. if no Medicare No.)

4. FACILITY PROVIDER NO.
   Federal No.

5. GENDER   1. Male   2. Female

6. RACE/ETHNICITY
   1. American Indian/Alaskan Native   4. Hispanic
   2. Asian/Pacific Islander   5. White, not of Hispanic origin
   3. Black, not of Hispanic origin

7. BIRTHDATE   Month — Day — Year

8. LIFETIME OCCUPATION

9. PRIMARY LANGUAGE   Resident's primary language is a language other than English.   0. No   1. Yes _____ (Specify)

10. RESIDENTIAL HISTORY PAST 5 YEARS   *(Check all settings resident lived in during 5 years prior to admission)*
    a. Prior stay at this nursing home   a.
    b. Other nursing home/residential facility   b.
    c. MH/psychiatric setting   c.
    d. MR/DD setting   d.
    e. *NONE OF ABOVE*   e.

11. MENTAL HEALTH HISTORY   Does resident's RECORD indicate any history of mental retardation, mental illness, or any other mental health problem?   0. No   1. Yes

12. CONDITIONS RELATED TO MR/DD STATUS   **Check all conditions** that are related to MR/DD Status, that were manifested before age 22, and are likely to continue indefinitely.
    a. Not Applicable—no MR/DD (Skip to Item 13)   a.
    MR/DD with Organic Condition
    b. Cerebral palsy   b.
    c. Down's syndrome   c.
    d. Autism   d.
    e. Epilepsy   e.
    f. Other organic condition related to MR/DD   f.
    g. MR/DD with no organic condition   g.
    h. Unknown   h.

13. MARITAL STATUS
    1. Never Married   3. Widowed   5. Divorced
    2. Married   4. Separated

14. ADMITTED FROM
    1. Private home or apt.   3. Acute care hospital
    2. Nursing facility   4. Other

15. LIVED ALONE   0. No   1. Yes   2. In other facility

[ ] = Code the appropriate response   [b.] = Check (✓) if response is applicable

16. ADMISSION INFORMATION AMENDED   *(Check all that apply)*
    a. Accurate information unavailable earlier   a.
    b. Observation revealed additional information   b.
    c. Resident unstable at admission   c.

II. BACKGROUND INFORMATION AT RETURN/READMISSION

1. DATE OF CURRENT READMISSION   Month — Day — Year

2. MARITAL STATUS
   1. Never Married   3. Widowed   5. Divorced
   2. Married   4. Separated

3. ADMITTED FROM
   1. Private home or apt.   3. Acute care hospital
   2. Nursing facility   4. Other

4. LIVED ALONE   0. No   1. Yes   2. In other facility

5. ADMISSION INFORMATION AMENDED   *(Check all that apply)*
   a. Accurate information unavailable earlier   a.
   b. Observation revealed additional information   b.
   c. Resident unstable at admission   c.

III. CUSTOMARY ROUTINE (ONLY AT FIRST ADMISSION)

1. CUSTOMARY ROUTINE (Year prior to first admission to a nursing home)   *(Check all that apply. If all information UNKNOWN, check last box only.)*

CYCLE OF DAILY EVENTS
a. Stays up late at night (e.g., after 9 pm)   a.
b. Naps regularly during day (at least 1 hour)   b.
c. Goes out 1+ days a week   c.
d. Stays busy with hobbies, reading, or fixed daily routine   d.
e. Spends most time alone or watching TV   e.
f. Moves independently indoors (with appliances, if used)   f.
g. *NONE OF ABOVE*   g.

EATING PATTERNS
h. Distinct food preferences   h.
i. Eats between meals all or most days   i.
j. Use of alcoholic beverage(s) at least weekly   j.
k. *NONE OF ABOVE*   k.

ADL PATTERNS
l. In bedclothes much of day   l.
m. Wakens to toilet all or most nights   m.
n. Has irregular bowel movement pattern   n.
o. Prefers showers for bathing   o.
p. *NONE OF ABOVE*   p.

INVOLVEMENT PATTERNS
q. Daily contact with relatives/close friends   q.
r. Usually attends church, temple, synagogue (etc.)   r.
s. Finds strength in faith   s.
t. Daily animal companion/presence   t.
u. Involved in group activities   u.
v. *NONE OF ABOVE*   v.
w. UNKNOWN—Resident/family unable to provide information   w.

Signature and Date of RN Assessment Coordinator: _____
Signatures and Dates of Others Who Completed Part of the Assessment:

_____   _____   _____

_____   _____   _____

END

Form 1827HF   BRIGGS, Des Moines, IA 50306 (800) 247-2343 PRINTED IN U.S.A.   (9-90)

PART TWO

Ethical and Governmental Issues Associated with Nursing Care of the Elderly

Ethical, legal, and policy issues form a pervasive influence on much of nursing practice and health care for older people. The availability of biomedical technology, varying philosophies about individuals' and families' rights to choose, malpractice factors, and limitations on financial resources make the delivery of nursing care to this population increasingly complex. Chapter 4 examines ethical and legal issues and explores some of the common areas with which nurses need to concern themselves, including Living Wills, Durable Power of Attorney, and Patient Self-determination Act.

Chapter 5, "Governmental Policies," was written by an experienced nursing home administrator and gerontological nurse practitioner. This chapter gives an historical background on laws that have affected many of the current policies related to the elderly. To provide the best nursing care possible, nurses need expert working knowledge of the resources and constraints or structure inherent in governmental policies. A section on acquired immunodeficiency syndrome (AIDS), is included in this chapter as a policy issue, not because it is a common problem for the elderly at present, but because nurses need to be aware of the increasing competition for scarce health care resources and long-term care placement associated with the growing population of AIDS patients.

4
Ethical Issues

THOMAS R. McCORMICK

It is commonly expected that most inhabitants of the United States will live beyond the age of 70 years. The demographics of the aging population are well documented. There are 33 million people in the United States over the age of 65. The great majority of these persons are active and healthy. Improvements in wellness lifestyles, including attention to exercise, nutrition, the avoidance of tobacco, and moderate alcohol use, along with developments in health care have contributed to longevity and a high quality of life for many older citizens. After achieving their major life goals most people look forward to the satisfaction of increased leisure time and independence from the workplace. A surprisingly high percentage will live out the last years of their lives in their own homes, carrying out the activities of daily living independently, or with a minimum of support.

On the other hand, the increasing numbers of elderly persons implies that a significant percentage of these individuals will need health care. Approximately 23% of persons over the age of 65 have one or more aspects of disability in self-care, while 40% over the age of 75 years have a multiple chronic illness (Special Report, N Engl J Med, 1991). Especially, as the end of life approaches, intensive medical and nursing care may be sought. Many of the health problems of the elderly are of a chronic nature and demand continuity of care. Others may expect to die from the rather sudden onset of symptoms of cancer, heart or vascular disease, or

other organ system failures. Unfortunately, with advancing age there is an increased risk for the development of Alzheimer's disease, a lingering degenerative process. Currently it is estimated that 40% of those over the age of 75 years have dementia (Special Report, N Engl J Med, 1991). This is unfortunate because those 85 years and older make up a category of the population that is growing at a rate six times that of the population as a whole.

The one fact that is clearer to this generation of persons than any other age group is the certainty of death. No one escapes old age alive. Many older patients have achieved a general acceptance of death and its inevitability. They do not fear death itself and often find solace in their religious beliefs, the support of their faith community, family, friends, and the achievement of their major life goals. Others may even look forward to death as a final rest from their labors and a relief from suffering.

Most elderly persons, however, admit to fear and anxiety about the circumstances of their dying. Common concerns center around the appropriate use of the health care system as life draws to a close. Some are fearful that they may be denied access to the health care that is needed to restore them to health or to alleviate their suffering. Still others are anxious that they will lose control and be placed on life-prolonging technology that will keep their bodies alive long past the survival of their minds and spirits.

53

Thus, a cluster of complex ethical issues surround the elderly person concerning the appropriate use of health care in the final stages of life. Nurses caring for the older patient often have opportunities to provide support for the patient's preferences and can be powerful advocates for the values of the patient at a time of vulnerability or diminished capacity. Too frequently in this society, some of the most crucial decisions regarding health care arise at a time when the patient's decision-making capacities may be most threatened by mental and physical impairment and suffering.

Patient Rights

Health care professionals, by virtue of training, possess a superior body of knowledge about health and disease. When combined with the virtue of benevolence, physicians and nurses may appropriately recommend a course of action that is designed to promote the apparent best interests of the patient. It must never be minimized, however, that the best interests of any particular patient are determined by the values or preferences of that patient. Competent adult patients have the right to make their own health care decisions. This includes the right to refuse treatment, even lifesaving or life-prolonging treatment. This right is not lost when the patient experiences diminished capacity or even loses mental competency for decision making.

There are several ways in which the patient's wishes may be served:

1. The competent patient may establish his preference through verbal communication with the health care provider before the loss of competency.
2. The patient's preferences may be preserved in a Living Will or Natural Death Act Directive to Physicians.
3. The patient's wishes may be carried out through the appointment of a guardian.
4. The patient may designate a legal surrogate, who is apprised beforehand of the desires and values of the patient and is given Durable Power of Attorney for Health Care.
5. The wishes of an unconscious or incompetent patient may also be communicated by the legal next of kin. Increasing numbers of states have recognized a hierarchy of decision makers by listing in order those with the

power to exercise choices on behalf of the incompetent patient, such as the following:
   a. the patient's spouse,
   b. children of the patient who are at least 18 years of age,
   c. parents of the patient, and
   d. adult brothers and sisters of the patient who are reasonably situated to participate in the decision-making process (Revised Code of Washington State Law).

Autonomy

The right of patients to be self-determining in their health care is well established in both ethical principles and legal precedents. From an ethical perspective, there is general agreement that such rights are based on our society's high regard for patient autonomy or self-rule. Ethicists remind us of the evolution away from physician paternalism, a practice that was encouraged in the Hippocratic tradition, and toward the self-determination of the modern, enlightened, autonomous patient.

There are numerous legal cases supporting patient autonomy. In one of the earliest cases, decided in 1914 by Justice Cardozo in *Scholendorf v Society of New York Hospital*, the judge asserted "Every human being of adult years and of sound mind has a right to determine what shall be done with his body" (Jonsen et al, 1982).

While there is general agreement and respect for the principle of patient autonomy, in actual nursing practice, the application of this principle frequently is problematic. The most common application of the autonomy principle is through the notion of the informed consent of a competent adult patient, or conversely, the refusal of consent for treatment. The patient must be assumed to be competent, a legal term, unless there is persuasive evidence to the contrary. In that case, to declare a patient legally incompetent requires a psychiatric examination and a competency hearing by the court. The judge must issue a ruling declaring the patient incompetent and a guardian must be appointed, or recognized, by the court as the bona fide surrogate decision maker on the patient's behalf.

It is often the case in the clinical setting that the elderly patient has diminished capacity for decision making, but is not incompetent, or the patient's capacity may wax and wane with changes in the current health status. In such cases, the status of the patient may change from moment to moment, hour to hour, or day to day. These changes require appropriate assessment by the health care professionals toward the end that the integrity of the patient may be served. The patient may not have the capacity to perform some tasks, such as accurately balancing a checkbook, but may clearly have the capacity to refuse renal dialysis, chemotherapy, or a particularly invasive procedure.

In such cases, the guidance of an ethical principle may be much more practically useful than resorting to the courts each time the patient's mental status changes. Appropriate use of the principle of patient autonomy is to a large degree dependent on the commitment of the health care professionals in responding to individual patients. For example, the behavior of one elderly patient who spends a great deal of time alone may simply be the choice of one who relishes privacy and introspection. The same behavior in a different patient may signal the onset of clinical depression, and further investigation may reveal a constellation of vegetative symptoms that indicate the need for antidepressants. Our society places great trust in the integrity of the health care professionals in respecting and protecting the rights and interests of the vulnerable elderly under these circumstances.

Decision-making Challenges

Physicians and nurses who are committed to following the preferences of their patients to the best of their ability find it particularly vexing when urgent decisions must be made at a time when the patient is of diminished capacity. Under such circumstances it is easy to see that treatment decisions might be made that are contrary to the patient's desires. The conservative ethic of erring on the side of life when the patient's wishes are doubtful or unknown usually prevails, particularly in an emergency. Therefore, patients may be subjected to more aggressive intervention in the last stage of life than they would have desired (see Display 4–1).

Elderly patients who are unexpectedly confronted with treatment decisions with profound implications often find themselves overwhelmed in attempting to comprehend what it will mean to be placed on a respirator or to refuse a respirator when they are in respiratory distress. For example, consider the 84-year-old patient with emphysema, who has made it abundantly clear that he did not want to spend his last days on a respirator. Now, however, his dyspnea worsens and he becomes increasingly anxious about his shortness of breath and asks the nurse if she thinks he should go on the ventilator. The nurse, acting as his advocate, will assure him that if he chooses he can receive ventilator assistance. She will also assure him that she remembers his earlier request not to be placed on a respirator. The nurse might say "I remember that on several occasions you told us you absolutely did not want to be placed on a ventilator. Now that you are having more difficulty breathing it is only natural that you feel anxious. Many patients at times like this are so anxious about breathing that they may feel the respirator is their only choice. I want to remind you as we said in our earlier discussion that you do have another choice. We have good medications to help treat the discomfort you are feeling about your shortness of breath. We can give you some medication to help you relax. With the medication, you will not feel so anxious about your breathing. You may be wondering, what would that be like, or what would happen then. Many patients simply go to sleep, their respirations gradually become lighter, and they are able then to die peacefully in their sleep, without resorting to the use of a respirator."

In this case, it may be easier to simply intubate the ambivalent patient and provide respiratory support, thus avoiding a possibly stressful conversation. However, the role of advocacy suggests that the nurse find ways to support the authentic values of the patient by providing leadership in such crucial moments of decision making.

The formerly able patient who was clear that he wanted to be a no-code, may agree to a code designation from a persuasive nurse or physician while in a more vulnerable state as an inpatient. As in the previously mentioned case, the nurse-advocate will find ways to address the anxiety and ambivalence of the patient so that his *authentic* wishes may be carried out.

It should be borne in mind that the patient may not know what his authentic values are until he is actually faced with dying or "doing nothing more" to prolong his life. Patients in general often become distressed and anguished when it is disclosed that nothing more can be done medically to prolong their lives. Exceptions to this are individuals who have passed through the transition in which they have relinquished hope in a curative model and have come to accept palliative measures and the inevitability of death.

Advanced Directives

Much of the uncertainty regarding the patient's wishes can be overcome by the use of advanced directives. Currently, 47 states and the District of Columbia have passed Natural Death Acts (also popularly called Living Wills) and/or Durable Power of Attorney for Health Care Acts (41 states have Natural Death Act Laws). Both of these legally affirm the right of competent adult patients to declare in advance their wishes regarding refusal of aggressive treatment in the face of a terminal illness when death is imminent. The Natural Death Act Directive to Physicians is intended to stand as the patient's final word in the event that the patient should become incompetent. Some states provide further opportunity for patients to exclude particular interventions by listing on the Living Will exclusions such as respirators, dialysis, or artificially administered nutrition or hydration. The Nevada Supreme Court outlined a process whereby a terminally ill patient or a nonterminally ill patient may discontinue life-support systems (Medical Ethics Advisor, 1991).

The first state to pass Natural Death Act Legislation was California in 1976, with many other states following shortly thereafter. In spite of this, the percentage of the population who have actually signed a directive has remained very small, probably fewer than 10%. An even smaller number have provided a copy of the Living Will to their primary physician. This is due, no doubt, to a variety of reasons, including the denial of death and the hesitancy to consider morbid ideas. However, the largest single factor has been the lack of public awareness about the need for taking this action and the availability of this legal document to protect their values when they are unable to communicate their wishes. To address the issue of public awareness, Senators Danforth and Moynihan sponsored the Patient Self-determination Act (PSD), which was included in the Omnibus Budget Reconciliation Act of 1990 and was passed with little notice or notoriety.

This landmark federal legislation, although passed in 1990, was scheduled to take effect in December 1991. The Patient Self-Determination Act places new demands on health care providers to act on behalf of patients. In order to be eligible to receive Medicare and Medicaid payments, health care institutions must now explain to all patients on admission to a health care facility their right to make decisions concerning medical care, "including the right to accept or refuse medical or surgical treatment and the right to formulate advanced directives" (Omnibus Budget Reconciliation Act, 1990).

The written information described in the Patient Self-Determination Act is to be provided to adult individuals in the following circumstances:

- In the case of a hospital, at the time of the individual's admission as an inpatient.
- In the case of a skilled nursing facility, at the time of the individual's admission as a resident.
- In the case of a home health agency, in advance of the individual coming under the care of the agency.
- In the case of a hospice program, at the time of initial receipt of hospice care by the individual from the program.
- In the case of an eligible managed care program, at the time of enrollment of the individual with the organization (Omnibus Budget Reconciliation Act, 1990).

It is anticipated that the 1990s will give rise to a dramatic increase in the use and implementation of Living Wills or Natural Death Act Directives as more and more elderly patients discover that they can convey their wishes even beyond the loss of consciousness or lucidity (see Display 4–2).

DURABLE POWER OF ATTORNEY FOR HEALTH CARE

Although the Living Will is a legal document in most states, some health care providers may be uncomfortable implementing its directives to withhold aggressive treatment if they believe such treatment would benefit the patient, or if a significant amount of time has passed since the document was signed. If, in addition to the Living Will, the patient has executed a Durable Power of Attorney for Health Care (see Display 4–3), these problems can usually be overcome quite simply. The patient's legally appointed representative can declare and interpret the patient's wishes and values. This agent is chosen because he is perceived to be sufficiently familiar with the patient so as to accurately reflect the unique values of the patient. The intent behind the Living Will can be disclosed and affirmed, thus reassuring the physicians and nurses that the actual wishes of the patient are being served.

This action of the surrogate in representing the wishes of the patient is called *substituted judgment.* It means that the surrogate is standing in for the incompetent patient and providing the judgment he believes the patient would have made for himself had the patient the capacity to do so. For example, the person holding Durable Power of Attorney for Health Care for an elderly Jehovah's Witness might refuse, on the patient's behalf, a blood transfusion that is judged by the physician to be an essential lifesaving procedure. In such a case, one may disagree with the values of the patient (regarding blood transfusions) while upholding the authentic preference of the patient to refuse blood (substituted judgment).

Physicians and nurses are by training, and by commitment to the codes of the professions, morally obligated to act in the best interests of the patient. In most cases it is ethically correct to follow the best interest principle as a guiding ethical principle. This is particularly true when patients are unable to decide for themselves. In the case of the elderly Jehovah's Witness, however, following the best interest principle in a strict medical sense would be the wrong thing to do since it would be a violation of a sincerely held religious belief. Following the substituted judgment of the patient as articulated by the chosen representative would be ethically correct.

Cases such as those cited remind us that the unconscious or incompetent patient often presents the health care team with several ethical issues surrounding his care. Frequently, two or more of the prima facie principles of medical and nursing ethics, such as autonomy and beneficence, come into play. It may be difficult to choose between them. In an emergency situation when the wishes of the patient are not clearly known, it is the general practice to follow the principle of do no harm or to provide the greatest benefit for the patient in terms of a reasonable medical or nursing judgment. On the other hand, when the patient's wishes are clearly known, or when a patient's surrogate decision maker can speak for the patient, the principle of autonomy may ethically take precedence. Such is our respect for the always fragile and often variable meaning of patient autonomy in the clinical setting.

DO NOT RESUSCITATE ORDERS: CODE OR NO-CODE?

The appropriate code designation is another perplexing ethical issue surrounding treatment decisions near the end of life. In the 1960s it became widely known that persons suffering cardiac or respiratory arrest could be resuscitated. At first, cardiopulmonary resuscitation (CPR) was performed on younger persons, usually with an acute, reversible illness. During the 1970s and 1980s CPR became a technical imperative. More and more hospitalized patients were routinely given CPR if they arrested in the hospital. Eventually, it came to be considered an ethical imperative to attempt to resuscitate every patient, unless they had previously requested that no code be called. Resuscitative attempts were made on older patients, some with sepsis, multiorgan system failure, and even metastatic cancer.

By the beginning of the 1990s it became clinically apparent that many such resuscitative attempts were futile and very costly. With increasing frequency, more and more patients were requesting do not resuscitate orders (see Display 4–4). Many expressed fear of having their lives prolonged unnecessarily under conditions that they considered highly objectionable. Two cases in particular, those of Karen Ann Quinlan (1976) and Nancy Cruzan (1990), received widespread attention in the national news media. The plight of these two unfortunate patients, both in a persistent vegetative state as a result of neurologic insult, led to increased awareness on the part of the public. Many elderly patients in particular felt anxious about the possible loss of control over decisions about CPR and other forms of aggressive intervention that might result in their survival with an extremely poor quality of life.

The need for research into the outcomes of CPR in the hospital was apparent by the beginning of the 1990s. Investigation reveals that of the approximately 220 million people who die each year in the United States, CPR is performed on about one third of that number. Roughly one third of those receiving CPR in the hospital are revived, yet only a small fraction of those actually survive that hospitalization. Several studies seemed to confirm the hypothesis that if the patient is elderly, suffering from severe pneumonia, metastasized cancer, sepsis, acute stroke, or multiorgan system failure, then CPR is virtually a futile treatment.

It is now clear that code status needs to be discussed with the patient as early as possible. It is ideal for the primary care physician to have annual discussions with elderly patients about their wishes. Certainly, at the time of admission, the physician should discuss the possibilities of arrest with elderly patients and enter their decision about CPR into the chart. This is especially important because many patients who are sick enough to be hospitalized have a serious illness that erodes their capacity to make decisions as the illness progresses. Thus, it is most respectful of the patient's autonomy to discuss the issue of CPR so that the informed patient can make his own decision. Often, the nurse can be a special advocate for patients in such cases by helping them understand the nature of their illness and whether CPR appears to be appropriate in the light of their medical prognosis. The nurse, due to her close working relationship with patients, may also be the person with the best information about the values of the patient. Is Mr. Jones hanging on until his grandson arrives, and might he want CPR even if there was small likelihood of him leaving the hospital alive? Is Mrs. Smith adamant about not having CPR performed on her, even if her physician thinks there is a slim chance that she might survive this hospitalization?

Sometimes the patient is incapacitated or incompetent to make a decision about code status at the time of admission. In such cases, a legitimate proxy should assume the task of making a code designation that represents either the substituted judgment of the patient when he was rational or that is in the current best interests of the patient, if the former is unknown. The usual hierarchy of decision making by proxy is (1) legal guardian, (2) person holding Durable Power of Attorney for Health Care, (3) spouse, (4) adult children, and (5) siblings. Frequently, the nurse will be able to examine the chart and talk with those closest to the incapacitated patient. In her role as advocate of the patient, she can encourage and facilitate the process of getting the appropriate party to communicate the surrogate decision regarding CPR to the physician and recorded in the patient's chart.

Thus, the chart may indicate do not resuscitate orders by request of the patient or by request of the legitimate proxy. Still another category of code designation exists in current practice in many states: do not resuscitate by reason of medical futility. Since research has clarified the situations in which CPR is reasonably expected to be ineffective, it is important to recognize that there is no moral obligation to offer a medically futile procedure. In fact, there is growing consensus among health care professionals that it is morally obligatory to not offer medically futile treatments.

Nurses encountering such a situation find themselves on the cutting edge of ethical decision making. The most usual situation in which the futility designation is used is in the case of the very ill patient where CPR would be medically futile, who is incompetent to speak for himself, and who has not authorized proxy or family member to represent him. It should be noted, that if there is disagreement among the staff about his prognosis or the likelihood of futility, then such cases should be reviewed by the hospital or nursing home ethics committee. The nurse, as advocate for the patient, may at times be the one who would initiate a case of this nature with the hospital ethics committee and should have a role in the discussion of the case with the committee.

Another type of case that is perhaps the most psychologically vexing, if not ethically perplexing, is that of the terminally ill elderly patient for whom it is determined that CPR would be futile, yet the patient is competent and demands that everything humanly possible be done to preserve and prolong life, including CPR in the event that his or her heart stops. Many hospital ethics committees have found that there is no moral requirement to provide a futile medical intervention, even if it is desired or demanded by the patient. These controversies are on the edge of nursing ethics and push us to clarify the distinction between the provision of health care as a professional enterprise rather than a free market enterprise.

ARTIFICIALLY ADMINISTERED NUTRITION AND HYDRATION

Since the case of Karen Quinlan in 1976, there has been a broad acceptance of the fact that patients have the right to refuse a respirator or to discontinue the use of a respirator. The use of a respirator is usually seen as unwarranted in the case of a patient in a persistent vegetative state, or in the case of a patient who cannot be weaned from the respirator and does not wish to spend the remainder of his life tethered to an artificial breathing machine. The patient's right to refuse or to discontinue such treatment has been tested in the courts and affirmed.

The question of artificially administered nutrition and hydration has traditionally been judged differently than respirators. The provision of food and water has long been held as the basic requirements of primary care for any patient. Furthermore, the use of a nasogastric tube or intravenous line for fluids has been so technically simple to provide that in many cases it has been assumed to be an ordinary requirement of ethical nursing care.

On the other hand, it has long been observed that persons in the terminal phase of illness often become anorexic and simply do not want to eat. Oncology nurses state that cancer patients often lose their appetite near the end of life and die more comfortably if food and fluids are not provided by artificial means. Competent elderly patients in the terminal phase of life have often stopped eating and have refused artificially administered nutrition and hydration. It is important in nursing ethics to recognize that this is the right of a competent patient. In fact, the right of a patient to refuse unwanted medical interventions continues, even when competency is lost. Therefore, a patient can specify in an Advance Directive that he does not want artificially administered nutrition or hydration, or the patient can specify this with the agent serving as Durable Power of Attorney for Health Care.

One of the important outgrowths of the decision made in the Nancy Cruzan case by the Supreme Court of the United States was the court's definition of the provision of nutrition and hydration as a medical treatment. The court affirmed the right of states to pass legislation requiring "clear and convincing evidence" of the patient's wishes to have nutrition and hydration withheld. Following the higher court's judgment, the lower court in Missouri reopened the Cruzan case and new witnesses testified that Nancy had on several occasions given verbal testimony that she would not want to live in a vegetative state. The lower court found this to be clear and convincing evidence and allowed the removal of the tubes that had been sustaining her life for 6 years in a persistent vegetative condition. Nancy Cruzan died on December 26, 1990.

Since nurses are intimately involved in the care and comfort of patients, and since providing food and fluid is such an integral part of any care plan, this may be still another vexing issue in nursing ethics. Although the provision of nutrition and hydration is standard procedure in the vast majority of cases, it should be recognized that there are at least three categories of cases in which it is ethically justifiable to withhold nutrition and hydration: (1) when the competent patient refuses either oral or artificially administered nutrition and hydration; (2) when the patient is incompetent to communicate, but has left instructions in a qualified Advance Directive or with a Durable Power of Attorney for Health Care; and (3) when the provision of nutrition and hydration is considered futile and will not benefit the patient, but in fact may be disproportionately burdensome.

Some nurses have argued that while it is ethically justifiable to withhold certain interventions, once started, it is not ethically right to discontinue them. They argue that it is more difficult psychologically to discontinue a respirator or to discontinue the use of a nasogastric or gastrostomy tube for feeding. While recognizing that such actions may present psychological difficulty, especially for nurses new to the profession, it is generally held that it is more ethically justifiable to begin such interventions, knowing they can be discontinued if unwarranted, than not to initiate them for fear of never being able to stop.

Pain Management

Many of the health problems of the elderly place them at risk for pain and discomfort. Some forms of pain are chronic in nature and erode the patient's quality of life by limiting activities, thus reducing also the positive pleasures of life. Such patients may be forced to adapt their behavior to minimize pain and cope each day with some forms of discomfort that are not relieved by medication. Since physicians are primarily concerned with life-threatening illness and major disability, the nurse will often be attuned to the elements of pain and disability that, though not life threatening, are major factors in the patient's suffering.

The diseases of the elderly also put them at risk for high levels of distress from acute pain. Elderly patients are often fearful of excruciating or intractable pain. Many have seen family members and friends dying of an illness such as cancer in which the pain has been only poorly controlled. Almost universally, such patients state that they fear pain far more than they fear death itself and would rather die than to have their lives prolonged in agony.

The administration of appropriate pain control is an essential requisite of moral health care in this population. Although some dying patients surprisingly prefer to endure significant levels of pain in order to remain lucid and in contact with family members, most patients are anxious that they will suffer unnecessarily. Ordinarily the provision of pain medication is not morally problematic and is one of the avenues for beneficent nursing care. Sometimes, however, in caring for terminally ill patients who require high doses of pain medication, nurses fear that they might be culpable in causing the patient's death. This is another type of problem in nursing that can be ethically vexing.

In such cases, there are actually two nursing goals: (1) protecting the life of the patient and (2) alleviating the pain and suffering of the patient. Ordinarily, protecting or prolonging the life of the patient is the foremost goal. However, when the patient is terminally ill, and death is imminent, the goal of prolonging life will often take second place to the now primary goal of alleviating the patient's pain and suffering. Even if the administration of adequate pain medication will shorten the life of the patient by a few hours or days, if pain control is the goal of the patient, it is ethically justifiable. This concept is sometimes referred to by ethicists as the principle of *double effect*. The administration of morphine in sufficient dosages to relieve the pain of a cancer patient may decrease respiration and contribute in part to the hastening of death. Although both results are predictable, hence the double effect, only one is intended, the alleviation of pain and suffering. Here, motive and intention are also important ingredients, as the nurse is properly motivated by compassion for the suffering patient and intends to relieve that suffering through adequate medication. The cause of the patient's inevitable death stems from the underlying disease, in this case, cancer.

Quality of Life Issues

In commonplace transactions between health care providers and competent patients, the patient's presenting problem(s) elicits a recommendation for medical or nursing intervention. Once the patient understands the goals of the intervention, possible side effects, as well as the implications of foregoing the intervention, he can give informed consent for treatment or informed refusal.

In some cases, however, treatment options may never be offered to a particular patient based on quality of life considerations. Many nurses in geriatrics have heard explanations such as "her quality of life does not justify our offering this procedure at this time," as justification for not recommending a hip socket replacement, an aortic valve replacement, or coronary artery bypass surgery for an elderly patient.

It is often unclear, in such cases, just what quality of life means. It could mean that this is an expensive procedure, paid for by public funds, and in view of the patient's advanced age it is not cost effective. In reality, this is a resource allocation or cost containment issue. It could mean that the physician does not find much to value in the attributes and activities of this particular patient, according to her personal value system. This would be a second-party judgment on the value of the life of another individual. It could mean that the patient has expressed a sense of dissatisfaction with the conditions of his existence, even with the predicted benefit of the intervention, and wishes for only palliative care and comfort measures to be taken. The true locus of judgment about quality of life lies with the competent patient.

Appreciation of a patient's quality of life in medical decision-making should lead to care that is designed to improve or maintain quality of life. In this context, quality of life is considered as the benchmark from which to measure the potential benefit of a recommended intervention. However, if a patient's quality of life is used for interpersonal comparisons, as a measure of "value of life," or as a justification to withhold treatment, then dangerous consequences may be anticipated. The inappropriate application of quality of life principles to medical decisions may encourage prejudicial treatment toward selected classes of people, diminished respect for the sanctity of human life, and diminished trust in the medical profession's ability to provide "just" care to those in need (Pearlman, 1987).

Quality of life is also a factor in surrogate decision making. Unfortunately, by the time surrogacy is needed and the patient is incompetent, it is too late to ascertain the features or attributes that compose a minimally acceptable quality of life for the patient. Such a situation is a problem, both for the patient in protecting his autonomy, and for the surrogate in achieving the goal of representing the best interests of the patient.

This problem has been addressed by faculty at the Center for Health Law and Ethics, Institute of Public Law, University of New Mexico Law School, who have developed a "Values History" form to enable prior discussion of the values of the patient. Information gleaned through the judicious use of this form will prove invaluable to any surrogate decision maker since it represents the patient's values and feelings about quality of life issues (Lambert et al, 1990) (see Appendix 4–1).

RECOGNIZING OUR MORTALITY

Discussions that might be elicited through the use of the values history form, or any other useful approaches, contribute in a positive way toward helping individuals face their mortality. Facing one's mortality and recognizing the likely decisions that may confront us is a major first step in preparing to grapple with the many issues surrounding medical and nursing care at the end of life. Although it is human to deny death and to avoid thoughts about the end of life, it is also a part of human nature to engage our best rational thinking in preparing to cope with the end of life, which naturally comes to all persons. The nurse, in both the institutional and the home care setting, is well situated to assist elderly persons in confronting these issues.

ACCEPTANCE OF DEATH

Clinical observation indicates that elderly persons who reflect on their values and changing goals in the later stages of life are often able to face treatment decisions in the light of their own subjective meaning of life. The acceptance of death as a natural part of life appears to be more common in the elderly and often helps individuals face the inevitability of death with less anxiety and trepidation.

Since open discussion about issues related to death and dying is still avoided by many laypersons and family members, the nurse in geriatrics will want to develop communications skills related to such issues in the advocacy role.

ASSISTING ONE'S SURVIVORS BY PREPARING FOR DEATH

Grief is a natural and appropriate response to loss. Healthy grieving over the loss of an aging family member can be facilitated when there is not a backlog of unfinished family agendas, and the treatment decisions at the end of life were in keeping with the authentic values of the deceased. If the patient is able to provide some guidance regarding funeral arrangements and preferences regarding burial or cremation, it is very helpful for the survivors and avoids a sense of guilt that stems from not knowing what should be done. Nurses often play a key role in bridging the communication gaps between family members. Understanding family dynamics will facilitate the nurse's role as an enabling third party to a family impasse.

Conclusion

In summary, ethical issues arising in the care of the elderly are increasingly being recognized. Nurses are on the forefront of identifying ethical dilemmas facing individual patients as well as those common to geriatric nursing. The nature of the nurse–patient relationship in both home care and inpatient settings provides unique opportunities to serve as an advocate for this vulnerable population. Although the rights of elderly patients to actively participate in health care decisions are established in both legal precept and ethical principle, in actual practice they may be too easily overridden in the clinical setting. Elderly patients are susceptible to confusion, periods of incapacity, intimidation from those in authority, as well as weakness or pain associated with their health problems. The sensitivity of the geriatric nurse to these ethical issues and her or his commitment to serve as an advocate for the patient will provide challenges at the cutting edge of the nursing profession.

References and Other Readings

Beauchamp TL, Childress JF. Principle of biomedical ethics. 3rd ed. New York: Oxford University Press, 1989.

Finucaine TE, Boyer JT, Bulmash J, et al. The incidence of attempted CPR in nursing homes. J Am Ger Soc 1991; 39:624.

Jonsen AR, Siegler M, Winslade WJ. Clinical ethics. New York: Macmillan, 1982:52.

Lambert P, McIver Gibson J, Nathanson P. The values history: an innovation in surrogate medical decision-making. Law medicine & health care (law and aging). A Journal of the American Society of Law and Medicine 1990; 18:203.

Medical Ethics Advisor. 1991; 7:53.

Omnibus Budget Reconciliation Act of 1990. The Patient Self-Determination Act, 123, 776.

Pearlman RA. Quality of life: a complex factor in caring for older persons. Clinical Report on Aging 1987; 1:12.

Revised Code of Washington State Law. RCW 7.780.065.

Special report: a national agenda for research on aging. N Engl J Med 1991; 324:1825.

Veatch RM, Fry ST. Case studies in nursing ethics. Philadelphia: JB Lippincott, 1987.

APPENDIX 4–1
Values History Form

NAME: _____
DATE: _____

If someone assisted you in completing this form, please fill in his or her name, address, and relationship to you.

Name: _____
Address: _____
_____
Relationship: _____

The purpose of this form is to assist you in thinking about and writing down what is important to you about your health. If you should at some time become unable to make health care decisions for yourself, your thoughts as expressed on this form may help others make a decision for you in accordance with what you would have chosen.

The first section of this form asks whether you have already expressed your wishes concerning medical treatment through either written or oral communications and if not, whether you would like to do so now. The second section of this form provides an opportunity for you to discuss your values, wishes, and preferences in a number of different areas, such as your personal relationships, your overall attitude toward life, and your thoughts about illness.

Courtesy of University of New Mexico, Center for Health Law and Ethics, Institute of Public Law, School of Law, Albuquerque, NM 87131.

Section 1

A. WRITTEN LEGAL DOCUMENTS

Have your written any of the following legal documents? _____
If so, please complete the requested information.

Living Will
Date written: _____
Document location: _____
Comments: (e.g., any limitations, special requests, etc.) _____
_____
_____

Durable Power of Attorney
Date written: _____
Document location: _____
Comments: (e.g., whom have you named to be your decision maker?) _____
_____
_____

Durable Power of Attorney for Health Care Decisions
Date written: _____
Document location: _____
Comments: (e.g., whom have you named to be your decision maker?) _____
_____
_____

Organ Donations
Date written: _____
Document location: _____

Comments: (e.g., any limitations on which organs you would like to donate?) _____
_____
_____
_____

B. WISHES CONCERNING SPECIFIC MEDICAL PROCEDURES

If you have ever expressed your wishes, either written or orally, concerning any of the following medical procedures, please complete the requested information. If you have not previously indicated your wishes on these procedures and would like to do so now, please complete this information.

Organ Donation
To whom expressed: _____
If oral, when? _____
If written, when? _____
Document location: _____
Comments: _____
_____
_____

Kidney Dialysis
To whom expressed: _____
If oral, when? _____
If written, when? _____
Document location: _____
Comments: _____
_____
_____

Cardiopulmonary Resuscitation (CPR)
To whom expressed: _____
If oral, when? _____
If written, when? _____
Document location: _____
Comments: _____
_____
_____
_____

Respirators
To whom expressed: _____
If oral, when? _____
If written, when? _____
Document location: _____
Comments: _____
_____
_____
_____

Artificial Nutrition
To whom expressed: _____
If oral, when? _____
If written, when? _____
Document location: _____
Comments: _____
_____
_____
_____

Artificial Hydration
To whom expressed: _____
If oral, when? _____
If written, when? _____
Document location: _____
Comments: _____
_____
_____
_____

C. GENERAL COMMENTS

Do you wish to make any general comments about the information you provided in this section? _____
_____
_____
_____

Section 2

A. YOUR OVERALL ATTITUDE TOWARD YOUR HEALTH

1. How would you describe your current health status? If you currently have any medical problems, how would you describe them?
_____
_____
_____

2. If you have current medical problems, in what ways, if any, do they affect your ability to function? _____
_____
_____
_____

3. How do you feel about your current health status? _____
_____
_____
_____
_____

4. How well are you able to meet the basic necessities of life—eating, food preparation, sleeping, personal hygiene, etc.? _____
_____
_____

5. Do you wish to make any general comments about your overall health? _____
_____
_____
_____

B. YOUR PERCEPTION OF THE ROLE OF YOUR DOCTOR AND OTHER HEALTH CAREGIVERS

1. Do you like your doctors? _____
_____
_____

2. Do you trust your doctors? _____
_____
_____

3. Do you think your doctors should make the final decision concerning any treatment you might need? _____
_____
_____

4. How do you relate to your caregivers, including nurses, therapists, chaplains, social workers, etc.? _____
_____
_____

5. Do you wish to make any general comments about your doctor and other health caregivers? _____
_____
_____

C. YOUR THOUGHTS ABOUT INDEPENDENCE AND CONTROL

1. How important is independence and self-sufficiency in your life? _____
_____
_____

2. If you were to experience decreased physical and mental abilities, how would that affect your attitude toward independence and self-sufficiency? _____
_____

3. Do you wish to make any general comments about the value of independence and control in your life? _____
_____
_____

D. YOUR PERSONAL RELATIONSHIPS

1. Do you expect that your friends, family and/or others will support your decisions regarding medical treatment you may need now or in the future? _____
_____
_____
_____

2. Have you made any arrangements for your family or friends to make medical treatment decisions on your behalf? If so, who has agreed to make decisions for you and in what circumstances? _____
_____
_____
_____

3. What, if any, unfinished business from the past are you concerned about (e.g., personal and family relationships, business and legal matters)? _____
_____
_____

4. What role do your friends and family play in your life? _____
_____
_____

5. Do you wish to make any general comments about the personal relationships in your life? _____
_____
_____
_____

E. YOUR OVERALL ATTITUDE TOWARD LIFE

1. What activities do you enjoy (e.g., hobbies, watching TV, etc.)? _____
_____
_____

2. Are you happy to be alive? _____
_____
_____

3. Do you feel that life is worth living?

_____

_____

4. How satisfied are you with what you have achieved in your life? _____

_____

_____

5. What makes you laugh/cry? _____

_____

_____

6. What do you fear most? What frightens or upsets you? _____

_____

_____

7. What goals do you have for the future?

_____

_____

8. Do you wish to make any general comments about your attitude toward life? _____

_____

_____

F.   YOUR ATTITUDE TOWARD ILLNESS, DYING, AND DEATH

1. What will be important to you when you are dying (e.g., physical comfort, no pain, family members present, etc.)? _____

_____

_____

_____

2. Where would you prefer to die? _____

_____

_____

3. What is your attitude toward death?

_____

_____

4. How do you feel about the use of life-sustaining measures in the face of:
   terminal illness? _____

_____

   permanent coma? _____

_____

   irreversible chronic illness (e.g., Alzheimer's disease)? _____

_____

5. Do you wish to make any general comments about your attitude toward illness, dying, and death? _____

_____

_____

G.   YOUR RELIGIOUS BACKGROUND AND BELIEFS

1. What is your religious background?

_____

_____

2. How do your religious beliefs affect your attitude toward serious or terminal illness? _____

_____

_____

3. Does your attitude toward death find support in your religion? _____

_____

_____

4. How does your faith community, church, or synagogue view the role of prayer or religious sacraments in an illness? _____

_____

_____

5. Do you wish to make any general comments about your religious background and beliefs? _____

_____

_____

H.   YOUR LIVING ENVIRONMENT

1. What has been your living situation over the last 10 years (e.g., lived alone, lived with others, etc.)? _____

_____

_____

2. How difficult is it for you to maintain the kind of environment for yourself that you find comfortable? Does any illness or medical problem you have now mean that it will be harder in the future? _____

_____

_____

_____

3. Do you wish to make any general comments about your living environment? _____

_____
_____
_____

I. YOUR ATTITUDE CONCERNING FINANCES

1. How much do you worry about having enough money to provide for your care? _____

_____
_____
_____

2. Would you prefer to spend less money on your care so that more money can be saved for the benefit of your relatives and/or friends? _____

_____
_____
_____

3. Do you wish to make any general comments concerning your finances and the cost of health care? _____

_____
_____
_____

J. YOUR WISHES CONCERNING YOUR FUNERAL

1. What are your wishes concerning your funeral and burial or cremation? _____

_____
_____
_____

2. Have you made your funeral arrangements? If so, with whom? _____

_____
_____
_____

3. Do you wish to make any general comments about how you would like your funeral and burial or cremation to be arranged or conducted? _____

_____
_____
_____
_____
_____

Optional Questions

1. How would you like your obituary (announcement of your death) to read? _____

_____
_____
_____
_____
_____
_____

2. Write yourself a brief eulogy (a statement about yourself to be read at your funeral). _____

_____
_____
_____
_____
_____
_____

Suggestions for Use

After you have completed this form, you may wish to provide copies to your doctors and other health caregivers, your family, your friends, and your attorney. If you have a Living Will or Durable Power of Attorney for Health Care Decisions, you may wish to attach a copy of this form to those documents.

Display 4–1 Policy and guiding philosophy. (With permission of King County Medical Society, Seattle, WA, 1991.)

APPENDIX

This Appendix is for special application for long term care facilities including Nursing Homes, Home Health Agencies, Hospices, Assisted Living Facilities, Retirement Homes, Adult Family Homes, and Congregate Care Facilities.

POLICY AND GUIDING PHILOSOPHY
Regarding Health Care Directives
to Physicians for Individuals Residing
in a Long-Term Care Setting

1. Each individual whose care is coordinated by health care personnel shall be asked to express personal preferences regarding the following end-of-life issues:
   a. What to do in the event of cardiac arrest (resuscitate or not to resuscitate)?
   b. What to do in the event of serious medical illness?
   c. Who should make decisions on the individual's behalf if he or she becomes mentally incapacitated?

2. Care directed at promoting well-being and maintaining comfort and dignity will always be provided. Procedures or treatments which are known to be unnecessary or of no appreciable benefit to the individual will not be performed.

3. A surrogate decision-maker will be sought if the individual is unable to comprehend the questions or their implications; or if otherwise unable to express his or her own wishes.

4. Information regarding cardiac arrest, cardiopulmonary resuscitation (CPR), likelihood of survival, and potential complications is to be given to the individual or surrogate. A member of the health care team, who is comfortable and knowledgeable in discussion of end-of-life issues, should be available to answer questions. This person should be a nurse, social worker, or physician.

5. Documentation of the individual's preferences shall be kept in an accessible part of the medical record. The directives may be changed at any time, and should be reviewed yearly or when there has been a significant change of condition.

Display 4–1 (*Continued*)

PROCEDURES
For individuals <u>able</u> to make their own decisions:

1. Approved forms addressing the following material shall be part of the admission packet and given to individuals at or near the time of admission.
   a. What to do in case of cardiac arrest.
      (*Directive to Physicians and Caregivers*)
   b. What to do in event of serious medical problems.
      (*Expression of Intent to Physicians and Caregivers: Approach to Serious Medical Problems*)
   c. Who should make decisions on behalf of the individual when that person is incapable of making his or her own decisions?
      (*Explanation of Washington State Laws with Respect to End-of-Life Issues (see page 2*).)

   Educational materials explaining the directives should be provided. The forms should be completed within 30 days of admission.

2. A designated member of the ongoing healthcare team (nurse, social worker, or physician) shall:
   a. Discuss the directives with the individual and be available to answer questions. The discussion should include a description of CPR, the probable outcome and possible complications of this procedure, and the consequences of not initiating CPR.
   b. Ask the individual to designate his or her personal preferences and sign and date the directives.
   c. Document in the medical record the discussion and preferences that were indicated, including feelings, opinions, and reason given by the individual.

3. The attending physician shall acknowledge the choices made by signing the directives. The physician is to be encouraged to discuss the end-of-life issues with the individual and document this in the medical record as a progress note.

4. The signed directives and supporting documentation shall be kept in an easily accessible part of the medical record, such as immediately under the face sheet.

5. The indicated preferences may be changed at any time by the individual. The directives should be reviewed annually or after a significant change in medical condition.

For individuals who are <u>unable</u> to make their own decisions:

1. The individual shall be considered mentally incapacitated if, in the opinion of the nurses and physicians, he or she cannot understand the issues discussed in the directives and their implications.

   a. There should be objective findings on which to base this opinion such as:
      i. Inability to demonstrate understanding of issues discussed;
      ii. Grossly abnormal mental status as determined by an exam such as 'Fromage' or Mini Mental state exam.
      iii. Severe clinical depression or other major psychiatric or medical disorder which interferes with making the specific decisions.
      iv. Inability to communicate or make wishes known.

2. Once the determination of incompetency has been made you should determine whether there is a guardian of the person, having been appointed by the Superior Court of the State. If so, this person has power to be the surrogate decisionmaker. If not, you should determine whether there is a person holding a Durable Power of Attorney for Health Care which has been executed by the incompetent patient. If there is, this person has the power of the surrogate decisionmaker.

   In the event that there is neither a guardian nor a person holding a Durable Power of Attorney for Health Care, then Washington state law, RCW 7.70.065 provides the following classes of individuals who have the power to be the surrogate decisionmaker. They are listed in order of those having first choice to exercise the power:
   1. The patient's spouse.
   2. Children of the patient who are at least eighteen years of age.
   3. Parents of the patient.
   4. Adult brothers and sisters of the patient.

3. The surrogate decisionmaker shall be asked to designate preferences regarding CPR, and serious medical illness as described in 1. (a) (b) (c).

4. If no surrogate is available, a care conference should be held with the attending physician, nurse, and a third caregiver such as a social worker. Information from previous caregivers and other sources should be gathered. Prognosis, quality of life, and potential outcome of possible interventions should be reviewed.

   a. If all participants agree, they should make appropriate designations for the impaired individual. The attending physician shall document the result of the care conference and rationale for the choices in the medical record. All participants of the care conference should sign the directives. Choices should always attempt to reflect the best interests of the individual.

   b. If participants of the care conference disagree, the highest agreed upon level of care should be chosen. Guardianship procedure should then be initiated.

Display 4–2 Living will. (With permission of King County Medical Society, Seattle, WA, 1991.)

DIRECTIVE TO PHYSICIANS
(Living Will)

Directive made this _____ day of _____ (month, year).

I, _____ being
of sound mind, wilfully, and voluntarily make known my desire that my
life shall not be artificially prolonged under the circumstances set forth
below, and do hereby declare that:

1. (You may choose to check, *by initialing,* either one of the following
   options or both in order to provide direction to your physician.)

(a) _____ If I should be in an incurable or irreversible condition with
no expectation of recovery, I do not want any treatment that
will merely prolong my dying. Thus I want my treatment
limited to medical and nursing measures that are intended
to keep me comfortable, to relieve pain, and to maintain my
dignity.

(b) _____ If I am in a coma, which my doctors reasonably believe to
be permanent, or a persistent vegetative state I do not want
any life-prolonging treatment to be provided or continued,
including artificially provided nutrition and/or hydration.

(c) Additionally, I _____
_____
_____
_____

2. In the absence of my ability to give directions regarding the use of life-
   sustaining procedures, it is my intention that this directive shall be

---

Display 4–2 *(Continued)*

honored by my family and physician(s) as the final expression of my
legal right to refuse medical or surgical treatment and I accept the
consequences from such refusal.

3. If I have been diagnosed as pregnant and that diagnosis is known to
   my physician, this directive shall have no force or effect during the
   course of my pregnancy.

4. I understand the full import of this directive and I am emotionally
   and mentally competent to make this directive.

Signed _____

_____
City, County and State of Residence

The declarer has been personally known to me and I believe
him or her to be of sound mind.

Witness _____

Witness _____

Durable Power of Attorney for Health Care
(Designation of Agent for Health Care Decisions)

1.   I, _____
        (YOUR NAME)

as principal, designate and appoint the person listed below as my attorney-in-fact for health care decisions (hereafter, Agent).

Designee: Name _____

Address _____

City/State _____ Telephone _____

2.   Powers Related to Health Care Decisions

My agent for health care decisions shall have the following powers:

To make health care decisions on my behalf if I am unable to do so, including giving informed consent to health care providers. Included in this power is the authority to make decisions about life-prolonging medical procedures, such as (but not limited to) a respirator, placement or removal of tubes to provide nutrition or hydration, antibiotics, and cardiopulmonary resuscitation.

I intend my agent to have the authority to consent to giving, withholding or stopping my health care treatment, service or diagnostic procedure. All of this is to be in keeping with my instructions below or in my Directive to Physicians (Living Will).

Instructions: _____

_____

_____

Display 4-3   *(Continued)*

By completing this document, I intend to create a durable power of attorney for health care under chapter 11.94 of the Revised Code of Washington. It shall take effect upon my incapacity to make my own health care decisions and shall continue during that incapacity to the extent permitted by law or until I revoke it.

By signing this document, I indicate that I understand the purpose and effect of this durable power of attorney for health care.

(You must sign this in the presence of a Notary Public for it to be valid.)

Dated this _____ day of _____ , 19_____

Signed _____

STATE OF WASHINGTON

County of _____

On this day personally appeared before me, _____
_____ to me known to be the individual described in and who executed the within and foregoing instrument, and acknowledged that he/she signed the same as his/her free and voluntary act and deed for the uses and purposes therein mentioned.

Given under my hand and official seal this _____
day of _____ , 19_____

_____
Notary Public in and for the State of Washington,

residing in _____

My appointment expires _____

Display 4–4 Patient directive to physicians and caregivers. (With permission of King County Medical Society, Seattle, WA, 1991.)

PATIENT DIRECTIVE TO PHYSICIANS AND CAREGIVERS
Concerning Sudden Death or Cardiac Arrest

_____ INITIATE CARDIOPULMONARY RESUSCITATION (CPR) (full code)
All efforts should be made at resuscitation in the event of sudden death or cardiac arrest.

_____ NO CPR (no code)
No efforts at resuscitation should be made in the event of sudden death. I will accept sudden death as the end of my natural life. I request that my physician will write NO CPR in my medical records.

THIS DECISION MAY BE CHANGED AT ANY TIME.

Name (please print) _____

Signature of Patient or Surrogate _____ Date _____

(Print name) _____

If Surrogate, Relationship to Patient _____

Physician's Signature _____ Date _____

(Print name) _____

5

Governmental Policies Affecting Care of the Elderly and Acquired Immunodeficiency Syndrome

MARIAN CAUDILL

Health care of the elderly is affected by a variety of governmental policies. Those issues generally fall into categories of health maintenance, access to care, funding, and establishing and enforcing standards of care. Since the passage of the Social Security Act in 1935, the federal government has become increasingly involved in provision of services to the elderly (Allen, 1987). The involvement of the government in health care for our aging population means that professionals practicing in the field of gerontologic nursing are affected by numerous regulations, rules, guidelines, and laws.

Social Security Act of 1935

In 1935 the United States Congress passed the Social Security Act, which was intended to be an old-age insurance policy. The original design was to provide cash assistance to the elderly to help with health care costs. The Social Security monthly check was to be the total extent of governmental support or participation. The support did not originally cover those elderly who were institutionalized. Care for aging persons who were institutionalized was left solely to the individual state and county governments. Federal monies were available for long-term care for chronically ill and disabled persons. Over time, several court cases were filed by states that had placed long-term residents in private homes in attempts to force the federal government to pay for their health care services. The states were successful in their suits; thus shifting the source of payment to the federal government. Those successful court cases marked the beginning of the nursing home industry and the expansion of government involvement in long-term health care for the elderly.

In 1935, 50% of the elderly were indigent; that number rose to 66% by 1940 (Clement, 1985). By 1959 the number of indigent elderly had decreased to 35%, then dropped to 14% in 1978 because of the expansion of Social Security benefits. In 1981 one of every five elderly Americans depended almost exclusively on Social Security for their entire income (Kaplan, 1985).

There were 11 titles in the original Act that defined the program, established administrative guidelines, and authorized necessary taxes for support. In 1950 additions to the Act provided for matching federal monies to individual states to support funding for medical care for those persons who were receiving public assistance. That provision was the forerunner of the Medicaid program, which today supports the majority of residents in nursing homes throughout the nation.

The Kerr-Mills Act of 1960 provided for medical assistance to the aged in the form of matching federal funds, varying between 50% and 83%, to individual states. The program began slowly, with only half of the states taking advantage of it during the first 5 years of its implementation.

Title XVIII, Medicare, and Title XIX, Medicaid, were added to the original Social Security Act in 1965 and 1966, respectively. By 1967 control of programs and services within nursing homes began in the form of a requirement that facilities participating in the Medicare/Medicaid programs have licensed administrators. Title XX was added to the Social Security Act in 1974. Its purpose was to provide for in-home services for the elderly.

From 1935 until 1975 there was continuing expansion of benefits under the Social Security Act. In 1975 that focus changed. The control and reduction of costs to Medicare/Medicaid ensued. Since that time the government has been pursuing efforts to reduce expenditures and/or shift financial responsibility for services back to the states.

TITLE XVIII: MEDICARE, PART A

Medicare, Part A, is automatically available to each recipient of Social Security benefits. It is primarily focused on hospital-related services. However, it does cover both nursing home costs and home health care costs for those aging persons who qualify. Requirements for use of Medicare benefits change regularly and frequently, making it difficult for health care professionals to maintain current expertise. Frequent changes make it difficult for the elderly themselves to learn how to access and use the benefits.

Many elderly persons believe that Medicare is an insurance program that will meet all their health care needs. Nurses working in geriatric settings frequently must interpret and explain to their patients the complicated issues of increasing deductibles, exclusions, limitations, and restrictions placed on hospital admissions and discharges. Nurses who work in long-term care settings are often confronted by anxious patients or their relatives who learn for the first time that Medicare does not cover routine and ongoing nursing home services.

TITLE XVIII: MEDICARE, PART B

Participation in Part B of the Medicare program is voluntary. For a monthly payment, the subscriber may have half of the costs for selected services paid by Medicare. Physician services, many outpatient services, and most laboratory, health specialist, and medical equipment used in the home are covered under Medicare, Part B. Many services needed by the elderly, which would assist them to remain independent in activities of daily living, are not covered under Part B. Services not covered, but required for independence include eye examinations and eyeglasses, hearing examinations and hearing aids, and foot care and supportive and corrective devices to enable ambulation. Dental care is also excluded from the Medicare program. There is no provision for preventive dental care, fillings, removal or replacement of teeth, or dental devices. Services that are covered under Part B have an increasing annual premium and an increasing deductible amount that shifts greater and greater amounts of program costs back to the participant.

There has been a substantial tightening of Medicare, Part B benefits since October 1, 1990. There was a 2% cut to providers for such services between October 31, 1990 and January 1, 1991 in order to meet the federal deficit reduction target. During 1990 Medicare made cuts of as much as 15% for 244 services that were defined as "overpriced." An additional 6.5% reduction occurred January 1, 1991, for surgical and technical services not reduced earlier. Cuts to providers of services under Medicare, Part B were excluded in radiology, anesthesiology, pathology, and preventive medicine, psychiatric, emergency, and critical care services. The only increase in prevailing charges in 1991 were for services in the primary care area.

Hospitals were also affected by cuts in Medicare after January 1, 1991. Reimbursement for capital expenditures associated with outpatient services were cut by 15% in 1991 and 10% in each year until 1995 (Grimaldi, 1991). Hospital outpatient diagnostic services and other professional services rendered on an outpatient basis will also be cut progressively through 1995.

Efforts to reduce the federal deficit have a direct effect on health care for the elderly. Federal planners expect that Medicare fees and rate increases to providers will continue to be low, and the beneficiaries of Medicare services will be required to absorb greater proportions of the costs. The Social Security taxes may also increase for the long-term survival of the entire Medicare program.

TITLE XIX: MEDICAID

Medicaid is an entirely different program from Medicare. While Medicare is an insurance program, Medicaid is a program that provides for medical care for persons of all ages on welfare programs or who are medically indigent. Medicaid is a program of funding to states in the form of grants from the federal government that provides variably 50% to 83% of costs. The amount of federal support is dependent on the average per capita income of each individual state. The method used in setting the percentage of participation by the federal government was questioned in the 1991 Congress. Several states that have low populations are asking that there be a consideration given to the number of state residents who are supporting a given number of Medicaid recipients. The ratio of supporters to recipients varies greatly among the states.

The individual states control the Medicaid expenditures and determine most eligibility requirements. Some states have required counties to also participate in funding their Medicaid programs. Since determination of eligibility is at the level of the local Department of Health and Human Services, there is a great deal of community control of benefits and eligibility.

Services that are typically covered under the Medicaid program after the patient spends down to the eligibility requirement are inpatient hospital services, outpatient services, nursing home care, limited home health care, laboratory tests, and radiology services. Other services covered vary from state to state. These other services include medications, dental care, eyeglasses, prostheses, medical transportation, and home health care.

Approximately 55% of Medicaid costs nationally are provided by the federal government. During fiscal year 1990 the program exceeded $70 billion. The method used by the Government Accounting Office for setting the percentage of individual state's portion of the Medicaid cost is considered inequitable. States such as Pennsylvania, New Hampshire, Rhode Island, Florida, and Maryland have high average per capita incomes that exaggerate the state's funding capabilities. The method used by the Government Accounting Office to set the percentage state match for Medicaid ignores the number of residents living at or below poverty level and ignores the corporate incomes. Others, such as Nevada and the District of Columbia, have a very high rate of poverty.

A proposal by the Government Accounting Office to establish a more equitable method of Medicaid funding would base the formula on the total taxable resources of the state. The proposal would also reduce the federal matching lower limit to 40%. The proposal to change the funding formula is not supported by the Health Care Financing Administration management (Contemporary Long Term Care, 1991b). During 1991 the Health Care Financing Administration worked on a comprehensive reform of the entire Medicaid program. Changing the method of funding was viewed by the administration to be counterproductive to the total reform planning.

Hospitals and nursing homes in 13 states have filed lawsuits claiming payment rates are inadequate, according to Schwartz (1991). Physicians are also withdrawing from providing services to Medicaid recipients because of low reimbursement rates. In New York up to 85% of physicians no longer participate in the program. The lawsuits follow passage of the Boren Amendment that requires individual states to reimburse providers for reasonable and adequate rates to carry out the Medicaid program. Lawsuits have been filed in several states against the state agencies to recover actual costs of providing services. One of the first suits to be settled under the Boren Amendment was in Michigan where providers received gross adjustments for reimbursement rates during 1990 (Contemporary Long Term Care, 1991a).

Funding is crucial to ensure participation by providers of health care to the elderly receiving services under the program. During 1990 the Medicaid program costs rose 11%, to approximately 14% of the total state budgets nationally. Medicaid program costs were second only to funding for elementary and secondary education. Costs have been exaggerated by the changes required under the Omnibus Budget Reconciliation Act of 1987 (OBRA 1987). By 1995 the Medicaid portion of state budgets is expected to increase to 17%. It is projected that $3.5 billion of that increase is directly attributable to implementing OBRA 1990, according to Schwartz (1991).

Congress reached a budget compromise with President Bush during its 1990 session. The compromise was that budget additions would be offset with subtractions someplace else. The compromise came at a time when the country was in a recession, had just finished a war in the Middle East, was implementing OBRA 1987 and OBRA 1990, and was experiencing increasing numbers of elderly eligible for services under the Medicaid program.

In spite of the increasing costs at both the state and federal levels for the Medicaid and Medicare programs for the elderly, it is wise to keep in mind that the individual elderly patient is paying out of pocket about the same proportion of his or her mean annual income in 1985 as in 1965 when the program began. The amount paid out of pocket averages about 15% (Kane and Kane, 1990).

TITLE XX: SOCIAL SERVICES BLOCK GRANT

The Social Services Block Grant is also known as Title XX of the Social Security Act. It provides for home-based services, employment, education and training, information and referral, day services, legal services, as well as home-delivered and congregate meals. Fees for services are charged to those participants in the program with incomes greater than 80% of the state's median income.

Gerontologic nurses who practice in the home-based setting need to become familiar with the programs and services available in their community. Programs such as Meals on Wheels, Choreworker, and Homemaker services are available to support elderly in their own homes as long as functionally possible. Other services that can be provided at the home of the recipient are controlled at different levels of government.

Local area on aging offices
    Friendly visiting volunteers
    Home rehabilitation and protective services
    Congregate meals
    Senior citizen centers
Medicare
    Hospice
    Home health and respite care
Local department of social and health services
    Social workers and home health aides
    Adult day care centers
Local department of mental health
    Geriatric mental health services

Older Americans Act of 1965

The Older Americans Act of 1965 focused on the provision of services in the noninstitutional setting. It provides for services to those citizens over the age of 60 through a variety of agencies. To date the Older Americans Act is the strongest governmental policy in demonstrating national commitment to the elderly. It is based on the philosophy that health care throughout life is essential for healthy old age (Davis, 1985). Health care financing should be continuous, tailored to specific needs of the elderly, and should be provided without regard to age, race, or prior work record. The act acknowledges that services for the elderly should be aimed at prevention and restoration, as well as acute care. Under the act the right to self-determination, choice, and alternatives for the elderly are supported through financing from federal, state, and local resources.

The Older Americans Act of 1965 provides for cost controls and encourages low-cost, yet optimal quality of care. The act specifically targets persons over the age of 60 who are low income, minority, and isolated. There is no financial means test for access to programs covered by the act.

Title I of the Older Americans Act states the goals of the program to be equal opportunity for every older individual for the full and free enjoyment of affordable housing, retirement in health, adequate income, optimal physical and mental health (which science can offer without regard to economic status), employment, freedom of independence and self-determination in planning and managing one's own life, efficient community services such as low-cost transportation, coordinated social services, access to civic, cultural, educational, and recreational opportunities, and full restorative services for elderly needing institutional care.

Title II of the act established the Administration on Aging as a part of the Department of Health and Human Services. A commissioner is empowered to administer the act and to report directly to the Secretary of the Department of Health and Human Services.

Title III is the part of the Older Americans Act that covers major service provision. It directs the Area Agencies on Aging to be responsible for needs assessment and plan development at the local level. The Area Agencies on Aging do not deliver direct services except for information and referral. They administer the local plan and serve as advocates and enter into contracts for services within the community. Services that are contracted by the Area Agencies on Aging are social services, nutrition services for those over 60 and their spouses, and home-delivered meals.

Title III was amended in 1978 to provide for the Ombudsman Program. The purpose of the program is to investigate and resolve complaints on behalf of nursing home residents; monitor, develop, and ensure implementation of federal, state, and local laws governing long-term care facilities; give public agencies information about problems of residents in long-term care facilities; and train volunteers for the program.

States are required to develop procedures to allow ombudsmen access to residents' and facility records without disclosing the identity of the person filing the complaint. The states must develop and maintain a system of reporting and recording complaints and must ensure security of ombudsman records. The ombudsman program has no legal authority over the long-term care facilities, but does have the authority to communicate information to state licensing and certification agencies.

The local Area Agencies on Aging may enter into contracts that cover a broad range of activities that include health services, transportation, housing, education, and recreation. The Area Agencies on Aging are charged with provision of services to help the individual avoid institutionalization. They may also cover legal services, counseling, and physical exercise programs.

Title IV provides for mental health services. Though these services were identified as a priority in the preamble, they were not given great priority until 1981. In that year Title IV provided for discretionary demonstration grant programs for mental health services. In 1984, families of the victims of Alzheimer's disease and related disorders were made a priority under Title III. Despite provisions within both titles of the Older Americans Act, mental health services were never emphasized as a core support service in the local areas (Cohen and Hastings, 1989).

Title V of the Older Americans Act provides for community service employment for older persons. It is the only portion of the Older Americans Act that is not administered by the Administration on Aging or the Department of Health and Human Services. Title V provides for senior employment programs that are actually administered by the US Department of Labor. The Department of Labor implements the employment program by direct funding to both public and private organizations.

Title VI was added to the Older Americans Act in 1978 as an amendment. It was implemented in response to pressure from Native Americans and provides for grants to Indian tribes. The definition of outcomes expected by this portion of the act is vague. In essence, there is a clearer definition for reporting of data about numbers of programs being developed and groups being served than there is definition of benefits and outcomes from such programs.

Title VII of the Older Americans Act was added in 1984. The provision under Title VII is specifically for health education and health training for older individuals.

According to Allen (1987), nationally the cost per older adult for the supportive and senior centers has been approximately $13 per year or $91 per year for the older adult in poverty. Similar costs exist for congregate meals. The cost for home-delivered meals averages about $2.50 per older adult, or $15.50 per person living in poverty. The total program cost for all of the services covered in the Older Americans Act averages $28.50 per older adult or $200 per adult living in poverty. The costs to the federal government seem small when evaluated on the per participant basis. Since there is no requirement for financial means test for the programs it seems quite economical. Perhaps one reason for such small per participant cost is that the local Area Agencies on Aging do actually target most services to the economically needy.

The full intent of the act has never been implemented because of budget constraints. The area of greatest need is in the inability of Area Agencies on Aging to coordinate a service system in the local community. Some networking in the community does occur, but the full intent has never been achieved. The primary reason for failure is in the lack of funding and also the lack, in some cases, of the legal authority to implement all titles of the act.

Negotiating the Continuum of Care

Clinical nurse specialists in gerontology and gerontologic nurse practitioners often are employed in intensive care settings or institutional care settings for the elderly. The most intense type of care for the elderly is provided in the acute care setting, which is extremely well controlled by the federal government by means of Medicare and Medicaid requirements for program participation. Hospitals are generally very compliant in meeting requirements for reimbursement. Because of the control of payment to hospitals and other providers of services, the federal government sets criteria for admission, controls the types of services that can be provided, and dictates time intervals for discharge of Medicare patients. Nurses working in the acute care setting are required to learn and update their knowledge of such requirements. They must learn how to negotiate the Medicare/Medicaid system, use it to its best advantage, and teach and counsel patients regarding coverage of services.

At the opposite end of the care continuum are the care settings varying from totally independent living for the elderly, to group homes, foster homes, and assisted living or congregate care communities. In these settings the nurse in gerontology will find that services that are available to the elderly are well controlled by the federal or state government by virtue of requirements for provider payment, licensing requirement for the facility, and the federal mandate covering the provider of service. The hospice and home health programs are but two examples of services that are very well controlled by Medicare regulation covering types of services, frequency or duration of services, qualifications of persons providing the services, and the amount of reimbursement that will ultimately be paid.

Professional nursing in the community-based setting is again controlled in many services by the state or federal government. Programs such as adult day care are controlled by state Medicaid rules, while respite care for hospice is controlled by Medicare regulations.

At the end of the long-term care continuum is the licensed nursing facility described as either skilled or intermediate until October 1990, and since that time referred to simply as nursing facilities. Nurses working in such institutional settings find that Medicare and/or Medicaid regulations control most of their nursing practice and delivery of services of all types to the elderly. Even in those nursing facilities that are completely private (do not participate in either Medicaid or Medicare programs) find that they too must meet the same requirements as program participants because their licensing inspections are done by the same team using the same criteria for licensure as are used for program participants.

In virtually all care settings (home-based, community-based, and institutional), the state and federal government control the provision of services to the elderly by definition of criteria for access, funding, and setting standards of care and qualifications for providers of services. As in programs other than health care, whenever the government provides the funding, it also provides the control of the program.

Omnibus Budget Reconciliation Act

The Omnibus Budget Reconciliation Act of 1981 (OBRA 1981) brought a major change in the number of uninsured persons nationwide. That change in policy allowed individual states to reduce Medicaid eligibility (Allen, 1987). When added to the Medicaid cutbacks that occurred in the late 1970s and up to 1983, it meant that the percentage of low income persons insured by the Medicaid program decreased from 63% to 46%. Groups that were particularly affected were women below age 65 and children. Low income elderly were also affected.

A second group of elderly affected by OBRA 1981 was the mentally ill aged. Because of this act, individual states are permitted to set limits for community-based services and determine mandatory and optional services. As a result, the services provided for the elderly in the arena of mental health vary tremendously from state to state.

OBRA 1987 brought multiple changes in provision of services to the elderly. Perhaps the most significant changes occurred in the nursing home industry. OBRA 1987 required changes in delivery of services that had to be implemented by October 1, 1990. Some of the types of changes that were required established criteria for quality of care and quality of life in the nursing home. The act ensured full access of the ombudsman to a nursing facility and unannounced survey inspections that would focus on the residents. OBRA 1987 set standards for nursing staffing and staff training and certification, as well as ongoing education. It required the following:

Full-time social workers in nursing homes with more than 120 beds

Resident participation in planning his own care

Resident rights in the nursing home

Resident assessment for mental illness/mental retardation before admission

Major interdisciplinary assessment and development of a plan of care for the resident within a specified time frame

Establishment of facility-wide quality assessment and assurance committees.

The state agencies responsible for implementing the Medicaid program were targeted under OBRA 1987 as well. The state agencies were allowed to increase staffing to monitor nursing home complaints and to increase their enforcement capabilities. Individual states were required under the act to pay for the implementation of OBRA 1987 and to supply cost reports to the public that would document how an individual nursing facility spends its Medicaid monies.

Nursing homes nationwide began to be surveyed for compliance with the OBRA guidelines in October 1990. The implementation of the act has varied from state to state. California was one state that refused to implement OBRA 1987 based upon the state's position that its present regulatory system met the intent of the 1987 OBRA (Contemporary Long-Term Care, 1991c). The case is in the courts.

The Omnibus Budget Reconciliation Act of 1990 also brought policy changes that affect the health care of the elderly. OBRA 1990 provides for the following:

Direct reimbursement of all nurse practitioners and specialists in rural areas for services that they "are authorized to perform under state law" (Geriatric Nursing, 1991);

Nursing facilities' obligation to give written information at the time of admission about

The resident's right under state law to accept or refuse medical treatment,

The right to determine advance directives such as Durable Powers of Attorney for Health Care and Living Wills,

The right to refuse intrafacility transfer if the main purpose for the transfer is to remove the person from an area of the facility reserved for Medicare-skilled nursing care.

Under OBRA 1990 the Secretary of Health and Human Services is required to propose a plan to replace the current reimbursement system for nursing facilities with a prospective type of payment system. The plan would necessarily take into account the numbers of low income senior citizens, the case mix and volume, and the patient characteristics.

The act makes the provision that individual states help pay the private insurance premiums of an adult child if the child's insurance plan would cover the parents and the cost of coverage would be lower than covering the parents under Medicaid.

Current Factors Affecting Long-term Care

Demographic changes affect health care for the elderly, particularly long-term health care. The US Census Bureau predicts between 1984 and 1999 the number of people aged 75 to 84 will increase by 58% (Griffin et al, 1989). Those elderly above age 85 years are projected to increase 132% during that same period. Generally, the need for medical care does not increase dramatically until the eighth and ninth decade of life. Those over age 85 are approximately 18 times more likely to require nursing home care as their peers in the 65 to 74 age group.

Medical professionals and paraprofessionals are in greater demand. Nursing homes are expected to need more than 1 million registered nurses by the year 2000, which is double the number needed in 1990. The labor shortage in nursing homes is expected to decline until 1996 because of the decline in birthrate between 1958 and 1976. The scarcity of new workers available to work in long-term care will drive up wages for entry-level employees.

Increasing costs for health care and the reduction in reimbursement for health services will affect delivery of care to the elderly. In 1984 the national health expenditures were approximately 10.6% of the gross national product. The percentage is expected to be 15.3% of the gross national product by 1993. At the same time that health care costs are increasing, there has been a federal policy for cost containment and cutbacks in funding. The government has contained Medicaid expenditures for nursing homes by keeping the reimbursement rate low. That cost containment effort has resulted in nursing homes reduction in net income from +4.4% to a loss of 0.9% from 1985 to 1987, according to a survey by the American Health Care Association.

Implementation of the requirements of OBRA 1987 is expected to affect costs for delivery of care. The requirements for 24-hour licensed nursing, training, and certification for nursing assistants and new staffing will add to the cost of care. The requirements for training nursing assistants alone is projected to cost over $100 million per year.

There is a trend toward growth in consumer education. Consumers are learning that they have choices in health care and a right to participate in personal health decisions. Under OBRA 1987 residents in nursing facilities must be educated about their rights, the provision of restorative services, and restrictions on transfers. Residents in nursing facilities are also becoming familiar with programs for infection control, quality assurance, and other types of safety standards. Not only are consumers becoming knowledgeable about rights and services, they are becoming aware of their right to refuse care.

The pressures brought to bear on the current health care system by factors such as changing demographics, increases in costs and reduction in reimbursement, shortage of health care personnel, and increasing knowledge of the consumer are causing a reevaluation of the health care delivery system in the United States. The current system of health care is inadequate to meet the needs of all citizens. Since the fastest growing segment of the population is among those over age 85, the impact of the current system has the greatest potential to affect the older age groups.

Summary

Governmental policies affect the clinical practice of gerontologic nurses in all practice settings. Whether the nurse is working in home-based, community-based, or an institutional setting, the state and federal government affects access to care, funding, and establishment and enforcement of standards for delivery of care. Nurses are required to be knowledgeable about the regulations, rules, and guidelines placed on them by the regulatory

agencies. Additionally, nurses must be knowledgeable about programs, resources, community agencies, and their requirements in order to educate patients and help them access care.

Since the implementation of the Social Security Act in 1935 there has been governmental intrusion in and control of health care in this country. That control grew with the addition of the Medicare and Medicaid programs as state and federal government defined criteria for definition of services, funding, licensing, access, and limitations to services.

Looking forward to 1993 to 1994, nurses in gerontology will be practicing in all settings under new rules and regulations as a reformed system for health care delivery, where the government has total control of the system, is implemented. Nurses will not only become the providers of services under the new system, but will be beneficiaries of that system as well.

AIDS and the Elderly

The acquired immunodeficiency syndrome (AIDS) epidemic impacts older people (over 50) in three ways: as persons with AIDS, as care givers of other persons with AIDS, and as competitors in long-term care for limited dollars and personnel.

THE ELDERLY WITH AIDS

In 1989 there were 167,000 cases of AIDS in people over 50; over half have died. Most new cases of AIDS in people over 50 (1988) were in gay and bisexual men (65.8%). The next largest group was people who had received transfusions (17.3%). Heterosexual transmission made up 4.6% of new cases. There are more women with AIDS in older age groups and more whites. The only age category to have shown an increase in AIDS in heterosexual transmission is people over 50 (Table 5–1). In the future it is predicted that there will be an increase in both heterosexual and transfusion transmission of AIDS, with a decrease in number of new cases in gay and bisexual men (Riley, 1991).

In 1987, 10% of AIDS diagnoses were in people over age 50, but predicting how many human immunodeficiency virus (HIV) seropositive people over 50 will be diagnosed with AIDS or AIDS-related complex is difficult. A study in San Francisco (Hessel, 1988) of gay men found that in 9 years 42% had been diag-

TABLE 5–1   *New Cases of AIDS in People Aged 50 and Older*

Group	Percent
Gay/bisexual men	65.8
Transfused patients	17.3
Intravenous drug users	8.3
Heterosexuals	4.6
Hemophiliacs	2.0
Gay and bisexual intravenous drug users	1.9

From the Centers for Disease Control, Surveillance Data, January 1988.

nosed as having AIDS and another 47% had symptoms associated with AIDS-related complex. Based on this, the incubation period is up to 10 years, but it may be shorter among older persons. The epidemic is different for subgroups; the epidemic for gay men in San Francisco is different from those in Africa and probably from older Americans.

Biologic changes with age may increase the HIV transmission among older individuals because of decreases in immune system function. With age there appears to be a decline in primary antibody response. The progression of HIV is faster in old people than in younger people. There is a lower medial HIV incubation time (5.8 versus 7.3 years) in older adults than in younger adults. Older sex partners of HIV-infected transfusion recipients are more likely to seroconvert than younger people. Postmenopausal women have a thinning of the vaginal wall, leading to vaginal mucosal disruption during coitus. Tears in the vaginal wall, causing a genital lesion, can contribute to HIV infection, and this places older heterosexual women at increased risk.

Large studies in New York and San Francisco have shown decreased survival time for patients over 40 with AIDS. The reason for this is not known (Bacchetti et al, 1988; Rothenberg et al, 1987).

There are certain diseases more likely to occur in older AIDS patients: influenza, bacterial pneumonia, tuberculosis, and neurologic diseases (Kendig and Adler, 1990). Immunization against influenza is recommended, but

this may not be protective since their immune response is often inadequate. The tuberculin test may show a false-negative on the Mantoux test because HIV-1 induced dysfunction and age both may result in allergy to the test. About two thirds of all AIDS patients develop clinical evidence of AIDS dementia complex (Price et al, 1988). Older patients can be thought to have Alzheimer's disease or parkinsonism rather than HIV-1 induced neurologic disease. Correct and early diagnosis of these conditions is important to stop progression with early treatment.

At present, treatment for HIV infection is the same for all ages of people with AIDS— azidothymidine. The drug may improve survival but it has side effects that make it necessary to stop the drug or decrease the dose. There have been no comparisons by different ages on response to therapy (Kendig and Adler, 1990).

There is little information about age-related sexual behavior and lifestyles that could be related to HIV infection. Studies are old or biased. Older people tend to be monogamous but this does not rule out the use of prostitutes of both sexes, about which little is known.

Older people do have more misconceptions about AIDS; more believe the disease can be transmitted by eating utensils and toilet seats. A study of 885 people over 50 found that 43% had never heard of the HIV antibody test compared with 24% of younger people (Dawson, Cynamon, Fetti, 1987).

THE ELDERLY AS CARE GIVERS

The second area where HIV infection affects older people is as care givers to their children and grandchildren affected with AIDS. This illness creates financial hardships on the care giver. It also demands knowledge and skill in dealing with the many aspects of the disease and creates worry for the parent. Caregiving responsibility frequently falls to a parent about the time of retirement. Families contribute greatly to the care of AIDS patients—that often means the parents. Fifty percent of persons with AIDS (PWA) live with and receive care from parents (Ory and Zablotsky, 1989). This can be traumatic if parents learn for the first time as a result of this illness that their son is gay. The long course of the illness permits time to work out the relationship. However, the illness is devastating to the patient, making it hard on the parent to see the daily suffering and ultimately accept their death.

Grandparents may be the only caregiver for a child or baby with AIDS. The mother may be ill herself with AIDS or be unable to care for her child because of lack of funds or drug use. Children with grandparents able and willing to care for them are fortunate.

COMPETITION FOR HEALTH CARE RESOURCES

The third area in which AIDS affects older adults is in the allocation of limited resources, people, and money, particularly as it relates to long-term care. Some state laws require people with AIDS be admitted to nursing homes. With most beds occupied by the elderly and a projected increase in need for beds in long-term care there is no space for persons with AIDS. The nursing home staff is not prepared to care for acutely ill younger patients. Rather, staff education is in geriatrics and chronic disease, not AIDS and its many severe complications. The reimbursement rates do not adequately cover costs of patients in nursing homes now, so adding high technology, drugs, and high levels of care needed for AIDS patients will strain the existing resources. Cognitively impaired elderly patients with depressed immune systems and increased vulnerability to infections could wander into the rooms of persons with AIDS, and this could increase the elderly persons' risks for acquiring an infection from a person with AIDS. Likewise the person with AIDS could also get infections from the elderly patients.

In a study of 110 nursing homes in a state not requiring admission of AIDS patients, the reasons for not admitting those with AIDS who have applied for admission were (1) no isolation area, (2) concern for staff and patient safety, (3) fear of being infected with AIDS, (4) lack of staff education concerning AIDS, (5) inappropriate reimbursement, (6) fear of losing future admissions, and (7) a union problem with staffing (Carner and Bressler, 1990). Sixty-one percent of administrators felt comfortable admitting AIDS patients compared with 70% of paraprofessional staff, those who give the care. Eighty-five percent of administrators said families of patients would not support admitting AIDS patients, and there was concern that private paying patients would transfer out of the facility that accepted AIDS patients. Only 8% of the nursing homes had or were developing a policy on AIDS.

Few nursing homes in the sample (11%) said they would ever be willing to admit AIDS patients. Those that said they would limited the number (1) they would admit. They agreed that one day they would have to admit AIDS patients to nursing homes.

Certainly persons with AIDS have the right to the best care. The question arises, is the nursing home whose residents average over 85 years, the place to provide the care? Those who are writing on the subject think that what is learned about the care of persons with AIDS is transferable to the elderly. It may be, but it raises ethical and medical issues. Care may be different for persons with AIDS than for elderly people based on stigma attached to how AIDS was contracted: intravenous drug use, transfusions, homosexual or heterosexual contact, or some combination.

REQUIRED TESTING

Legislators are writing laws to require all physicians, dentists, nurses, and other health care workers to be tested for AIDS and if HIV seropositive to report it. If these laws are passed it may decrease the already shrinking pool of aides and others who presently seek employment in nursing homes or want to enter long-term care. This is an emotional issue and people on both sides of the question strongly support their opinions.

GERIATRICS AND AIDS

The following are some things to remember about geriatrics and AIDS:

1. The need for care requires a multidisciplinary team.
2. Those who give the care need to be involved in all aspects of decision making.
3. Both the cognitive and functional status of the older patient should be assessed.
4. Care requires using many tiers of the health care system.
5. If an elderly patient presents with an unusual course to his or her illness, think of HIV.
6. In older patients who are HIV positive, continue to look for usual diseases; do not attribute all illness to HIV.

References and Other Readings

Allen JE. Nursing home administration. New York: Springer, 1987.

American Association of Homes for the Aging Provider News. Key Bush advisor predicts delay in national long-term care policy. 1991; 6:1.

Bacchetti P, Osmond D, Chaisson RE, et al. Survival patterns of the first 500 patients with AIDS in San Francisco. J Infect Dis 1988; 107:1.

Benjamin AE. Long term care and AIDS: Perspectives from experiences with the elderly. Milbank Quarterly 1988; 66:415.

Carner E, Bressler J. AIDS and the long-term care system. The Journal of Long-Term Care Administration 1990; 18:13.

Clement PF. History of U.S. aged's proverty shows welfare program changes. Perspectives on Aging 1985; 9:4.

Cohen D, Hastings MM. Mental health in the elderly. In: Eisdorfer C, Kessler DA, Spector AH, eds. Caring for the elderly: developing health policy. Baltimore, MD: The Johns Hopkins University Press, 1989:364.

Contemporary Long-Term Care. Boren suit begins in Kansas ends in Michigan. 1991a; 14:12.

Contemporary Long-Term Care. Imbalanced Medicaid formula assailed by GAO. 1991b; 14:10.

Contemporary Long-Term Care. Judge to California: comply with OBRA regulations. 1991c; 14:10.

Davis K. Health care policies and the aged: observations from the United States. In: Binstock RH, Shanas E, eds. The handbook of aging and the social sciences. New York: Van Nostrand Reinhold, 1985:740.

Dawson D, Cynamon M, Fitti. AIDS knowledge and attitudes. Advanced data, vital, and health statistics of National Center for Health Statistics. DHHS, No. 146, Nov. 19, 1987.

Griffin KN, et al. Current forces shaping long-term care in the 1990's. The Journal of Long-Term Care Administration 1989; 17:8.

Grimaldi PL. Congress slices Medicare physicians fees. Nursing Management 1991; 22:22.

Hessel NG, Ruthorford G, O'Malley P. The natural history of human immunodeficiency virus infection in a cohort of homosexual and bisexual men: a 7-year prospective study. Paper presented at the IV International AIDS conference, Stockholm, Sweden, 1988.

Kane RL, Kane RA. Health care for older people: organizational and policy issues. In: Binstock RH, George LK, eds. The handbook of aging and the social sciences. New York: Academic Press, 1990:419.

Kaplan B. Social Security: 50 years later. Perspectives on Aging 1985; 9:4.

Kendig N, Adler W. The implications of the acquired immunodeficiency syndrome for gerontology research and geriatric medicine. J Gerontol 1990; 45:77.

OBRA '90 cuts Medicare, calls for living wills, sets Sept. 1991 deadline for PPS in nursing homes. Geriatric Nursing 1991; 12:6.

Ory M, Zablotsky D. Notes for the future: research, prevention, care, public policy. In M. Riley, M. Ory, D. Zablotsky, AIDS in an aging society. New York: Springer-Verlag, 1989, pp. 202–216.

Paulsen LG. The Oregon experiment. J Am Ger Soc 1991; 39:620.

Price RW, Brew B, Sidis J, et al. The brain in AIDS: central nervous system HIV-1 infection and AIDS dementia complex. Science 1988; 239:586.

Riley M, Ory MG, Zablotsky D. Aids in an aging society. New York: Springer, 1989.

Rothenberg R, Woelfel M, Stoneburner R, et al. Survival with the acquired immunodeficiency syndrome. Experience with 5833 cases in New York City. N Engl J Med 1987; 317:1297.

Schwartz R. Governors press for relief. Contemporary Long-Term Care 1991; 14:24.

PART THREE

Normal Aging

The third part of the book is the last section dealing with background knowledge that is basic to all gerontological nursing practice. Nine different aspects of aging or managing daily living as an older person are addressed.

Chapter 6 deals with the characteristics of the aged population as a group in the 1990s. This lends a general perspective within which to view the specifics of the individual older person.

Chapter 7 examines the tasks associated with managing living after the age of 70. The roles of the adult years undergo transition and relationships are altered. There are also specific tasks associated with preparation for dying and death. Knowledge about these role alterations and tasks is essential to diagnose and treat individuals and their families.

In Chapter 8 the normal changes in structure and functioning that occur with aging are examined. While these may predispose to pathology, such problems and the associated nursing care are not discussed here. This chapter is limited to discussing normal physiological changes, as a baseline for alterations in functional capacities that occur with pathology and its treatment.

Chapter 9 presents normal laboratory values in the elderly. Some of these values are the same for all ages; others change with age. It is important for nurses to know these differences so as to be able to assess the meaning of any laboratory value in the elderly. These values have been arranged in table form, alphabetically by category to make them easy to locate. The content includes both common and specialized laboratory tests.

In Chapter 10, Medications and the Elderly, pharmacokinetics and pharmacodynamics are discussed in relationship to aging. Drug use and abuse as well as approaches to drug therapy are presented.

Chapter 11 focuses on normal age-related changes in the teeth, supporting structures, and salivary glands and the resultant pathology that can occur. The authors have been teaching dental students and providing dental care to nursing home residents for many years and reflect on their perspective of the nurse's role in maintaining oral health for fragile, dependent elderly.

Chapter 12 presents the nutritional issues associated with living in the later years. Both the current standards for nutritional intake and the barriers to achieving them are discussed. Problems in daily living associated with eating, shopping, and food preparation are also considered.

Chapter 13 focuses on the dynamics and issues associated with families of the elderly. As individuals are living longer, families are facing the challenges of helping their older members manage their daily living with decreasing personal and external resources—even as their own lives increase in complexity.

The final chapter in this section, Chapter 14, addresses the challenges older individuals face and the responses they make to living with diminishing resources.

6
Characteristics of Older People and Introduction to Theories of Aging

MAXINE PATRICK

It is not unusual to find individuals who are in their 80s and 90s doing the same things as well as people a decade or two younger, though perhaps a bit more slowly. Too often sick and institutionalized elderly people are seen as the norm of old age. Although it is true that the risk of disease and disability increases with age, older persons are not necessarily incapacitated. At the same time, over 75% of all the health care today is given to people age 65 and over. Thus, knowledge of geriatrics and gerontology is basic for all health care providers.

Geriatrics (from the Greek *geras,* old age, and *iatrikos,* healing) is defined as "the branch of medicine concerned with medical problems and care of old people" (Stedman's, 1990). Geriatrics, like pediatrics, is not limited to physicians even though "medicine" is contained in the definition. Nurses, physical therapists, dietitians, and dentists all practice geriatrics. Knowledge of pathophysiologic changes of age and the illness and disease that can accompany these changes is used by all professionals who care for old people.

Gerontology covers a broader field of aging, including all academic disciplines and areas of professional practice. Gerontology is defined as the scientific study of the process and problems of aging (Stedman's, 1990). It includes (1) scientific studies of processes associated with aging;

(2) scientific studies of mature and aged adults; (3) studies from the humanities; and (4) applications of knowledge for the benefit of mature and aged adults. Gerontology focuses on the biological, psychological, and social aspects of normal aging. The nurse needs this knowledge in order to help the older person deal with normal changes that come with age. For example, normal eye changes lead to decreased vision, which predisposes to falls and fractures. Some memory loss is normal, but intelligence remains intact, so older people can be taught about care of their illness.

Kastenbaum suggests that it would be most straightforward to apply the word *geriatrics* to caregivers and restrict *gerontology* to the study of aging and the aged. However, he concedes that the two are hard to separate, since both scholarly and applied dimensions continue to form, interact, and change (Maddox, 1987).

This book is organized to combine gerontology and geriatrics into one framework. Chapters on normal age functioning and changes (gerontology) precede those on high-risk health problems (geriatrics). This chapter begins the gerontologic approach by discussing the characteristics and resources of the aged population and theories of aging.

In order to use the daily living–functional health status model discussed in Chapter 1, the nurse needs data on the gender, family situation, housing, leisure activities, and other demographic characteristics of the patient and family relevant to the current health situation.

Life Expectancy and Life Span

Life expectancy and life span are two different concepts. It is important for the nurse to be able to differentiate them.

LIFE SPAN

Life span is the average age to which an individual might live if entirely free from disease or accidents, the potential number of years a member of the species might live. For humans it has been estimated to be 110 to 115 years, with some estimates as high as 130 years. Inherent in the definition of life span are factors that make it difficult to reach the upper limits. Environmental factors such as air and water quality and chemical pollution are as important in determining life span as the incidence of disease.

LIFE EXPECTANCY

Life expectancy is the number of years a particular individual can be expected to live, calculated on the basis of age, with variation by sex, race, and the factors that prevail in the individual's country, such as infant mortality, wars, famine, and disease.

The average life expectancy for Americans is 75 years (Centers for Disease Control, 1990). The United States ranks 17th in life expectancy among 33 developed countries. Japan has the highest life expectancy (79.1 years). Hungary has the lowest (69.7), and the former Soviet Union the next to lowest (69.8 years). Although the United States has the highest gross national product per capita and spends the largest amount on health per capita in the world, longevity is decreased by factors including the failure to allocate resources effectively or possibly the American lifestyle.

Sixty-five is often the age considered as old. This book has selected age 70 and older to define the aged. Neugarten (1982) defined "young old" as 65 to 74, "middle old" as 75 to 84, and "oldest old" as 85 and older.

Olshansky and Cassel (1990) reported that if major fatal diseases were eliminated, life expectancy would not increase much. Eliminating all forms of cancer, which cause one fifth of all deaths in the United States, would increase life expectancy at birth by 3.17 years for women and 3.2 years for men.

Table 6–1 shows that women at birth and at age 65 have a longer life expectancy than men and that African-Americans have a shorter life expectancy than whites. Life expectancy at birth and age 65 for African-Americans and whites is projected to be equal in 2080.

EFFECTS OF LIFE EXPECTANCY ON SOCIETY

Researchers at the National Institute of Aging and University of Southern California predict that in 50 years life expectancy at birth will be 8 to 10 years more than forecast by the Census Bureau (Fields, 1989). According to their calculations, based on decreased mortality and advancements in medicine, women could expect to live to 92 rather than 83; men would live to 85.9 instead of 75 years. This prediction would mean that in 2040 there would be 20 million more persons over 65 than the government estimates, three times the current level. These researchers also point out that no one predicted the great number of people over age 85 in 1988.

TABLE 6–1 *Life Expectancy at Birth and at Age 65*

	1986	2005*	2025*
AT BIRTH			
White			
Male	72.2	74.6	75.5
Female	79.1	81.5	82.4
Black			
Male	66.8	72.0	72.8
Female	74.2	78.1	79.9
AT AGE 65			
White			
Male	14.9	16.1	16.9
Female	19.1	20.9	21.7
Black			
Male	13.5	15.2	16.2
Female	17.6	19.7	20.9

*Projections
From Life expectancy at birth and age 65 by race and sex 1950 to 2080. Middle mortality assumption. US Bureau of Census Pop Report Series P. 25, no. 1018, 1989:153.

These projected larger numbers of elderly would have a major effect on Social Security and Medicare programs and heavily impact the already strained health care system (US Bureau of the Census, 1989).

PERCENTAGE OF POPULATION OVER 65

The percentage of the population aged 65 and older is 12.4%. According to the Bureau of the Census (1989), the proportion of the population 65 and older is predicted to remain at 13.1% to 13.2% between 1995 and 2005 and to increase markedly to 22% of the total population from 2010 to 2030.

The white population after 1990 will grow more slowly than before and in 40 years will begin to decline compared with African-American and other races, which will have a greater growth rate. The African-American population is projected to increase 50% by 2030. Asians, Pacific Islanders, and Native American populations are projected to triple in size by 2040 (Bureau of the Census, 1989).

FASTEST GROWING SEGMENT

Of those over 65, the fastest growing age group is aged 85 and over. According to the Bureau of Census 1989 projections the number will double from 1980 to 2000 and redouble from 2000 to 2040. The population over 85, the very old, will benefit most from future decreases in mortality. Presently 1% of the population of the United States is over 85. This percentage is projected to increase to 5% in 2050.

THE OLDEST SEGMENT

Presently there are 46,000 people 100 years and older (US Bureau of the Census, 1989). These numbers are projected to increase to 1,440,000 by 2080 in the total US population. Clearly we are an aging society. Those who will be 100 in 2080 are 11 years old in 1991. Those who will be 85 in 2050 were born in 1965 and are 27 in 1991. People who will be the oldest citizens of the United States in the next century are today's children and young adults.

Aging in the World

Sixty is the age used to compute information about old people in the world. In 1950, the people in the world over 60 equalled the popula-

tion of the former Soviet Union. By 2000 that group is projected to equal the population of Europe and by 2050 to equal the population of the entire Western Hemisphere (Aging in All Nations, 1982).

Table 6–2 shows how the ranking of the nations by populations over age 60 is projected to change from 1950 to 2025. The only European country projected to be ranked in the top 10 is the former Soviet Union. The nations with the greatest change are poorer ones—India, Mexico, Nigeria, and Brazil.

Concern about this "graying population" has been voiced in the United Nations for many years. In 1982, 120 nations attended a United Nations sponsored World Assembly on Aging. This assembly alerted the world to the impact of the predicted increases in aging, with the greatest increases occurring in the developing countries. The political and economic issues of these increases have not been addressed by many countries because other crises seem more pressing, but unless they are addressed there will be physical and psychological suffering for older people and their families (Tout, 1989).

TABLE 6–2   *Change in the Population of Countries That Will Have More Than 15 Million People Aged 60 and Older in 2025*

Country	Rank in 1950	Rank in 2025
China	1	1
India	2	2
Former USSR	4	3
USA	3	4
Japan	8	5
Brazil	16	6
Indonesia	10	7
Pakistan	11	8
Mexico	25	9
Bangladesh	14	10
Nigeria	27	11

Based on estimates and projections of population by sex and age, 1950 to 2025, prepared by the Population Division of the United Nations. UN Document A/CONF.113/4, March 1982.

The Dependency Ratio

The total dependency ratio is the sum of young people (usually under 18) and elderly people (usually 65 and older) who are dependent on the number of people between ages 19 and 64. The ratio is a crude index of the total burden on the working population, who support the young and the old. This burden has implications for retirement, economic policies, housing, health care facilities, types of personnel and products, and recreational and social facilities.

Both fertility rates and mortality influence the dependency ratio. Fertility rates have changed; more women over 35 are starting families. African-Americans and Hispanics are projected to have increased numbers of children due to the increased numbers of women in the child-bearing age.

Shifts in the dependency ratio tend to affect policy decisions. For example, in the United States, Social Security benefits will be delayed according to the Social Security Amendment of 1983. The present retirement age of 65 at which full benefits can be received will increase to 66 in the year 2000 and to 67 in 2027. Chen (1987) determined that, with the use of 65 as the retirement age, the dependency ratio increased from 1940 to 1964, dropped in 1965, and will continue to drop until 2000; the next 40 years will show marked increases because retirement ages will be adjusted for the mortality gain. In contrast, using an equivalent retirement age calculation, dependency ratios increase little, from 53.8% in 1985 to 57.7% in 2040 (Chen, 1987).

The median age of the US population is projected to increase (US Bureau of the Census, 1989).

Year	Median Age
1987	32.1
2000	36.0
2030	42.0
2080	44.0

The smaller numbers of younger people and increased numbers of older people is a worldwide trend. The ages used to calculate the support group in the dependency ratio worldwide are different (ages 15 to 59). The group providing the most support will increase in less developed regions and decrease or remain the same in other regions. The lesser developed areas of the world will still have to deal with larger numbers of elderly (over age 60) in the future beyond 2025.

Educational Levels among Older People

The number of years of formal education of older people is increasing (Table 6–3). The gap in education between people over 65 and over 25 is narrowing (Kart, 1990). The percentage of people over 65 who complete high school is projected to increase from 46.2% in 1985 to 63.7% in 2000. The median years of school completed in 2000 for all ages is projected to be over 12 years.

There are great disparities in educational levels of various ethnic and cultural groups in the United States. Educational opportunities did not exist for many of today's elderly African-American people. Only 17% of African-Americans over 65 completed high school compared with 41% of white elderly. Hispanic elderly are the least educated; the number with no formal education is eight times greater than for whites. Asian and Pacific Islander elderly are the best educated minority. Many immigrants to the United States from these areas were professionals in their country of origin. Twenty-six percent are high school graduates compared with 41% of white elderly (AARP, 1980). Native American elderly have received

---

TABLE 6–3   *Educational Attainment of the Population 65 Years and Over and 25 Years and Over in 1975, 1985, and 2000*

Both Sexes	1975 (%)	1985 (%)	2000 (%)
Median school years completed			
65+	9.0	11.3	12.4
25+	12.3	12.6	12.8
Percent high school graduates			
65+	35.2	46.2	63.7
25+	62.5	72.3	80.4

From the US Bureau of the Census. Current Population Report Series p. 23, no. 138. Demographic and socioeconomic aspects of aging in the US by Seigel J, Davidson M. Washington, DC: US Government Printing Office, 1984.

poor education, both on and off the reservations, and about 12% have no formal education.

As older people become better educated they have different expectations of what they want in health care. They know their rights to access programs and want to participate more in health care decisions, especially in quality of life and right to die issues. Their years of education, maintenance of alertness and culture, and ability to learn into old age have implications for health teaching and other nursing care issues.

Marital Status

The marital status of older women and men is different. The 1980 US Census figures show that almost three fourths of white men over 75 are married. In contrast, the number of married women markedly declines with age; 70% of women are married at ages 55 to 64, but only 20% are married when they are over 75. These statistics have remained stable over the years (Table 6–4).

Divorce rates for people over 65 have risen, but decline the older people become. They are higher for women than men. African-Americans have higher divorce rates than whites and other minority groups. Asian and Pacific Is-

lander elderly have the lowest percentage of single women of all races, but the highest percentage of single men. The largest number of elderly widows and widowers are elderly African-Americans (Table 6–5).

Some of this information could be inferred because men marry younger women and have shorter life expectancies and life spans than women. Men tend to remarry more than women. Marital status is an important factor in health and has an influence on income, housing, care givers, support during times of crisis, and loneliness.

WIDOWS

In *Growing Old*, a study of disengagement, researchers found that widows tended to adapt successfully to aging and to integrate well into the social system of a peer group of other widows (Cummings and Henry, 1961). Other researchers have reported similar findings. Studies have not supported widowhood as a cause for mental illness in older women. If in good health, married and widowed women differed little in psychiatric impairment, regardless of socioeconomic status. Risk factors for psychiatric impairment were contingent on the number of deprivations associated with widowhood, particularly poor physical health and low socioeconomic status (Lowenthal et al, 1967).

TABLE 6–4 *Distribution of Male and Female Population Aged 55 Years and Over by Marital Status and Age*

Marital Status	Age 55–64 (%)		Age 65–74 (%)		Age 75+ (%)	
	Men	Women	Men	Women	Men	Women
1981						
Single	5.1	4.2	4.9	5.4	3.5	6.2
Married	84.7	70.3	83.0	50.1	72.0	23.3
Widowed	4.0	18.4	8.2	40.1	22.1	68.2
Divorced	6.1	7.1	3.9	4.4	2.5	2.3
1995						
Single	4.4	3.1	5.3	5.3	4.7	5.4
Married	81.1	71.8	78.4	48.8	70.9	20.5
Divorced and widowed	14.5	25.1	16.3	45.9	24.5	70.2

From the US Bureau of Census. Current Population Reports, Series p. 23, no. 138. Demographic and Socioeconomic aspects of aging. Washington, DC: US Government Printing Office, 1984.

TABLE 6–5   *Marital Status of Persons Aged 65 and Older by Race and Sex in 1980 by Percent*

Race and Sex	Married	Widowed	Divorced or Separated	Single, Never Married
White				
Men	74.2	13.9	6.6	5.4
Women	36.1	51.1	6.0	6.8
African-American				
Men	56.9	21.1	14.7	6.3
Women	25.0	57.7	11.6	5.6
Hispanic				
Men	65.0	16.0	12.8	6.3
Women	30.8	49.9	12.3	7.1
Asian/Pacific Islander				
Men	65.4	12.9	14.2	7.5
Women	30.2	55.6	10.1	4.1
Native American				
Men	59.7	20.6	13.6	6.1
Women	31.1	55.1	10.3	3.6

From A Portrait of Older Minorities, Washington, DC, AARP, 1980.

WIDOWERS

Men who are widowed experience greater difficulties than widows. The absence of someone to help them accommodate to the culture and deal with relatives affects their capacities to adjust to being alone. They are less likely than are women to have developed confidants outside the marriage (Cummings and Henry, 1961).

Income and the Elderly

Social Security benefits are the largest single source of income for elderly people. These benefits constituted 40% of the income of old people in 1988. Earnings, property income, and pensions follow in that order as income sources (Gilford, 1988). Social Security benefits are not fixed, but since 1975 have been indexed to the consumer price index so that there have been cost-of-living adjustments when the consumer price index increases more than 3%. Older people have been better able to keep up with costs than some younger families. For this reason, some people in Congress and elsewhere have questioned the degree of poverty of elderly people.

While many old people are poor, there are many who are not. The national average net worth of all people over 65 in 1984 was $32,700. The median net worth of those over 75 was $55,200. Seven percent of those 65 and over had net worth of over $250,000 (American Association of Retired Persons, 1990).

But for many old people poverty is real. The median yearly income for older men in 1989 was $13,107 and was $7655 for women. Households headed by someone 65 or over reported a median income of $23,179. This median varied by race: whites, $23,817; African-Americans, $15,766; and Hispanics, $19,310. (US Census Bureau, 1990). The poverty rate rose to 12.2% of the elderly in 1990. Among African-Americans it rose to 31.9% and among Hispanic elderly it was 28.1% (US Department of Commerce, 1990).

POVERTY LEVEL

The poverty level was established in 1961 by nutritionists and economists at the US Department of Agriculture and statisticians at the Social Security Administration and Census Bureau. They calculated that the average family spends one third of its income on food and arrived at the total family need by multiplying food costs by three. However, the poverty level for people over 65 is set 10% lower than the family level. Under this definition, 12% of people over 65 are at or below the poverty level, compared with 13.1% of the general population. If, however, the poverty level was the same for elderly as for all other people, 14.4% of the population 65 and over would be at or below the poverty level.

There are concerns about this method of calculating the poverty level for the elderly. The present calculation assumes that older people need 10% less income because they need 10% less food. While they may not need as many calories, calories are only one part of nutrition. The required dietary allowance of Americans shows that older people may actually require a higher quality of diet than some of the other age groups. Moreover, the amount of income spent on food, fuel, and shelter must be recalculated, since the other costs have risen faster than those of food. In 1991 congressional committees held hearings asking the Census Bureau to justify the age differences in setting the poverty level (Margolis, 1990).

RELATIONSHIP OF LIVING ALONE TO POVERTY

Elderly people living alone or with nonrelatives had the lowest incomes. In the United States 22% of people living alone were in poverty compared with 6% living in families. The median income of the total group of elderly living alone in 1989 was $9638; for whites it was $10,086, Hispanics $6762, and African-Americans $6035.

According to 1982 government figures, women were more likely to be living in poverty than men. Over one third of all elderly African-Americans were poor compared with one fifth of Hispanics, and one tenth of all whites. The highest risk for poverty was for African-American women living alone (Table 6–6).

These figures take on added meaning with increasing numbers of older African-Americans and Hispanics projected for the future. Ideally, interventions should increase minorities' opportunities for jobs that contribute to better income, Social Security benefits, and pensions during years while they are working. However, these interventions are not being made to the

TABLE 6–6 *Poverty Rates for Selected Elderly Subgroups in 1982*

	Percent below Poverty Level
All elderly	15
Elderly women	18
Elderly women living alone	28
Elderly African-Americans	42
Elderly African-American women living alone	66

From Tomorrow's Elderly Issues for Congress. Report for the House Select Committee on Aging. Comm. Pub. No. 98–457. Washington, DC: US Government Printing Office, 1984.

extent necessary; poverty for elderly people in minority groups will clearly continue.

Health Status and Limitations on Activities

The National Health Survey on Aging (1984) shows that the majority (67.5%) of people 65 and over report that their health is good or excellent. More African-Americans and those with lower income report their health as poor or fair than do white older people and those with higher incomes.

Eighty percent of the noninstitutionalized elderly report at least one chronic condition. The number of chronic conditions, even though some may be disabling, is not a measurement of functional status. The ability to function has more to do with self-assessment of health rather than the number of diagnosed conditions. Self-assessment of health correlates with other measures of health status and health behavior.

FUNCTIONAL AND INSTRUMENTAL ACTIVITIES OF DAILY LIVING

Functional ability is usually classified by activities of daily living (ADLs) and instrumental activities of daily living (IADLs). Functional status includes at least three domains: physical, social, and psychological. ADLs designed by

Katz and others (1963) include assessing basic hygiene and managing self-care such as walking, bathing, eating, and dressing. IADLs include household chores related to social tasks such as shopping, cooking, laundry, and managing money (Lawton and Brody, 1969). These measurements used to describe service needs of the elderly are more important in assessing independent living ability than estimates of disease or numbers of chronic conditions. Functional status measures are used for determining compensation for disability and eligibility for insurance and government assistance programs.

In a large sample (27,909) it was found that the older people get, the more difficulty they have with at least one ADL and/or IADL. This study showed more women over 85 have difficulty with at least one ADL (38.4%) and IADL (56.4%) than men (26.3% and 50.5%). African-Americans have more difficulty with ADLs (15.5%) and IADLs (23.5%) than whites or Hispanics. A later study also reported more African-American and Hispanic noninstitutionalized elderly have difficulty with IADLs than ADLs (Leon and Lair, 1990).

ACTIVITIES OF DAILY LIVING

Table 6–7 shows that noninstitutionalized persons 65 and over with ADL difficulty had the greatest difficulty with bathing, followed by walking, bed and chair transfer, and dressing and the least difficulty with eating. A total of 11.1% of noninstitutionalized elderly with any ADL or walking difficulty received help.

TABLE 6–7   *Functional Status of the Noninstitutionalized Population Aged 65 and Older: Estimates of Persons with ADL and Mobility Difficulties as a Percent of the Total Population Aged 65 and Older in the United States in 1987*

Population Characteristic	Total Population Aged 65 or Older	Walking or at Least One ADL*	Bathing	Bed/Chair Transfer	Dressing	Toileting	Feeding	Walking
POPULATION WITH ADL AND WALKING DIFFICULTIES								
Number (in thousands)	27,909	3601	2492	1635	1437	975	316	2152
Percent		12.9	8.9	5.9	5.1	3.5	1.1	7.7
PERCENT OF TOTAL POPULATION BY LEVEL OF DIFFICULTY AND DEPENDENCE								
Functioning without help[†]		1.8	0.9	1.4	0.6	0.2	0.1[‡]	0.6
Functioning with help[†]								
Equipment only		2.9	1.1	1.1	0.1[‡]	0.9	0.0[‡]	3.6
Personal assistance only		3.5	4.5	1.7	4.1	0.9	0.6	0.6
Both		4.7	2.4	1.2	0.3	1.0	0.1[‡]	1.5
Unable to perform activity with or without help[†]		NA	NA	0.5	NA	0.5	0.3	1.4
PERCENT OF TOTAL POPULATION BY DURATION OF PROBLEM								
More than 3 months		11.7	0.8	5.1	4.5	3.0	0.9	6.8
More than 3 months and functioning without help		1.6	0.8	1.3	0.5	0.2	0.1[‡]	0.5

*Persons with more than one difficulty are assigned to the category representing the highest level of dependence.
†The levels indicate increasing dependence and are mutually exclusive.
‡Relative standard error is equal to or greater than 30%.
NA, question on total dependence for these items not collected since inappropriate.
From the Agency for Health Care Policy and Research: National Medical Expenditure Survey—Household Survey, round 1.

INSTRUMENTAL ACTIVITIES OF DAILY LIVING

At least 17.5% of the 65 and over noninstitutionalized persons in 1987 reported they had difficulty with one IADL. Getting around the community was the activity reported by the largest percentage (13.5%) as being difficult. Shopping and doing light housework was the next highest percentage (Table 6–8). A smaller percentage of older people who lived with a spouse reported difficulty with one or more ADL or IADL. Those who lived with other relatives had more limitations than people who lived alone.

Theories of Aging

Gerontology is not a single unified discipline. It is a multidisciplinary assembly of explanatory schemes, each using its own theoretical terms, each based on different conceptual universes. The theoretical terms at all levels differ significantly. Theories of aging have been formulated in biology, psychology, and sociology; the logical relationships among them is not clear (Moody, 1988).

McKee (1982) calls for an elucidation of the philosophical foundations of gerontology that would clarify the relationships among the different domains and theoretical levels of explanation. What is at stake is the relationship between theory and practice, between what we know or think we know and how we act and choose (Moody, 1988).

BIOLOGICAL THEORIES OF AGING

Cristalfo (1988) believes that there is no good definition of the biology of aging and no explanation of why aging begins. Theories of the biology of aging try to explain a progression of disease and death related to the process of aging, but how these elements are related is obscure. There is no adequate theory of biologic aging.

TABLE 6–8 *Functional Status of the Noninstitutionalized Population Aged 65 and Older: Estimates of Persons with IADL Difficulties as a Percent of the Total Population Aged 65 or Older in the United States in 1987*

Population Characteristic	Total Population Aged 65 or Older	At Least One IADL*	Use of Telephone	Handling Money	Shopping	Getting about the Community	Preparing Meals	Doing Light House-work
POPULATION WITH IDAL AND WALKING DIFFICULTIES								
Number (in thousands)	27,909	4884	1237	1758	3072	3774	2090	2823
Percent		17.5	4.4	6.3	11.0	13.5	7.5	10.1
PERCENT OF TOTAL POPULATION BY LEVEL OF DIFFICULTY AND DEPENDENCE								
Difficulty but functioning with help[†]		1.3	1.1	0.3	0.3	0.6	0.5	0.8
Functioning with help[†]		6.8	1.7	2.8	3.9	8.9	1.9	3.3
Unable to perform activity with or without help[†]		9.4	1.6	3.2	6.8	4.0	5.1	6.0
PERCENT OF TOTAL POPULATION BY DURATION OF PROBLEM								
More than 3 months		16.4	4.1	5.9	10.2	12.5	6.7	9.0

*Persons with more than one difficulty are assigned to the category representing the highest level of dependence.
[†]The levels indicate increasing dependence and are mutually exclusive.
From the Agency for Health Care Policy and Research: National Medical Expenditure Survey—Household Survey, round 1.

There are two major classes of biologic theories, stochastic and developmental-genetic. Examples of the former are somatic mutation and error. Developmental-genetic theories include neuroendocrine, intrinsic mutagenesis, immunologic, and free radical theories* (Christafalo, 1988). These theories are only mentioned here, because at this time they are not helpful in nursing management. Interested readers may learn more about these biological theories in articles and books on gerontology (Schneider and Rowe, 1990).

CONCEPTUAL BASES FOR PSYCHOLOGICAL AND SOCIOLOGICAL THEORIES OF AGING

Social sciences use concepts of culture, social structure, and socialization as the structure for their theories on aging. Psychology's approach lies somewhere between biology and other social sciences, dealing primarily with the organization of behavior in the adult years. Organisms grow up and grow old as a consequence of their heredity and environment (Birren, 1988). However, theories must also include people's everyday experiences, which psychological theories of aging fail to cover.

PSYCHOLOGICAL THEORIES

One major psychological theory that includes late adulthood (not defined by years) was developed by Erickson as a part of his eight stages of ego development. The stage that is applicable to the elderly is ego integrity: a basic acceptance of one's life as having been inevitable, appropriate, and meaningful, and acceptance of death as a part of life; versus despair, a failure to accept one's life as appropriate and meaningful, accompanied by a fear of death (Erickson, 1950).

SOCIOLOGICAL THEORIES

Many sociological theories on aging are not theories in the strictest sense. They are descriptions or perspectives based on major sociological theories, but not systematically organized theories in themselves. Few studies have tested them. Some studies report that their findings support or reject a given theory, but the studies

*At this time (June 1992) there is increased interest in free radicals as a cause of aging in research centers in Europe and the United States.

were not designed to test the theories on which they comment. Researchers in social gerontology seem to want to conceptualize, but not to formulate and test explicit theoretical statements. Different classification systems and definition of terms are used; thus data cannot be compared across studies or progress made toward development of theories on aging.

Existing theories have been classified by Kart (1990) under the headings *aging and the individual* (role theory, activity theory, disengagement, socioenvironmental, exchange and aging, and symbolic interactionism) and *aging and society* (subculture, modernization, age stratification, and political economy of aging). Table 6–9 and Figure 6–1 show sociological theories and how they have influenced social theories of aging.

Birren and Bengtson (1988) groups the sociological theories similarly. Structural functionalism argues that social behavior is best understood from the perspective of the equilibrium needs of the social system. The concepts are role, norms, and socialization, with a focus on consensus and conformity rather than conflict. Theories of aging in this category are disengagement, modernization, and age stratification. Symbolic interactionism influences activity theory, social competence/breakdown, and subculture theories. These theories emphasize processes of social interaction. Individuals develop a sense of self through interpreting others' responses to their behavior (Birren and Bengtson, 1988). The third category, exchange theory, states that interactions between individuals are attempts to maximize rewards and reduce costs (Dowd, 1975). Marxism is a political theory of social distribution in a capitalist society based on social relations of production (Birren, 1988.). Rather than addressing biological or psychological issues, aging is assessed in terms of inequities in power and income, whether capitalism is supportive of the needs of the elderly. Lastly, the social phenomenological theory of aging covers phenomenology and ethnomethodology theories, examining the process of social construction.

USE OF THEORIES IN NURSING

Nurses should read original theories rather than condensed versions or someone else's interpretation. Most work on sociological theories of aging was done in the 1960s and 1970s and was aimed at predicting successful aging. Increasing numbers of people study, research,

TABLE 6–9 *Sociological Theories of Aging*

Activity (Cavan, 1949; Havighurst and Albrecht, 1953)	The more active elderly persons are, the greater life satisfaction. Self concept is related to roles and previous roles must be replaced with new ones to remain active.
Disengagement (Cummings and Henry, 1961)	Society withdraws from the aging person to the same extent as the person withdraws from society. Mutual withdrawal.
Exchange (Dowd, 1975)	Interaction between individuals is an attempt to maximize rewards and reduce costs. Balancing between rewards and costs are by withdrawal, extension of power network, emergence of status, and coalition formation. When rewards and costs are not balanced, one party becomes more powerful as happens in aging.
Continuity (Atchley, 1972)	In the process of becoming an adult, the individual develops habits, commitments, preferences, and a host of other dispositions that become part of his personality. As the person ages these are maintained. In the life cycle these predispositions constantly evolve from interactions among personal preferences and experiences and biological and psychological capacities.
Symbolic interactionism (Blumer, 1969; Mead, 1934)	Human beings in interacting with one another have to take account of what each is doing or is about to do; one has to fit one's own line of activity in some manner to the actions of others.

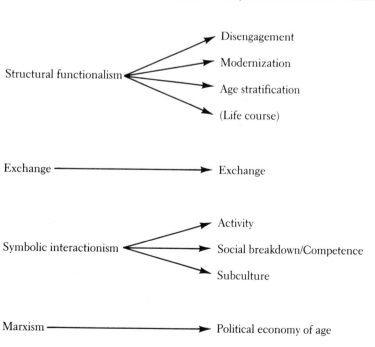

FIGURE 6–1 The influence of sociological theories on theories of aging. (From Birren JE, Bengtson eds., Emergent theories of aging. New York: Springer Publishing Company, 1988, p. 335; with permission.)

and work in the field of gerontology, but little progress seems to be made in theory development.

In spite of the lack of overall theories in gerontology, nurses will find theoretical issues thought provoking and helpful in making decisions about patient care.

References and Other Readings

Aging in all nations. A special report on the UN World Assembly on aging. Vienna, Austria: National Council on Aging, 1982.

American Association of Retired Persons. A portrait of older minorities. Washington, DC, 1990.

American Association of Retired Persons. A portrait of older minorities. Long Beach, CA, 1985.

American Association of Retired Persons. A profile of older Americans. Long Beach, CA, 1990.

Atchley RC. The social forces in later life. Florence, KY: Wadsworth, 1972.

Birren J. A contribution to the theory of the psychology of aging in emergent theories of aging. In: Birren J, Bengtson V. Emergent theories of aging. New York: Springer, 1988:153.

Blumer H. Symbolic interactionism. Englewood Cliffs, NJ: Prentice Hall, 1969.

Cavan RS. Self and role in adjustment during old age. In: A. Rose (ed.), Human behavior and social processes. Boston: Houghton Mifflin, 1962.

Centers for Disease Control, Atlanta, Georgia. Life expectancy in 33 developing countries. April 7, 1990.

Chen Y-P. Making assets out of tomorrow's elderly. The Gerontologist 1987; 27:410.

Christafalo V. An overview of the theories of biological aging. In: Birren, Bengtson, eds. Emergent theories of aging. New York: Springer, 1988:118.

Cummings E, Henry W. Growing old. New York: Basic Books, 1961.

Dowd J. Aging as exchange: A preface to theory. Gerontol 1975; 30:584.

Erickson E. Childhood and society. 2nd ed. New York: W.W. Norton, 1950.

Fields H. New study using census figures. Modern Maturity Bulletin, AARP, Long Beach, CA, 1989.

Gilford D. The aging population in the twenty-first century. Committee on National Statistics, Commission on Behavioral and Social Sciences and Education, National Research Council. Washington, DC: National Academy Press, 1988.

Havighurst RJ, Albrecht R. Older people. NY: Longmans, Green, 1953.

Kart CS. The realities of aging. 3rd ed. Boston: Allyn & Bacon, 1990.

Katz S, Ford AB, Moskowitz RW, et al. Studies of illness in the aged. The index of ADL: a standardized measure of biological and psychosocial function. JAMA 1963; 185:914.

Lawton MP, Brody W. Assessment of older people: self-maintaining and instrumental activities of daily living. The Gerontologist 1969; 9:179.

Leon J, Lair T. Functional status of the non-institutionalized elderly: estimates of ADL and IADL difficulties. DHHS publication no. (PHS) 90-3462. National Medical Expenditure Survey Research Findings 4, Agency for Health Care Policy and Research. Rockville, MD: Public Health Service, 1990.

Lowenthal M, Berkman P, et al. Aging and mental disorder. San Francisco: Jossey-Bass, 1967.

Maddox G. The encyclopedia of aging. Spring, 1987.

Margolis R. Risking old age in America. Boulder, CO: Westview Press, 1990.

McKee PL. Philosophical foundations of gerontology. Human Sciences Press, 1982.

Mead GH. Mind, self and society. University of Chicago Press, 1934.

Moody HR. Toward a critical gerontology. In: Birren, Bengtson, eds. Emergent theories of aging. New York: Springer, 1988.

Neugarten B. Policy for the 1980's: age or need entitlement? In: Neugarten BL, ed. Age and need. Sage Publications, 1982.

Olshansky SJ, Carnes B, Cassell C. In search of Methuselah: Estimating the upper limits to human longevity. Science 1990; 250:634.

Rasenwaike I. The extreme aged in America. Westport, CT: Greenwood Press 1985.

Schneider E, Rowe J. Handbook of the Biology of Aging, 3rd Ed. San Diego: Academic Press, 1990.

Stedman's medical dictionary. 25 ed. Baltimore, MD: Williams & Wilkins, 1990.

Tout IK. Aging in developing countries. New York: Oxford University Press, 1989.

US Bureau of the Census. Current population. Report series, p. 23, no. 138, Demographic and socioeconomic aspects of aging in the US, by Seigel J, Davidson M. Washington, DC: US Government Printing Office, 1984.

US Bureau of the Census. Population report series, p. 25, no. 1018. Projections of the population of the US by age, sex and race 1988 to 2080, by Spencer G. Washington, DC: US Government Printing Office, 1989.

US Department of Commerce, Public Information Office, Census Bureau Reports 1990. p. 60, no. 174, 175, 176RD. Washington, DC: US Department of Commerce Census Bureau.

7
Challenges of Daily Living and Development in Later Life Stages

MAXINE PATRICK

Much attention has been focused on the developmental tasks and challenges of the first two decades of life. The tasks and challenges facing those who survive to the seventh, eighth, and ninth decades are at least as demanding and perhaps more formidable than the first two.

The older person's perspective of the growth and development tasks of old age constitute an ongoing frame of reference for going about the tasks of daily living. This perspective determines a person's basic approach and outlook. People who live into their 70s and 80s will have suffered many losses, yet a perspective of developmental tasks that emphasizes the integration and management of loss is essentially negative. Those who survive most successfully approach daily living with zest and fortitude. Their goal is not merely to adjust to losses, but to live life fully as it exists, i.e., to continue to grow within the realities of their lives. Nurses can support older people in their quest for continued growth and a positive way of life. Nurses may also be able to help those older persons who tend to see the bleaker side of life, particularly when they experience setbacks in their health, to find personal satisfactions and ways of maintaining quality of life.

The way the older person views life sets a tone that pervades not only all of the ongoing tasks of life, but also those special larger tasks that must be dealt with in old age. The older person must approach and address these special tasks effectively in order to manage life successfully.

Ongoing tasks of daily living in the seventh decade and beyond include role changes and modifications, alterations in control over decision making and independence, assuming responsibility for unfamiliar activities, maintaining oneself in the face of losses, finding new sources of support, and preparing for death and dying. Although these tasks are not peculiar to older people, they take on unique features when addressed in the late years.

Role Changes

A variety of role changes occur in old age, with some new roles, some changes in the way old roles are carried out, and even role reversals.

RETIREMENT

Often the first role changes in old age are associated with retirement. Retirement is a modern industrial phenomenon, accepted today as a reward for a lifetime of work. For many people it comprises almost one third of their life (25 years). It is no longer viewed as something for those no longer able to work, but as an active, independent, healthy time of life. Sufficient income and good health are important factors in adjusting to retirement, but these qualities are important for any age and any stage of life.

Until recently, most research on retirement from the work force focused on men. However, women now comprise 45% of the work force. Their patterns of entry and reentry into the labor market may make their adjustment to retirement different from men's adjustment. Additionally, women never retire from many of their household roles.

Research literature tends to assume retirement means complete cessation of work. In reality, many people do not abruptly stop work and fully retire. Instead they have done some previous planning, and they work part time, change jobs, become self-employed, or become volunteers.

EARLY RETIREMENT

People now tend to retire before the age of 65, many in their late 50s or early 60s. Retirement decisions are usually based on expected income. In some instances continuing to work can actually reduce income or fail to add to it. Usually, income is reduced by one third in retirement. However, studies have shown that most retired elderly feel that their income is adequate for their needs. Expenses associated with work are reduced and income is spent in different ways.

Mandatory retirement at a set age is gradually being eliminated except for a few jobs. More and more it is up to the individual to decide when to retire. Elimination of mandatory retirement policies is predicted to have little influence on retirement decisions. People seem to decide when they wish to retire and hold to that decision.

RESPONSES TO RETIREMENT

Some researchers have compared retirement in men to widowhood for women as a stressful time; however, these findings have not been supported. Retirement is not necessarily a stressful time. It has been found that those who wait until the last possible moment to retire find initial response to retirement more stressful than those who chose to retire before it was required.

Anticipation of retirement was viewed by elderly men as worse than the actual event. When men in their late 50s or early 60s were asked about retirement their responses were negative; however, after a few years of retirement these same men viewed it positively, if their health was good.

A longitudinal study of four generations found that the oldest retired men and women had few difficulties in their lives from friends, family, work (if still working), money, or health (Fiske and Chiriboga, 1990). In contrast younger old people reported many difficulties in these areas.

RETIREMENT EFFECTS ON WIVES WHO ARE HOMEMAKERS

Men's retirement affects the lifestyle of the wives who never worked outside of the home. Patterns in daily living have been built around the absence of the husband during the day. After the husband's retirement, the wife's sense of freedom and control is diminished by the need to accommodate the husband's presence and expectations. Some wives give up volunteering and seeing friends. Retired men who are "lost" in their retirement, whose work was their life, tend to present the greatest challenge to their wives.

HOUSING AND LIVING ARRANGEMENTS

Perhaps the most significant change in the life of the older person is the move to different housing or living arrangements. This change can signal a loss of independence and a break with associations of the past.

Many factors determine where and with whom an older person will live: marital status, gender, children, siblings, health, and income. There are many kinds of housing, but frequently it is hard to find the right place for an older person to live. The options are limited by whether or not the kind of housing desired or needed is available, whether the family knows about it, the cost, and the match between the services needed and those provided. The goal is for the elderly to live in the least restrictive housing available based on the individual's functional status.

The environment where one lives should include places to shop for groceries and needed supplies; medical, dental, and pharmaceutical services; recreation and social opportunities; and transportation to them. All of these elements should match what the older person wants and needs. Little has changed over the years in the housing needs of the elderly. As the number of old people increases, specialized housing requirements will increase. There is little to suggest that old people in the future will have more income to afford better housing. Another concern is the likelihood of deterioration in health, with increased risk for the need to change to a long-term care facility or to use a large number of community resources to maintain the elderly in their current residences.

INDEPENDENT LIVING

There are many kinds of housing available to the elderly, but most old people, given a choice, prefer to live in independent households. Of those who do, 75% are homeowners and 25% are renters. Among those who own their own homes, 86% have them fully paid for.

Older people living independently eventually may have to make a change in living. They may seek to change their housing when it becomes too costly to maintain the home; they are displaced by changes in the neighborhood; they fear to remain in the home; or they become too ill or fragile to live independently.

The United States provides few supports to help keep older people in their own homes. European countries do a better job than the United States in helping maintain this first choice in housing for the elderly. European social services are based on the belief that it is humane and economical to provide services to maintain older individuals in their own homes, even though the services needed are expensive. In Sweden, for example, one fifth of those over 65 receive some home help (Thorslund et al, 1991).

HOME SHARING

Sometimes older people are able to remain in their own homes by sharing their homes. Compatibility is essential, but often the arrangement must be tried before it is known if it will work. The combinations may be old–old, old–young, or old and a family. There are situations where two or three widows could live together in one of their homes, reduce expenses, and provide each other with companionship. The most difficult aspect of this kind of living arrangement may be that each person has to give up some independence; this drawback may be balanced if each person has some need for assistance that can be provided by another. In some areas organizations are set up to match older individuals who wish to share their homes with others who would like to move in.

ACCESSORY APARTMENTS

Accessory apartments constructed within the same house or close by the home of a family member allow closeness and privacy for the older individual and for the younger family. Many states and cities have passed zoning ordinances allowing such units to be built. They seem to be more popular in California and Hawaii than in other states. They are called "second units" or "chana" (extended family) units in Hawaii. Older people can have their own cooking facilities or share meal times. There can be as much togetherness or aloneness as each party desires. This living arrangement allows grandchildren and grandparents to be near each other, a highly desirable intergenerational exchange. It also provides a degree of independence for both groups while reducing the worry and guilt of younger people, who feel responsible for their parents' well-being yet find it difficult to travel to visit them.

RETIREMENT FACILITIES

The development of specialized housing and care for older people has become a growing industry. Both private and public resources are involved. Types of retirement facilities range from whole communities to special buildings, from nursing homes and assisted care facilities to boarding homes. Recently, "catered living" units are being developed by a hotel chain.

Many older people realize that they may have to move out of their homes or apartments one day. The affluent have more options. They can afford to pay for services that permit them to remain in their own homes so that a move may not be necessary. If they choose eventually to move to a retirement home or to a continuing care retirement community (CCRC), they may select one, put their names on a waiting list, and even make a downpayment years in advance of an anticipated move. When the need arises, they move into the place they have chosen. For those with limited incomes the choices are more restricted, as is seen in the following discussion of retirement facilities.

People are waiting until they are quite old to move into the place they select to retire. One retirement home reported that 90 is now the average age of the new resident. Pynos (1985) gave 75 as the average age of moving into a CCRC. In either case, these people are old and may soon be in need of considerable assistance for activities of daily living and health care.

Continuing Care Retirement Communities

CCRCs are life care communities. They consist of independent living units, assisted living sections where people live independently but receive assistance with personal and health care, and skilled nursing care units.

These communities usually require an entrance fee ranging from $20,000 to over $60,000 and a monthly maintenance fee that depends on the size of the unit. The entrance fee may be on a sliding scale based on financial status, and may not be refundable. Monthly maintenance fees can increase when there is an increase in costs of the CCRC. The resident does not own a percentage of the building; however, in some states property taxes are being charged to people living in such units since they are not considered to be nonprofit enterprises, even though many CCRCs are owned by churches. Thus, a state increases revenue at the expense of older people. Anyone considering a move to a CCRC should investigate the ongoing and probably increasing monthly costs.

Retirement Subdivisions

Retirement subdivisions have long been established in some cities. In addition there are entire retirement cities, such as Sun City, Arizona and Leisure World, California. The residents in these communities (minimum age, 55) tend to be younger than residents of CCRCs. They buy their home, cooperative unit, or condominium. The communities provide the same services as any town. In addition, they feature many recreational facilities, e.g., golf courses, bowling greens, and swimming pools. There are lectures, games, courses, and professional and amateur entertainment. In Sun City life is designed to be busy and entertaining. This kind of community attracts those who seek planned activities. Some people find it a disadvantage that all of the people living here are old; contacts with younger people may be limited to employees of the bank, gas station, and stores.

Mobile Home Parks

For middle and upper income people who want to live in their own homes and want to be more mobile, there are mobile homes and mobile home parks. Some people move their homes back and forth from the north to the south each year, whereas others leave their homes parked in the south and return to them each year. Mobile home communities also appeal to those who want an active lifestyle. There is usually a common area for arts and crafts activities in addition to options for travel and entertainment.

Hotel Communities

The Marriott Corporation entered the housing market for frail elderly in 1988. Its Brighton Garden Homes are based on a "catered living" concept, offering housing to people who do not require nursing home care, but who do need assistance with personal care, e.g., dressing, grooming, bathing, and medication. The housing consists of 85 rental living units and a 30-bed nursing center. Thirty of these communities are planned by 1994, the first of them on the east coast. Thus, a corporation has used the demographics of an aging population and an interest in health care as a basis to expand its business. It will be interesting to see if other hotel corporations follow this pattern.

Congregate Housing

Congregate housing is defined by the International Center for Social Gerontology as "a type of multi-family dwelling in which there is a central dining facility with or without a central kitchen." This definition is sometimes expanded to cover similar living arrangements. Often these units are government subsidized, so that the rent is a percentage of income. Because low income housing is so limited, many older people wait for years for admission to congregate housing.

The Congregate Housing Services Program requires an assessment of the applicant's need for assistance with activities in daily living, e.g., with eating. All residents pay for rent and meals on a sliding scale. These units keep people out of institutions and reduce costs, but not enough units are available. There is little money in state or federal budgets to build more of them, and private builders are not interested in such construction (Nachison, 1985).

Many congregate housing units are projects of the Department of Housing and Urban Development and by law cannot limit the residents to just the elderly. The mix of younger families, teen-aged people with physical handicaps, and frail elderly has brought some conflict and fear for safety. There are reports that older people have been robbed and beaten by younger residents.

Board and Care Chronically impaired, dependent elderly and disabled individuals often use board and care housing, also known as residential care facilities, community care facilities, personal care homes, domiciliary care homes, adult factor care, family homes, group homes, and halfway houses. These facilities provide food, shelter, some degree of protective oversight, and generally nonmedical personal care by a nonrelative (McCoy, 1983). Assistance with health care, such as giving an insulin injection, is not permitted by a nonrelative.

The federal government does not directly regulate these homes but requires states to set and enforce standards. Although all states have regulations, not many states implement them. A large number of board and care facilities operate without licenses and thus avoid all state supervision of care. Board and care housing could prevent improper placement that would also be more costly, such as a nursing home for elderly who do not need full-time care. However, without licensing and inspection to ensure a safe environment, the quality of care in these facilities is largely dependent on management.

NURSING HOMES

Nursing homes are caregiving facilities developed to provide long-term care to chronically ill or dependent individuals. Nursing homes are licensed by the state and are inspected by both state and federal teams. Costs for nursing home care are high and usually are not well covered by insurance.

The average age of residents in nursing homes is the middle 80s. The percent of people 65 and over living in nursing homes is declining. It was 5% until 1977, when it decreased to 4.8%. In 1985 it decreased to 4.6% and is projected to be 4.0% in 2000 (Clinical Report on Aging, 1988). However, the chance of spending some time in a nursing home for those over 65 is much higher. These percentages do not show what is happening in different stages of old age, i.e., 22% of people over 85 are living in nursing homes. It is estimated that, with the proper assistance, 16% to 35% of the elderly living in institutions could live in the community.

RESPITE CARE

Respite care is not a form of housing, but a temporary method to provide support to an individual or family caring for an older family member in the home. Respite services are usually provided in reserved beds or rooms in an existing nursing home. The caregivers are regular staff and all services are part of the existing facility. The charges vary and are paid by the patient or family. Respite care service may also be provided to frail elderly within their homes. Insurance coverage or some stable funding is needed to increase the number of respite care beds and services available to all the elderly population.

Respite care can be offered for a night (so that caregivers can get some much needed sleep), for a day, weekends, or several weeks. In the latter case, the caregivers may take a vacation, may be ill themselves, or may require an extended respite from caregiving responsibilities for some other reason.

WIDOWHOOD

Modern science has made old age a woman's world. Over age 75, 68.2% of women are widows compared with 22.1% of men who are widowers. Since there are more women than men in the population, the actual number of women who are widows is even greater.

There are reasons for this disparity. Women usually marry older men. Men have 9 years less life expectancy than women; some diseases with no cure have a higher incidence among men, e.g., cancer of the lung and heart disease. Further, when women are widowed they tend to remain single because there are fewer men available to marry. In contrast, widowed older men tend to marry again; they have more choices.

Cummings and Henry (1960) state that widowhood is an honored state that society affords to women. Widowhood is not comparable to retirement, but the role change can be difficult because of loneliness and reduced income.

ADAPTATION TO WIDOWHOOD

Women seem better able to adapt to living alone than men. The tasks of daily domestic living, cooking, shopping, and cleaning, are activities that women do routinely whether they are alone or living with others. Most men have to learn or relearn these activities. On the other hand, adapting to living alone after years of living with someone and to the lower income that is common for widows is difficult. Some women have great difficulty accepting their husband's death and some may never adjust. Those people may need professional assistance.

If the widow was the primary caregiver for an ailing, dependent spouse, she may actually feel relieved to be free of this burden (Gaynor, 1990). The spouse's death may allow the woman to rejoin friends, travel, or participate in daily living with fewer constraints.

WIDOWS AND THEIR ADULT CHILDREN

Some widows become dependent on grown children and in-laws, expecting them to take over the duties of the husband. They expect children to include them in all activities. This situation may arise when the woman was dependent on her husband for social activities, household and car maintenance, and finances or if he maintained control over all aspects of their lives.

White widows and African-American widows have been found to tend to live alone. Hispanic and Asian widows live with others. White widows had the fewest children and lived in the smallest households, while Hispanic widows lived in the largest households (Pehlam and Clark, 1987).

SOCIAL LIFE FOR WIDOWS

The common stereotype that women are more sociable than men throughout their lives has not been supported in recent studies (Fiske and Chiriboga, 1990). Where the husband's friends were the couple's social friends, the widow finds it more difficult to continue in these groups once the husband dies. She becomes the unattached woman, pitied by others, perceived as a threat or someone for whom one must find a companion. These situations can make the widow uncomfortable in the group.

On the other hand, many women who live alone in their older years have a variety of acceptable social options. Since there are many widows, they form social groups. Women who worked outside the home develop a circle of friends from this group. Other women find support and social groups from church and volunteer activities.

WIDOWERS

Little is known about widowers. Adjustment to living alone after years of marriage may depend on how domestic the man was in marriage, whether he has hobbies to occupy his time, and how much and in what ways the couple relied on each other. Couples may have appeared to be independent and functioning adequately because they compensated for each other's deficits or there was a clear and comfortable division of labor. In this case the surviving spouse would be ill-prepared to assume the functions of the deceased. Together they made a whole. The loss of either partner would reveal a dependent person.

Older widowers often are treated with care by widows. They may, in fact, receive more attention than they want. Old men have many dancing and card playing partners. If they live in their own home, goodies and hot dishes are brought in by the widowed neighbors. Often these are friendly gestures, particularly if the neighbor knew the wife of the widower. It is natural to cook for someone and this task helps the lonely widow as well.

Some studies show that widowers have more problems than widows. They suffer more health problems, become more socially isolated, fail to maintain family ties, and are less likely to have a confidant (Bengston et al, 1990).

GRANDPARENTING

In the past the situation of grandparents was simple. Each grandchild had four or fewer grandparents. The grandchildren may not have known all of them because the grandparent may have died before the grandchild was born or the grandparents lived in another city or country and did not visit. The grandparent also could have been institutionalized and not visited by the grandchild. Today there are all kinds of grandparent–grandchild relationships as people live longer and lifestyles have changed. Four and five generation families are common. A child may have up to 50 years of contact with a grandparent. Divorce and remarriage, several times over, can mean that a grandparent will have generations of in-laws or step-grandchildren.

The role of grandparents has no fixed entry or exit points. It depends on the age, gender, race, and role of the parents. Grandparents serve as alternate role models for their grandchildren. They provide continuity with the past. Because they have a different set of responsibilities for the children from the parents, they have different relationships that

Styles of Grandparenting

STYLE	BEHAVIOR
Formal	Does not interfere with parents. Provides treats for children but no advice to parents
Fun seeker	Enjoys playing with grandchildren with mutual satisfaction for both
Surrogate	Provides care for the children when parents are working or unavailable for other reasons, e.g., social activities
Reservoir of family wisdom	Has special skills or memories that are shared with the children
Distant figure	Sees grandchildren only on special occasions, events, holidays, birthdays

Grandparents may engage in more than one style of grandparenting.
Adapted from Neugarten B, Weinstein K. The changing American grandparent. Journal of Marriage and Family 1964; 26:199.

often meet an important need in the grandchildren. Grandparents are a valuable resource in the family. The role of grandparent can give the older person an important source of affection, responsibility, and status in the family.

STYLES OF GRANDPARENTING

Neugarten and Weinstein (1964) identified five styles of grandparenting: formal, fun seeker, surrogate parent, reservoir of family wisdom, and distant figure. Formal grandparents tend to be older and do not interfere with the younger family. They provide treats for the grandchild but no advice to their children. The fun seeker enjoys playing with the grandchild, with mutual satisfaction to both. Surrogate grandparents take care of the child, usually when the parents work. Grandparents with special skills are the reservoir of family wisdom. The distant figure grandparent may only see the grandchild on special events, holidays, or birthdays.

GRANDPARENTS AS PARENTS

Grandparents of single parent children or chemically addicted children can find themselves assuming full parental responsibility for their grandchildren (Bengston et al, 1990). In the United States 3.2 million children live with

their grandparents, and this figure probably represents underreporting. Grandparental assumption of the role of parent seems to occur more frequently in African-American families: 4% of all white children and 12% of all African-American children now live with grandparents. Grandparents are also assuming responsibility for grandchildren with aquired immunodeficiency syndrome when the parent is unable or unwilling to accept this responsibility.

PARENT–CHILD ROLES

The roles between parents and their adult children eventually tend to reverse. This is particularly true if the parents become physically or mentally dependent. The changes usually are slow and subtle, as elderly people gradually move to more peripheral positions, e.g., in conversations, in decision making, and perhaps physical presense. The older person's ideas may still be valid, but somehow they do not seem to carry the same weight. The aging parents begin to be treated in "special" ways because of their age.

The most difficult time of transition may be when the aging parents actually begin to lose their capacity for making sound judgments about their safety and their capacity for self-care and independent living. Just as at one time these parents may have felt that "parents know what is best for their children," so now their children feel they know what is best for their parents. Sometimes the role reversal is allowed to take place, but at other times parents exert their independence and continue to make their own decisions. In any case, if the parents live long enough, some role alterations can be anticipated.

PATIENT ROLES

The patient role is certainly not new for many older persons. However, here too there are often subtle but noticeable changes with advanced age. One of the most difficult to tolerate is the increasing loss of credibility as historian and reporter of one's own subjective health experience. Often physicians or nurses do not take complaints seriously because they may think whatever the old person says is due to age or confusion.

The older patient is in a vulnerable position because chronic illness may not respond to medical therapies. This vulnerability makes the older person dependent on the decisions of the health care provider. There are risks of rejection and loss of care associated with noncompliance that strongly affect the older patient's relationship to the caregiver.

One of the characteristics attributed to the patient role is the obligation to give it up and return to a nonpatient status (Parson and Fox, 1953). Chronic illness in the aged provides little opportunity to give up the patient role; it is ongoing. Older patients need special skills, status, and assistance in negotiating with health care providers to compensate for the stereotypic low-power position to which they may be relegated. Health care providers need to be better informed about aging, take the patient seriously, and teach the skills the patient needs to maintain some control.

PRIMARY CAREGIVER AND CARE-RECIPIENT ROLES

Another set of roles often associated with the later years is that of primary caregiver and care recipient. These have a major effect on day-to-day living.

Spouses, male or female, tend to be expected to assume the primary caregiver role, even if there are some limitations in their own physical status. Wives often hold tenaciously to the role, even to the point where their own physical and emotional health is compromised

and the care deteriorates. Sisters and daughters (particularly single daughters) who live in the same area as their dependent, aging relatives tend to be expected by other family members and society to assume the primary caregiver role on a regular basis (Brody, 1985). These same people who designate the caregiver also tend to evaluate that person's performance in the role.

Until recently care usually had to be provided for parents and spouses, but the acquired immunodeficiency syndrome epidemic has placed many parents in the position of caring for their children once again, this time as adults.

Certainly, moving into primary caregiver and care recipient roles alters former marital, sibling, and child–parent roles. For the caregiver the associated physical and emotional burden of giving care, in addition to having to relate to family members, health care personnel, and representatives of bureaucracies, is a task that can tremendously alter daily living and may yield more or less satisfaction. For the care recipient who maintains awareness of what is happening, the role change and associated daily living may be both difficult and unsatisfying. Nurses can play a major role in helping both the givers and receivers of care to deal with the demands of daily living and find support and satisfactions (see the discussion of high-risk areas of acting as primary caregiver to the elderly in Chapter 13).

ROLE OF DECISION MAKER

For some who survive into the seventh, eighth, and ninth decades there comes a time when their role as decision maker over their own lives and property changes. Others (often adult children) begin to send signals that perhaps the older person is losing some ability to make appropriate decisions about life, environment, and resources. In the classic situation, the older person wishes to continue to live independently but others decide it is time to change to a more dependent lifestyle. Covert or overt cues regarding the older person's decision-making control can undermine self-esteem, self-worth, and confidence.

For those who continue to be mentally competent, relinquishing the role of decision maker is hard, even when its legitimacy may be realized (Pallett, 1990). Planning ahead intellectually for this time may remove the surprise; it may not reduce the discomfort. Perhaps the greatest threat is that any initial loosening of control over one's daily living portends a trajectory for diminishing control. Care providers should develop strategies that enable the older person to engage in informed decision making and to negotiate the future actively. In this way some of the personally destructive influences associated with feeling powerless may be minimized.

REPEOPLING ONE'S WORLD

Maintaining well-being in later years depends on contact with human beings and animals. Older persons who have no one to depend on and no one who depends on them experience more difficulty as they age. Patterns of isolation that are built over time do not change in old age; they create a reality that persists. Nurses need to be aware of past patterns when they contemplate interventions related to social support systems in older persons.

In one study of people over age 90, all had excellent social skills for repeopling their worlds. There are many resources for adding new people to one's life. These include senior citizen groups, churches and community organizations, pets, volunteer work, moving to a more populous area, sharing one's housing, joining a friendly phone group, and expanding one's correspondence.

MAINTAINING ONESELF IN THE FACE OF LOSSES

One of the tasks requiring adjustment in daily living is that of maintaining oneself in the face of losses. Many older survivors manage this well, others do not. There are many losses as one ages; few are predictable. As one ages there is a gradual slowing down in all aspects of living, which helps minimize the impact of the losses that occur. The individual can adjust to a gradual loss of physical functioning, such as decrease in sight, and not even realize it until the ophthalmologist tells them they are blind in one eye and only have sight in the other one, or following a cataract removal, when they realize how little they saw before. The same thing can occur with diminished cardiac function; the person adjusts to decreased energy levels and shortness of breath and denies there is a problem that needs medical attention.

Illness and incapacitation can make other losses harder to bear. Dependency increases the suffering at crucial times; the world may seem to have come to an end for that person.

Memory loss is normal with aging as described in Chapter 15. Even in middle age people have adopted ways of assisting with remembering; appointment books and lists are common in all age groups. As one ages it is necessary to develop more ways to help jog the memory or use compensatory mechanisms, such as always putting things in the same place.

Losses of spouse, sibling, child, and friends are to be expected, yet even after a lengthy illness death is still a shock to the survivor. If the quality of the relationship was positive, the loss is most severe. However, even the death of someone who seems incompatible can cause major problems. Arguing and fighting do not always mean what they seem. Just having another person available sets the pattern for activities and demands of daily living and may provide more support than appeared on the surface.

A change in residence for any reason is a loss. There is disagreement as to whether or not moves increase mortality (Borup, 1981). There is agreement that it is stressful to move, whether to a new living arrangement or a new area within an existing facility, whether planned or unplanned. People who have cognitive disorders don't do as well when moved than those not so impaired. In one study of first admission of patients over 65 to a psychiatric hospital, 26% died within 6 months (Lowenthal et al, 1967). Deaths also increased during the first few months of moving to a nursing home.

Many older people fear moving in with their children, and for some this is a valid concern. They must adjust to someone else's household where they may not be wanted. They have to give up freedom and control. But if alternative forms of housing are not possible and the older person is not ill, living with children is a logical option.

Giving up driving is hard, especially in a city or an area where there is no other form of transportation. Some people keep a car in the garage for years, even after they no longer have a driver's license, as a kind of tie to the past, a security blanket, a sign of their former independence and control of mobility. It takes stamina, experience, and patience to ride the bus; some people have none of the above when they can no longer drive. Learning to ride the bus is not easy when you are old.

Some of the older population experience loss differently because they have lived isolated lives. Many of these are professional women. They may also have small families or no relatives. They may have never joined clubs or had many friends or social interactions. When they move to a nursing home where sociability is a measure of adjustment, these people will have trouble because they don't participate. They may have protected themselves from losses by not getting close to others. It may be harder for nurses to deal with these old people because they cannot use the usual management techniques.

SEXUALITY, INTIMACY, AND AFFECTION

Manifestations of sexuality, intimacy, and affection may change with time or circumstances, but there is no reason that sexuality and intimacy cannot be important throughout a lifetime. Sexual interest and desire, like many other areas of life, can be important to some older people and boring to others. The attitude and activities can be dependent on: the quality of earlier sexual experiences and relationships; thoughts, values, and beliefs about sexuality; present health status; and presence or absence of a spouse or companion.

Nurses and physicians working with the elderly are frequently uncomfortable discussing sexual issues or fail to acknowledge that sexuality and intimacy are still needs in an older person's life. Health care professionals who provide care to the elderly should be aware of their own beliefs about the nature and place of sexuality in old age. Biases, stereotyping, and conflicting values or expectations can create difficulties for their patients.

It is agreed that sexual history should be a part of a general evaluation of the older person. Further follow-up may be indicated when the patient gives cues indicating some problem with sexuality; the pathophysiology or its treatment will generate fears of alteration of sexual capacity, e.g., hysterectomy, prostatectomy, chemotherapy. The pathophysiology or its treatment actually does diminish or eliminate sexual capacity, e.g., pelvic radiation, radical prostatectomy, chronic obstructive pulmonary disease, or congestive heart failure. Impotence can be a side effect of medications.

PHYSICAL CHANGES

Sexual change in old age involves both tissue and response changes. Response shows a gradual slowing (Bulter and Lewis, 1990). The increased time needed for sexual arousal and climax means that the man and woman are more likely to respond at the same time, a difference from younger years. Men may experience reduced preejaculatory fluid and reduced force in ejaculation. Women experience drying of vaginal membranes.

Men remain fertile as long as they live. Older men are concerned about their ability to maintain sexual potency and performance. While problems in these areas can occur at any age, among the elderly the factors that diminish sexual capability include fatigue, anxiety, alcohol consumption, and medications.

Older women can continue patterns of sexual functioning throughout their lives. Pleasure in sexual intercourse may depend on successful adaptations to maintain comfort with vaginal drying, decreased male lubricity, and increased fragility of mucosal membranes. Frequency of intercourse may depend on the availability of a partner.

ELDERLY HOMOSEXUALS

It is estimated that 10% of older adults are homosexual. Long-term relationships in gay couples are common, but little is known about these relationships because many have not been open about them. Professional sensitivity to the needs and difficulties of lesbian and gay couples should be the same as for any other couple.

MANIFESTATIONS OF AFFECTION

While the need for sexual intercourse may diminish among some elderly, the ongoing need for intimacy and affection do not. Among older adults when needs for intimacy (interpersonal relationships providing well-being) are met, both psychologic and physical well-being were found to be enhanced. Couples whose sexual performance is impaired may maintain their closeness and sexuality by increasingly communicating their affection for each other in speech and touching.

Failure to thrive because of lack of affection is a high-risk syndrome, among the elderly as well as infants. Older individuals who are aware of the risk can foster situations that satisfy their need for touch and positive human contact. Where the older person is in an institution, responsibility for prevention of failure to thrive syndrome rests in the hands of the health care providers who have become the resident's or patient's day-to-day family. The staff should provide affectionate, nonprocedural touch—hugging, patting, touching, and holding hands—and eye contact. They should show by the way they talk to their patients that they value and like them (Poznanski-Hutchinson and Bahr, 1991).

Experiencing affection and intimacy in day-to-day living is important to health and well-being. More is being learned about the high risk of deficits or deprivation in these dimensions of caring in the lives of the elderly. Nurses in all settings have major responsibilities to foster environments and interventions to promote well-being and prevent this deficiency syndrome.

PREPARATION FOR DEATH AND DYING

Death, like birth, is a natural component of living. Planning for dying requires an acceptance that death is indeed a part of life. A nurse who understands her legal responsibility to know about the patient's wishes about dying and who has a positive attitude about the person's right to make decisions about death can help the older person. To be of greatest assistance nurses should examine their own philosophy of death and life and should understand different cultural and religious beliefs about death and dying. They should be able to interpret state laws about patients' rights to participate in decisions about their lives.

ESTATE PLANNING AND FUNERAL ARRANGEMENTS

Preparing for death includes some concrete tasks and negotiations. Some of the tasks include making plans for transfer of one's possessions (estate planning and drawing up a will) and making arrangements for a funeral and disposal of one's remains (see Display 7–1). Those who accept death as a natural element of life and who prefer orderliness in transitions make these arrangements. Estate planning may

---

Documents Needed by Survivors to Care for an Estate

The following types of documents should be assembled and placed in a fire-resistant document box. A list of the documents and their location should be attached to one's estate planning material. The designated executors should be made aware of the location of materials needed to carry out their tasks.

_____ Automobile title

_____ Birth certificate

_____ Bank books, certificates of deposit, annuities, IRA/Keogh plans

_____ Citizenship papers

_____ Contractual agreements

_____ Deed to home and title insurance

_____ Discharge papers from the service

_____ Income tax reports and receipts

_____ Insurance policies—home/auto/life/other

_____ Marriage license/divorce decrees

_____ Mortgage

_____ Negotiable papers

_____ Promissory notes

_____ Social Security information

_____ Stocks and bonds

_____ Trust fund data

_____ Wills

_____ Other important information or papers

---

be as simple as taping the name of the desired recipient on the bottom of items or as complex as multiple visits to an attorney and establishing trusts.

Every person should have a will stating intentions about the disposition of property and giving directions about funeral services and disposition of the body. Because state laws vary about wills, legal assistance is advisable; drawing up a will can be quite inexpensive. It is necessary to keep the original in a safe place and to be sure that the executor is aware of its location. Because there are so many items, tasks, and records associated with this preparation, lists and packets have been made available to assist in planning and communicating one's last wishes.

ADVANCE DIRECTIVES ABOUT HEALTH CARE

In many states Living Wills may be drawn up to instruct family and physicians that one's life should not be artificially prolonged under circumstances of imminent death. All states provide some form of Durable Power of Attorney for Health Care to designate a surrogate decision maker to help ensure that wishes are carried out if one is unable to communicate. These documents can assist the older person toward autonomy in end-of-life decisions. Examples are given in Chapter 4.

Two recent studies of older persons' use of advance directive shows that, although a majority of people state that they would be willing to have life-sustaining treatment removed should they become incompetent, a very small percentage have signed Living Wills. Only a small percentage of those who have signed such documents have shared them with their physicians. Understanding of the use of these documents is limited, in both physicians and patients; often information is not readily available to patients through health care providers. Physicians, not sure about their responsibilities in relation to Living Wills, may nevertheless make life decisions without knowing whether the patient has signed a Living Will. Tramm (1990) and Henry (1991) indicate the important role nurses can play in learning a patient's wishes concerning health care decisions, educating patients, families, and colleagues about advance directives, and becoming advocates for the patient's autonomy in health care decision making.

Conclusion

Every stage of life carries certain very basic tasks. The later decades are no exception. The majority of older people manage these tasks effectively with minimal assistance. For some,

circumstances or preferences necessitate that nurses serve as a major resource in enabling them to engage in these tasks in positive, satisfying ways. Nurses' expertise and attitudes to growing old are important elements of their therapeutic interventions.

References and Other Readings

Bengston V, Rosenthal C, Burton L. Families and aging. In: Benstock R, George L, eds. Handbook of aging and the social sciences. 3rd ed. San Diego, CA: Academic Press, 1990:263.

Borup JH. Relocation, attitudes, information network and problems encountered. Gerontologist 1981; 5:501.

Brody E. Patient care as a normative family stress. Gerontologist 1985; 25:19.

Butler R, Lewis M. Merck manual of geriatrics. Merck Sharp & Dohme Research Laboratories, 1990:631.

Clinical report on aging. American Geriatric Society, 1988; 2:3.

Cummings E, Henry W. Growing old. New York: Basic Book, 1961:293.

Fiske M, Chiriboga D. Change and continuity in adult life. San Francisco, CA: Jossey-Bass, 1990: 342.

Gaynor SE. The long haul: the effects of home care on care givers. Image 1990; 22:208.

Henry JL. Autonomy in medical decision-making and use of advance directives by the elderly [Master Thesis]. Seattle, Washington: University of Washington, 1991.

King County Medical Society. Healthcare decisions about the end of life. Seattle, Washington, 1991:16.

Lowenthal M, Berkman P, et al. Aging and mental disorders in San Francisco. San Francisco, CA: Jossey-Bass, 1967:10.

McCoy JL. Overview of available data relating to board and care homes and residents. Washington, DC: US Department of Health and Human Services, 1983.

Nachison J. Who pays? The congregate housing question. Generations 1985; 9:34.

Neugarten B, Weinstein K. The changing American grandparent. Journal of Marriage and Family 1964; 26:199.

Pallett PJ. A conceptual framework for studying family care giver burden in Alzheimer's type dementia. Image 1990; 22:52.

Parson T, Fox R. Illness, theory and the modern urban American family. Journal of Social Issues 1953; 8:31.

Pelham AO, Clark WF. Widowhood among low income racial and ethnic groups in California. In:

Lopata H, ed. Widows. Durham, NC: Duke University Press, 1987:191.

Poznanski-Hutchinson C, Bahr RT. Types and meanings of caring behaviors among elderly nursing home residents. Image 1991; 23:85.

Pynos J. Options for mid-upper-income elders. Generations 1985; 9:31.

Thorslund M, Norstrom T, Kerstin W. The utilization of home help in Sweden. Gerontologist 1991; 31:116.

Tramm JM. Health care decision making and use of advance directives by the elderly [Masters Thesis]. Seattle, Washington: University of Washington, 1990.

Display 7-1 Putting my house in order. (With permission from People's Memorial Association, Inc., Seattle, WA 98102.)

PLEASE KEEP THIS PAGE

PUTTING MY HOUSE IN ORDER

Information for Family, Executor, and Friends (Personal Representative)
Please complete both sides

This is to notify my family, executor, and close friends of my wishes regarding the disposal of my remains and the following arrangements that have been made through

THE PEOPLES MEMORIAL ASSOCIATION, INC. OF SEATTLE, WASHINGTON

To fulfill my wishes and complete these arrangements when my death occurs, please notify

BLEITZ FUNERAL HOME
Seattle - (206) 282-5220

Do not hesitate to consult your religious leader or funeral director for guidance in completing this form, if you wish. Print the word or words necessary to complete the statements to express your wishes and provide the additional information requested.

Name _____ PMA number _____

It is my wish that my remains be _____ cremated, buried, entombed

It is my wish that the ashes be _____ scattered, buried, given to next of kin, executor (personal representative) or friend
(Funeral Director will be responsible for storage of ashes for 2 months only)

If burial preferred, cemetery arrangements _____ should be. have been _____ made. If already arranged,

fill in: _____   _____   _____   _____
       name of cemetery   city or place of cemetery   section   plot

I _____ want a service. If a service is held, prefer _____
   do, do not   *memorial or funeral

If a service is held, I would like it held in a _____ church, mortuary chapel, residence, (other place-please state)

If a church is preferred, give: _____   _____   _____   _____
                                name of church   address of church   city or place   postal code

I _____ want newspaper notices published.
   do, do not

I _____ prefer memorial gifts in lieu of flowers. If memorial gifts in lieu of flowers pre-
   do, do not
ferred, I would request that donations be sent to the following organization:

_____   _____   _____   _____
name of organization or charity   street address   city or place   postal code

I _____ wish to donate my eyes, at time of death, to the eye bank.
   do, do not

I _____ wish to donate such other organs, bone or tissue, at the time of death as may be
   do, do not
considered medically useful. This also authorizes donations of pace maker, if applicable.

I _____ wish to donate my body, at time of death, to closest Medical Teaching Facility.
   do, do not

_____   _____
name of next of kin, or executor, to indicate his/her knowledge   signature of member
and approval of plan.

_____   _____   _____
next of kin or executor's street address   city   date

*Memorial Service without the deceased present. - Funeral Service with deceased present.

PMA- 1989   OVER

Display 7-1 *(Continued)*

Keep this section with your personal papers for use by your survivors.

Location of my will _____

Location of Insurance Policies _____

Executor (personal representative) named _____

My Attorney is _____

I have Bank Accounts at: _____
       location _____ acct.#
       location _____ acct.#
       location _____ acct.#

Safety Deposit Box Numbers _____ Banks _____

Location of Safety Deposit Box Key _____

Real Estate Owned _____
_____
_____

Location of Deeds _____

I have the following stocks, bonds, contracts or other valuables at: _____
_____
_____

My social security number _____

Other information _____
_____
_____
_____

Signature _____

Address _____

My phone is _____

Date compiled _____
(change as revised)

8

Aging Changes in Structure and Function

MARSHA D. FRETWELL

Aging is a phenomenon that is experienced by all living organisms. Encompassing that period in the life span that follows growth and maturity and precedes death, it has presumably been a reality for individuals since the evolutionary beginnings of humans. Depending on the individual genetic endowments, there has always been a tremendous variation in the length and nature of the experience of aging in different individuals, families, and societies of the world, i.e., since recorded history, there have been individuals who have succeeded in extending the time after physical maturity by decades, thereby approaching the apparent biologic limit of 115 years of life for *Homo sapiens*. The most remarkable aspect of aging in the late twentieth century is the increase in the number of individuals who are successfully extending the years between maturity and death.

The art of providing excellent nursing or medical care for the older patients is best described as the "art of the possible." Each patient presents to the clinician with a complex mixture of influences that have been operating subtly over time: genetic endowment, environmental stresses, the normal changes of aging, and the pathophysiologic changes of disease. Critical to achieving an appropriate and optimal outcome for each patient is our ability to discern within this mixture of influences those

Parts of this chapter were taken from the Second Edition and written by Ralph Goldman, MD (deceased).

factors that are amenable to our therapeutic efforts. Aging has been described by Strehler (1977) as having four characteristics: it is universal, progressive, decremental, and intrinsic. Presumably, those changes or influences related to the normative process of aging may be impervious to our efforts. The assignment of any of our patient's problems to "old age," unless based in a clear understanding of the normal changes in structure and function that can be expected over the lifetime of an individual, represents therapeutic nihilism.

In this chapter, we first present a conceptual framework for understanding the biology of normal aging that is useful to clinical practice. We then review the major changes associated with aging in the structure and function of the cells, tissues, and organ systems of human beings.

The Biology of Aging

The hallmark of aging is a reduced ability to respond adaptively to environmental change. Thus, the changes of aging are not so much in the resting pulse or the fasting blood sugar, but in the ability to return these parameters to normal after a physiologic or psychological stress, such as running up three flights of stairs or giving a piano recital. This reduced ability to respond adaptively to environmental change can be demonstrated at all levels of biologic organization from the molecule to an organ system to

113

the entire organism. This reduced ability to respond to environmental changes represents the substrate within which age-associated disease can flourish. Alternatively, in very old individuals without chronic disease, this reduced ability to respond to environmental change or stress underlies their enhanced mortality from treatable disorders such as pneumonia or a fractured hip.

One approach to understanding the biology of aging is to define the tasks of the mature organism (after growth and reproduction) as *maintenance tasks.* Because many cells and body components are specialized for particular functions and cannot be replaced when they eventually lose function, the aging organism becomes increasingly less effective in the maintenance tasks and eventually meets the environmental challenge that is sufficient to cause death. Holliday (1988) supports this approach by pointing out that each of the theories of aging can be effectively restated as a mechanism involving the maintenance of the organism. For instance, the somatic mutation theory of aging proposes that mechanisms for the repair of DNA eventually break down or are overwhelmed by environmental insult (e.g., ionizing radiation), leading to inaccurate genetic templates and errors in the production of cellular proteins. Ultimately, the process of aging and dying may be best viewed as a failure of maintenance. The maximum lifespan for *Homo sapiens* is estimated at approximately 115 years. We can view that as an end against which our efforts at self-maintenance are balanced. Eventually, the adult organism is unable to cope with the accumulation of environmental damages and resultant defects in cells, tissues, and organ systems. Disease and death occur. Our tasks as clinicians and health professionals may be seen as assisting older individuals in their self-maintenance. This effort begins with health education and disease prevention. When disease does occur, understanding the complexity of factors underlying it will improve our ability to diagnose and treat it effectively.

CELLULAR CHANGES

There is a gradual loss of cells as a person ages. This has been documented by changes in organ weights and total cell counts and by determinations of changes in the amount of potassium, DNA, intracellular water, and nitrogen in the aged compared with the young organism. The somatic cells of the body can be characterized as those capable of reproduction (known as mitotic cells) and those, primarily nerve and muscle cells, incapable of reproduction (known as postmitotic cells). The postmitotic cells cannot survive forever because sooner or later damaging cellular events occur. These postmitotic cells appear to be one of the critical elements necessary for the evolution of complex organisms and, by their inability to indefinitely review and repair themselves, contribute to the inevitability of the aging of the entire organism. When lost, for whatever reason, postmitotic cells are not replaced and their number decreases with age. Those cells that remain show age-related changes. The most characteristic change is the accumulation of a pigment within the storage granules of the cytoplasm. There is also electron microscopic evidence of changes in the other cellular organelles such as distortion in structure and reduction in number of mitochondria and fragmentation of chromosomes. Hayflick (1965) has shown that contrary to the previous belief that mitotic cells are immortal, these cells have a finite capacity for reproduction and, thus, for replacement. Human embryonal cells in tissue culture are capable of approximately 50 divisions; the rate of replacement decreases as the cell line ages, and eventually the line dies. The number of residual generations is inversely related to the age of the individual supplying the cells. The same phenomenon is seen in all vertebrates studied, and the potential number of cell generations is directly correlated with the life span of the species.

The remaining cells, on histologic examination, tend to be larger and the structural pattern of the tissues is increasingly irregular. As a result, although the total number of cells may decrease 30% between youth and old age, the cellular mass decreases by a somewhat smaller amount. The decrease in metabolically active cells is paralleled by a decrease in intracellular water, although the extracellular water and plasma volume remain constant (Fig. 8–1). There is an increase in body fat with age that equals or exceeds the decrease in cell mass and may obscure this change in compositional distribution.

EXTRACELLULAR MATRICES

A fairly uniform series of age-related changes is found in the extracellular matrices of the connective tissue. Most important are changes occurring in collagen, which is a relatively inert

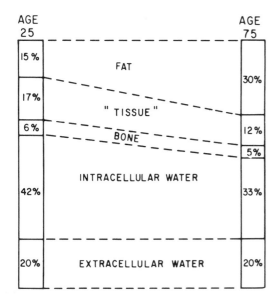

FIGURE 8-1 Distribution of major body components with age. (From Goldman R. Speculations on vascular changes with age. J Am Geriatr Soc 1970; 18:765; with permission.)

long-chain macromolecule produced by the fibroblasts. There is little evidence that, once formed, collagen fibers are either altered or reabsorbed. New fibers are produced that form bundles with the older fibers and cross-link chemically. The increased density of this widespread tissue component undoubtedly affects diffusion of nutrients and wastes and impairs function, as by reducing pulmonary compliance and vascular elasticity. It is this increase in collagen that affects the culinary tenderness of an old laying hen as compared with a fryer, mutton with lamb, and beef with veal. Elastin, another component of the connective tissue matrix, becomes fragmented and calcified with age, also reducing tissue elasticity. The matrix of cartilage becomes brittle, more easily disrupted, and, as a result, contributes to the progressive increase in arthritis. Changes in bone are significant, but cannot be so directly related to specific changes in the matrix. Bone changes are discussed in more detail later.

EXTRACELLULAR FLUID AND SOLUTES

Although the decrease in intracellular water reflects the changes in cell mass, there is no associated change in the extracellular water. In addition, there are few changes in the solute content of the extracellular fluid, and these

changes are so small as to be evident only on statistical analysis. There is a progressive decrease in the serum albumin and an increase in the globulin, with the total protein remaining relatively constant. The serum cholesterol increases slowly until about age 65; then it stabilizes or decreases slightly. In the frail or medically ill older patient, very low cholesterol levels may be seen. These are the result of the stress and malnutrition often associated with the treatment of an acute illness. The fasting blood glucose is unchanged, but the levels following a glucose challenge increase progressively and significantly with age. The other routine determinations show little age-related change.

PROBLEMS WITH RESEARCH ON AGING

There are many problems inherent in research on aging that must be recognized in evaluating the data. Figure 8-2 shows the reduction in total body water and oxygen consumption at rest with age. When body water is equated to cell mass, there is no change in relative oxygen consumption, implying that there is no alteration in the function of the tissues that remain. Further investigators are necessary to determine if the metabolic process has been altered and, especially, if the functional reserve has been impaired.

Another problem with research on aging is shown in Figures 8-3A and B. Figure 8-3A shows a decrease in the resting cardiac output

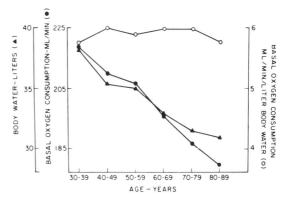

FIGURE 8-2 Relationship of age to total body water (antipyrine space), basal oxygen consumption, and basal oxygen consumption per unit of body water. Drawn from data presented by Shock and colleagues, 1963. (From Gregerman RL. In Gitman L (ed). Endocrines and aging. Springfield, IL: Charles C. Thomas, 1967; with permission.)

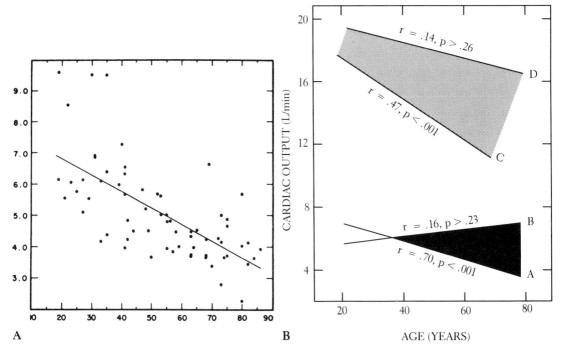

FIGURE 8–3 A, The relationship between resting cardiac output and age in 67 men without circulatory disorders. The line represents the linear regression on age. (From Brandfronbrener M, Landowne M, Shock NW. Changes in cardiac output with age. Circulation 1955; 12:557. Reprinted with permission.) B, Cardiac output measured at rest and during exercise at exhaustion in the upright position versus age. (From Schneider EL, Rowe JW, eds., Heart and circulation. In: Handbook of biology of aging, 3rd ed. Orlando, FL: Academic, 1990.) (Line A [least squares linear regression] from Brandfronbrener, 1955; lines B and D from Rodeheffer et al, 1984; line C from Julius et al, 1967.)

with age. Figure 8–3B incorporates the data from graph A into line A, which, with data from other studies, shows cardiac output measured at rest and during exercise at exhaustion in the upright position versus age. Line B, in contrast to line A, shows no reduction or even an increase in cardiac output with age. The variation in the results of this research likely stems from heterogeneity of selection criteria among the various studies. Line B data (least square linear regression) are from a study that carefully removes those subjects with occult coronary disease from their pool of subjects for the study of normal aging.

When comparing subjects of different ages (the cross-sectional approach), there are two other potential sources of confusion: the various cohorts have had different exposures and the survivors represent a selected group. Without longitudinal studies it is not possible to determine if the change was protective, or if the more severely affected persons had a higher mortality, thus hiding an even greater average trend.

Body Systems

CARDIOVASCULAR SYSTEM

At least 40% of all individuals over the age of 65 die of cardiac disease, 15% of cerebrovascular disease, and possibly another 5% secondary to other types of vascular impairment. Because well over one half of all deaths are due to defects of the cardiovascular system, it is important to identify those changes that are age-related as opposed to those that are pathologic in origin. However, because, as will be seen later, the frequency of cardiovascular complications can be mathematically related to age, a number of gerontologists now question whether all cardiovascular "disease" that follows this pattern may not, in fact, be a manifestation of differential rates of aging. Other specialists in the changes in cardiovascular function with age point out how powerful the influence of differing life-styles (diet, exercise, smoking, and coping styles) is on the lifetime incidence of cardiovascular disease and suggest that these variables have not yet been adequately controlled for in the studies. Thus, as we review the changes in cardiovascular structure and function, both disease and life-style, as well as aging, must be considered as etiologic factors.

HEART

Size   The concept that cardiac enlargement with age must indicate an underlying pathologic process has clouded the determination of actual aging change. It is now the consensus that there is myocardial hypertrophy with age per se. This amounts to an 8% to 15% increase in 24-month-old as compared to 12-month-old rats. In humans the left ventricular wall may be 25% thicker at age 80 than at age 30 years.

Areas of fibrosis are present and the overall collagen content is increased according to most, but not all, studies. In rats, there may be subendocardial and subepicardial concentrations of connective tissue, perhaps corresponding to subendocardial localization in humans. The heart valves become thicker and stiffer with age. Since myocardial cells are postmitotic, replacement of lost fibers, as well as the increase in total muscle mass, is accomplished by hypertrophy of the residual bundles. In rats there is sclerosis of the coronary arteries, manifest by fibrosis of the media, thickening of the wall, and elastocalcinosis, but there is no narrowing of the lumina or artherosclerotic changes. In senile rats there is a reduction in the capillary to muscle fiber ratio and a decreased capillary density; however, this can be increased by exercise.

Cells   The previously noted increase in volume of lipofuscin pigment may be appreciable, but its effect on cardiodynamics is unknown. On electron microscopic studies old hearts contained autophagic vacuoles, rarely seen in the myocardium of young animals, and some observers have noted changes in the myofibers and the mitochondria.

Heart Rate   The resting heart rate in humans essentially is unchanged with age. The magnitude of sinus arrhythmia decreases, apparently due to muscular rather than autonomic neural change. Variation in sinus rate with respiration is diminished as is the spontaneous variation in heart rate monitored over a 24-hour period in stress or any coronary artery disease.

Cardiac Output at Rest   The net result of the age-associated changes in heart architecture and contractile properties permit the aged heart to function normally at rest, in spite of changes in aortic distensibility. Arterial stiffening in the aorta (reflected in the age-associated increase in systolic blood pressure) increases the afterload (resistance to outflow) to left-ventricular ejection, but in healthy individuals, this is compensated for by the age-associated left-ventricular hypertrophy. With the extra contractile force, the aging left ventricle succeeds in ejecting a fraction of end-diastolic volume that is similar in younger individuals.

Coronary Blood Flow   There are no data in normal humans regarding the effect of age on coronary blood flow. Studies of coronary flow in a group of rats showed that the maximal flow was decreased by an amount proportional to the degree of myocardial hypertrophy. Maximal oxygen extraction (86%) was identical in both young and old. Studies on oxidative phosphorylation are inconclusive. There is no evidence that the observed anatomic and physiologic changes can be attributed to a reduction in vascular perfusion.

Electrocardiographic Changes   The normal electrocardiograph shows little change with age. There are small, inconspicuous but statistically significant increases in the PR, QRS, and QT intervals. There is also a decrease in the amplitude of the QRS complex, and, probably as a result of the noted left-ventricular thickening, a left shift in the QRS axis. Since pathologic changes in the heart accumulate with age, comparable changes are increasingly seen in the electrocardiograph, but these should not be considered normal manifestations of aging.

Cardiac Response to Stress   Three factors are involved in the cardiac response to stress: an increase in the heart rate, an increase in myocardial contractibility, and the Frank-Starling mechanism (an increase in myofibrillar length with increased efficiency and increased ventricular volume). The cardiac response of an older person to stress is most similar to that of younger subjects who are exercising in the presence of beta-adrenergic blockade. Beta-adrenergic stimulation that occurs under stress modulates the heart rate, arterial tone, and myocardial contractility. In older individuals, the effect of bolus infusion of beta-adrenergic agonists to increase heart rate diminishes with advancing age. Both arterial and venous dilitation responses to beta-adrenergic stimulation (to reduce afterload under stress) declines with age. Finally, while there is little support for a reduction of intrinsic contractile reserve of cardiac muscle in aging, the beta-adrenergic modulation of the mechanisms that govern the effectiveness of myocardial excitation-contraction coupling decreases in advanced age. Recent evidence indicates a decrease in the number of catecholamine receptors on the myofibers, which may have some relationship to the reduced rate response. Further, with age, the refractory interval between stimuli-causing mechanical response increases, although there is no increase in the electrical refractory interval.

A number of studies have suggested that with age both the isometric contraction and relaxation times are prolonged. Recent studies indicate that contraction depends on the release of calcium from the sarcoplasmic reticulum to act on the contractile proteins, and relaxation requires that the calcium be removed from these proteins and taken up again by the sarcoplasmic reticulum. The release of calcium is slowed in age, as a result not of inadequate catecholamine concentration but of apparent lack of response, perhaps due to the reduced number of receptors. The uptake of calcium during diastole is slowed by an age-related deficiency in the sarcoplasmic reticulum. Under these conditions a prolonged refractory period, and some limitation in cardiac rate, is understandable.

Studies of rat trabecula carnea, paced at 24 beats per minute in vitro in an isometric system, showed *no significant age-related difference in active tension or maximum rate of tension development*. Because there was no age difference in the active tension curves at all lengths up to that at which contraction tension was maximal, the Frank-Starling mechanism seems to be intact. There is evidence that there is less compliance, or relaxation of tension, with age. This stiffness may result from increased connective tissue or from changes in the myocardium itself; obviously it decreases myocardial efficiency.

In summary, although older individuals have a diminished heart rate response to exhaustive exercise, some older subjects are able to use the Frank-Starling mechanism to increase stroke volume in compensation for the heart rate deficit. Thus, the hearts of these elderly subjects are able to preserve cardiac output during exercise in the presence of a reduced heart rate.

Physical Work Capacity and Oxygen Uptake A standardized measure of the limit of performance capacity is the maximal oxygen consumption (VO_2 max). Under stress, this can increase to greater than ninefold over the basal level. While the maximal oxygen consumption rate is limited in individuals of greater age, it is not clear exactly what mechanisms are most influential: changes in central circulatory function versus some peripheral factor such as the changes in muscle mass. In fact, the extent of the decline in the maximal work capacity, VO_2 max, and maximal cardiac output with increasing age varies significantly with life-style factors such as physical conditioning and the presence of occult or clinical cardiovascular disease.

BLOOD VESSELS

Elastin gives the arteries their resiliency, a property that diminishes with aging, independent of atherosclerotic processes. The elastic fibers progressively straighten, fray, split, and fragment. These changes are associated with increasing deposition of calcium, which has been termed *elastocalcinosis*. Both the media of the elastic arteries and the elastic lamina of the muscular arteries are involved in this process. At the same time, the increasing absolute amount of collagen in the vessels and the cross-linkage of collagen fibers into bundles of larger and larger size further compromises the vascular distensibility. In young arteries half the collagen is at maximum length with a 60% stretch, whereas in old arteries only a 30% stretch is possible. The increased volume of the aorta compensates in part for this lack of elasticity. However, the intra-aortic systolic pressure increases more abruptly as an increasing amount of blood is forced into the vessel during increased activity.

Pulse–Wave Velocity The pulse-wave velocity reflects the decreasing elasticity of the blood vessels. The aortic pulse-wave velocity increases from 4.1 m/s at age 5 years to 10.5 m/s at age 65 years. The radial pulse-wave velocity is greater than the aortic pulse-wave velocity until age 65; thereafter the order is reversed. This change in velocity is independent of atherosclerosis, but Simonson and Nakagawa (1960) showed that pulse-wave velocity changes in patients with coronary artery disease were greater than were to be expected by age alone. This accelerated change could be due to the complicating effects of atherosclerosis or it could indicate that acceleration of the normal vascular changes predisposed to atherosclerosis. The aortic pulse pressure increases from the arch to the bifurcation in children but remains unchanged in old age. O'Rourke and his associates (1968) estimate that in youth 8% of the heart energy is lost in pulsatile work and that this increases to 17% in the aged because of the diminished elasticity.

There is reduced blood flow to the various organs with age, but this reduction is not symmetric. Flow to the brain and the coronary vessels is reduced proportionately less than is the total cardiac output, but flow to most other tissues (particularly the kidneys) is reduced more. The status of the splanchnic blood flow is uncertain, with values showing both a lesser and a greater than average reduction (Table 8–1).

The altered distribution of blood flow, as well as the increased peripheral resistance with age, could derive from either anatomic or physiologic causes. Anatomic changes that disproportionately reduce flow through a tissue

increase peripheral resistance. The usual mechanism, which regulates local blood flow and controls peripheral resistance, is variation in arteriolar tone.

Studies of age-related changes in adrenergic responsiveness of the vascular smooth muscle have produced interesting results. As discussed previously, there is a decline in the beta-adrenergic responsiveness of the vascular smooth muscle with age, with a consequent decrease in the relaxation of vascular smooth muscle. On the other hand, the responsiveness of the vascular smooth muscle is not greatly changed with age. Abrass (1986) has suggested that the increase in peripheral resistance in older persons may be due to the persistence of alpha-adrenergic vasoconstriction in the face of diminished beta-adrenergic vasodilatation.

It is not unexpected that with increasing vascular rigidity the systolic blood pressure increases with age. When a pressure pulse is applied to a rigid instead of an elastic tube in experimental systems the diastolic pressure decreases proportionately and the mean pressure is unchanged. However, the diastolic pressure actually increases slightly. This is compatible with the observed increase in peripheral resistance and is necessary to maintain the blood pressure despite the reduced cardiac output.

There are significant changes in the capillary walls. The capillary endothelial cells lie on a layer of collagen-like material, the basement membrane, which separates these cells from those of the tissues. The basement membrane gradually thickens from about 700 nm in youth to 1100 nm in old age. There are no direct physiologic data to correlate with this change, but it is not unreasonable to suspect that there is resultant slowing in the exchange of nutrients and waste products across the capillary wall.

TABLE 8–1 *Age Changes in Regional Perfusion*

	Bender[*]	Landowne and Stanley[†]
Cardiac output	−0.75	−1.01
Cerebral flow	−0.35	−0.5
Coronary flow	−0.5	
Visceral flow (liver)	−1.1	−0.3 (−0.36)[‡]
Renal flow	−1.1	−1.9
Remainder (by difference)		−1.3

Columns under heading: Approximate Average Rate of Change (% per year)

[*]Bender AD. The effect of increasing age on the distribution of peripheral blood flow in man. J Am Geriatr Soc 1965;131:192.
[†]Landowne M, Stanley J. Aging of the cardiovascular system. In: Shock NW, ed: Aging—some social and biological aspects. Washington DC: American Association for the Advancement of Science, 1960.
[‡]Flood C, et al. The metabolism and secretion of aldosterone in elderly subjects.

URINARY SYSTEM

KIDNEY STRUCTURE

Each human kidney contains approximately 1 million nephrons at birth. These increase in size, but not in number, until maturity. A few nephrons normally are lost during maturation, but then the loss accelerates, so that between ages 25 and 85 the number decreases by 30% to 40%. Recent microdissection studies show that the obsolescence starts as a sclerosis or scarring of the glomeruli, followed by atrophy of the afferent arterioles. These studies demonstrate that this process is not primary to the large vessels. In fact, the glomeruli in the deep cortex near the medulla (the juxtamedullary glomeruli) retain one capillary, which enlarges as the remainder of the glomerulus atrophies and becomes a shunt between the afferent and efferent arterioles. These become the vasa recta, supplying the renal medullae. The atrophic nephrons are not replaced. The compensation that occurs results from enlargement of the residual nephrons. Despite this, the net weight of the kidney decreases about 30% from maturity to old age.

KIDNEY FUNCTION

Because the number of functional units in the kidney is reduced with age, it is not unexpected that function also declines. Shock and his associates showed that the glomerular filtration rate (GFR) decreased 46% from age 20 to age 90 (Rowe, 1976). At the same time the renal plasma flow decreased 53%. The ratio between

the filtration rate and the plasma flow, the filtration fraction, increased as a result. In Figures 8–4 and 8–5 Wesson (1969) has collected the results of a number of different studies, showing the decreases in the GFR and the renal plasma flow. Calculation of the filtration fraction from these data indicate that the increase may not occur until the sixth or seventh decades (Table 8–2). The data show that some quite old persons may have better function than others considerably younger. In a recent longitudinal study of a large number of subjects, the individual trends paralleled those of the group; persons with extreme values had been at the extreme at earlier ages as well.

The fractional extraction of low concentrations of para-aminohippuric acid show no age-related decrease. The concentration of para-aminohippuric acid is determined simultaneously in the renal arterial and venous blood and the fractional removal is calculated. The average ratios were 91.8% and 91.1% in youth and old age, respectively. Thus, the ratio of the

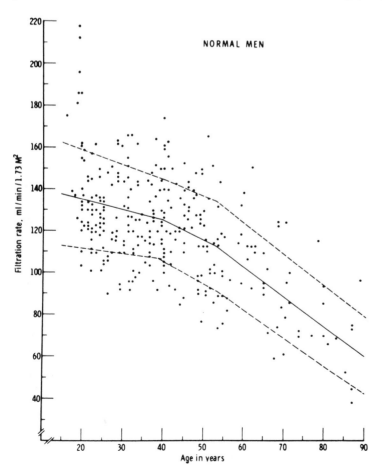

FIGURE 8–4 Age changes in glomerular filtration rate (Cin) of normal men (mean and one standard deviation). (From Wesson LG. Physiology of the human kidney. New York: Grune & Stratton, 1969; with permission.)

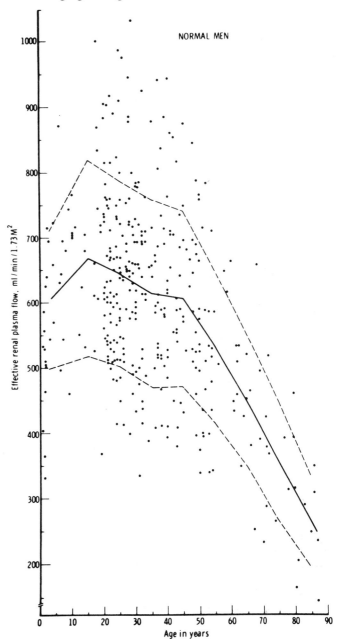

NORMAL MEN

FIGURE 8-5 Age changes in effective renal plasma flow (PAH or diodrast) of normal men (mean and one standard deviation). (From Wesson LG. Physiology of the human kidney. New York: Grune & Stratton, 1969; with permission.)

blood supply to the nephrons and to the parenchymal tissue remains constant despite the reduction in tissue supplied.

The reduced renal tubular cell mass is reflected by reduced maximal tubular functions. The reabsorption of glucose from the filtrate (Tm_G) is decreased 43.5% and the maximum secretion of Diodrast (iodopyracet) (Tm_D) decreased 47.6% and that of para-aminohippurate (Tm_{PAH}) by a similar amount, values that closely parallel the filtration rate. Thus, the reduction reflects a reduced number, not a reduced function, of the individual cells. The ability to concentrate the urine declines moderately. The usual value for maximum specific gravity in youth is 1.032, which decreases to 1.024 at age 80. A similar decline in maximum osmolality is noted from 1040 to 750 mOs/L between ages 20 and 80 years. Studies of urinary dilution reveal a decreasing C_{H_2O}, but when the C_{H_2O} is di-

TABLE 8–2   ***Average Values for GFR, Renal Plasma Flow, and Filtration Fraction by Age and Sex***[*]

	Women			Men		
Age	GFR	RPF	FF	GFR	RPF	FF
15	123	655	0.188	138	665	0.208
25	119	585	0.203	132	650	0.203
35	117	575	0.203	128	615	0.208
45	112	570	0.196	121	610	0.198
55	105	480	0.219	110	530	0.208
65	94	425	0.221	96	445	0.216
75	84	300	0.280	80	350	0.229
85				66	250	0.264

[*]The individual GFR and RPF values are derived from Figures 8–4 and 8–5 and are approximations. The filtration fractions are computed from these data.

vided by the residual GFR, the value is constant, again reflecting a reduced cell mass. The administration of acid load produces a comparable reduction in the serum bicarbonate and urinary pH at all ages. The rate at which the acid load is excreted is proportional to the residual GFR. There is a slight relative decrease in ammonia production, with a proportionate increase in the titratable acidity. The response to base loads is also delayed and prolonged.

CLINICAL IMPLICATIONS

There is concern about the possible effects of the age-related reduction in renal function, especially in relation to drugs primarily dependent on renal excretion. However, *50% residual function is quite adequate*, when it is realized that renal patients can be managed with functions as low as 5% and 10% of normal. It is important to realize that less creatinine is produced because of the reduced muscle mass and, as a result, the serum creatinine does not increase in proportion to the decrease in renal function. Therefore, when dosage is critical, *a creatinine clearance, not the serum creatinine alone, should be the criterion for renal function.*

Because of the time and logistical difficulties in collecting complete 24-hour urine specimens

to calculate creatinine clearance, several authors have developed formulas or normograms to predict creatinine clearance from steady-state serum creatinine concentration. The most widely used is that of Cockcroft and Gault (1976):

$$\frac{\text{Creatinine}}{\text{clearance}} = \frac{(140 - \text{age in years})\,(\text{weight in kg})}{72 \times (\text{serum creatinine in mg/dL})}$$

RESPIRATORY SYSTEM

STRUCTURE

With age, the respiratory or lung function changes in two specific ways. First, the ability to generate a forced expiratory flow rate peaks between the ages of 20 and 25 years and then declines by about 25 cc/yr. Until the age of 40, this attrition is thought to be secondary to changes in body weight and strength rather than loss of tissue. Second, there is an increase in the residual volume of air left in the lungs after a maximal exhalation. This residual volume is determined by a balance between the inward elastic tissue forces of the lung tissue and the outward forces of the ribs and muscles of respiration. The anteroposterior diameter of the chest increases with age. There may be progressive kyphosis, complicated by osteoporosis and vertebral collapse, calcification of costal cartilages, reduced mobility of ribs, and partial contraction of inspiratory muscles. These factors reduce the compliance of the chest wall and the force of the expiratory muscles.

The aging lung becomes increasingly rigid and less likely to collapse when the chest cavity is opened. The inward elastic recoil of the lung results from the combination of elastic fibers, which help to keep the airways open under conditions of low lung volumes, and the surfactant, which works at the air–fluid interface. There is no evidence for a change in the length or diameter of these fibers with aging, but there does appear to be an age-associated disruption in their attachment to the walls of the alveoli and the small airways. There is no evidence for a change in the effectiveness of the surfactant system.

FUNCTION

The elevation of the ribs and flattening of the diaphragm result in a 50% increase in the functional residual capacity between the third and the ninth decades, and the residual volume increases 100%. As a result there is a partial inflation of the lungs at rest when compared with younger ages. Nevertheless, there is no significant change in total lung capacity. The dead space ventilation increases and approximately balances the decrease in oxygen requirement. As a result the resting tidal volume remains constant (Fig. 8–6). These changes are not sufficient to produce subjective or objective manifestations at rest or to predict the ability to cope with stress.

There is a nearly linear decrease in the maximal breathing capacity between the third and ninth decades. This test is difficult to perform and is affected by poor motivation. The forced expiratory volume correlates well and is a satisfactory substitute. Both tests depend on the ability to move air out of the lungs and on such factors as airway resistance, the compliance of the lung itself, and the characteristics of the thoracic cage, including rigidity, loss of muscular strength, and velocity of contraction. A simple but useful test is the ability to blow out a bookmatch at 6 inches with the mouth wide open. Failure indicates advanced functional impairment requiring further evaluation (Fig. 8–7).

Blood Gases There is no change in the arterial pressure of carbon dioxide between the ages of 20 and 80, but there is a 10% to 15% decrease in the pressure of oxygen. The oxygen saturation decreases about 5%. In the past, the decrease in arterial oxygen pressure has been attributed to a decrease in pulmonary diffusing capacity. This would be compatible with the observed thickening of the basement membranes. Recently, it has been proposed that if there were ventilation–perfusion mismatching, unventilated capillaries would not be exposed to oxygen. The higher diffusibility of carbon dioxide would maintain its pressure constancy. In the low-pressure pulmonary system, gravity might cause dependent, basilar localization of blood flow. The basal portion of the lung is the best ventilated in the young, and there is correspondence between ventilation and perfusion. Later, the increasing lung rigidity improves apical ventilation, there is relative basal alveolar collapse, and ventilation–perfusion mismatching results. The constancy of the partial pressure of carbon dioxide suggests that alveolar ventilation is adequate. The extent to which the decreased arterial oxygen pressure is due to reduced diffusing capacity, to ventilation–perfusion mismatching, and to increased dead space will undoubtedly be resolved.

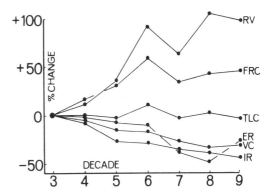

FIGURE 8–6 Percentage changes in static lung volumes in normal subjects at various ages compared with values found in the third decade of life. RV, residual volume; FRC, functional residual capacity; TLC, total lung capacity; ER, expiratory reserve; VC, vital capacity; IR, inspiratory reserve. (From Mithoefer JC, Karetzky MS. In: Powers JD (ed.): Surgery of the aged and debilitated patient. Philadelphia: WB Saunders, 1968; with permission.)

OXYGEN USE

The maximal amount of oxygen used under stress is reduced 50% by age 80. Alveolar ventilation is adequate, because the partial pressure of carbon dioxide does not increase. However, the arteriovenous oxygen difference does not increase to the expected degree. Because this indicates underutilization of oxygen already in the circulation, it cannot be due to failure at the pulmonary level. Possible causes include failure of perfusion, delayed oxygen diffusion,

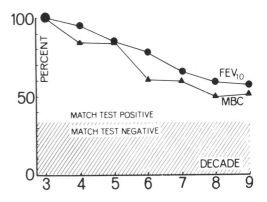

FIGURE 8–7 Percentage change in maximal breathing capacity (MBC) and forced expiratory volume (FEV) with age in normal subjects. (From Mithoefer JC, Karetzky MS. In: Powers JD (ed.): Surgery of the aged and debilitated patient. Philadelphia: WB Saunders, 1968; with permission.)

and impaired oxygen utilization of the stressed tissues.

Emphysema has much in common with the aging lung. The maximum breathing capacity and forced expiratory volume are decreased in both, the residual volume and the functional residual capacity are increased, the lungs are rigid and distended on autopsy, and the microscopic changes may be similar. However, the normal aged individual does not have the elevations in blood carbon dioxide and bicarbonate that are found in emphysema as a result of the functional obstruction.

CLINICAL IMPLICATIONS

The increased rigidity of the thoracic wall and the decreased strength of the expiratory muscles decrease the propulsive effectiveness of a cough, an extremely important clinical consideration. The reduced cough efficiency, decreased ciliary activity in the bronchial lining, and the increased dead space all enhance the potential for mechanical and infectious respiratory complications of surgery and enforced bed rest in the aged person. Because of their potential severity, it is necessary to anticipate and prevent these complications whenever possible.

GASTROINTESTINAL SYSTEM

STRUCTURE

Despite a wide variety of functional changes described or implied, description of anatomic change in the gastrointestinal tract is limited. In studies of morphologic changes with age in the musculature of the esophagus, age-associated decrease in the numbers of slow-acting type 1 muscle fibers were noted in both the pharyngeal constrictor muscle (skeletal muscle under voluntary control) and in the skeletal and smooth muscle of the esophagus. In general, there is a decrease in the density or numbers of fibers and a trend toward hypertrophy of remaining individual fibers. One study also noted a decrease in the number of myenteric ganglion cells, along with thickening of the smooth muscle layer. It is important to note that these purported changes are based on cross-sectional studies comparing different individuals, and there was no clear reference to controlling for underlying disorders.

Age-associated gastric mucosa atrophy has been reported by several studies. It is usually at-tributed to accelerated cell death or a slowing of the renewal process of gastric mucosal cells and is thought to underlie the achlorhydria observed with aging. Several studies dispute that there is a relationship between age and the degree of atrophy, and one study reports near normal histology in up to one third of patients with achlorhydria over 80 years. As in other structural changes thought to be secondary to aging alone, the discovery of increasing antibodies to *Campylobacter pyloris* with age complicates our interpretation of the gastric mucosa changes with age.

Although it is believed there is atrophy of the small intestine, there is no documentation. What little information is available suggests a drop-off in the number of neurons along with an increase in thickness and cross-sectional area of the muscle coat with age. Small bowel radiographic studies are reported to show a coarser outline. One study showed no variation in the average villus height and height of the individual entrocyte between 10 young and 10 old individuals. There may be a reduction in mucosal surface area. On the other hand, one postmortem study of jejunum specimens found the villus height to be shorter in older individuals.

Both arterial and venous varicosities are not uncommon and may represent unrecognized sites of bleeding. The number of Peyer's patches, and the number of follicles within them, decreases.

In the vermiform appendix there is fibrous atrophy of what was originally a large amount of lymphoid tissue, and the lumen becomes progressively obliterated from tip to base. In contrast to the unatrophied condition of small intestinal smooth muscle, atrophy of the muscularis externa develops in the colon. Additionally, there is an increase in the connective tissue component, some mucosal atrophy, abnormalities of the mucosal glands, cellular infiltration of the mucosa and lamina propria, and hypertrophy of the muscularis mucosa.

Diverticulosis of the sigmoid colon becomes common, and it is present in at least one third of all individuals over age 60 and perhaps two thirds of people over age 80. In diverticulosis, there is an increase in the number of elastin fibers in the taeniae coli, with an increase in the thickness of taenia and circular smooth muscle. These structural changes may lead to a shortening of the colon and higher intraluminal pressures.

MOTILITY

In studies that exclude older individuals with diabetes or neuropathy, there is a normal frequency of peristaltic contractions and lower esophageal sphincter relaxation occurring after a swallow. While the number of spontaneous contractions did not differ between the two groups, there was an age-related reduction in the amplitude of esophageal contractions in a subgroup of 80-year-old subjects. This implies that in the very old, there may be a weakening in smooth muscle contraction, but not in the neural system innervating the muscles.

Few reports of age-related changes in gastric and small intestinal motility were found, and studies in large bowel motility appear to be limited, despite the general assumption that constipation in the aged is due to decreased colonic peristalsis and possibly to decreased abdominal muscle tone.

Fecal incontinence increases in frequency with age and may occur in 20% of hospitalized geriatric patients. Brocklehurst (1951) found that one third of these patients had organic neurologic changes and another third were confused without neurologic signs. Rectal awareness of balloon distention was diminished in many of the incontinent patients, despite the increased frequency of evacuation. The sphincter appeared to have decreased tone by digital examination and the stool was frequently semiliquid.

Manometric examinations of the reflex responses of the internal and external sphincters have been performed. The internal sphincter is strongly contracted in the normal state and the external sphincter much less so. Older, incontinent persons had normal internal sphincter reflexes, but the external sphincter reflexes were absent and were thought to be the major factor in incontinence. Normally, the two sphincters function complementarily, which, for example, allows for the passage of gas without the loss of stool. This competence obviously fails when incontinence appears.

SECRETION

Recent studies have revealed that in healthy older adults there is no reduction in the volume of saliva produced. Unstimulated and stimulated parotid fluid outputs among nonmedicated healthy adults of different ages are not different.

Gastric Acid The secretion of both free and total gastric acid decreases with age. Since this is most marked in association with atrophic gastritis, and the incidence of atrophic gastritis increases with age, this type of gastritis could be either an aging or a pathologic process. Gastric atrophy also results in a decrease in the production of intrinsic factor; however, this is rarely sufficiently complete to cause pernicious anemia. The gastric secretion drops markedly between ages 40 and 60 to about one fifth of earlier values; then it becomes stable.

Pancreatic Enzymes Pancreatic amylase in fasting duodenal juice is decreased, but normal amounts are available after stimulation. Since older persons often rely on high carbohydrate diets, it is important to note that the pancreatic amylase, even in the absence of salivary amylase, seems adequate for carbohydrate digestion. The amount of pancreatic trypsin is also reduced, but the lipase appears to be relatively stable. Thus, the older person should, in most instances, be capable of digesting a normal dietary intake. However, the reported studies are by no means consistent, and further studies are necessary. Also, there is little clinical evidence that the stool contains significant amounts of undigested nutrients, although further studies are warranted.

ABSORPTION

Absorption is the most critical function of the gastrointestinal tract. A number of established and possible age-related factors could influence this function, such as the rate and degree of digestion, the integrity of the absorbing surface, the efficiency of the transport mechanisms, gastrointestinal motility, and alterations in vascular perfusion.

There is little information on *protein* absorption, although selective defects in amino acid absorption have been suggested. Glucose is absorbed by an active transport mechanism. *Glucose* absorption studies have been difficult to interpret because of changing glucose–insulin relationships. Determinations of the rate of decrease of residual glucose in the rat intestine indicate a slower rate of absorption. This is supported by an apparent delay in the absorption of 3-methyl glucose and galactose. Xylose, which is absorbed by passive transport, also exhibits imparied absorption, although possibly not until very late in life. Two studies that showed that fat absorption was delayed, also showed that absorption could be accelerated by adding lipase to the fat meal, thus suggesting that the decreased rate is due to deficient lipase secretion. Persistently elevated chylomicron counts may be due to inactivity rather than age. Radioactive fat tolerance tests found no significant difference in fat absorption between healthy young and old subjects.

Calcium absorption occurs in the proximal small intestine and may correlate with the secretion of gastric acid. There is agreement that *calcium absorption becomes impaired as a result of decreased active transport.* Iron is also absorbed in the proximal portion of the small intestine and also depends on gastric acid secretion. Iron absorption appears to remain intact except in the presence of achlorhydria, which reduces the absorption of nonheme iron found in food. Vitamin A tolerance curves are unchanged, although the peak blood level may be later, suggesting delayed absorption. It is probable that vitamins B_1 and B_{12} are less well absorbed in old age, but there is no evidence that absorption is inadequate except in overt cases of pernicious anemia.

LIVER

Calloway and coworkers (1965) documented the known decrease in liver size by examining 400 livers obtained at autopsy. The peak average weight of 1929 g in the fourth decade declined to 1000 g in the tenth, with the most marked decline after the sixth decade. It remained constant at 2.5% of total body weight until the seventh decade and then dropped to 1.6% by the tenth. Cellular changes are so characteristic that in 46 of 50 attempts it was possible to identify young and old livers.

The liver undergoes several changes with this reduction in size. There is a reduction in blood flow, alteration in hepatocyte size and ultrastructural features, including increased aneuploidy, ductular proliferation, and liver cell necrosis, reduced protein synthesis, and a reduction in metabolism of a number of drugs.

The clearance of bilirubin is not affected by age and there are no significant differences in the total serum bilirubin, SGOT, SGPT, and alkaline phosphatase values in young and old persons. Although there is an insignificant decrease in the total serum protein from 7.40 to 7.04 g/100 mL, there was a significant difference in the albumin/globulin (A/G) ratio, which was 4.04/3.06 g/100 mL in the young subjects (average age, 23) and 3.26/3.76 g/100 mL in the old subjects (average age, 79). The reduced serum albumin in most cases is related to an underlying chronic disease or associated malnutrition and should not be assumed to be part of normal aging.

Dynamic tests of liver function include the clearance of anionic dyes such as sulfobromophthalein. In this test there is a storage phase, splanchnic blood flow phase, and a secretory phase. In older individuals, there is a linearly decreased storage capacity, some decrease in blood flow, but no reduction in secretory capacity. Other studies using antipyrine demonstrate an age-associated reduction in clearance of this drug. The liver enzymes of older individuals may be less inducible than those of younger individuals, and ascorbic acid deficiency may potentiate the reduction in antipyrine metabolism.

The most important aspect of these complex impairments in live enzyme function is their propensity to contribute to adverse drug reactions in older ill patients. We have no formula to calculate the clearance capacity of an individual's liver. One approach is to first count the number of drugs that an older individual is on that are metabolized in the liver. If that number is three or more, frequent blood levels of those medications should be made to ascertain whether there is a drug interaction that is further impairing the clearance of these potentially harmful agents.

GALLBLADDER

Biliary stones are estimated to be present in 10% of men and 20% of women between the ages of 55 and 65 years and to approach 40% by the eighth decade. The mechanism of formation is probably the same as at all ages, but obviously the normal mechanisms of cholesterol stabilization and absorption become progressively less efficient.

PANCREAS

The weight of the adult human pancreas averages 95 g. Several reports indicate that there is no significant decrease in pancreas weight whether expressed as absolute weight or as a percentage of total body weight. However, it has been reported that the fat content of the pancreas increases, which may mask loss of functional tissue. Microscopic and electron microscopic studies have shown metaplasia and proliferation of ductile cells, irregularities of size, arrangement, and staining of parenchymal cells, and alterations in subcellular organelles. As noted in the studies of pancreatic secretions, there is generally a decreased volume and concentration of enzymes, but they remain sufficient for normal digestive functions. A study by Laugier and Sanles (1985), who performed duodenal aspirates in patients of a wide age range, found pancreatic volume and bicarbonate concentration peak in the fourth decade, then decline. In contrast, outputs of lipase, phospholipase, and trypsin declined linearly with age. Decreased outputs of volume and protein or lipase in response to secretin or cholecystokinin were observed, particularly in those individuals over 65 years.

NERVOUS SYSTEM

CHANGES IN BRAIN STRUCTURE

Neurons are postmitotic and, when lost from any cause, are not replaced. In contrast to the irreplaceable neurons, the glial cells that surround and support the neurons not only go through cell division and reproduction, they can proliferate in response to injury or loss. Longitudinal studies of brain structure by computed tomographic scanning demonstrate highly selected atrophy of brain tissue in restricted areas with aging rather than a global reduction. Most evidence indicates some neuronal loss (10% to 60%) with normal aging in the neocortex, cerebellum, and the hippocampus. This atrophy is accompanied by a net reduction in the blood flow that reaches 10% to 15%, while the capillary network of cerebral cortex appears to increase in diameter, volume, and length. Cell loss is less striking in the subcortical structures. There is increased dendritic growth in some neurons of the cerebral cortex and hippocampus of aging individuals.

The chemical constituents of the aging brain—the proteins, nucleic acids, and lipids—each show changes that correlate with the gradual loss in the weight of the brain with aging. With the reduction in normal protein content, the accumulation of abnormal proteins in the tangles and plaques is seen. Enzymes associated with glucose metabolism are reduced. While there is little or no change in the DNA content of neurons of the central nervous system, the RNA changes dramatically, with reductions in some areas of the brain and increases in other parts.

At the cellular level many changes have been documented. The most extensively studied has been the intracellular accumulation of lipofuscin pigment. This major accumulation occurs in storage vacuoles and is quantitatively highly correlated with age. The amount per cell varies, but can be sufficient to fill the cytoplasm and force the nucleus into an eccentric position. Despite the obvious and apparently significant nature of this material and the interest that it has engendered, it is not known if its presence has any actual effect on cell function.

There are several anatomic lesions that have a high correlation with senile dementia, regardless of the age of onset. The most common are senile plaques and neurofibrillary tangles. The question of whether senile dementia is a manifestation of aging or a disease process has not been resolved. Age unquestionably is a major factor, since the age-specific incidence increases geometrically. It is a major problem, with over 1 million persons requiring custodial care at the present time. Although it is not generally recognized, dementia is associated with a high mortality and might legitimately be considered a major cause of age-related death.

NEUROTRANSMITTERS

Perhaps the most active area of interest and study at present is the neurotransmitters. Neurotransmitters are chemicals that are responsible for the transmission of information from one neuron to another and include the following major groups: catecholamines and serotonin, acetylcholine, gamma-aminobutyric acid, and glutamic acid. The catecholamines include dopamine, norepinephrine, and epinephrine, and they are mostly involved in the control and modulation of visceral functions, emotions, and attention. During aging in apparently normal individuals, there is a significant reduction in the synthetic capacity of certain catecholaminergic neurons, leading to lower levels of dopamine (especially in the striatum), norepinephrine, and epinephrine. Similarly, levels of serotonin, which is involved in central regulatory activities such as drinking, respiration, heart beat, thermoregulation, sleep, and memory, are also reduced. It is likely that these reductions in the pivotal regulatory neurotransmitters play a role in the overall reduction in the aging individual's capacity to respond to physical and emotional stress in an efficient and effective manner. Recent investigations have shown that levels of monoamine oxidase

(MAO), the enzyme responsible for the breakdown of the catecholamines, increase with age in the human brain.

Current treatment of depression is based on the hypothesis, supported by considerable data, that depression is associated with decreased stores of catechols in the brain, and the use of MAO inhibitors, which block the MAO breakdown of catechols, is based on this rationale. The reciprocal increase of MAO and decrease of norepinephrine may explain the depression and apathy so often associated with aging. It also appears that steroid sex hormones are necessary for adequate catechol function, and it is possible that the symptomatology of menopause may be related to the abrupt reduction of estrogen production.

Parkinson's disease, or paralysis agitans, increases in frequency with age. Chemical studies show a decrease in dopamine, another epinephrine precursor, in the midbrains of these patients. This has been the rationale for the use of L-dopa, which has had considerable success in controlling symptoms. It is obvious that expansion of this type of information will help explain and ameliorate aging phenomena.

Acetylcholine metabolism and activity appear to change little with normal aging. The enzymes for the production of acetylcholine appear to be reduced in the cerebral cortex, but are unchanged in the striatum of the basal ganglia. Loss of cholinergic function with aging is controversial because of concern that brains of individuals with unrecognized Alzheimer's disease may have been included in the studies.

Gamma-aminobutyric acid operates mostly as an inhibitory neurotransmitter and glutamic acid as a stimulatory neurotransmitter. The enzyme responsible for converting the glutamic acid into the gamma-aminobutyric acid decreases 20% to 30% with age in the human cortex, basal ganglia, and thalamus. Although there is speculation that this shift toward glutamic acid may play a role in the increased sensitivity of older individuals to benzodiazepines (both bind to the same cell surface receptors), this has not been confirmed by studies.

NERVE CONDUCTION VELOCITY

The extensive use of electromyography as a diagnostic procedure has produced a mass of clinical data showing age-related changes in nerve conduction velocity. Nerve conduction velocity is most rapid in myelinated fibers and is roughly proportional to the diameter of the neuron. Most of the reported studies have been made of the motor conduction of the ulnar nerve. The velocity is quite slow in the newborn infant and averages 30 m/s. This increases rapidly so that at approximately 3 years of age almost all values are at the lower range of adult normal and maximal adult levels are achieved by age 5. There is a variation between individual studies, but young adults have an average conduction velocity of slightly less than 60 m/s.

From maturity the velocity decreases with age, especially after the fifth decade. By the eighth or ninth decade, values of approximately 50 m/s are generally reported. This represents a decrease of approximately 15%. The conduction velocity is slightly greater in women than in men. No statistically significant difference has been noted between the dominant and nondominant extremities. One study of sensory conduction in the median nerve reported a 30% decrease in conduction velocity between the ages of 20 and 95 years. A significant decrease was also noted in both the motor and sensory latency between 20 and 80 years.

SLEEP

Sleep is a phenomenon of great biologic and clinical importance. Four levels of increasing depth can be identified by electroencephalographic criteria and are numbered in increasing order. An additional level associated with rapid eye movements, known as REM sleep, is borderline in depth but is associated with the majority of dreams and has multiple unique physiologic characteristics. In infancy, deep levels 3 and 4 predominate and arousal is rare throughout the sleep cycle. With aging, levels 3 and 4 become less prominent and brief arousals more frequent. By old age, there is little level 4 sleep and there may be numerous brief arousals, although the total sleep time is only slightly reduced from young adulthood (Fig. 8–8). It is this frequent arousal that gives the impression of sleeplessness, even though in most instances actual sleep loss is minimal. Sedatives reduce latency to the onset of sleep and decrease the number of arousals. However, after a few days the pattern characteristic of the individual usually recurs and the sedative becomes ineffective. At this point, withdrawal may produce adverse effects even though the drug has lost its therapeutic value. With rare exceptions, seda-

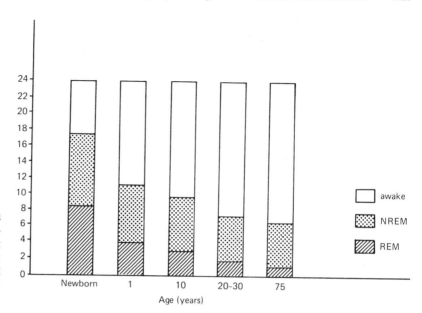

FIGURE 8–8 Changes in sleep pattern with development. (From Lee K. Rest and comfort status. In: Concepts basic to nursing practice, 3rd ed. St. Louis: C. V. Mosby, 1981, p. 607.)

tives should be used only briefly for specific situations. As noted previously, the neurotransmitter serotonin, which is important in sleep regulation, is diminished with aging and clearly reduced in states of clinical depression. Any evaluation of sleep disorder should clearly consider anxiety and depression as factors interacting with the normal changes of aging.

BRAIN CIRCULATION AND OXYGEN USE

The circulation and oxygen use of the cerebrum, are important physiologic components that have been well studied. The parameters generally examined include the cerebral blood flow (CBF) in mL/min/100 g of brain tissue, mean arterial pressure (MAP) in mm Hg, cerebral oxygen consumption rate ($CMRO_2$) as mL O_2/min/100 g of brain tissue, and cerebrovascular resistance (CVR) expressed as mm Hg/mL blood flow/min/100 g of brain. The cerebrovascular resistance is equal to the mean arterial pressure divided by the cerebral blood flow. A summary of data is presented in Table 8–3.

These studies by various authors are remarkably consistent, and there is a progression of values from age 17 to age 80. During this period the mean arterial pressure remained at 90 to 100 mm Hg. The cerebral blood flow declined from 79 to 46 mL/min/100 g of brain tissue. The cerebral oxygen consumption rate declined from 3.6 to 2.7 mL O_2/min/100 g of brain. The derived cerebrovascular resistance

showed a reciprocal increase from 1.3 to 2.1 mm Hg/mL blood/min/100 g of brain. Hypertension increased the cerebrovascular resistance but had little effect on oxygen use. There is a significant reduction in cerebral blood flow and metabolism with aging. Patients with dementia cluster at the lowest values of blood flow and oxygen use. Yet on an individual basis there is much overlap, and subjects without overt intellectual deterioration may be comparable with some who are totally incapacitated.

ENDOCRINE SYSTEM

The relationship between aging and the structure and function of the endocrine system cannot be easily separated from the changes in the central nervous system, which are discussed in a subsequent section. Deep in the center of the brain are the cells of the hypothalamus that release several types of hypothalamic-releasing hormones episodically, which in turn influence the release of anterior pituitary hormones, which influence the end-organ function of the adrenal gland, thyroid gland, pancreas, gonads, and kidney. The neurons where this cascade of hormonal secretion is initiated are influenced by a complex neural network of neurons from the brain stem, limbic system, diencephalon, and neocortex. The system is autoregulated by a series of feedback loops that are, in general, inhibitory. Thus, once the cascade is set off, it is the level of the end-organ product, for in-

TABLE 8–3 *Effect of Aging on Cerebral Hemodynamics and Metabolism**

	No. of Observations	Age Range (yr)	Mean Age (yr)	MAP	CBF	CVR	CMRO$_2$
1*	4	17–18	17	97	79.3	1.3	3.6
2†	19	18–36		85	65.3	1.3	3.8
3‡	25	20–44	29	91	52.0	1.8	3.1
4	12	18–40	30	91	53.0	1.8	3.4
5*	12	18–47	32	94	57.5	1.7	3.2
6†	15	38–55		96	60.5	1.6	4.0
7‡	23	45–75	56	101	46.0	2.2	2.9
8†	17	56–79	63	97	50.6	2.0	3.3
9§	23	45–86	68	95	46.0	2.1	2.7
10*	13	57–99	80	94	47.7	2.1	2.7

*Fazekas JF, Kleh J, Finnerty FA. Influence of age and vascular disease on cerebral hemodynamics and metabolism. Am J Med 1955; 18:477.
†Scheinberg P, et al. Effects of aging on cerebral circulation and metabolism. Arch Neurol Psychiatr 1953; 70:77.
‡Heyman A, et al. The cerebral circulation and metabolism in arteriosclerotic and hypertensive cerebrovascular disease. N Engl J Med 1953; 249:233.
§Shenkin HA, et al. The effects of aging, arteriosclerosis, and hypertension upon the cerebral circulation. J Clin Invest 1953; 32:459.

stance, the corticosteroids or thyroid hormone, that actually becomes the turn-off switch. In this way homeostasis or the internal hormonal balance is maintained. In addition to the morphologic and neurotransmitter changes of the central nervous system associated with aging, this neuroendocrine system is influenced by internal oscillators or biologic clocks, stress, exercise, and depression.

As previously stated, the hallmark of the aging organism is a progressive reduction in its capacity to maintain homeostasis in the face of environmental stress. The overall effect of the changes in aging in the neuroendocrine system is a progressive resistance to the inhibitory feedback of the end-organ hormonal secretion. Thus, even though the initial response to a stressful stimuli may be appropriate, as the organism ages there is an increased likelihood that the response may be persistent and ultimately inappropriate and even harmful to the organism.

PITUITARY GLAND

The weight of the pituitary gland may decrease 20% in extreme old age, but the significance cannot be determined because the patients ex-amined also had prolonged terminal illnesses. However, there is a marked decrease in the number of mitoses, decreased vascularity, increased connective tissue, a change in the proportion of cell types, and definite disorganization of the cellular organelles.

Growth Hormone Several recent experiments in humans and animals clearly demonstrate that growth hormone secretion declines progressively in aging men. This decline is most evident during sleep. In addition, the circadian variation of growth hormone is blunted with age (Carlson, 1972).

Thyroid-Stimulating Hormone Plasma thyroid-stimulating hormone (TSH) does not decrease with age, but several studies indicate that there is reduced TSH release on stimulation by thyrotropin-releasing hormone. This probably is due to impairment of the TSH release mechanism, because the pituitary content of TSH is normal. Again, there is a blunting of circadian variation (Barracet, 1985).

Adrenocorticotropic Hormone A reduction in feedback inhibition of adrenocorticotropic hormone and/or its hypothalamic-releasing hormone, corticotropin-releasing hormone by glucocorticoids is the most clearly demonstrable age-associated change in the hypothalmic–pituitary axis.

Follicle-stimulating Hormone and Luteinizing Hormone The amount of follicle-stimulating hormone in the postmenopausal pituitary is clearly elevated, but the status of luteinizing hormone is less clear. The blood level of follicle-stimulating hormone increases 15-fold and that of luteinizing hormone threefold. In the postmenopausal state estrogens appear to have an impaired negative-feedback effect, and the elevated gonadotropins are not suppressed completely except with unphysiologically high doses. The gonadotropins increase much more slowly and less significantly in men. Apparently the feedback mechanism remains more intact in men than in women.

Antidiuretic Hormone Although studies in rats show a decrease in antidiuretic hormone with age, there is no such evidence for humans. There does seem to be an increased frequency of the syndrome of inappropriate secretion of antidiuretic hormone particularly under the stress of acute physical and emotional illness.

THYROID GLAND

The thyroid gland probably does not change weight with age, although the frequency of clinical nodularity is increased. Microscopically there is fibrosis, cellular infiltration, and micronodularity as well as macronodularity.

The plasma thyroxine (T_4), both protein-bound and free, is unaffected by age, but the plasma triiodothyronine (T_3) decreases 25% to 40% after the sixth decade. Thyroxine-binding globulin increases slightly and thyroxine-binding prealbumin decreases. As noted, TSH levels are unchanged.

The rate of radioiodine accumulation in the thyroid gland decreases with age at the 6-hour determination, but the differences at 24 hours are less clear. It is now believed that the reduced renal function of older persons results in longer retention of radioiodine, with a greater opportunity for late accumulation in the thyroid gland. Prolonged exposure thus compensates for a slower rate of uptake.

The normal plasma T_4 concentration and the reduced radioiodine uptake by the gland suggest that the rates of destruction and replacement of thyroid hormone are slowed pro-

portionately. Gregerman and his associates (1962) showed that the hormone degradation decreased 50% in the six decades between 20 and 80 years. The turnover rate averaged approximately 88 ng/d at age 20 and decreased to 42 ng/d at age 80. The reduced rate of T_4 disposal probably is due to slowed hepatic metabolism, although reduced physical activity may also be a factor.

The thyroid response both to stress and to exogenous TSH is comparable at all ages. This ability of the aged thyroid to respond normally to stress implies that the age-related decrease in normal T_4 turnover results from reduced peripheral need rather than from failure of thyroid response. The normal blood levels of both T_4 and TSH indicate a physiologic balance and are evidence against either thyroid or pituitary insufficiency. However, the decrease in the plasma T_3 presents a theoretic problem. If T_3 is the effective hormone, the failure of TSH to respond to the age-related decline is inconsistent. Yet the correlation of decreased oxygen consumption with decreased cell mass and the absence of clinical manifestations make the concept of age-associated hypothyroidism as a routine phenomenon difficult to accept.

PARATHYROID GLANDS

Past difficulties with parathyroid hormone (PTH) assay have resulted in conflicting interpretations of bone and renal stone disease. One recent report suggests that PTH decreases with age except in cases of osteoporosis, where it is increased. Estrogen is believed to protect against the demineralizing effects of PTH, and the postmenopausal decrease in estrogens may heighten the physiologic sensitivity to PTH.

PANCREAS

Insulin Studies by Andres (1967) indicate that there is constant decrease in the glucose tolerance with age. The average 2-hour serum glucose value is 30 mg/dL higher at 75 years than the values derived from young adults. By such standards, more than half of these individuals must be considered diabetic. This phenomenon seems to be independent of age-related obesity, despite the fact that fat impairs the hypoglycemic effect of insulin. Andres suggests that arbitrarily, and until better information is available, an age-determined rating be established and that the top 7 percentile at each age be considered diabetic and the next 7 percentile potentially diabetic (Fig. 8–9).

The impairment in these tests may be the result of either a reduced insulin release from the pancreas or a reduced peripheral sensitivity to circulating insulin. Earlier studies suggested that the defect was a failure of peripheral utilization. Evidence has accumulated more recently indicating that there may be a delay in insulin release by the beta cells and that, because higher blood glucose levels result, there eventually may be higher blood levels of insulin as well.

It is of interest that while the usual insulin assay at basal conditions shows similar total insulin levels, recent studies demonstrate that the less active proinsulin is a larger fraction of the whole in the older person. The implications of this observation need further study.

Glucagon   Glucagon, which causes an increase in blood glucose, could have an effect on the glucose tolerance. One study on the effect of glucagon administration showed a delayed and reduced response with age. Another showed no difference in fasting levels or in response to intravenous arginine stimulation.

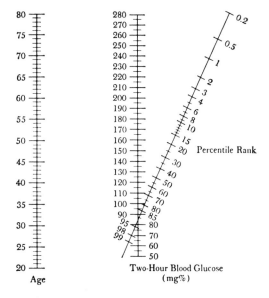

FIGURE 8–9   This nomogram enables the clinician to rank a response to the oral glucose tolerance test against the response of other people of the same age. (From Andrew R. Diabetes and aging. Hosp Pract 1967; 2:63; with permission.)

ADRENAL GLANDS

The human adrenal gland shows no major gross changes with age, but microscopic alterations include cortical nodule formation, increased connective tissue and pigment, reduced lipid, and changes in intracellular organelles. There may be vascular dilatation and hemorrhages.

Glucocorticoids   The plasma level of cortisol and the normal diurnal cycle, high in the morning and low at night, persist at all ages. However, a variety of diseases abolish the diurnal rhythm and, because multiple diseases are common with age, abnormal cycles may be more frequent. The secretion rate of cortisol is reduced 25% in old men, and there is a comparable decrease in the urinary excretion rate. The disposal rate of cortisol in elderly subjects was prolonged 40%, which is compatible with the constant blood level and reduced excretion. The combination of normal blood levels, reduced production rate, delayed degradation, and normal adrenocorticotropic hormone levels is comparable to the change in T_4.

Several experiments have been performed to test the ability of the aging adrenal to respond to stress. The results have been variable, about equally divided between a normal and a reduced response.

Aldosterone   Both the blood levels and the urinary excretion of aldosterone decrease about 50% between youth and old age. The metabolic clearance rate drops 20% and the splanchnic extraction decreases from 96.3% to 89.7%. The increase in urinary excretion following sodium depletion is only 30% to 40% of the response in young adults, and the secretion of renin shows a parallel age-related decrease. In a third of the women over the age of 70 the plasma and urine levels are low, and there is no response to sodium deprivation, postural change, or exercise.

Adrenal Androgens   The adrenal androgens make up the largest component of adrenal steroid hormone production, but their function is not known. The urinary excretion of 17-ketosteroids decreases progressively to about one half of the values in youth. The adrenal androgens, primarily dihydroepiandrosterone, decrease more rapidly than the total ketosteroids in both blood and urine. It is possible that this decrease is due to a reduced rate of production rather than to altered removal.

GONADS

Estrogens Following ovarian atrophy after menopause, there is no ovarian estrogen produced, and the remaining estrogens are adrenal in origin. Despite a decrease in the metabolic clearance rate, the plasma estradiol level decreases to between 5% and 10% of prior levels, and the estrone to 25%, indicating an even lower rate of production. In men, estrogens are produced by the adrenal cortex and there is little age-related change.

Progestins Progesterone is produced primarily by the ovary and placenta and to a lesser extent by the testis and adrenal cortex. The production and excretion decrease abruptly after the reproductive period. The production rate decreases about 60% between youth and old age. Pincus and associates (1955) proposed that because progesterone is a precursor of cortisol, adrenal production can be sustained.

Testosterone Blood levels of testosterone probably decrease, but the reports are not unanimous. However, there is agreement that the metabolic clearance rate and the production rate have declined and circadian variation is blunted (Marrama, 1982). The capacity of testosterone-binding globulin increases with age, further lowering the free testosterone.

THE BLOOD

Remarkably little change with age has been reported for blood and its components. Until at least age 80 there is no decrease in the blood volume, despite the decrease in active cell mass of the body. There are only very subtle changes in the red blood cells. Although anemia is frequent it appears not to be a consequence of normal aging, but rather a response to stress, which would be unlikely to cause a hematologic problem in a younger patient. One recent study of carefully selected healthy young and old persons, who were clearly hematologically normal, showed no significant differences in peripheral blood or ferrokinetic data. Quantitation of bone marrow hematopoietic stem cells and differentiated precursors revealed no significant differences.

The number and distribution of the neutrophils are unchanged. Neutrophil function can be assessed by measuring the ability of the neutrophils to phagocytose and kill bacteria. Another approach is to evaluate the respiratory burst and secretion of enzymes following exposure of the neutrophils to stimulatory agents. In neutrophils from young and old subjects, secretion of enzymes in the basal state is similar, but following stimulation the rate and total amount of enzyme released is clearly reduced in the older individuals. Of particular interest is the fact that, at least in mice, malnutrition mimics these reductions in reserve capacity in neutrophils seen with aging. The synergy between the changes of aging and the malnutrition seen in our hospitalized older patients may explain their higher morbidity and mortality from bacterial infections.

No change in platelet structure, number, and function has been observed, except for a possible increase in adhesiveness. The results of the few available studies of hemostasis and coagulation conflict, and most aged persons probably fall within the normal range for younger persons. Fibrinogen does seem to be increased, but the evidence for hypercoagulability is not conclusive. There is, at the same time, no evidence of inadequate clotting factors.

The erythrocyte sedimentation rate can be accelerated even in the absence of any evidence of disease. Values up to 40 mm/h (Westergren method) are not unusual (normal is <5 mm for men and 15 mm for women). This may be due to the age changes in plasma proteins, particularly the increase in fibrinogen.

IMMUNE FUNCTION

The determination of the effects of age on immune function and host defense is difficult because there are so many external and individual factors besides age that are influential. Nutrition, environmental pollution, prior illnesses, influences of the endocrine and neurochemical systems, and chemicals can all subtly influence host defense and therefore make it difficult to isolate the role of age. Even in the oldest old, one can find individuals with no alterations in their immune function. In general, however, function decreases with aging.

The thymus gland is essential to the differentiation of marrow lymphocytes into thymic or T-lymphocytes, needed for both humoral and cellular immunity. The thymus starts to involute at sexual maturity and is only 5% to

10% of maximal mass by age 45 to 50 years. No thymic hormones are detectable by age 60. Although the number of T-lymphocytes appears unchanged, more cells are immature and the ratio of helper cells to suppressor cells is increased. Most important, there is a 50% to 80% reduction in response to antigenic stimuli.

The total amount of circulating immunoglobulin is unchanged, but there is an increase in IgA and IgG at the expense of a decreased IgM. There is also a decrease in the amount of natural antibodies and an increased frequency of autoantibodies. The antibody response to antigens is decreased owing to the improper processing of the antigen by T cells, particularly helper T cells. This can be reversed, at least in part, by the administration of thymic hormone or young lymphocytes.

Cell-mediated immunity is similarly impaired, apparently by the same mechanisms. Fewer cells are available to mediate the reaction, and in the case of graft rejection, there are fewer cytotoxic T cells. Sensitization to appropriate antigens is less universal. Transfer of lymphocytes from older to younger syngeneic mice produces a graft-versus-host reaction, not manifested with the opposite transfer, indicating that the age-related increase in autoimmune activity is both a cellular and a humoral phenomenon.

Limited studies suggest that reduced humoral and cellular immunocompetence, reduced suppressor cell activity, and increased autoantibody activity are all associated with reduced survival.

MUSCULOSKELETAL SYSTEM

MUSCLES

Muscles are composed of postmitotic cells and are dependent on intact motor neuron innervation for survival. A gradual loss of muscle strength is a characteristic of aging. Careful studies reveal that there is a significant linear decrease in the number of muscle cells with age and that this decrease actually exceeds the loss of essential neural components. The loss exceeds the relative loss of total body mass as well. Some of this change is masked by an extracellular increase in interstitial fluid, fat, and collagen. Ultrastructural changes are extensive and complex. Lipofuscin deposition is marked. The density of capillaries per motor unit is decreased.

Although oxygen use per unit of tissue is essentially unchanged, there is a significant reduction in the activity of half of the enzyme systems so far studied. There is a prolongation of contraction time, latency period, and relaxation period by about 13% and a decrease in the maximal rate of tension development.

Fortunately, recent studies using regular exercise programs in individuals over 70 years and in nursing home patients over the age of 90 years have demonstrated 10% to 15% increases in muscle mass and an increased capacity for resynthesis of adenosine triphosphate and glycolytic activity. There is a growing realization that many of the physiologic changes said to be associated with aging, such as cardiovascular, biochemical, musculoskeletal, and psychological changes, as well as the decrease in muscle mass, may be associated with inactivity.

JOINTS

Joints are covered with cartilage, avascular tissue that shows major changes in structure as early as the third decade. Aging cartilage has impaired mechanical properties, attributable to altered structure of the proteoglycans and collagen in the matrix surrounding the chondrocytes. The entrapment and release of water from these large macromolecules forms the lubrication for the cartilage's mechanical stress-reducing system. When these molecules are altered with age, the water content of the cartilage is decreased, protection of the cartilage is impaired, and injury is possible. As the cartilage is eroded, bone makes direct contact with bone and results in one form of degenerative arthritis, with resulting pain, crepitation, and limitation of movement. Loss of water from the cartilage results in narrowing of the joint spaces, particularly of the intervertebral disks, and contributes to the loss of height. Although epidemiologic studies relate osteoarthritis to aging, biochemical studies distinguish changes in aging cartilage from those in osteoarthritic cartilage. For instance, the water content of cartilage in osteoarthritis is increased in contrast to the decrease noted in aging.

In another form of degenerative joint disease, there is an irregular bony overgrowth at the edges of joints, presumably at sites of trauma. When this occurs on the fingers, usually in women, it may be only unsightly. When it occurs about the hip, the femoral head may become trapped, painful, and immobile. This is the most common cause for hip replacement. When it occurs on the vertebrae it may impinge on spinal nerves as they penetrate the intervertebral foraminae, causing severe pain (sciatica is a common example) and often a corresponding muscle weakness.

BONE

Bone is a complex tissue that undergoes change throughout life. Starting before the age of 40 years in both sexes, there is a shift from an increase in bone mass to a progressive decrease. This is characterized by gradual reabsorption of the interior surface of long and flat bones and a slower accretion of new bone on the outside surface. Thus, the long bones are externally enlarged but internally hollowed out, the vertebral end plates are thinned, and the skull becomes slightly enlarged. At the same time there is a loss of the trabeculae. The end result is weaker bone that is subject to fracture.

Roentgen examination then shows the characteristic features of reduced bone mass, or osteoporosis, which is characterized microscopically by a loss of both bone salts and the supporting protein matrix. Modern experimental methods have established that aging bone loss is a universal phenomenon. Bone loss in women is approximately 25% and in men is 12%. Since in women this represents a 750-g loss from an original 3000 g in the skeleton whereas in men it is only a 450-g loss from 4000 g, it is obvious why osteoporosis is more apparent in women.

Osteoporosis may result from immobilization, failure to absorb calcium, excessive calcium loss from the bowel or the kidney, or a number of endocrine disorders that affect the protein matrix. None of these is demonstrably the cause of aging osteoporosis. Ovariectomy may accelerate and estrogen supplement may delay the process, but only for relatively short periods. There is little relationship to calcium intake. Changes in calcium balance are hard to detect, and balance is achieved on the normal intake of 8 to 12 mg/kg body weight per day.

Thinning of bone predisposes to fracture, particularly of the hip, vertebral body, shoulder, and wrist, and particularly in women. The most serious is fracture of the hip, which leads to immobilization and increased mortality. The cumulative risk of hip fracture at age 90 is 32% in women and 17% in men. Vertebral fractures with collapse cause back pain that usually resolves in several months. Shoulder and wrist fractures result from falls on the outthrust arm; they are inconvenient but usually heal well.

It is possible that there is progressive bone loss with age and that the most marked osteoporosis is seen in those with the least bone mass at the start. Thus, what is perceived as osteoporosis is the lower end of a distribution curve that is shifting to a reduced density. If this is the case, it is not surprising that the results of therapy are equivocal.

There is considerable loss of height with age that is difficult to evaluate without longitudinal data. If the span of the outstretched arms, which does not change with age, is used to estimate mature height, it has been estimated that the average loss is 1.5 inches between ages 65 to 74, increasing to 3 inches by ages 85 to 94. This loss is due to multiple factors, such as decrease in intervertebral disk height, vertebral osteoporosis and collapse, kyphosis resulting from both these factors, and a characteristic knee flexion. Thus, the musculoskeletal system contributes greatly to the appearance of age.

SKIN, HAIR, AND NAILS

Wrinkling of the skin and graying of the hair are the most universally recognized manifestations of aging. They are most readily apparent in the exposed areas, but are present in all the protected areas as well.

The cell layers of the epidermis are thinned, and the remaining cells reproduce more slowly and are larger and more irregular. Normal cell replacement is reduced by 50%, and healing is significantly delayed. There is a decrease in the number of melanocytes present in whites, resulting in reduced tanning on solar exposure. Epidermal macrophages are reduced 70% and may contribute to the reduced cutaneous cellular immunity and sensitivity to antigens.

The epidermis rests on the dermis, with the dermal papillae rising up as mounds containing capillaries to which the equally irregular epidermal rete pegs conform. With age both layers become thinner, and the papillae and rete become less prominent. The flattening of the dermal papillae is due to loss of capillaries from the central core. As a result, there may be a greater tendency for the epidermis to slide over the dermis, which may be a mechanism for formation of the frequent "senile purpura," bruises that appear just under the skin, especially in women. An increased vascular fragility contributes to the increased frequency of purpura. Elastin loses its elastic characteristics and collagen bundles become larger and stiffer. These changes are responsible for the wrinkling and sagging of aging skin, but the exact mechanism is not known.

There is also a marked loss of subcutaneous fat. This change is greatest in the extremities and in men. Skinfold thickness decreases from an average of 1.2 cm in men aged 25 to 29 to 1 cm at ages 65 to 79 and 0.9 cm over the age of 80 years. In women the average decrease from 1.5 to 1.4 cm may lack statistical significance. The thinning of the skin, the slowed cellular turnover, the loss of subcutaneous cushioning, and the reduced blood supply all contribute to increased frequency of decubitus ulcers in the immobilized older person.

The sweat glands decrease in size, number, and function, contributing to skin dryness. Function of apocrine and sebaceous glands decreases. Although sebaceous glands are said not to atrophy with age, the loss of some hair follicles must result in a decrease in their number. Although the mammary glands involute, the loss of breast fat makes the glandular component more prominent. The epidermal glands are under variable endocrine control, but responsivity decreases with age.

The rate of active hair growth decreases with age. Graying is due to the reduction of melanin production by the melanocytes of the hair follicle. Genetic factors control the age of onset, with great individual variation. The total amount of visible hair is determined primarily by the ratio of active to resting follicles. In white men age may cause a decrease in scalp hair and no change in the beard, but an increase in the hair of the ears and eyebrows. Axillary and pubic hair decrease after the climacteric, but white women may have increased facial hair, possibly in response to unopposed adrenal androgens.

The rate of nail growth decreases from 0.83 mm per week in the third decade to 0.52 mm per week in the ninth decade. The more rapid rate in men is reversed in the sixth decade. Localized injuries to the nail matrix result in altered nail production, manifested by longitudinal ridges that cause increased visible striation with age.

SENSORY ORGANS AND SENSATION

THE EYE

Visual acuity decreases with age. Friedenwald (1952) estimated, based on projections from available data, that blindness would be universal if survival were extended to 130 years. The actual amount of visual loss is variable. The major amount is due to cumulative damage to the transparent portions of the ocular system. However, there is also loss of the extent of the visual fields, decrease in the speed of dark adaptation, elevation in the minimal threshold of light perception, a greater proportionate loss of visual acuity in dim illumination, and reduction in the critical speed of flicker fusion.

The lens is formed by cells that, as they mature, lose their nuclei and cell membranes, while their cytoplasm becomes crystalline and transparent. The lens continues to grow throughout life, although at a decreasing pace, as new cells develop surrounding the transparent nuclear region. Thus, the lens material in the core approaches the age of the individual, while the outer layers are progressively younger. With age the crystalline nucleus becomes progressively more rigid and discolored. Only the more recent portion near the surface is sufficiently soft and deformable to participate in accommodations, and as the ratio of the cortex to the nucleus becomes smaller, the ability to accommodate decreases. This process is remarkably uniform and predictable. Between ages 40 and 45 years, almost all persons require corrective lenses to read and perform tasks requiring accommodation (Fig. 8–10). Whether the more or less complete opacification that occurs in cataract formation, and that markedly increases in frequency with age, is a pathologic process or a manifestation of differential aging, cannot be answered.

As the person ages, a tilting of the lens above the vertical axis increases the power of the horizontal meridian, resulting in astigmatism with the major axis horizontal. The continued lens growth causes it to enlarge progressively toward the posterior surface of the cornea, reducing the depth of the anterior chamber. The resulting change in the optical nodal point, along with the continued growth and increased density of the lens nucleus, increases the refractive power of the lens and produces a relative myopia. The efficiency of the mechanism for reabsorption of the intraocular fluid decreases and, with the decreasing depth of the anterior chamber, may contribute to the increased frequency of chronic glaucoma in older persons.

A well-known phenomenon, arcus senilis, is an age-related deposition of lipid that forms a white circle at the outer edge of the iris. Although it appears earlier in persons with hyper-

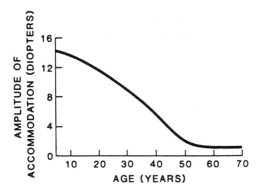

FIGURE 8–10   Amplitude of accommodation versus age. (From Rich LF. Ophthalmology. In: Cassel CK, et al (eds.), Geriatric medicine. New York: Springer-Verlag, 1990.)

lipidemia, the impression that it is correlated with atherosclerosis has not been established.

The pupil becomes smaller and response to light and accommodation decreases. According to Howell (1949), by age 85 only one third of subjects respond to light and none respond to accommodation. The ability to visualize the optic fundi becomes increasingly important with age, yet retinal examination becomes progressively more difficult.

THE EAR

More than one third of individuals over the age of 75 years experience a loss of hearing. Audiometric studies indicate that the mean puretone threshold increases with age at all frequencies and for both sexes. Until the ninth decade there is little loss in threshold sensitivity of frequencies of 250 to 1000 cycles per second, and then only for men. There is a marked increase in the threshold at higher frequencies, again more significant for men, particularly after the age of 60. Most individuals over 60 have lost their serviceable hearing for frequencies above 4000 cycles. The historical correlate of this sensory presbycusis is degeneration of the organ of Corti at the basal end of the cochlea. The restriction of these changes to a few millimeters of the basilar turn of the organ explains the abrupt high-tone loss.

The ability to hear and understand speech is more important than hearing pure tones. Although speech frequencies are relatively low, the ability to identify words is affected more than would be expected. This loss of speech

understanding with age is referred to as neural presbycusis and is characterized by a reduction in the population of cochlear neurons in the presence of a functional organ of Corti. Welch et al (1985) suggest that there may also be decrements involving a central integrative and synthesizing hearing disability and have called this phenomenon *central presbycusis*. In this case, older individuals have greater difficulty than younger people in understanding rapid speech, foreign accents, and speech transmitted via poor transmitting equipment. These difficulties are accentuated when background noise or competing speech are present, as in group situations.

Tinnitus does not seem to correlate with actual measured hearing loss. The auditory reaction time increases and becomes significant after 70 years. Age changes in vestibular function have not been studied.

TASTE AND SMELL

There is no evidence that the number of lingual taste buds declines with age. Earlier studies suggesting that there are higher frequency of taste complaints among older people examined institutionalized persons rather than healthy ambulatory older persons. Several recent, carefully controlled studies find only modest and quality-specific decremental changes in gustatory function in older persons. For example, the ability of older persons to detect salt decreased slightly with age, while no change in the detection threshold for sweet was noted. The importance of medication usage in raising the taste thresholds of older patients was highlighted in one study.

On the other hand, while there is no clear evidence in humans for changes in olfactory innervation with age, there is general agreement that elderly individuals show reduced ability for odor recognition.

TOUCH

No data could be found on changes in dermal sensation with age. However, histologic studies show a highly age-correlated decrease in the number of pacinian, Merkel's, and Meissner's corpuscles. Many of the remaining corpuscles showed marked disorganization and change. On the basis of these observations it would be reasonable to assume some reduction in the acuity of touch sensation. On the other hand, the free nerve endings underwent very little change, and the dermal sensation pain should be relatively much more intact.

PERSPECTIVE

It was noted at the beginning of this chapter that survival to maturity is followed by a decreasing frequency of acute disease and an increase in chronic processes. Although myocardial and cerebral infarction are acute episodes and are frequent causes of disability and death, they follow on the time-dependent development of atherosclerosis and other vascular changes. It was also noted that there is a growing conviction among gerontologists that the aging process is intrinsic and is independent of extrinsic (environmental) factors that may, however, accelerate the process. If this concept is true, it is necessary to reorient some aspects of social and research policy.

There is a consistent decrease in mortality at early ages and an increase into the postreproductive ages. However, while there is what is termed a squaring of the curve, the upper limits of survivorship have not been significantly altered. The magnitude of the change is shown in Table 8–4. Only 18% of women in 1600 survived to the reproductive age of 20, 11% completed the period, and approximately 3% reached age 65. In the developed countries today, over 97% reach age 20, 96% reach 40, 82% reach age 65, and 62% reach age 75. After this age, however, mortality increases rapidly.

An important concept was introduced by Benjamin Gompertz, a British actuary, in 1825. Strangely, it was not until a short time ago that his observation was recognized by biologists. His concept was that after a high neonatal mortality the death rate dropped to a nadir at the onset of puberty, and then increased. The important component was that at some point past maturity the risk of death increased geometrically; when age was plotted on a regular scale, but risk of death was plotted on a logarithmic scale, the result was a straight line. Thus, in advanced age the risk of death is related to age and is independent of specific cause.

The fact of the Gompertz observation is well established and is true, with little modification, for almost all living organisms. The interpretation is subject to some variation. Many theories of aging have been proposed and are under investigation. Although interesting, it is not possible to examine these theories in this short chapter.

If aging is universal, why is there a variety in the causes of senescent death? It was postulated initially that after maturity the decremental changes exceeded the incremental changes in structure and function. We have seen a wide variety of such changes in the cells and in all organ systems. If we postulate that species survival depends on reproduction and survival in a limited ecologic niche, then there would be an advantage if young persons could compete successfully with older persons once successful reproduction had taken place. Thus, aging need have no program, but rather, the exhaustion of a finely tuned program of repair. When we examine most chronic conditions and diseases of the aged, their morbidities and mortalities can be plotted in individual curves identical with the Gompertz curve, i.e., they show an age-related increase with a slope below, but parallel with, the overall curve. This

TABLE 8–4   *Survivorship of White Women (%)*

	Age				
	1	20	40	65	75
Townswomen, York, 16th century	45	18	11	3	
Aristocrats, England, 16th century	82	70	58	11	
United States, 1900	89	79	68	44	7
United States, 1972	99	98	97	85	69

Data from Cowgill UM. The people of York: 1538–1812. Sci Am 1970; 222:104; and the Monthly Vital Statistics Report, Vol 33, No 3. Supplement, June 22, 1984, Hyattsville, MD.

observation is true for all of the vascular dependent conditions (i.e., heart disease, stroke, ischemic gangrene) as well as for cancer, senile dementia, arthritis, osteoporosis, and diabetes mellitus. It probably would be true of other age-related conditions if the data were available.

As a result of variations in constitution, plus the factor of specific environmental exposure, the rate of deterioration of each system will be different. For example, it is known that the level of blood pressure is associated with mortal risk and that, at any age, the lower the blood pressure, even within the so-called normal range, the longer the life expectancy. If the force of each systolic impact produces damage to the vascular wall, it is not unreasonable to anticipate an earlier manifestation of vascular decline with each increment in this force. The same would be true for each of the risk factors. Similarly, if neoplasia is due to a decrease in immune protection, which is known to decline with age, then the increased incidence of cancer with age is explicable. If a carcinogenic factor were added from the environment, then the manifestation of neoplasia would be earlier.

Thus, the cause of death could vary, even though its specific manifestation was closely related to the aging process. It should be realized that, because of the geometric increase in frequency of each potential cause, the older the person the more likely that if one cause is avoided (or successfully treated) another will shortly appear.

References and Other Readings

Abrass IB. Catecholamine levels and vascular responsiveness in aging. In: Horan MJ, ed. Blood pressure regulation and aging. New York: Biomedical Information Corp., 1986

Andrew R. Diabetes and aging. Hosp Pract 1967; 2:63.

Aniansson A, Grimby G, Rundgren A, et al. Physical training in old men. Age Aging 1980; 9:186.

Barreca T, Franceschini R, Messina V, Bottaro L, Rolandi E. 24 hour thyroid stimulating hormone secretory pattern in elderly men. Gerontology 1985; 31:119.

Bartoshuk LB, Rifken B, Marks LE, et al. Taste and aging. J Gerontol 1986; 41:51.

Baum BJ. Salivary gland function during aging. Gerodontics 1986; 2:61.

Bender AD. The effect of increasing age on the distribution of peripheral blood flow in man. J Am Geriatr Soc 1965; 13:192.

Bird T, Hall MRP, Schade ROK. Gastric histology and its relation to anemia in the elderly. Gerontology 1977; 23:309.

Brocklehurst JC. A study of the bladder, rectum and anal sphincter in senile incontinent patients. In: Incontinence in old people. Edinburgh: Livingstone, 1951.

Brocklehurst JC, ed. Textbook of geriatric medicine and gerontology. 3rd ed. Edinburgh, Churchill Livingstone, 1985.

Calloway NO, Foley CF, Lagebloom P. Uncertainties in geriatric data II organ size. J Am Geriatric Soc 1965; 13:20.

Carlson HE, Gillin JC, Gorden P, Snyder F. Absence of sleep related growth hormone peaks in aged normal subjects and in acromegaly. J Clin Endocrinol Metab 1972; 34:1102.

Cassel CK, Riesenberg DE, Sorenson LB, Walsh JR. Geriatric medicine, 2nd ed. New York: Springer-Verlag, 1990.

Cockcroft DW, Gaulet HM. Prediction of creatinine clearance from serum creatinine. Nephron 1976; 16:31.

Cowgill UM. The people of York: 1538–1812. Sci Am 1970; 222:104.

Dockery DW, Speizer FE, Ferris BG Jr, et al. Cumulative and reversible effects of lifetime smoking on simple tests of lung function in adults. Am Rev Respir Dis 1988; 137:286.

Fazekas JF, Kleh J, Finnerty FA. Influence of age and vascular disease on cerebral hemodynamics and metabolism. Am J Med 1955; 18:477.

Finch CE, Hayflick L, eds. Handbook of the biology of aging. New York: Van Nostrand Reinhold, 1977.

Flood D, Gherondache C, Pincus G, et al. The metabolism and secretion of aldosterone in elderly subjects. J Clin Invest 1967; 46:960.

Friedenwald JS. The eye. In: Lansing AI, ed. Cowdry's problems of aging: biological and medical aspects. 3rd ed. Baltimore: Williams & Wilkins, 1952.

Geokas MC, Centeas CN, Majumdar APN. The aging gastrointestinal tract, liver and pancreas. Clin Geriatr Med 1985; 1:177.

Gilchrest BA. Age-associated changes in the skin. J Am Geriatr Soc 1982; 30:139.

Gregerman RI, Gaffney G, Shock N. Thyroxine turnover in euthyroid men with special reference to changes with age. J Clin Invest 1962; 41:2065.

Hayflick L. The limited in vitro lifetime of human diploid cell strains. Exp Cell Res 1965; 37:614.

Hazzard WR, Andres R, Bierman EL, et al. Principles of geriatric medicine and gerontology. 2nd ed. New York: McGraw Hill, 1990.

Heyman A, Patterson JL, Duke W, Bottey L. The cerebral circulation and metabolism in arteriosclerotic and hypertensive cerebrovascular disease. N Engl J Med 1953; 249:223.

Holliday R. Toward a biological understanding of the aging process. Perspect Biol Med 1988; 32:109.

Hollis JB. Castel DO. Esophageal function in elderly

men. A new look at presbyesophagus. Ann Intern Med 1974; 80:371.

Holt PR. Intestinal absorption and malabsorption. In: Texter EC Jr, ed. The aging gut. New York: Masson, 1983.

Howell TH. Senile deterioration of the central nervous system. Br Med J 1949; 1:56.

Hrushesky WJM, Fader D, Schmitt O, et al. The respiratory sinus arrhythmia: a measure of cardiac age. Science 1984; 224:1001.

Kenney RA. Physiology of aging: a synopsis. Chicago: Year Book Medical, 1982.

Lakatta EG, Gerstenblith G. Alterations in circulatory function. In: Hazzard, ed. Principles of geriatric medicine and gerontology. 2nd ed. New York: McGraw Hill, 1990.

Landowne M, Stanley J. Aging of the cardiovascular system. In: Shock NW, ed. Aging—some social and biological aspects. Washington, DC: American Association for the Advancement of Science, 1960.

Laugier R, Sanles H. The pancreas. Clin Gastroenterol 1985; 14:749.

Leese G, Hopwood D. Muscle fibre typing in the human pharyngeal constrictors and esophagus: the effect of aging. Acta Anat 1986; 127:77.

Lipschitz DA, Udupa KB, Milton KY, et al. Effect of age on hematoporesis in man. Blood 1984; 63:502.

Lipschitz DA, Udupa KB, Boxer LA. The role of calcium in the age related decline of neutrophil function. Blood 1988; 71:659.

Marrama P, Carine C, Baraghini GF, et al. Circadian rhythm in testosterone and prolactin in the aging. Mauritas 1982; 4:131.

Martin JB, Reichlin S. Clinical neuroendocrinology. 2nd ed. Philadelphia: Davis, 1987.

McDonald RK, Solomon DH, Shock NW. Aging as a factor in the renal hemodynamic changes induced by standardized pyrogen. J Clin Invest 1951; 30:457.

Miller IJ, Jr. Human taste bud density across adult age groups. J Gerontol 1988; 43:326.

Murphy C. Taste and smell in the elderly. In: Meiselmen HL, Riclin RS, eds. Clinical measurements of taste and smell. New York: Macmillan, 1986:343.

Murray JF. Aging. In: Murray JF, ed. The normal lung: the basic for diagnosis and treatment of pulmonary disease. Philadelphia: WB Saunders, 1976.

Navab F. Mechanisms of absorption of protein breakdown and some aspects of enteral hyperalimentation. In: Texter EC Jr, ed. The aging gut. New York: Masson, 1983.

Nelson JB, Castell DO, Dunlop CE. Histologic changes associated with aging in rat ileal smooth muscle: correlation with physiologic data. Gastroenterology 1987; 92:1551.

Niewoehner DE, Kleinerman J. Morphometric study of elastic fibers in normal and emphysematous human lungs. Am Rev Respir Dis 1977; 115:15.

O'Rourke MF, Blazek J, Morrels C, et al. Pressure wave transmission along the human aorta. Changes with age and in arterial degenerative disease. Circ Res 1968; 23:567.

Peck WA, et al. Osteoporosis. National Institutes of Health Consensus Development Conference Statement, vol. 5, no. 3. Bethesda, MD: NIH, 1984.

Petty TL, Silver GW, Stanford RE. Mild emphysema is associated with reduced elastic recoil and increased lung size but not with air-flow limitation. Am Rev Respir Dis 1987; 136:867.

Pincus G, Dorfman R, Romanoff L, Rubin B. Steroid metabolism in aging men and women. Recent Prog Horm Res 1955; 11:307.

Port S, Cobb FR, Coleman RE, et al. Effect of age on the response of the left ventricular ejection fraction to exercise. N Engl J Med 1980; 303:1133.

Pradhan SN. Central neurotransmitters and aging. Life Sci 1980; 26:1643.

Reichel W, ed. Clinical aspects of aging. 3rd ed. Baltimore: Williams & Wilkins, 1989.

Rossman I, ed. Clinical geriatrics. 3rd ed. Philadelphia: JB Lippincott, 1986.

Rowe JW, Andres R, Tobin JD, Norris AH, Shock N. The effects of age on creatinine clearance in man: A cross sectional and longitudinal study. Gerontol 1976; 31:155.

Scheinberg P, Blackburn I, Rich M, Saslow M. Effects of aging on cerebral circulation and metabolism. Arch Neurol Psychiatr 1953; 70:77.

Schneider EL, Rowe JW. Handbook of the biology of aging, 3rd ed. Orlando, FL: Academic Press, 1990.

Shenkin HA, Novack P, Galuboff B, Soffe A, Bartin L. The effects of aging, arteriosclerosis, and hypertension upon the cerebral circulation. J Clin Invest 1953; 32:459.

Simonson E, Nakagawa K. Effect of age on pulse wave velocity and aortic ejection time in healthy men and men with coronary artery disease. Circulation 1960; 22:126.

Stafford JL. Age-related differences in CT scan measurements. Adv Neurol 1988; 45:409.

Strehler BL. Time, cells and aging. 2nd ed. New York: Academic Press, 1977.

Warren PM, Pepperman MA, Montgomery RD. Age changes in small intestine mucosa. Lancet 1978; 2:849.

Weksler ME. Senescence of the immune system. Med Clin North Am 1983; 67:263.

Welsh LW, Welsh J, Healy M. Central presbycusis. Laryngoscope 1985; 95:128.

Wesson LG. Physiology of the human kidney. New York: Grune & Stratton, 1969.

Whiteway J, Morson BC. Pathology of aging—diverticular disease. Clin Gastroenterol 1985; 14:829.

9
Laboratory Values for the Elderly

CONNIE DAVIS

One of the more difficult aspects of providing health care for the elderly is the interpretation of laboratory test results. Aging, in the absence of disease, produces many changes in organ systems. It is therefore reasonable to expect that at least some of the laboratory values for healthy elderly persons will differ from those of the healthy younger adult population. Although some authors have shown valid reasons for continuing to consider these values as "abnormal" (Freedman and Marcus, 1980; Harnes, 1980), it seems essential that health care providers be able to discriminate values associated with the normal aging process from those accompanying disease. Such discrimination is possible only if the standards for comparison reflect, as nearly as possible, a similar population.

Most reputable laboratories determine their own reference values. For this chapter, Henry's text, *Clinical Diagnosis and Management*, 18th edition, 1991 was used as a source for standard values. Other standards can be found in texts by Tietz, Miale, Williams, Wintrobe, and Thompson (see the references at the end of this chapter for full citation).

Dybkaer's review of over 300 reported studies and his team's normalization[*] of values is an important reference for comparison of numerous studies of laboratory values in the elderly.

Perspectives and Limitations

In practice, the designation normal range is being amended in favor of the term reference interval to provide a concept of values more closely associated with the population they describe (Rock, 1984; Butts and Lilje, 1982). A valid perspective must also include several categories of specific values when considering geriatric data (Dybkaer et al, 1981; Sunderman, 1975).

POPULATION

The reference population and the way it was chosen are key factors in viewing the data. Definitions of *healthy population* vary widely. The rationale for use of in-house patients, geriatric home residents, or unselected populations as reference groups generates ongoing debate (Garry et al, 1983; Vogel, 1980). Use of alcohol or tobacco by the reference population has been shown to affect laboratory values (Chan-Yeung et al, 1981). The use of prescription medications by the aged is frequent and can also affect test results (Lamb, 1983; Vestal and Dawson, 1985). The number of individuals used in the data set is also important; geriatric values have been slow to evolve for lack of enough subjects for adequate statistical defini-

[*]*Normalization* was accomplished by comparing reference values relatively rather than directly. The values reported for subjects between ages 20 and 40 were assigned a value of 1. All data for other age groups were reported as decimals in comparison with that value of 1 (Dybkaer et al, 1981).

141

tion (Rock, 1984). Other factors such as sex differences, diet, ethnic differences, and differences in body build and activity level that apply to younger populations seem to magnify variability when the elderly are considered.

DIFFERENCES IN LABORATORY METHODS

Differences in values are introduced by the methods used. Instruments vary, and although protocols for standardization have been established, laboratory to laboratory variations due to methods and instruments used may be considerable. Tests may be performed under differing conditions, e.g., enzyme analysis conducted at different temperatures (Butts and Lilje, 1982). Values for similar tests may be reported in differing units—a prime example is the eventual conversion of all units to Systéme Internationale (SI) units (Henry, 1991; Kaplan and Szabo, 1988). Finally, tests used may have differing capabilities for sensitivity, precision, and specificity (Rock, 1984).

OTHER FACTORS

As with other research the collection and preparation of specimens and the types of specimens affect the values reported. These can vary considerably. Study designs also affect findings. Both longitudinal and cross-sectional studies have been used to define parameters for the elderly and both have merits (Jernigan, 1980). Statistical methods also can influence the interpretation of results (Butts and Lilje, 1982). Circadian, or daily, rhythms underlie physiologic processes and must be considered when interpreting laboratory values. The concept of homeostasis does not encompass the temporal structure of physiology. Small variations, such as a 10% variation in plasma potassium throughout the day, would be unremarkable within a reference interval for a laboratory value, but other variations, such as plasma cortisol, which can vary normally between 2 μg/100 mL and 15 μg/100 mL within a few hours, may lead to a misinterpretation of results (Moore-Ede et al, 1983). Clinical chemistry and chronobiology are beginning to provide information that will greatly increase the knowledge obtained from laboratory values (Halberg and Montalbetti, 1983).

SPECIAL CONSIDERATIONS

Special problems arise when one attempts to compare values from the elderly with reference data. Pathology in the aged may not manifest classic signs and symptoms. Biochemical individuality—variation for the individual over time—may be more important in indicating abnormalities (Steel, 1978; Rock, 1984).

Conversely, a reference range for the elderly that indicates significant differences from the younger adult populations' values may serve to hide those with true disease. This is one of the problems with establishing separate reference ranges for the aged (Freedman and Marcus, 1980; Harnes, 1980).

As with so many other facets of health care for the elderly, the interpretation of laboratory data is complex. The ideas and values discussed in this chapter as well as the laboratory data from an elderly clientele require evaluation in the light of these constraints.

Organization of Information on Laboratory Tests

The remainder of this chapter divides laboratory tests into three categories: hematology, blood chemistry (including arterial blood gases and enzymes), and urinalysis. Each individual test is arranged alphabetically, with other common names for the test in parentheses. Reference intervals for the elderly reported from research are listed and standard values for adults from Henry (1991) are printed in italics for comparison with the values for the elderly. Male and female values are given when variance is expected. Readers are encouraged to consult a text with nursing implications for procedures on obtaining specimens. The column *Purpose of Test* provides the clinician with a quick overview of information that can be obtained from each laboratory value. Clinical conditions that may increase or decrease the laboratory value follow. General references for this material are *Diagnostic Tests Handbook* (1987) and *Merck Manual of Geriatrics* (Abramson and Berkow, 1990). The final column titled *notes* relates the physiologic background of the test or laboratory value and comments on age-related changes and clinical guidelines for further testing.

TABLE 9-1 Laboratory Values for the Elderly

Name of Test	Reference Interval	Purpose of Test	Decreased Indicates	Increased Indicates	Notes
HEMATOLOGY					
Activated partial thromboplastin time (APTT)	25–36 seconds 1.5–2.5 × control indicates therapeutic effect (*Diagnostic Tests*, 1987)	Screen for deficiencies of clotting factors in intrinsic pathways except VII and XIII, monitor heparin therapy		Deficiency of clotting factors; presence of heparin, fibrin split products, fibrinolysins or circulating anticoagulants that are antibodies to specific clotting factors	Activated partial thromboplastin time is more sensitive than prothrombin time (PT). Unaffected by age
Erythrocyte sedimentation rate (ESR)	M: 3–74 mm/h F: 3–78 mm/h (Sharland, 1980) M: <20 mm/h (50–85 years old) F: <30 mm/h (50–85 years old) M: <30 mm/h (over 85 years old) F: <42 mm/h (over 85 years old)	Monitor inflammatory or malignant disease, aid detection of occult conditions like tuberculosis, tissue necrosis, connective tissue disease	Polycythemia, sickle cell anemia, hyperviscosity, low plasma protein	Acute or chronic inflammation, tuberculosis, paraproteinemias, rheumatoid fever, rheumatoid arthritis, some malignancies, anemia, monoclonal gammopathy, elevated fibrinogen, osteomyelitis	Limited usefulness due to interference of anemia, hypoalbuminemia, nonspecific for disease. Values >19 (men) >22 (women) may indicate illness (Beers and Besdine, 1987). Isolated ESR up to 50 mm/hr is not significant unless clinical symptoms are present (Gambert and Duthie, 1983)
Fibrinogen (factor I)	200–400 mg/dL	Differentiation of suspected bleeding disorders	Hypo- or dysfibrinogenemia; disseminated intravascular coagulopathy; fibrinolysis; severe hepatic disease; cancer of prostate, pancreas, or lung; bone marrow lesions; recent trauma	Cancer of stomach, breast, or kidney, inflammatory disorders such as membranous glomerulonephritis, pneumonia	Age-related increases parallel ESR (Vogel, 1980)

(Continued)

143

TABLE 9–1 (Continued)

Name of Test	Reference Interval	Purpose of Test	Decreased Indicates	Increased Indicates	Notes
Hematocrit (Hct, Ht)	M: 42–48% F: 39–45% (Garry et al, 1983) M: 40–54% F: 38–47%	Part of complete blood count (CBC). Diagnosis of hydration status, anemia, polycythemia	Anemia, hemodilution	Polycythemia, hemoconcentration due to blood loss	
Hemoglobin (Hgb, Hb)	M: 12.3–16.4 g/dL F: 11.6–14.3 g/dL (67–70 years old) Decreasing to: M: 9.0–13.4 g/dL F: 10.4–12.4 g/dL (91–100 years old) (Besa, 1988) M: 15.0–17.0 g/dL F: 13.8–15.6 g/dL (Garry et al, 1983) M: 13.5–18.0 g/dL F: 12.0–16.0 g/dL	Screen for anemia or polycythemia, monitor response to therapy	Anemia, recent hemorrhage, hemodilution from fluid retention. Refer to MCV, MCH, MCHC to determine type of anemia	Hemoconcentration from polycythemia or dehydration	Vogel (1980) puts low value at 11.5 g/dL in men, 11.0 g/dL in women. Lower values could be due to decreased RBC survival, decreased RBC production, or enzyme changes that decrease viability of RBCs (Vogel, 1980)
Iron and total iron binding capacity (TIBC)	Iron: M: 73–143 μg/dL F: 76–122 μg/dL TIBC: M: 291–387 μg/dL F: 293–355 μg/dL (Garry, 1983) Iron: 60–150 μg/dL TIBC: 250–400 μg/dL	Estimate total iron storage, aid diagnosis of hemochromatosis, distinguish between iron deficiency anemia and anemia of chronic disease, assess nutritional status	Decrease in both iron and TIBC indicates iron deficiency. Decrease in iron and normal or slight decrease in TIBC suggests chronic inflammation, chronic renal failure, chronic tuberculosis, mycotic infection, suppurative infection, metastatic cancer, anemia of chronic disease	Increased iron and normal TIBC suggests iron overload, thalassemia or lead poisoning. Increased TIBC may be found in iron deficiency states (Besa, 1988)	Hematinics have no effect on anemia caused by chronic disease. Control of chronic disease will correct anemia (Howe, 1983)

Name of Test	Reference Interval	Purpose of Test	Decreased Indicates	Increased Indicates	Notes
Osmotic fragility	Refer to values by individual lab. Increases with age. (Rate of hemolysis is slower) (Araki and Rifkind, 1980)	Confirm morphologic red cell abnormalities, contribute to diagnosis of spherocytosis	Increased resistance to hemolysis from thalassemia, sickle cell anemia, postsplenectomy, red cell disorders in which codocytes or leptocytes are found	Increased tendency to hemolysis from hereditary spherocytosis, spherocytosis from autoimmune hemolytic anemia, severe burns, chemical poisoning	Cells have a more asymmetric distribution in aging (Howe, 1983)
Platelet count	150,000–400,000/μL No significant change in count with age	Part of CBC. Evaluate platelet production, aid diagnosis of thrombocytopenia and thrombocytosis	Aplastic or hypoplastic bone marrow, infiltrative bone disease such as cancer, leukemia, disseminated infection, megakaryocytic hypoplasia, ineffective thrombopoeisis due to folic acid or vitamin B_{12} deficiency, pooling in enlarged spleen, increased destruction due to drugs or immune disorders, disseminated intravascular coagulopathy, mechanical injury to platelets, severe burns, massive blood transfusions, kidney or liver disease	Hemorrhage, infectious disease, malignancies, iron deficiency anemias, recent surgery, splenectomy, inflammatory disorders, such as collagen vascular disease, rheumatoid arthritis, primary thrombocytosis, polycythemia vera, chronic myelogenous leukemia, pulmonary embolism, metastatic cancer, cirrhosis, tuberculosis, reticulocytosis, acute infection, cardiac disease, chronic pancreatitis, myeloproliferative disorders, fractures, high elevation	Counts <100,000 indicate that bleeding is likely. Counts <50,000 can cause spontaneous bleeding, <5000 can be fatal. Decrease in granular constituents (Sie, 1981), increase plasma platelet release factors are found in old age (Zaino, 1981)

(Continued)

TABLE 9–1 *(Continued)*

Name of Test	Reference Interval	Purpose of Test	Decreased Indicates	Increased Indicates	Notes
Prothrombin time, protime (PT)	9.5–12 s Unaffected by age. Varies by lab and testing equipment	Evaluate liver function and extrinsic coagulation system, monitor response to oral anticoagulants		Deficiency in fibrinogen, prothrombin, or factors V, VII, X; vitamin K deficiency, hepatic disease, ongoing oral anticoagulant therapy	When receiving oral anticoagulants, PT is titrated to a level determined by condition requiring anticoagulation therapy (Hirsh et al, 1989; Ruben et al, 1990)
Red blood cell count, erythrocyte count (RBC)	M: 3.67–5.69 million/mm³ F: 3.33–5.57 million/mm³ (Htoo et al, 1979) M: 4.6–6.2 million/μL F: 4.2–5.4 million/μL	Part of CBC. Diagnosis of anemia and polycythemia	Anemia, fluid overload, hemorrhage	Primary or secondary polycythemia, dehydration	Values are higher at greater altitude, women have lower values than men throughout life
Red Cell Indices, Erythrocyte Indices					
Mean corpuscular volume (MCV)	M: 73.1–106.9 μ³ F: 74.8–105.7 μ³ (Htoo, et al, 1979) 80–96 μm³	Part of CBC. Differentiate types of anemia	Microcytic, hypochromic anemias caused by iron deficiency, pyridoxine responsive anemia, thalassemia. Test iron, transferrin, and heavy metals to further differentiate	Macrocytic anemias caused by megaloblastic anemias, disorders of DNA synthesis caused by drugs, reticulocytosis, deficiency of folic acid or vitamin B_{12} (test to confirm), chronic liver disease	MCV measures the ratio of Hct to RBC count, thereby determining RBC size. Besa (1988) states values lower than 80 μm³ indicate deficiency
Mean corpuscular hemoglobin (MCH)	M: 24.1–36.5 mmg F: 25.2–35.4 mmg (Htoo et al, 1979) 27–31 pg	Part of CBC. Differentiate types of anemia, see MCV	Microcytic anemia	Macrocytic anemia (see above)	MCH gives weight of Hgb in average RBC

Name of Test	Reference Interval	Purpose of Test	Decreased Indicates	Increased Indicates	Notes
Mean corpuscular hemoglobin concentration (MCHC)	M: 30.6–36.2 gm% F: 30.9–35.9 gm% (Htoo et al, 1979) 32–36%	Part of CBC. Differentiate types of anemia, see MCV	See MCV	Spherocytosis	MCHC determines color of RBC (hypochromic or normochromic). When MCH, MCV, and MCHC are normal but Hgb is low, normochromic normocytic anemia (from underproduction, hemolysis, or blood loss) is diagnosed. See osmotic fragility, WBC count
Reticulocyte count	0.5–1.5% (of total RBC) No change with age	Aid in diagnosis of hypoproliferative or hyperproliferative anemias, assess blood loss, bone marrow response to anemia	Anemia of underproduction, such as hypoplastic or pernicious anemia. Review WBC count for further diagnostic information. Serum iron and TIBC assist determination of contribution of chronic illness to underproduction anemias (Howe, 1983)	Bone marrow response to anemia from either hemolysis or blood loss. If blood loss is ruled out, a Coombs' test can determine cause of hemolysis. Coombs' test is positive in immune anemias such as erythroblastosis, acquired hemolytic anemia, incompatible transfusion. Negative Coombs' test indicates	Reticulocytes are immature RBCs. Watch for trends

(Continued)

TABLE 9–1 *(Continued)*

Name of Test	Reference Interval	Purpose of Test	Decreased Indicates	Increased Indicates	Notes
				corpuscular defect: vasculitis, intravascular coagulation, infection, spherocytosis, malfunctioning spleen, enzymopathy (Howe, 1983)	
White blood cell count, leukocyte count (WBC)	3100–8900/mL (Caird, 1973)	Part of CBC. Determine presence of infection or inflammation, determine need for further tests, monitor response to chemotherapy or radiation therapy	Bone marrow depression, influenza, mononucleosis, infectious hepatitis	Infection or inflammation, leukemia, tissue necrosis due to burns, myocardial infarction, gangrene	Conflicting reports regarding age changes. No gross changes (Zaino, 1981), slight decrease (Caird, 1973; Dybkaer et al, 1981)

White Blood Cell Differential

Name of Test	Reference Interval	Purpose of Test	Decreased Indicates	Increased Indicates	Notes
Neutrophils, total	45.0–85.9% (Caird, 1973) *Mean* 59% 0–5% Poly's (bands, immature) *mean* 3% 50–65% segmented (segs, mature) *mean* 56% (Lee and Hayes, 1990)	Part of CBC. Evaluate capacity to resist and overcome infection. Diagnosis of leukemia, allergic reactions, and parasitic infection	Bone marrow depression, infections (hepatitis, influenza, mononucleosis), hypersplenism, collagen vascular disease, deficiency of folic acid or B_{12}	Certain infections (osteomyelitis, septicemia, herpes), ischemic necrosis, metabolic disorders, stress response, inflammatory disease. Increase neutrophils and bands with acute infection or injury	A granulocyte
Eosinophils	0–8.0% (Caird, 1973) *Mean,* 2.7%	Same as above	Stress response, Cushing's syndrome	Allergic disorders, parasitic infections, skin diseases, neoplastic disease	A granulocyte. Diurnal variations opposite monocytes (Casale and deNicola, 1984)

Name of Test	Reference Interval	Purpose of Test	Decreased Indicates	Increased Indicates	Notes
Basophils	0.3–2% *Mean*, 0.3% (Diagnostic Tests, 1987)	Same as above	Hyperthyroidism, stress	Chronic myelocytic leukemia, polycythemia vera, some chronic hemolytic anemias, Hodgkin's disease, myxedema, ulcerative colitis, chronic hypersensitivity states, nephrosis	A granulocyte
Lymphocytes	10.0–50.0% (Caird, 1973) *Mean*, 34%	Same as above	Severe debilitating illness (such as congestive heart failure [CHF], renal failure, advanced tuberculosis), defective lymph circulation, high levels of adrenal corticosteroids, immunosuppression	Infections (syphilis, tuberculosis, hepatitis, infectious mononucleosis, cytomegalovirus), thyrotoxicosis, hypoadrenalism, ulcerative colitis, lymphocytic leukemia. Increased in chronic and viral infections	Nongranulocyte. Diurnal variations prevalent, maximum at 2000 h (Casale and deNicola, 1984)
Monocytes	0–8.0% (Caird, 1973) *Mean*, 4%	Same as above		Infections (subacute bacterial endocarditis, tuberculosis, hepatitis), collagen vascular disease, systemic lupus erythromatosus, polyarteritis nodosa, carcinomas, lymphomas, monocytic leukemia	Nongranulocyte. Diurnal variations prevalent, peak at noon (Casale and deNicola, 1984). Ingest bacteria and tissue debris

(Continued)

TABLE 9-1 (Continued)

Name of Test	Reference Interval	Purpose of Test	Decreased Indicates	Increased Indicates	Notes
BLOOD CHEMISTRY					
Acid phospha-tase	0.0–1.6 IU/L (Jernigan, 1980) 0.13–0.63 U/L	Crude screen for prostatic cancer, monitor response to therapy for prostate cancer		Marked increase in-dicates a tumor that has spread beyond prostatic capsule. Moderate increase indicates prostatic infarction, Paget's disease, Gaucher's disease, multiple myeloma. A decline from a high indi-cates successful treatment of pros-tate cancer	Acid phosphatase is an enzyme found primarily in prostate and semen, some found in liver, spleen, RBCs, bone marrow, and platelets. Prostate specific antigen (PSA) has replaced acid phosphatase as screening test for prostatic can-cer. (See PSA)
Alanine amino transferase (ALAT, ALT) formerly: Serum glu-tamic pyruvic transaminase (SGPT)	0–56 IU/L (Jernigan, 1980) M: 0–45 IU/L F: 20–37 IU/L (Rej, 1989) 4–36 μ/L	A liver enzyme test. Detect and evaluate treatment of acute hepatic disease, es-pecially hepatitis or cirrhosis without jaundice, distin-guish between he-patic and myocar-dial tissue damage, assess hepatotoxic-ity of medications	Vitamin B$_6$ defi-ciency (Rej, 1989)	Very high (up to 50 × norm) indicates viral or severe drug-induced hepatitis or other hepatic dis-ease with extensive necrosis. Moder-ately high to high: infectious mononu-cleosis, chronic hep-atitis, intrahepatic cholestasis, chole-cystitis, early or im-proving viral hepati-tis, severe hepatic congestion due to heart failure. Slight to moderately high: active cirrhosis, drug-induced alco-	Enzyme necessary for tissue energy production. Ap-pears in hepato-cellular cytoplasm. Some found in kid-neys, heart, skele-tal muscle. See AST/ALT ratio. Peaks at age 50 in men, by age 65 ALAT is lower than in young adults

Name of Test	Reference Interval	Purpose of Test	Decreased Indicates	Increased Indicates	Notes
				holic cirrhosis, and similar causes of hepatic injury. Marginal elevations found in acute myocardial infarction (MI)	
Alkaline phosphatase (AP, ALP)	45–160 IU/L (Jernigan, 1980) 15–20 K-A units indicates borderline elevation in elderly, >50 K-A units indicates Paget's or metastatic liver disease (Caird, 1973) 20–130 IU/L	A liver enzyme test. Detect and identify skeletal diseases, primarily those with osteoblastic activity. Detects focal hepatic lesions causing biliary obstruction, such as tumors or abscesses, assess response to vitamin D in treatment of deficiency induced rickets	Hypophosphatasia, protein deficiency, magnesium deficiency	Marked increase: severe biliary obstruction by gallstones, malignant or infectious infiltration, fibrosis, Paget's disease, bone metastasis, hyperparathyroidism. Moderate increase: cirrhosis, mononucleosis, viral hepatitis, osteomalacia, deficiency-induced rickets, minor bone trauma in osteoporotic patients, fracture (Beers and Besdine, 1987)	This enzyme influences bone calcification and lipid and metabolite transport. Compare with other enzymes. Increase with aging may be due to increased liver disease, renal changes in vitamin D metabolism, which cause demineralization (Kelly, 1979). Elevations above reference range are likely to be bone related (Beers and Besdine, 1987)
Amylase	30–220 U/L Lower in elderly (Jernigan, 1980)	Diagnosis of acute pancreatitis, distinguish between pancreatitis and other abdominal disorders associated with pain, detect pancreatic injury	Chronic pancreatitis, pancreatic cancer, cirrhosis, hepatitis	Marked increase: acute pancreatitis (4–12 h after onset). Moderate increase: biliary obstruction, pancreatic injury from perforated peptic ulcer, pancreatic cancer, acute salivary gland disease	This enzyme is synthesized in salivary glands and pancreas, digests starch and glycogen. Urine levels also used

(Continued)

TABLE 9–1 (Continued)

Name of Test	Reference Interval	Purpose of Test	Decreased Indicates	Increased Indicates	Notes
Arterial Blood Gas Analysis (ABG):					
PaO_2	80–100 mm Hg (Diagnostic Tests, 1987)	Indicates amount of oxygen lungs are delivering to blood	Impaired respiratory function, insufficient oxygen from inspired air		Elderly may have PaO_2 less than 80 mm Hg without hypoxemia (Diagnostic Tests, 1987). Not a reliable indicator of ventilatory status
$PaCO_2$	35–40 mm Hg	Indicates lung's capacity to eliminate carbon dioxide	Hyperventilation, respiratory alkalosis. Respiratory compensation for metabolic acidosis is indicated by low pH, bicarbonate, and $PaCO_2$	Impaired respiratory function, respiratory acidosis, or metabolic alkalosis if compensating (pH and bicarbonate elevations accompany increased $PaCO_2$)	End product of cell metabolism. Used as compensatory mechanism
pH	7.38–7.44	Acid–base level of blood	<7.35 is considered acidosis. Metabolic acidosis occurs in starvation, severe diarrhea, diabetic ketoacidosis, renal disease. Respiratory acidosis occurs in COPD, pneumonia, barbiturate or sedative overdose	>7.45 is considered alkalosis. Metabolic alkalosis occurs in severe vomiting, nasogastric intubation with suctioning, diuretic therapy, and excess bicarbonate intake. Respiratory alkalosis occurs in hyperventilation, fever, and mechanical overventilation	Metabolic acidosis: low pH and bicarbonate ion. Respiratory acidosis: low pH and increased $PaCO_2$. Metabolic alkalosis: high pH and bicarbonate. Respiratory alkalosis: high pH, high $PaCO_2$
O_2 content	15–23%	Measure volume of oxygen combined with HGB			

Name of Test	Reference Interval	Purpose of Test	Decreased Indicates	Increased Indicates	Notes
O_2 saturation	94–100%	% of HGB carrying oxygen			
HCO_3^- (bicarbonate ion)	21–28 mEq/L	pH as influenced by metabolism	Metabolic acidosis (see pH)	Metabolic alkalosis (see pH)	Used as compensatory mechanism
Aspartate aminotransferase (AST), asparate transaminase. Formerly: serum glutamic-oxaloacetic transaminase (SGOT)	10–65 IU/L (Jernigan, 1980) M: 15.2–64.8 IU/L F: 16.2–62.3 IU/L (O'Kell and Elliott, 1970) M: 20–55 U/L F: 20–35 U/L (Rej, 1989) 8–33 U/L	Part of cardiac profile. Detect recent MI. Used in conjunction with CPK and LDH to aid detection and differential diagnosis of acute hepatic disease, monitor progress and prognosis in cardiac and hepatic disease. Assess hepatotoxicity of drugs (Rej, 1989)	Vitamin B_6 deficiency (Rej, 1989)	(1) **Very high** (>20 × norm): acute viral hepatitis, severe skeletal muscle trauma, extensive surgery, drug-induced hepatic injury, severe passive liver congestion. (2) **High** (10–20 × norm): severe MI, mononucleosis, alcoholic cirrhosis, resolving or early 1. (3) **Moderately high to high** (5–10 × norm): dermatomyositis, chronic hepatitis and prodromal or resolving 2 (4) ***Slight to moderately high*** (2–5 × norm): hemolytic anemia, metastatic hepatic disease, tumors, acute pancreatitis, pulmonary emboli, delirium tremens, fatty liver, biliary	Enzyme found primarily in liver, heart, skeletal muscle, kidneys, pancreas. Minor amounts in RBC. Is released in proportion to cellular damage. In acute MI, AST rises 6–10 h after onset, peaks 24–48 h, returns to norm in 4–5 days. In hepatic disease, rises 4–8 h after onset, peaks 24–48 h, returns to norm 4–8 days. Liver involvement is indicated by higher and prolonged values (Lee and Hayes, 1990)

(Continued)

TABLE 9-1 (*Continued*)

Name of Test	Reference Interval	Purpose of Test	Decreased Indicates	Increased Indicates	Notes
AST/ALT Ratio	1.15 (Rej, 1989)		Extrahepatic biliary obstruction, acute viral hepatitis (Rej, 1989)	obstruction (1–3 days after), any preceding condition. Alcoholic liver disease, organic toxic hepatitis, cirrhosis, cholestasis, chronic active hepatitis (Rej, 1989)	
Bilirubin	M: 0.0–1.7 mg/dL F: 0.0–1.0 mg/dL (Wilding et al, 1972) M: 0.2–1.2 mg/dL F: 0.1–1.0 mg/dL (O'Kell and Elliott, 1970) 0.2–1.4 mg/dL (Jernigan, 1980) *Direct: up to 0.3 mg/dL Indirect: 0.1–1.0 mg/dL Total: 0.1–1.2 mg/dL*	Evaluate liver function, aid diagnosis and monitoring of jaundice, aid diagnosis of biliary obstruction and hemolytic anemia		Indirect (unconjugated, or prehepatic) hepatic damage, hemolytic anemia. Direct (conjugated, posthepatic): biliary obstruction. Increase in both: continued hemolysis, continued biliary obstruction with resultant hepatic damage	Bilirubin is major product of hemoglobin catabolism
Blood urea nitrogen (BUN)	M: 22.0–60.0 mg/dL (Caird, 1973) M: 7.6–35.5 mg/dL F: 5.9–31.6 mg/dL (O'Kell and Elliott, 1970) 9.0–33.0 mg/dL (Jernigan, 1980) *8–23 mg/dL*	Test renal function, aid diagnosis of renal disease, aid assessment of hydration	Severe hepatic damage, malnutrition, overhydration	Renal disease, reduced renal blood flow such as dehydration, urinary tract obstruction, increased protein catabolism	Measures nitrogen fraction of urea, the chief end product of protein metabolism. Reflects protein intake, renal capacity, and liver function. May overestimate renal function in elderly (Beers and Besdine, 1987). See creatinine

Name of Test	Reference Interval	Purpose of Test	Decreased Indicates	Increased Indicates	Notes
Calcium	F: 8.5–10.5 mg/dL (Caird, 1973) M and F: 8.0–10.2 mg/dL (O'Kell and Elliott, 1970) M: 8.9–10.9 mg/dL F: 9.1–10.9 mg/dL (Wilding et al, 1972) 9.2–11.0 mg/dL	Diagnosis of neuro-muscular, skeletal, and endocrine disorders; dysrhythmias, blood clotting deficiencies, acid–base imbalance	Hypoparathyroidism, total parathyroidectomy, malabsorption, Cushing's syndrome, renal failure, acute pancreatitis, peritonitis	Hyperparathyroidism, parathyroid tumors, Paget's disease, multiple myeloma, metastatic cancer, multiple fractures, prolonged immobilization, inadequate calcium secretion as in adrenal insufficiency and renal disease, excess calcium ingestion, overuse of antacids containing calcium carbonate	Vitamin D necessary for absorption. Varies inversely with phosphorus. Intestinal absorption decreases with age, possibly related to decrease in vitamin D metabolism (Gallagher et al, 1980). Age-related renal changes may contribute to decreased calcium (Jernigan, 1980)
Carbon dioxide, total (CO_2)	19–31 mEq/L (Caird, 1973) 24–30 mEq/L (Jernigan, 1980) 21–28 mM	Evaluate acid–base balance	Metabolic acidosis: diabetic acidosis, renal tubular acidosis, severe diarrhea, intestinal drainage respiratory alkalosis: hyperventilation	Metabolic alkalosis: severe vomiting, continuous gastric drainage respiratory acidosis: hypoventilation from emphysema or pneumonia. Also may occur in primary aldosteronism and Cushing's syndrome	
Chloride	96–108 mEq/L (Caird, 1973) 98–110 mEq/L (Jernigan, 1980) 95–103 mEq/L	Detect acid–base imbalance, aid evaluation of fluid status, and extracellular cations	Prolonged vomiting, gastric, suctioning, intestinal fistula, chronic renal failure, Addison's disease, dilution from CHF or edema	Severe dehydration, complete renal shutdown, head injury producing neurogenic hyperventilation, primary aldosteronism	Major extracellular cation, maintains osmotic pressure of blood

(Continued)

TABLE 9–1 (Continued)

Name of Test	Reference Interval	Purpose of Test	Decreased Indicates	Increased Indicates	Notes
Cholesterol, total (see also lipoprotein phenotyping)	142–324 mg/dL (Jernigan, 1980) <200 mg/dL = desirable 200–239 mg/dL = borderline high, if have two other risk factors, should have HDL and LDL tests >240 mg/dL = lipoprotein analysis is indicated. (National Cholesterol Education Program [NCEP], 1988) 150–250 mg/dL	Part of lipid profile. Assess risk of coronary disease, evaluate fat metabolism, aid in diagnosis of nephrotic syndrome, pancreatitis, hepatic disease, hypothyroidism and hyperthyroidism	Malnutrition, cellular necrosis of liver, hyperthyroidism	Risk of coronary artery disease, incipient hepatitis, lipid disorders, bile duct blockage, nephrotic syndrome, obstructive jaundice, pancreatitis, hypothyroidism	Cholesterol is absorbed from diet and synthesized in liver as a building block of steroid hormones, glucocorticoids, and bile acids. For each 1% increase in cholesterol there is a corresponding 2–3% increase in coronary artery disease. Levels >150 mg/dL significantly increase risk (Lamy, 1989)
Creatine kinase (CK), creatine phosphokinase (CPK)	Total: 18–392 IU/L (Jernigan, 1980) M: 55–170 IU/L F: 30–135 IU/L CPK-MM 94–100% CPK-MB 0–6% CPK-BB 0% (Lee and Hayes, 1990)	Part of cardiac profile. Detect and diagnose acute MI and reinfarction, evaluate chest pain, severity of myocardial ischemia, detect dermatomyositis	Sedentary lifestyle, immobility. Diagnosis of acute MI in immobile persons is difficult because baseline values are low (Lott and Stang, 1989)	Increase total CK: severe hypokalemia, CO poisoning, malignant hyperthermia, postconvulsion, alcoholic cardiomyopathy, occasionally in pulmonary or cerebral embolism. Increased CK-MB: myocardial infarction, cardiac surgery, muscular dystrophies, polymyositis, severe myoglobulinemia. Increased CK-MM: trauma to	Enzyme that catalyzes creatine-creatinine metabolic pathway in muscles and brain tissue. CK-BB found mainly in brain tissue. CK-MB: primarily in cardiac muscle, also in skeletal muscle. CK-MM: predominate type, found in skeletal muscle. Rises 6 hours after acute MI, peaks in 18–24 h, returns to nor-

Name of Test	Reference Interval	Purpose of Test	Decreased Indicates	Increased Indicates	Notes
				skeletal muscles, dermatomyositis, muscular dystrophy, hypothyroidism, increased muscular activity. Detectable CK-BB: brain tissue injury, certain widespread malignant tumors, severe shock, renal failure	mal in 3–4 days. IM injection or surgery damages muscle and may elevate CPK-MM and total CPK, confounding results (Lee and Hayes, 1990)
Creatinine	0.4–1.9 mg/dL (Caird, 1973) 0.7–1.7 mg/dL (Jernigan, 1980) 0.6–1.2 mg/dL	Assess renal glomerular filtration, screen for kidney damage. Creatinine clearance is considered before prescribing medications that are excreted by the kidney (Hering and Carlson, 1982)		Renal disease that has damaged more than half of nephrons, gigantism, acromegaly, diabetic nephropathy, renal insufficiency	More sensitive than BUN. Elderly may have normal values even when have disease. Lean body mass decreases in elderly, leading to decrease daily creatinine production, which may overestimate renal function. (Beers and Besdine, 1987). Creatinine clearance may be estimated with following equation:

$$\text{Creatinine clearance (mL/min)} = \frac{(140 - \text{age})(\text{body weight in kg})}{(72)(\text{serum creatinine in mg/dL})}$$

(Continued)

TABLE 9–1 (Continued)

Name of Test	Reference Interval	Purpose of Test	Decreased Indicates	Increased Indicates	Notes
					Women may have values 15% lower than that calculated with equation due to decreased muscle mass
Ferritin	M: 30–699 μg/L F: 27–392 μg/L (Garry et al, 1983) M: 15–200 μg/L F: 15–150 μg/L	Determine iron status and storage	Chronic iron deficiency, malnutrition, liver disease, nephrotic syndrome, malignancy (Besa, 1988)	Hepatic disease, iron overload, leukemia, acute or chronic infection or inflammation, Hodgkin's disease, chronic hemolytic anemia, chronic renal failure, malignant tumors	Ferritin is an iron storage protein, serum values reflect iron stores
Free thyroxine and free triiodothyronine (FT_4, FT_3)	Varies by lab: FT_4: 0.8–3.3 mg/dL FT_3: 0.2–0.6 mg/dL FT_4 may decrease slightly in elderly (Noth, 1985) FT_4: 0.9–2.3 ng/dL	Measure metabolically active form of thyroid hormones, aid in diagnosis and treatment of hypothyroidism	Decreased FT_4: hypothyroidism except when receiving T_3 replacement therapy	Increase in both: hyperthyroidism, increased FT_3 with low or normal FT_4: T_3 toxicosis	
Gamma glutamyltransferase (GGT) Gamma glutamyltranspeptidase	Varies with method 5–40 IU/L, commonly	Liver enzyme test. Provides information about hepatobiliary diseases, assess liver function, detect alcoholic ingestion, distinguish between skeletal disease and hepatic disease when serum AP is increased		Sharp increase: obstructive jaundice, hepatic metastasis. Increase: any acute hepatic disease, acute pancreatitis, renal disease, prostatic metastasis, postoperative status, alcohol ingestion. Possible increase: epilepsy, brain tumor, acute MI (5–10 days after)	GGT is more sensitive to hepatic necrosis than AST. Very sensitive to alcohol ingestion

Name of Test	Reference Interval	Purpose of Test	Decreased Indicates	Increased Indicates	Notes
Glycosylated hemoglobin, total fasting hemoglobin, glycohemoglobin	5.5–9% (*Diagnostic Tests,* 1987)	Assess long-term diabetic control		Poor diabetic control in preceding 60–90 days	Reflects average blood glucose. Not affected by current metabolic state
Glucose, fasting plasma glucose, fasting blood sugar (FBS)	M: 77–135 mg/dL F: 73–139 mg/dL (O'Kell and Elliott, 1970) M: 52–135 mg/dL F: 58–135 mg/dL (Wilding et al, 1972) 70–110 mg/dL	Screen for diabetes mellitus, monitor drug or dietary therapy for diabetes, indicator of hydration	Hyperinsulinism, insulinoma, Gierke's disease, functional or reactive hypoglycemia, myxedema, adrenal insufficiency, congenital adrenal hyperplasia, hypopituitarism, malabsorption syndrome, hepatic insufficiency	Diabetes mellitus, pancreatitis, recent acute illness, Cushing's syndrome, acromegaly, pheochromocytoma, hyperlipoproteinemia, chronic hepatic disease, nephrotic syndrome, brain tumor, sepsis, dumping syndrome, anoxia, convulsive disorders	Two FBS >140 mg/dL confirms diabetes. The hyperglycemia of aging may be due to decreased insulin biosynthesis and/or secretion, alteration in insulin action, decreased peripheral glucose utilization, changes in diet, decreased physical activity, increased adipose tissue (Trilling, 1990)
Lactic dehydrogenase (LD, LDH)	Total LD: M: 61–200 mU/L F: 71–206 mU/L (O'Kell and Elliott, 1970) LD_1: 17–27% LD_2: 27–37% LD_3: 18–25% LD_4: 3–8% LD_5: 0–5%	Part of cardiac profile and liver function tests. Aid in differential diagnosis of myocardial infarction, pulmonary infarction, hepatic disease, support CK studies, monitor response to some kinds of chemotherapy		Increased total LD: cardiac injury, hemolysis, megaloblastic anemia, advanced malignancy (leukemia, lymphoma). LD_1 greater than LD_2; acute myocardial infarction, necrosis of kidney cortex, advanced metastatic	LD_1 and $_2$: appear in heart, kidneys, RBCs. LD_3: lungs. LD_4 and $_5$: liver, skeletal muscles. LD_1 rises 12–24 h after MI, peaks in 2–5 days, returns to normal in 7–12 days (Lee and Hayes, 1990). LD_6: recently iden-

(Continued)

159

TABLE 9–1 (Continued)

Name of Test	Reference Interval	Purpose of Test	Decreased Indicates	Increased Indicates	Notes
				melanoma, ovarian or testicular cancer. LD_2 and LD_3; leukemia, lymphoma LD_3; lung, pancreatic cancer, and pulmonary infarction. LD_4 and LD_5; malignancies with metastases to liver. LD_5; severe CHF, skeletal muscle injury, hepatoma, prostate cancer, excess muscle activity. Increase in all LD: shock, response to treatment of Burkitt's lymphoma, Ewing's sarcoma, Hodgkin's, and non-Hodgkin's lymphoma (Wolf, 1989)	tified, seems indicative of severe CHF (Wolf, 1989)

Lipoprotein Phenotyping:

Name of Test	Reference Interval	Purpose of Test	Decreased Indicates	Increased Indicates	Notes
Low density lipoprotein (LDL)	< 130 mg/dL = desirable 130–159 mg/dL = borderline ≥ 160 mg/dL = high risk (NCEP, 1988)	Part of lipid profile. To assist in determination of cardiac risk		Increased risk of coronary artery disease	At ≥ 160 mg/dL if coronary artery disease and two risk factors are present or ≥ 190 mg/dL, drug therapy is recommended (NCEP, 1988)

Name of Test	Reference Interval	Purpose of Test	Decreased Indicates	Increased Indicates	Notes
High density lipoprotein (HDL)	>35–40 mg/dL (NCEP, 1988)	Cardiac risk	CHD, diabetes mellitus type I or II, uremia, obesity, smoking, diet high in polyunsaturated fat	Increased HDL is desirable. Alcohol intake, exercise, weight loss increase HDLs	"Good cholesterol" may predict longevity
LDL/HDL ratio	3: acceptable 2: better (NCEP, 1988)	Cardiac risk	Lower risk of cardiac disease	Increased risk of coronary artery disease	May be best overall indicator of risk (Fehily et al, 1982)
Total lipoproteins	400–800 mg/dL				
Osmolality	280–295 mOsm/L	Hydration status	Excess body fluids in vessels from overhydration or hypervolemia	>295 mOsm/L indicates fluid loss, hemoconcentration, dehydration, hypovolemia	Osmolality can be calculated using other lab values:

$$\text{Serum osmolality} = \text{serum sodium} \times 2 + \frac{\text{BUN}}{3} + \frac{\text{glucose}}{20}$$

Name of Test	Reference Interval	Purpose of Test	Decreased Indicates	Increased Indicates	Notes
Oral glucose tolerance test (OGTT)	Peaks 180–200 mg/100 mL in 1–2 h, declines slowly	Confirm diabetes mellitus in some cases, aid diagnosis of hypoglycemia, malabsorption syndrome	Normal until 2 h after glucose load then decreased: insulin shock, spontaneous hypoglycemia, hypoadrenalism. Little response to glucose: pituitary deficiency, myxedema	Sustained elevated glucose test confirms diabetes mellitus. Also increased in myasthenia gravis, brain injury, Cushing's syndrome, hemochromatosis	Currently considered superfluous in diagnosis of diabetes mellitus (ADA, 1988)

(Continued)

TABLE 9–1 (Continued)

Name of Test	Reference Interval	Purpose of Test	Decreased Indicates	Increased Indicates	Notes
Potassium (K+)	M: 3.7–5.6 mmol/L F: 3.5–5.3 mmol/L (Wilding et al, 1972) 3.0–5.9 mmol/L (Jernigan, 1980) 3.8–5.0 mEq/L	Part of cardiac profile. Evaluate clinical signs of electrolyte imbalance, monitor renal function, acid-base balance, and glucose metabolism, evaluate neuromuscular and endocrine disorders, detect origin of dysrhythmias	Aldosteronism, Cushing's syndrome, loss of body fluids, excess licorice ingestion are causes of hypokalemia. Hypokalemia can cause dysrhythmias. ECG also used to diagnose potassium imbalances. Flat or inverted T waves are indicative of low K+ (Lee and Hayes, 1990)	Burns, crushing injuries, diabetic ketoacidosis, MI, renal failure, Addison's disease caused hyperkalemia. Peaked T waves on ECG are indicators of hyperkalemia (Lee and Hayes, 1990)	K+ is major intracellular cation. K+ is included in cardiac profile because levels <2.5 mmol or >7 mmol could result in cardiac arrest (Lee and Hayes, 1990)
Prostate specific antigen	0.1–2.6 mg/mL (Oesterling, 1991)	Detect prostatic cancer		Increase with prostatic cancer. Temporary increases with: prostatic hypertrophy, recent digital rectal examinations, cystoscopic examinations, prostate needle biopsy, transurethral resection	PSA may not be present in all types of prostatic cancer. Its usefulness as a screening tool is still undergoing study (Oesterling, 1991)
Protein Electrophoresis					
Total serum protein	6.0–7.8 g/dL Slight decrease with age (Andreson, 1989)	Aid diagnosis of hepatic disease, protein deficiency, blood dyscrasias, renal disorders, GI and neoplastic disorders	Malnutrition, GI disease, blood dyscrasias, essential hypertension, Hodgkin's disease, uncontrolled diabetes, malabsorption, hepatic	Dehydration, vomiting, diarrhea, diabetic acidosis, fulminating and chronic infections, multiple myeloma, monocytic leukemia,	

Name of Test	Reference Interval	Purpose of Test	Decreased Indicates	Increased Indicates	Notes
			dysfunction, nephrosis, surgical and traumatic shock, severe burns, hemorrhage, hyperthyroidism, benzene and carbon tetrachloride poisoning, CHF, chronic infections	chronic inflammatory disease	
Albumin	M: 3.5–4.7 g/dL F: 3.7–4.6 g/dL (Wilding et al, 1972) 53% 3.2–4.5 g/dL	See above	Malnutrition, nephritis, nephrosis, diarrhea, burns, hepatic disease, Hodgkin's disease, hypogammaglobulinemia, peptic ulcer disease, acute cholecystitis, sarcoidosis, collagen diseases, systemic lupus erythematosus, rheumatoid arthritis, essential hypertension, metastatic cancer, hyperthyroidism	Multiple myeloma	Albumin maintains oncotic pressure, transports many substances including drugs. Decrease with age probably due to decrease liver function (See Fretwell, Chp. 8)
Globulins	2.0–4.1 g/dL (Leask et al, 1973) Up to 60% (Diagnostic Tests, 1987) 2.3–3.5 g/dL	See above, also immune system function	Varies with neoplastic and renal disease, hepatic dysfunction, and blood dyscrasias. Gamma globulins are increased in multiple myeloma	Chronic syphilis, tuberculosis, multiple myeloma, collagen diseases, systemic lupus erythematosus, rheumatoid arthritis, diabetes, Hodgkin's disease, subacute bacterial endocarditis	Alpha and beta globulins transport lipids, hormones and metals; gamma function as immunoglobulins

(Continued)

TABLE 9–1 (Continued)

Name of Test	Reference Interval	Purpose of Test	Decreased Indicates	Increased Indicates	Notes
Sodium (Na)	M: 134.0–146.6 mmol/L F: 134.7–146.8 mmol/L (Wilding et al, 1972) 135–146 mmol/L (Caird, 1973) 136–142 mEq/L	Evaluate fluid-electrolyte balance and acid–base balance. Assess related neuromuscular, renal and adrenal function	Inadequate sodium intake, excess sodium loss: prolonged sweating, GI suctioning, diuretic therapy, diarrhea, vomiting, adrenal insufficiency, burns, chronic renal insufficiency with acidosis	Inadequate water intake, excess sodium intake, water loss in excess of sodium: diabetes insipidus, impaired renal function, prolonged hyperventilation and occasionally severe vomiting or diarrhea. Sodium retention such as in aldosteronism	Must be interpreted in light of water balance. Na is major extracellular cation, maintains osmotic pressure for extracellular fluid. Influences K + and CI − levels. Absorbed by intestines, excreted by kidneys
Thyroid-stimulating hormone (TSH) Thyrotropin	0–15 μU/mL <5 μU/mL indicates adequate thyroid replacement (Noth, 1985). Up to 20 μU/mL may be normal (Feit, 1988) 0.5–5 μU/mL	Distinguish between primary and secondary hypothyroidism, confirm or rule out primary hypothyroidism, monitor drug therapy	Occasionally secondary to hypothyroidism, hyperthyroidism, thyroiditis. Undetectable TSH is considered normal	>20 μU/mL indicates primary hypothyroidism, endemic goiter. Slight increases are seen in euthyroid patients with thyroid cancer	Secreted by anterior pituitary through thyrotropin-releasing factor. TSH stimulates release of T_3 and T_4
Thyroxine (T_4)	5–13.5 μg/dL. Small decrease (Noth, 1985) or no change (Feit, 1988) 5.5–12.5 μg/dL	Evaluate thyroid function and aid diagnosis of hyperand hypothyroidism, monitor, replacement therapy	Primary or secondary hypothyroidism, T_4 suppression by normal, elevated, or replacement levels of T_3. Chronic illness (Feit, 1988)	Primary or secondary hyperthyroidism, including overreplacement therapy	FT_4, T_4, and TSH are required to diagnose hypothyroid states
Transferrin (siderophilin)	250–390 μg/dL of which 65–170 μg/dL are bound to iron (30% saturated). Decreases with age (Vogel, 1980)	Determine iron-transporting capacity of blood, evaluate iron metabolism in iron deficiency anemia	Hepatic damage, renal disease with extensive protein loss, acute or chronic infection, cancer, anemia, chronic disease	Severe iron deficiency	Formed in liver, it is a beta globulin, one of the serum proteins

Name of Test	Reference Interval	Purpose of Test	Decreased Indicates	Increased Indicates	Notes
			(infections, renal insufficiency, collagen vascular disease, malignancy)		
T_3, T_3 resin uptake, resin triiodothyronine uptake (T_3RU)	Mean in elderly: 2.2 ng/dL (Feit, 1988); 25–30% of radioactive T_3 binds to resin; 10–20% decrease in healthy elderly (Noth, 1985); 25–38%	Aid diagnosis of hypothyroidism when thyrobinding globulin (TBG) levels are normal. Aid in diagnosis of primary disorders of TBG levels	With a low T_4: hypothyroidism. With normal or increased FT_4 suggests increased TBG levels	In presence of high T_4: hyperthyroidism. With low or normal FT_4 suggests decreased TBG levels as in nephrotic syndrome, androgen excess, some medications	
Triglycerides	10–190 mg/dL; <250 mg/dL = low risk; 250–500 mg/dL = borderline risk; >500 mg = true hypertriglyceridemia (Avins et al, 1989); 38–345 mg/dL (Jernigan, 1980); 10–190 mg/dL	Part of the lipid profile. Screen for hyperlipidemia, help identify nephrotic syndrome, risk of coronary artery disease	Malnutrition, abetalipoproteinemia	Along with increased serum cholesterol, increases risk of coronary artery disease. Also biliary obstruction, diabetes, nephrotic syndrome, endocrinopathies, overconsumption of alcohol. Levels >1000 mg/dL indicate chylomicronemia	Both endogenous and exogenous sources exist. Values for women increase with age
Uric acid	M: 2.6–9.2 mg/dL; F: 1.9–8.5 mg/dL (O'Kell and Elliott, 1970); 3.1–7.9 mg/dL (Caird, 1973); M: 4.0–8.5 mg/dL; F: 2.7–7.3 mg/dL	Confirm diagnosis of gout, help detect kidney dysfunction	Acute hepatic nephropathy	Gout, impaired renal function, CHF, Gierke's disease, infections, hemolytic anemia, polycythemia, neoplasms, psoriasis	End product of purine metabolism, it is filtered in glomerulus and secreted by tubules. Thiazide diuretics are common cause of increase in

(Continued)

TABLE 9–1 *(Continued)*

Name of Test	Reference Interval	Purpose of Test	Decreased Indicates	Increased Indicates	Notes
					elderly. More than one test should be used to diagnose gout (Lee and Hayes, 1990)
Vitamin B_{12}	M: 136–807.5 pg/mL F: 120–712.5 pg/mL (Dybkaer et al, 1981) *160–950 pg/mL*	Distinguish forms of anemia	Strict vegetarian diet, GI malabsorption due to lack of intrinsic factor or loss of ileum		Schilling test may further differentiate cause of B_{12} deficiency
URINALYSIS					
Bacteria	*None*			Contamination (usually more than one organism), urinary tract infection. In the past $>10^5$ colony forming units/mL was considered significant for infection, but $>10^2$ CFU/mL has been shown to have sensitivity and specificity (Stamm et al, 1982)	10–50% of elderly have asymptomatic bacteriuria, which returns after treatment and rarely progresses to sepsis or decreased renal function (Beers and Besdine, 1987). Compare with blood and fecal tests
Bilirubin	*None*	To help identify causes of jaundice		Extrahepatic obstruction hepatocellular disorders, hepatocanalicular disorders, or intrahepatic obstruction	Destroyed by light. Must be tested in 10–30 minutes

166

Name of Test	Reference Interval	Purpose of Test	Decreased Indicates	Increased Indicates	Notes
Glucose	No glucose (Beers and Besdine, 1987) None	Detect glycosuria, monitor urine glucose. See note		Diabetes mellitus. Glycosuria can also occur in renal and thyroid disorders, hepatic disease, CNS disorders, conditions with low renal threshold, toxic renal tubular disease, heavy metal poisoning, glomerulonephritis, nephrosis, hyperalimentation, some medications	Unreliable for use in monitoring glycemic status due to variability of aged kidney reabsorption of glucose and altered renal blood flow (Beers and Besdine, 1987)
Ketones	No ketones (Beers and Besdine, 1987) None	Screen ketonuria, identify diabetic ketoacidosis and carbohydrate deprivation, distinguish between diabetic and nondiabetic coma, monitor diabetes and ketogenic weight reduction		Uncontrolled Type I diabetes, starvation, metabolic complications of hyperalimentation	
Leukocytes	0–4 HPF None			Urinary tract infection, kidney infection	If combined with bacteria and symptoms, treatment is recommended (Beers and Besdine, 1987)
pH	4.5–8.0	H + concentration of urine	Acidic: renal tuberculosis, pyrexia, phenylketonuria, acidosis	Alkalotic: urinary tract infection, metabolic or respiratory acidosis	

(Continued)

TABLE 9-1 *(Continued)*

Name of Test	Reference Interval	Purpose of Test	Decreased Indicates	Increased Indicates	Notes
Protein	0–1+ (up to 150 mg/24 h) (Shapiro et al, 1978; Beers and Besdine, 1987) *Negative*	Aid diagnosis of pathological states characterized by proteinuria, primarily renal disease		<0.5g/24 h indicates renal disease such as chronic pyelonephritis, 0.5–4 g/24 h indicates glomerulonephritis, amyloidosis, toxic nephropathies, renal failure from chronic illness such as CHF, diabetes >4g/24 h: nephrotic syndrome	Proteinuria is common in elderly, may be renal pathology or subclinical urinary tract infections (Dybkaer et al, 1981)
Specific gravity	1.005–1.020 Lower maximum in elderly 1.016–1.022		Diabetes insipidus, acute tubular necrosis, pyelonephritis, fluid excess	Nephrotic syndrome, dehydration, acute glomerulonephritis, CHF, liver failure, shock	Fixed specific gravity regardless of intake indicates chronic glomerulonephritis with severe renal damage

References and Other Readings

Abramson WG, Berkow R, eds. Merck manual of geriatrics. Rahway, NJ: Merck Sharp and Dohme Research Laboratories,1990.

American Diabetes Association. Physician's guide to non-insulin dependent (Type II) diabetes: diagnosis and treatment (2nd ed). Alexandria VA: American Diabetes Assoc., 1988 pp. 1–11.

Andreson GP. A fresh look at assessing the elderly. RN 1989; 52:28.

Araki K, Rifkind JM. Age-dependent changes in osmotic hemolysis of human erythrocytes. J Gerontol 1980; 35:499.

Avins AL, Haber RJ, Hulley SB. The status of hypertriglyceridemia as a risk factor for coronary heart disease. Clin Lab Med 1989; 9:153.

Beers M, Besdine R. Medical assessment of the elderly patient. Clin Geriatr Med 1987; 3:17.

Besa E. Approach to mild anemia in the elderly. Clin Geriatr Med 1988; 4:43.

Brenner M, Welliver J. Pulmonary and acid–base assessment. Nurs Clin North Am 1990; 25:761.

Butts W, Lilje D. Clinically significant reference intervals. Am J Med Technol 1982; 48:587.

Caird FI. Problems of interpretation of laboratory findings in the old. Br Med J 1973; 4:348.

Casale G, deNicola P. Circadian rhythms in the aged: a review. Arch Gerontol Geriatr 1984; 3:267.

Chan-Yeung M, et al. The effects of age, smoking and alcohol on routine laboratory tests. Am J Clin Pathol 1981; 75:320.

Craig JL, Bartholomew MD. Blood profile ranges by age decades in 7,337 male employees. In: Advances in automated analysis, vol III, Technicon International Congress, 1969, pp. 105–114. White Plains, NY, Mediad Inc, 1970. (7,337 male employees of the Tennessee Valley Authority)

Diagnostic tests handbook. Springhouse, PA: Springhouse Corp, 1987.

Dybkaer R, Lauritzen M, Krakauer R. Relative reference values for clinical chemical and hematological quantities in "healthy" elderly people. Acta Med Scand 1981; 209:1.

Fehily AM, et al. Dietary determinants of lipoproteins, total cholesterol, viscosity, fibrinogen and blood pressure. Am J Clin Nutr 1982; 36:890.

Feit H. Thyroid function in elderly. Clin Geriatr Med 1988; 4:151.

Freedman M, Marcus DL. Anemia and the elderly: is it physiology or pathology? Am J Med Sci 1980; 280:81.

Gallagher JC, et al. The effect of age on serum immunoreactive parathyroid hormone in normal and osteoporotic women. J Lab Clin Med 1980; 95:373.

Gambert S, Duthie EH. Laboratory testing in the elderly. Wis Med J 1983; 82:19.

Garry PJ, et al. Iron status and anemia in the elderly:

new findings and a review of previous studies. J Am Geriatr Soc 1983; 31:389.

Halberg F, Montalbetti N. Chronobiologic specification of reference values. Bull Mol Biol 1983; 8:75.

Harnes JR. Normal values with increasing age. J Chron Dis 1980; 33:593.

Henry JB. Clinical diagnosis and management. 18 ed. Philadelphia: WB Saunders, 1991.

Hering PJ, Carlson RE. Serum creatinine and renal function in the elderly. JAMA 1982; 248:31.

Hirsh J et al. Optimal therapeutic range for oral anticoagulants. Chest 1989; 95:55.

Howe RB. Anemia in the elderly: common causes and suggested diagnostic approach. Postgrad Med 1983; 73:153.

Htoo MS, et al. Erythrocyte parameters in the elderly: an argument against new geriatric normal values. J Am Geriatr Soc 1979; 27:547.

Jernigan JA. Reference values of blood findings in relatively fit elderly persons. J Am Geriatr Soc 1980; 28:308.

Kaplan A, Szabo L. Clinical chemistry: interpretation and techniques. 3rd ed. Philadelphia: Lea & Febiger, 1988.

Kelly A, et al. Patterns of change in selected serum chemical parameters of middle and later years. J Gerontol 1979; 34:37.

Lamb JO. Laboratory Tests for Clinical Nursing Bowie, MD: Robert Brady Co., 1983.

Lamy PP. Cholesterol: the beginning of a crusade. Center for Study of Pharmacy and Therapeutics for Elderly. Baltimore: University of Maryland, 1989.

Leask RGS, et al. Normal values of sixteen blood constituents in the elderly. Age Ageing 1973; 2:14.

Lee JL, Hayes ER. Assessment of patient laboratory data in the acutely ill. Nurs Clin North Am 1990; 25:751.

Lott JA, Stang JM. Differential diagnosis of patients with abnormal serum creatine kinase isoenzymes. Clin Lab Med 1989; 9:627.

Miale JB, ed: Laboratory medicine—hematology. 6th ed. St Louis: CV Mosby, 1982.

Moore-Ede MC, Czeisler CA, Richardson GS. Circadian timekeeping in health and disease. Part 2. Clinical implications of circadian rhythmicity. N Engl J Med 1983; 309:530.

National Cholesterol Education Program Expert Panel on Detection, Evaluation and Treatment of High Blood Cholesterol in Adults. Arch Intern Med 1988; 148:36.

National Heart, Lung and Blood Institute Consensus Development Panel. Treatment of hypertriglyceridemia. JAMA 1984; 251:1196.

Noth RH, Mazzaferri EL. Age and the endocrine system. Clin Geriatr Med 1985; 1:2232.

Oesterling JE. Prostate specific antigen: a critical assessment of the most useful tumor marker for adenocarcinoma of the prostate. J of Urol 1991; 145:907.

O'Kell RT, Elliott JR. Development of normal values for use in multitest biochemical screening of sera. Clin Chem 1970; 16:161.

Rej R. Aminotransferases in disease. Clin Lab Med 1989; 9:667.

Roben NJ, Kent DL, FIhn SD. Management of warfarin anticoagulation. Med Rounds 1990; 63.

Rock RC. Interpreting laboratory tests—a basic approach. Geriatrics 1984; 39:49.

Sharland DE. Erythrocyte sedimentation rate: the normal range in the elderly. J Am Geriatr Soc 1980; 28:346.

Sie P, et al. Evaluation of some platelet parameters in a group of elderly people. Thromb Haemost 1981; 45:197.

Silinsky JJ. What you can learn from the platelet count. RN 1985.

Stamm LE, et al. Diagnosis of coliform infection in actuely ill dysuric women. N Engl J Med 1982; 307:463.

Steel K. Evaluation of the geriatric patient. In: Reichel W, ed. Clinical aspects of aging. Baltimore: Williams & Wilkins, 1978.

Sunderman FW. Current concepts of "normal values," "references values," and "discrimination values" in clinical chemistry. Clin Chem 1975; 21:1873.

Thompson RB. A short textbook of hematology. 6th ed. Philadelphia: Pitman Medical Publishing, 1989.

Tietz NW. Clinical guide to laboratory tests. 2nd ed. Philadelphia: WB Saunders, 1990.

Trilling JS. Screening for non-insulin dependent diabetes mellitus in the elderly. Clin Geriatr Med 1990; 6:839.

Vestal RE, Dawson GW. Pharmacology and aging. In: Finch CE, Schneider EL, eds. Handbook of the biology of aging. 2nd ed. New York: Van Nostrand Reinhold, 1985; 744–819.

Vogel JM. Hematologic problems of the aged. Mt Sinai J Med 1980; 47:150.

Wilding P, Rollason JG, Robinson D. Patterns of change for various biochemical constituents detected in well population screening. Clin Chim Acta 1972; 41:375.

Williams WJ. Hematology in the aged. In: Williams WJ, et al, eds. Hematology. 4th ed. New York: McGraw-Hill, 1990.

Wintrobe M. Clinical hematology. 8th ed. Philadelphia: Lea & Febiger, 1981.

Wolf PL. Lactate dehydrogenase isoenzymes in myocardial disease. Clin Lab Med 1989; 9:655.

Zaino E. Blood counts in the nonagenarian. NY State J Med 1981; 81:1199.

10
Medications and the Elderly

CYNTHIA P. WHITE

Age-related changes in physiology and chronic disease states affect how medications act. This creates some special concerns about the older person taking both prescribed and over-the-counter medications. The available literature and clinical observations offer limited information on differences in medication efficacy and safety in the elderly. Clinical experience, however, indicates that the elderly do not respond to drug therapy in the same manner as younger adults. Based on current knowledge, there are some guidelines that can be used in working with elderly persons and their medication regimens.

Drug Use in the Elderly

PRESCRIPTION MEDICATIONS

The elderly account for about 35% of retail expenditures on prescription drugs and 40% of nonprescription drugs while representing only 12% of the population (Simpson, 1991). In 1987 at a symposium at Rutgers University it was estimated that persons 65 and older use 400 million prescriptions per year, filling twice as many as those under age 65. Others state 4.35 billion drugs are prescribed each year for the elderly (Simpson, 1991).

Most drugs prescribed are for cardiovascular conditions, 65% of all drugs used nationally. Another study reported cardiovascular drugs were

prescribed most, with central nervous system drugs second and analgesics third (Jones, 1989).

Ambulatory elderly persons living at home were found to use an average of two to four prescription drugs regularly (Hale et al, 1979; Cooper et al, 1982; Eberhardt and Robinson, 1979; Ostrom et al, 1985). Those residing in long-term care facilities receive even more medications than do persons living at home. In one study nursing home residents had from 7.9 to 10 drugs prescribed (Patrick, 1991). Other studies report 2.5 to 3.6 drugs prescribed.

NONPRESCRIPTION MEDICATIONS

Nonprescription over-the-counter drug use is common among the elderly (Knapp and Knapp, 1980; Baum et al, 1983). This self-medication trend is increasing because drugs that were formerly available by prescription only have been approved by the Food and Drug Administration for over-the-counter distribution (Simpson, 1991).

Pharmacokinetics and Pharmacodynamics

Physiologic changes that can affect therapeutics in the elderly do so in one of three ways:

1. The physiologic changes can affect drug action in the body (pharmacokinetics).

2. The changes can affect the ultimate effects of the drug once it reaches the receptor and acts (pharmacodynamics).
3. The changes can affect the adherence to a drug regimen. This includes a complex set of factors, such as remembering to take the drug and being able to swallow it.

PHARMACOKINETICS AND CHANGES WITH AGING

The Food and Drug Administration is beginning to move toward asking drug manufacturers to use elderly patients when they test drugs (American Pharmacy, 1984). However, the Food and Drug Administration is currently proposing publication of additional labeling requirements to include information on geriatric use under the precautionary category of the package insert required with each legend medication (Simpson, 1991). Studies in elderly persons are increasing, but most studies consist of comparisons of a group of young persons with a group of older persons, or patient selection may be biased by choosing a small number of elderly patients and including only those in good health, with no demonstrated evidence of cardiac, pulmonary, renal, or liver disease (Zaske and Hunter, 1985). This provides valuable information, but does not explain completely the changes associated with aging. The aging process involves continual functional and morphologic changes. The differences are not at the resting level of performance, but are in the body's ability to respond to stress (Abrass, 1988). Homeostatic mechanisms that control such functions as body temperature, electrolyte balance, pH, and osmotic processes show little change during the life span but the ability to recover from such metabolic imbalances slows dramatically.

With the physiologic changes of aging, there are changes in the manner in which the body handles drugs. Depending on the individual drug, there may be profound differences between young and old persons and in those elderly with chronic disease states and multiple medication use. Pharmacokinetics offers some explanations for the different responses and adverse effects. Pharmacokinetics is the study of the following:

Absorption: how the drug gets into the body
Distribution: where the drug goes in the body
Metabolism: how the drug is handled in the body
Excretion: how the drug is removed from the body (Table 10-1)

ABSORPTION

Absorption is the process by which a drug gets from the external environment into the body. Although most drug absorption takes place in the gastrointestinal tract since most drugs are taken by mouth, they can also be absorbed across the skin, through the lung, through the vaginal and rectal mucosa, and from the eye.

Alterations with Aging   With drugs taken by mouth there are a number of changes in the aging gastrointestinal tract that have the potential to affect absorption. Gastric pH increases, and there may be prolongation of gastric emptying (Evans et al, 1981). There is also some decrease in blood flow to the gastrointestinal tract (Mayersohn, 1982).

Some drugs and nutrients have been shown to have decreased absorption with age. These include calcium, iron, thiamine, and vitamin B_{12}. These nutrients are, however, absorbed by active processes, whereas most drugs are absorbed by passive diffusion (Vestal, 1990).

From the information so far available, for most drugs, there does not seem to be any significant difference in the rate or extent of absorption or in the time for maximal drug concentration to occur in the body (Plein and Plein, 1981). There is little evidence that the aging process alone has a significant effect on absorption (Henney, 1985).

DRUG DISTRIBUTION

Drug distribution is the process by which drugs move from the circulation system out into the tissues. Volume of distribution is a pharmacokinetic term that is not a physiologic parameter but is a theoretical means of describing how widely the drug is distributed throughout the body.

$$\text{Volume of distribution} = \frac{\text{Total amount of drug in the body}}{\text{Drug concentration in plasma}}$$

The volume of distribution of a drug is primarily dependent on lipid solubility, tissue binding, and plasma protein binding affinity.

Alterations with Aging   Factors that can affect the distribution of drugs are altered in aging. Since the volume of distribution of a drug is influenced by its ability to dissolve in adipose tissue as well as its binding to tissues at its site of action and complexation with plasma proteins, the changes in body composition as aging occurs significantly affect how medica-

TABLE 10–1 *Factors Affecting Drug Distribution in the Aging Process*

Pharmacokinetic Parameter	Age-related Physiologic Changes	Pathologic Conditions
Absorption	Increased gastric pH Decreased absorptive surface Decreased splanchnic blood flow Decreased gastrointestinal motility Decreased active transport Decreased gastric acid secretion	Achlorhydria Diarrhea Gastrectomy Malabsorption syndromes Pancreatitis
Distribution	Decreased cardiac output* Decreased total body water Decreased lean body mass Increased body fat	Congestive heart failure Dehydration Edema or ascites Malnutrition Renal failure
Metabolism	Decreased hepatic mass Decreased enzyme activity Decreased hepatic blood flow	Congestive heart failure Fever Hepatic insufficiency Malignancy Malnutrition Thyroid disease
Excretion	Decreased renal blood flow Decreased glomerular filtration rate* Decreased tubular secretion	Hypovolemia Renal insufficiency Dehydration Congestive heart failure Hypertension Atherosclerotic disease

*There is not agreement that these changes are age related.
Adapted from Schneider E, Rowe J (eds.). Handbook of biology of aging, 3rd ed. San Diego: Academic Press, 1990.

tions respond. Although total body weight remains relatively constant, aging brings a significant change in the weight of adipose (fat) tissue, with increases from about 14% to 30% of total body weight (Lamy, 1980). At the same time there is a loss of lean body mass (i.e., muscle tissue) of 25% to 30%. Because of these changes in percentage of body fat and a decrease in lean body mass, there are also changes in total body water by approximately 17% (see Chapter 8). Drugs that are highly water soluble decrease in volume of distribution because there is a greater concentration of drug in the plasma due to the decreased volume; however, the total amount of drug in the body remains unchanged. There is also a decrease in plasma concentrations of drugs that are highly fat soluble because the drug is absorbed in the fatty tissue, with a decrease in the volume of distribution. Composition changes in the body during the aging process cause resulting decreases in the volume of distribution for drugs that are distributed in body water and increases in volume for fat-soluble drugs. One would expect to see higher blood levels of water-soluble drugs and lower blood levels of fat-soluble drugs in the elderly (Mitchard, 1979).

The primary protein to which drugs bind in the plasma is albumin (Gibaldi, 1977). The total amount of protein in serum does not change significantly with age but the albumin/globulin ratio decreases with increasing age (see Chapter 8). After drugs enter the body and are distributed, they may attach to plasma and tissue proteins in such a way as to form a drug-protein complex. The two fit together like a lock and key and the bond created is reversible. The strength of the bond depends on the affinity of the medication for the protein.

Drug + protein ⇄ drug-protein complex

Albumin concentration is one of the factors determining how much of the drug will be bound to protein and how much will be unbound or free. A bound drug remains attached to protein and cannot cross membranes, whereas the free drug is available to diffuse out of the circulation and into the tissues to the various sites of action. It is this unbound, free drug that is pharmacologically active.

Changes in drug binding are most significant for highly protein-bound drugs (>90% protein bound). For example, warfarin is about 97% protein bound and with a decrease in serum albumin this leads to increases in free drug that is pharmacologically active to exert anticoagulant effects. Therefore, not only is it important to monitor this medication by evaluations of the prothrombin time, but determination of serum albumin should be done as well to help determine appropriate dosages. *Drug blood levels determined in laboratories generally measure total drug in the blood, both bound and free. In the elderly, the percentage of free drug may be significantly elevated for highly protein-bound drugs, increasing the risk of drug toxicity, even at therapeutic blood levels* (Greenblatt et al, 1982). For example, a formula has been developed for phenytoin, a highly protein-bound drug that is used to normalize and correct the observed drug levels based on the actual serum albumin.

$$C_{nl} = \frac{C_{obs}}{0.9 \times (alb/4.4) + 0.1}$$

C_{obs} = measured phenytoin concentration
C_{nl} = normalized phenytoin concentration
alb = serum albumin in g/100 mL

DRUG METABOLISM

Drug metabolism is the process by which drugs are chemically changed by enzymes. Most drug metabolism takes place in the liver, although there are other sites, such as the gastrointestinal tract and bloodstream. Although metabolism is often considered as a way to end drug action, some drugs have metabolites that also are active in the same way as the parent drug. There are also drugs that are not themselves active but are metabolized by the body into active compounds.

Alterations with Aging   Both the mass of the liver itself as well as its proportion of the body mass decrease with age. Regional blood flow to the liver also decreases (Geokas and

Haverback, 1969). Liver metabolism is divided into two main categories. Phase I is a preparative biotransformation reaction and phase II is a synthetic biotransformation reaction. In phase I reactions a compound is primarily made more water soluble and the metabolic activity of the parent compound is often retained (Sjoqvist and Alvan, 1983). Most tests of hepatic function, such as SGOT, SGPT, alkaline phosphatase, and total serum bilirubin are not changed with aging (see Chapter 9). There are some studies that suggest that the metabolizing capability of liver enzymes decreases with age, although the effect of age may be only one of many factors (Vestal and Dawson, 1984). The decrease in liver blood flow with age does appear to affect the metabolism of some drugs such as propranolol (Vestal and Wood, 1980). Cigarette smoking, which stimulates liver metabolism of some drugs, seems to have less effect in elderly people than in those who are younger (Vestal and Dawson, 1984). Neither a prolonged half-life nor a decreased clearance in elderly people can be consistently shown for drugs that are metabolized by the liver. At the present, there are no simple generalizations that can be made about the effects of aging on drug metabolism.

DRUG EXCRETION

After a drug is absorbed and has reached its site of action and produced the desired effect, there must be a way of eliminating it from the body. Clearance is another pharmacokinetic term that describes the elimination of a drug from the body. A drug is usually cleared from the body by liver metabolism, then it can be renally excreted. *Body clearance* is defined in terms of the volume of plasma or blood from which drug is completely removed per unit of time. *Half-life* defines the amount of time it takes to reduce the amount of drug in the body by 50%. With the changes of aging in liver metabolism and renal excretion, there is decreased drug clearance, leading to an increase in the half-life of a drug.

RENAL EXCRETION

Renal excretion is the process by which a drug is transferred from the circulation into the urine. The kidney can excrete both unchanged drug and active and inactive drug metabolites.

Alterations with Aging Glomerular filtration rate, creatinine clearance, and renal blood flow all decrease with age. Creatinine is a by-product of muscle and since in aging there is a decrease in lean body mass (muscle tissue) there is decreased production of creatinine. Therefore, in the elderly, corrections must be made based on various factors to accurately use creatinine clearance as a measure of renal function. Serum creatinine may remain normal in an elderly person even with significant declines in creatinine clearance and renal function (see Chapter 9). Drugs that are excreted to a significant extent in an unchanged state by the kidney are likely to be excreted more slowly in the elderly (a decreased clearance) and may have an increased half-life (Greenblatt et al, 1982). This is one of the most useful generalizations that can be made about changes with aging. If usual doses are given to elderly people, they may develop elevated blood levels and, depending on the drug, possible toxicity.

Creatinine clearance is an indicator of change in renal function, but it is not practical to use routinely in patient monitoring since it requires a 24-hour urine sample. Equations and nomograms are available that provide estimates of the person's creatinine clearance from age, sex, weight, and serum creatinine (see Chapters 8 and 9). The following equation can be used to estimate creatinine clearance for a patient with stable renal function (Lott and Hayton, 1978).

$$\frac{(140 - \text{age}) \times \text{lean body weight in kg}}{72 \times \text{serum creatinine}}$$

Comparing the estimated value with the normal value for young adults is a useful reminder of the decline in kidney function with aging. This can also help to identify patients most in need of smaller doses for renally excreted drugs (Gral and Young, 1980).

CHANGES IN PHARMACODYNAMICS WITH AGING

Apparent increases in adverse drug reactions and effects in the elderly can be explained by investigating pharmacokinetic changes. Reduced weight and age are risk factors for drug reactions at too high a dose. Elderly patients may have more adverse effects because they do not excrete drugs as effectively as young persons and thus are more likely to have higher drug levels if an average dose is given. However, age alone is not a cause for more drug reactions. There are not necessarily more adverse drug reactions in older people than in younger ones.

Another approach to understanding drug reactions is through the perspective of pharmacodynamics. This approach suggests that for some drugs, a given blood level or amount of drug at the site of action leads to a greater effect in elderly persons than in those who are younger. If the usual dose is given to an elderly person, the person may develop elevated blood levels and possible toxicity. The elderly are more susceptible to both therapeutic and toxic effects of drugs. Some studies suggest that elderly persons are more sensitive to the effects of certain antianxiety agents and sleeping medications (Plein and Plein, 1981). This hypothesis of increased sensitivity of the elderly to some drugs has found some support in clinical impressions; however, it is difficult to study. It could be a factor for certain drugs.

EFFECTS OF PATHOLOGY ON PHARMACOKINETICS

In addition to pharmacokinetic changes that take place as a result of normal, healthy aging, one must also consider the effects of pathology. Since chronic diseases are so prevalent in the elderly, their effects on pharmacokinetics must also be taken into account (see box on p. 176).

Drug Absorption Alterations Congestive heart failure leading to gastrointestinal edema and a decrease in blood flow to the gastrointestinal tract may cause a decrease in absorption of some drugs. Absorption may also be decreased in persons who have had bowel resections and changes in gastric emptying time (Mayersohn, 1982).

Alterations in the gastrointestinal tract in which insertion of an enteral feeding tube has become necessary will alter drug absorption. It is also necessary to consider the changes in bioavailability of solid versus liquid formulations of medications being used. If no liquid preparation is available, it must be determined how crushing the medication will affect its action. Various disease states and drug–drug interactions can also decrease absorption. The incidence of achlorhydria (decreased production of hydrochloric acid) is ten times greater in

Drugs with Additive Adverse Effects*

GASTROINTESTINAL IRRITATION

Salicylates: aspirin, diflunisal (Dolobid)
Nonsteroidal anti-inflammatory agents: ibuprofen (Motrin, Rufen), naproxen (Naprosyn, Anaprox), fenoprofen (Nalfon), sulindac (Clinoril), indomethacin (Indocin), tolmetin (Tolectin), meclofenamate (Meclomen), phenylbutazone (Butazolidin), piroxicam (Feldene)
Reserpine
Corticosteroids
Potassium chloride
Levodopa (Larodopa, Dopar)

SEDATION

Antihistamines: diphenhydramine (Benadryl), chlorpheniramine, meclizine (Antivert)
Tricyclic antidepressants
Antipsychotic agents
Sedatives, antianxiety agents: e.g., barbiturates, benzodiazepines such as diazepam (Valium), meprobamate
Skeletal muscle relaxants: methocarbamol (Robaxin), carisoprodol (Soma), cyclobenzaprine (Flexeril)
Hypnotics: flurazepam (Dalmane), chloral hydrate, barbiturates
Narcotic analgesics
Cold remedies containing antihistamines
Ethanol

ANTICHOLINERGIC EFFECTS

Antihistamines
Tricyclic antidepressants
Antipsychotic agents, particularly chlorpromazine (Thorazine), thioridazine (Mellaril)
Cold remedies containing antihistamines
Anticholinergic, antiparkinson agents: benztropine (Cogentin), trihexyphenidyl (Artane), procyclidine (Kemadrin), biperiden (Akineton)
Anticholinergic drugs used for gastrointestinal pain: propantheline (Pro-Banthine, Donnatal)

HYPOTENSION, PARTICULARLY POSTURAL HYPOTENSION

Diuretics
Nitrates
Antiadrenergic blood pressure medications: guanethidine (Ismelin),[+] reserpine, clonidine (Catapres), methyldopa (Aldomet)
Tricyclic antidepressants
Antipsychotic agents, particularly chlorpromazine (Thorazine) and thioridazine (Mellaril)
Levodopa (Larodopa, Sinemet)
Captopril (Capoten)
Nifedipine (Procardia)

Note: This is a partial list of drugs having additive adverse effects.
*These additive adverse effects tend to occur when the older person takes two or more medications with similar adverse effects. An additional risk is that some of these drugs appear in combination products and it may be difficult to remember all of the ingredients.
[+] The interaction between guanethidine or clonidine and the tricyclic antidepressants can cause an increase in blood pressure.

the elderly, resulting in decreased absorption of weakly acidic drugs such as barbiturates (Reidenberg, 1980; Gomolin and Chapron, 1983; Lamy, 1980). Drug–drug interactions also lead to decreased absorption of medications and is discussed later in the drug interaction section of this chapter.

Drug Distribution Alterations Albumin concentration can be severely decreased in persons with chronic liver failure, malnutrition, and renal failure. Albumin binding sites may also be altered in persons with renal failure (Wilkinson, 1980).

Drug distribution can be altered by solubility and binding capacity to tissues, but the ability of the heart to efficiently perfuse the liver and kidney will adversely affect drug distribution. As there is a decrease in cardiac output and greater rigidity in the arterial vasculature there is an increase in peripheral vascular resistance. These two factors lead to decreased regional blood flow, causing changes in distribution and clearance of drugs.

Metabolism Alterations Liver disease, especially chronic liver failure, may lead to a decrease in clearance of some drugs metabolized by the liver (Wilkinson, 1980). In some cases the metabolism of a drug in the liver is affected by liver blood flow if it has a high extraction ratio. The degree of the first pass effect also must be considered. In this instance much of the drug is removed by the liver before it can reach its site of action and there must be a dosage adjustment in medication.

Renal Excretion Alterations Renal failure may decrease or severely limit drug excretion with resulting accumulation of parent drugs or toxic metabolites. In addition to changes in renal function, chronic diseases (hypertension, diabetic nephropathy, atherosclerosis, and congestive heart failure) decrease renal excretion of medications by causing changes in glomerular filtration rate, tubular secretion, and a general decrease in renal blood flow.

Drug Misuse and Abuse

Elderly persons who are managing their own medications at home may misuse medication in one or more ways.

SHARING MEDICATIONS

One area that is difficult to estimate is the number of persons who share prescription and nonprescription medications. The underlying rationale for those who share drugs is often the desire to help out a friend by providing something that has, after all, given oneself symptom relief.

HOARDING MEDICATIONS

A related problem is the use of medications that have been prescribed at an earlier time. Saving prescription medications occurs commonly in the elderly (Ascione et al, 1980). There is risk associated with the use of outdated drugs.

SELF-MEDICATION

Persons may also medicate themselves with nonprescription drugs, vitamins, herbal remedies, or home remedies. These practices are not necessarily harmful, but may become so if they prevent the person from seeking or receiving needed medical evaluation and treatment. Although these practices may not be seen as drug therapy, such remedies do have the possibility of aggravating the underlying problem, affecting other current pathology, or interacting with prescribed drug therapy (Knapp and Knapp, 1980). In 1992 there are 57 drugs under consideration for a switch from prescription to over-the-counter status (Siegelman, 1990). They include nonsteroidal anti-inflammatory drugs, H_2 antagonists (cimetidine), new generation antihistamines (Seldane, Hisminal), various medications for the treatment of respiratory and allergic disorders (cromolyn, metaproterenol), and dermatologic products. This trend will lead to greater self-diagnosis and self-treatment.

DRUG STORAGE

Drug storage can be a factor in mismanagement. Many drugs are damaged by moisture, heat, and light. Prescription containers are designed to protect the drug product somewhat; therefore, even moving pills from one bottle to another may make deterioration more likely. The bathroom and kitchen, the two most common sites where drugs are stored in the home, are places where drugs tend to be exposed to changes in heat and moisture and are therefore not good sites for long-term storage of medications.

Mixing of medications in the same container and transfer of medications from one container to another also are problems that may lead to the use of the wrong medications. They become worthless for later use because they can no longer be identified. For the same reason, removal or damage of the label on the container may lead to adverse reactions.

MISUNDERSTANDING OF THE PURPOSE OF THE MEDICATION

A problem that cannot be defined strictly as misuse or abuse of medication is that of taking prescribed medication without understanding its purpose of action. Philosophically, in the past, medical care was sought when the patient needed emergent care; now medical advice is often sought in an effort to maintain health and prevent illness. Lack of medical knowledge by the elderly leaves them at greater risk for misuse of medications. This problem is increasingly likely when there are frequent medication changes such as when the person comes out of the hospital or long-term facility with new medications. But this can happen in ambulatory care as well. A project initiated at the University of Rhode Island College of Pharmacy in 1982 (Larrat, 1990) provides a review of a person's medications and determines the individual's understanding of those being taken. It is known as "the brown bag" prescription evaluation clinic because often medications are brought in to the review site in a brown bag (see Table 10–2).

DUPLICATE MEDICATIONS

Another consequence of ignorance about a medication regimen is an increased risk of taking duplicate medications. The person may take medications from two different containers that contain the same medication or may take pills that look different but contain the same ingredient in different brands. With the increasing availability of generic brands of medications, consumers can easily have medications that are different colors, sizes, and shapes, but contain the same active ingredient and dose (Simonson, 1984). Multiple health care providers and a lack of coordination of medication prescribing can also lead to duplication of medications.

TABLE 10–2   *Noncompliance Problems Identified by the "Brown Bag" Studies*

Lack of sufficient understanding of the medication regimen	19.1%
Over- or underutilization of medications	12.5%
Consumption of outdated medication	8.1%
Adverse effects	8.0%
Confusion due to a change in directions	6.8%
Taking the same medication under more than one name	5.9%
Taking medications improperly	5.6%
Problems due to a drug interaction or contraindication	5.5%
Confused by drugs with names that sound alike	0.6%

Adapted from Larrat EP: Patient's medication errors discovered by "brown bag" study. American Druggist 1990; 206:53.

Compliance

Health care providers tend to expect those who consult them to try to do exactly what they are told. Elderly persons comply as well as younger people with a prescribed regimen. They are, however, being asked to take multiple drugs over longer time spans, so that the problem of compliance is automatically magnified. Age alone is not a reason for noncompliance. Compliance is reduced if three drugs are ordered for someone over 65 (Jones, 1989).

REASONS FOR NONCOMPLIANCE

LACK OF UNDERSTANDING

One cause of noncompliance is lack of comprehension. A lack of knowledge and understanding of general health issues contributes to the misuse of medications. The person or primary caregiver does not understand the prescribed regimen due to a lack of communication by prescribers. There is often reluctance by older individuals to question physicians regarding their medical diagnosis and medications. Frequent alterations in medications, a common situation for many elderly persons, is a factor in misunderstanding the regimen as well.

ADVERSE DRUG REACTIONS

Adverse drug reactions may lead a person to stop taking a drug or to change the schedule of the prescribed medication. People may stop taking a medication or decrease the dose if they perceive no need for the medication, or they may increase the dose if they feel an increased need for the medication (Robinson, 1980; Cooper et al, 1982). The elderly, again, due to a lack of understanding regarding their medical condition and treatment, are less likely to actually report adverse medication effects. They merely stop taking their medications as prescribed or decrease the dosage without telling the prescriber. Patients believe that it is intelligent noncompliance to reduce the dose if there are adverse effects.

SCHEDULING DIFFICULTIES

Difficulties in scheduling times to take medications may be a cause of noncompliance for some persons, especially if there are multiple medications with different or conflicting schedules. Persons of all ages routinely alter dosing regimens to fit in with their own daily schedules (Weintraub, 1984). Health care workers do not bother to ask a patient about his normal eating or sleeping times and so create scheduling problems.

COST

The cost of medications may be a major factor in compliance because for many elderly people prescription medication is a large part of the monthly budget. Older persons may omit doses of medication to try to "stretch out" a prescription, delay having medications refilled when they run out, or not have prescriptions filled in the first place.

MEMORY DEFICITS

Poor memory is often blamed for noncompliance in the elderly. Although this is certainly the cause at times, most independent elderly persons who choose to are able to remember to take medications. It is possible that they may cite memory problems when they are unwilling to mention the real cause for noncompliance, such as cost or adverse effects.

PHYSICAL LIMITATIONS

Some people are physically unable to comply with medication regimens owing to lack of vision, inability to swallow medications, decreased hand strength for opening containers, or lack of strength and flexibility for handling a syringe, eyedroppers, or applying topical medications. Mobility problems may limit access to pharmacies so that the person is unable to refill medications when the current supply has run out.

GUIDELINES FOR ENHANCING COMPLIANCE

To enhance compliance and informed decision making regarding medications, it is important to gather data on problems the person may be having with their medications. Then it is possible to work with the person on ways to overcome the difficulties (see box on pp. 180–181). A review of drug use, including the pharmacist and other members of the health care team, can decrease drug-induced disease and noncompliance, and can inform the person about what to expect and the reactions to be reported (Morse, 1987).

The US Department of Health and Human Services (HHS, 1991) and the US Public Health Service have produced a report emphasizing health promotion and preventative medicine that proposes ways of decreasing medication complications. Three factors that contribute to the risk of avoidable adverse drug reactions are (1) inadequate compliance by patients with prescribed drug therapy; (2) multiple medicine use ("polypharmacy"); and (3) different health care providers prescribing medications for the same patient that interact and produce adverse reactions.

Adverse Drug Reactions

Adverse drug reactions are any undesirable effects that occur when drugs are used in the diagnosis and treatment of disease states. One of the difficulties in working with elderly people who may have multiple diseases is that the person most likely is receiving several drugs. This makes evaluation of adverse drug reactions difficult, since the reported symptoms may come from any of several drug responses or may not be a drug effect at all. Multiple chronic diseases increase the risk of adverse drug effects (Friesen, 1983) as do the psychologic changes of aging. Adverse drug reactions are a significant health problem, with serious consequences. In addition they can be expensive, often requiring return visits to the physician and purchase of

Guidelines to Assist in Effective Medication Taking

Promote under-standing	Offer information in language and manner appropriate to the person. Check understanding and offer information as often as needed
	Have medication prescribers add to the directions what the medications are being used for, e.g., hydrochlorothiazide, 50 mg, take one tablet daily for high blood pressure
Remain alert for adverse drug effects	Give specific information for each drug on signs and symptoms of adverse reactions
	Encourage older person to inform health care personnel if the person thinks he is having these signs and symptoms
	Be particularly observant when new drugs are added or dosages are changed
	Give data on any benefits being experienced from the medication
Simplify the regimen	Work with the older person's daily schedule to determine a feasible pattern for taking medications. Then work with the prescriber to try to fit the prescribed times into this schedule, e.g., taking two tablets twice a day is usually simpler than one tablet four times a day
	Ask the prescriber if any drugs can be eliminated; or if different medications can be taken at the same time
Decrease medication costs	Check the current Medicare manual at the local public library for current policy on payment for medications
	Encourage the older person to discuss cost concerns with prescriber
	Ask the prescriber to write prescriptions for generic forms of the drug; these are cheaper.* (Note, the name, color, and shape of the generic drug may be different from the other medication and this may need to be explained)
	Ask pharmacist if generic brands are available and can be used. If the generic substitution is made, the pharmacist should make sure that the products have bioequivalence. There are some medications such as phenytoin in which the brand name product (Dilantin) exhibits pharmacokinetic and bioavailability differences that can result in subtherapeutic or adverse reactions
	To get the benefit of pharmacy monitoring of medications purchase all prescriptions from one pharmacy
	When new drug therapy is tried, especially if there has been intolerance of such drugs in the past, ask the pharmacist if only a part of the prescription can be dispensed at first to see if it works and is tolerated
Manage physical barriers	Request nonchildproof caps on containers if there is difficulty in opening them. Either prescriber or purchaser may make this request (if, however, there are children in the household, consider the risks to them of accidental poisoning)
Memory aids: lists and calendars	Gather data on the memory system currently being used by the person

Guidelines to Assist in Effective Medication Taking (*Continued*)

	List the drugs to be taken, giving generic name, trade name, dose, description of tablet, and directions and reason taken
	A calendar, kept next to medication containers, can be used by marking off a dose when taken, writing down the dose when taken, or making small pouches from plastic wrap for individual doses and stapling them to a wall calendar
Special containers	Seven-day pill boxes have a lid, are portable and serve well if there are not too many medications
	Mediset containers are 7-day pill boxes with four compartments per day for four different dosing times. Drawbacks: bulky, requires some manual dexterity, and expensive. Useful for persons who are confused about drug regimen since a primary caregiver can fill the box for a week at a time
	Pharmacies may be able to dispense medications in blisterpacks similar to a unit dose. Each dose, individually packaged, has the name and strength of drug and the day and time it is to be taken. Drawbacks: expensive and not widely available
Coding prescription containers	Code container with symbols such as colored dots that indicate number of doses per day
	Wrap a rubber band around the container or turn the container upside down to indicate that the last dose has been taken
	Keep containers in a visible place where the person will see them in connection with the appropriate activity, e.g., leaving the bottle on the table where breakfast is eaten or at the bedside for bedtime medications

*In some states the prescriber can indicate permission for the pharmacist to substitute generic brands, even if the brand name is prescribed.

different medications or possible hospitalization (Williamson and Chopin, 1980).

Unfortunately, adverse drug reactions may be ignored by patients, family, and health care providers because they mimic certain stereotypes of aging. It may be assumed that confusion, falling, drowsiness, dizziness, or weakness are simply the consequences of aging rather than a possible adverse drug reaction. Adverse drug reactions cause 10% to 40% of all general hospital admissions and 16% of all psychiatric hospital admissions. In a recent study of 315 elderly patients admitted to an acute care hospital, 28% were drug related. Adverse drug reactions attributed to 16.8% of admissions and noncompliance with medication regimens accounted for 11.4% (Nananda et al, 1990). Another study found that the most common drugs causing hospital admissions were theophylline, digoxin, warfarin, aspirin, quinidine, furosemide, phenytoin, ibuprofen, verapamil, and procainamide (SASHPADR, 1991).

PERSONS AT RISK

Some risk factors associated with adverse reactions to drugs include being a woman (Domecq, 1980), taking a larger number of drugs (Jue, 1984), a higher drug dosage, a past history of drug reactions (Levy et al, 1980), and impaired renal or hepatic function (Jones, 1989).

Elderly patients in institutions, especially acute care hospitals, are at highest risk for experiencing an adverse reaction (Simonson, 1984). Adverse reactions also may prolong the hospital stay (Williamson and Chopin, 1980).

Certain medications are associated with higher risk of adverse reactions in the elderly. These are discussed in a later section of this chapter.

Several criteria for identifying persons at greater risk for adverse drug effects have been identified (Simonson and Pratt, 1981). These include

Age 75 years or older
Extremely small stature
An excessive number of medications
More than one chronic health condition requiring medication
New symptoms or changes in overall condition after modifications in drug therapy regimen
High-risk medications
Renal cardiac dysfunction

One of the most important contributions that a health care provider can make to an older person's well-being in terms of medications is to have a high index of suspicion about adverse drug reactions. *If one automatically questions whether any new symptoms could be due to drug therapy there is less chance of missing adverse drug effects.*

DRUGS WITH PARTICULAR RISKS FOR ADVERSE REACTIONS

It is tempting to advise health professionals to be cautious with every drug given to elderly persons. The following drugs are listed because (1) they are drugs whose clearance is decreased in the elderly, leading to an increased risk of adverse effects when given at average doses, (2) the elderly seem to be sensitive to the effects of the drug, and (3) the drugs have adverse effects that could be significant for many diseases commonly found in the elderly population. This chart contains some of the drugs used most commonly by elderly persons (see box on p. 183).

Drug Interactions

A drug interaction is the alteration of the effect of one drug by another. The most prevalent cause of altered absorption in the elderly is due to drug–drug interactions. There are a variety of mechanisms by which interactions can occur: there may be interference in the absorption, distribution, metabolism, or excretion of the drug or there may be additive or synergistic effects in drugs that have similar pharmacologic effects.

Drug interactions can be difficult to evaluate. There are a number of potential drug interactions; however, the actual incidence of clinically significant drug interactions identified is much lower (Gouveia and Miller, 1978). Furthermore, many factors affect the severity of a given drug interaction for a particular person. The effect of the drug interaction may be to increase the therapeutic effects of the drug, decrease the effects, or increase the risk of adverse drug reactions.

Elderly persons may be at higher risk for potentially serious drug interactions because they use more medications, they have altered physiology that may change how drugs are handled by the body, they have more chronic diseases, and they have decreased homeostatic mechanisms to adjust readily to drug effects. Older persons are also more likely to be taking medications that the prescribing physician is unaware of, either nonprescription drugs or those prescribed by another physician. They are also more likely to be taking certain medications such as cardiac, diabetic, or antiarthritic drugs that have the potential for serious drug interactions. Table 10–3 (p. 186) and its accompanying chart contain a list of some of the significant drug interactions.

Approaches to Drug Therapy in Elderly Persons

Guidelines for health care providers for optimizing drug therapy and minimizing problems follow.

1. Know the drug prescribed
2. Know the patient well
   a. Know the risk factors
   b. Adjust dose
   c. Know the cost of drugs
   d. Do not assume the patient understands
3. Inform the patient adequately
4. Have a systematic monitoring system
5. Consider all new events as possibly drug related (Jones, 1989)

DRUG HISTORY

An invaluable tool for working with older persons managing a medication regimen is the drug history. Given the complexity of medications for many elderly, this data base is crucial.

Common Drugs Used by Elderly and Their Risks

Digoxin (Lanoxin)	Significant renal excretion with decreased clearance in the elderly. Narrow therapeutic index, with therapeutic dose only slightly smaller than toxic dose Dosing based on lean body mass; another reason for decreasing average dose for the elderly. Common cause of serious adverse reactions. Signs and symptoms include loss of appetite, blurred vision, depression, confusion, bradycardia, and other arrhythmias. Note that these signs of toxicity are different from the usual signs listed for younger adults. Arrhythmias may occur with no other warning signs
Beta blockers	Potentially serious adverse effects such as bradycardia and hypotension. Can interact with a number of disease states. May cause or exacerbate congestive heart failure. Can aggravate asthma or chronic obstructive pulmonary disease. May cause hypoglycemia in diabetic patients on insulin while blocking the tachycardia that is one of the warning signs of hypoglycemia
Guanethidine (Ismelin)	An antihypertensive reserved for persons with severe hypertension. Commonly causes postural hypotension and impotence. Should be reserved for those who have been unresponsive to other medications
Reserpine	Can cause severe depression, especially at higher doses. Should not be given to depressed persons. Also causes diarrhea, nasal stuffiness, and reactivation of peptic ulcers
Warfarin (Coumadin)	Elderly may have increased sensitivity to warfarin (Vestal and Dawson, 1984), thus may require smaller doses. Need careful monitoring for bleeding and drug interactions
Cimetidine (Tagamet)	Clearance decreased in the elderly, thus need smaller doses. Use of full doses in the elderly, particularly those with impaired renal function, has caused drug-induced confusion
Laxatives	Abuse of laxatives by the elderly is a continuing and common problem despite publicity. Chronic use leads to dependency as well as dehydration and electrolyte loss. Avoid stimulant laxatives such as those containing phenolphthalein (found in many nonprescription laxatives such as Ex-Lax). Safer alternatives are bulk laxatives such as psyllium colloid (e.g., Metamucil) and stool softeners such as docusate (Colace, Surfak)
Levodopa (Larodopa, Dopar, Sinemet)	Doses need to be titrated carefully to the individual. Drug frequently causes dizziness and postural hypotension and can cause confusion and psychosis
Diuretics	Caution is advised in the elderly since they are at greater risk for dehydration and postural hypotension than younger people. Thiazides and loop diuretics (furosemide, Lasix; bumetanide, Bumex; and ethacrynic acid, Edecrin) can cause potassium and magnesium depletion. They also elevate serum glucose and may elevate serum uric acid, exacerbating gout. Potassium-

(Continued)

Common Drugs Used by Elderly and Their Risks (*Continued*)

	sparing diuretics (spironolactone, Aldactone; triamterene, Dyrenium; and amiloride, Midamor) may elevate serum potassium levels in persons with renal impairment
Anticholinergic agents	Drugs such as benztropine (Cogentin) and other antiparkinson drugs have multiple adverse effects including dry mouth, urinary retention, constipation, blurred vision, drug-induced confusion, and psychosis. Other drugs with such anticholinergic effects include the tricyclic antidepressants and some antipsychotic agents such as chlorpromazine (Thorazine) and thioridazine (Mellaril). The elderly are at particular risk for these adverse effects since they are more likely to have diseases with similar effects
Corticosteroids	Long-term use may have damaging effects on the elderly, including osteoporosis, cataract formation, increased risk of glaucoma in susceptible individuals, potassium loss, muscle wasting, and increases in serum glucose with loss of diabetic control, risk for GI ulceration
Nonsteroidal anti-inflammatory drugs	Phenylbutazone (Butazolidin) is the most toxic of these drugs and should not be used for elderly persons, particularly not on a long-term basis. They can cause fatal blood dyscrasias, fluid retention, and gastrointestinal irritation. Of the other agents, indomethacin (Indocin) has been most implicated in causing reactions such as headache and feelings of drunkenness or confusion. All of the drugs can cause sodium and fluid retention and may exacerbate hypertension or congestive heart failure. Like aspirin, these drugs can cause gastrointestinal irritation and bleeding and should be used cautiously in persons with a history of peptic ulcer disease
Tricyclic antidepressants	Elderly persons have greater risk of significant effects, including sedation, postural hypotension, anticholinergic effects, and confusion. Cardiac arrhythmias can occur. Doses should be small, especially initially, and should be increased slowly. It is also important to monitor for beneficial effects as well as for toxicity, and it may be necessary to increase the dose or switch to another drug if no improvement is noticed after several weeks on the drug
Antipsychotic agents	Drugs such as chlorpromazine (Thorazine), thioridazine (Mellaril), haloperidol (Haldol), and thiothixene (Navane) are often overused in the elderly. They can be useful to control unmanageable behavior in cognitively impaired older persons, but they do not result in improved memory. Doses should be very small. It is imperative to monitor for therapeutic effect. Extrapyramidal symptoms such as drug-induced parkinsonism occur more frequently with higher doses. These drugs are contraindicated in persons with idiopathic Parkinson's disease. Tardive dyskinesia, a possibly irreversible movement disorder caused by antipsychotic agents, is a greater risk for the elderly. For this reason these drugs should be used only when urgently needed and discontinued as soon as possible (Barnes and Raskind, 1980)

Common Drugs Used by Elderly and Their Risks (*Continued*)

Antianxiety agents, sedatives, hypnotics	This is another group of drugs overused with the elderly. This group includes barbiturates, benzodiazepines, and miscellaneous sedative and hypnotic agents. Barbiturates are to be avoided in the elderly because (1) they have high potential for addiction, (2) they may cause paradoxical agitation, (3) they have numerous drug interactions, (4) they often cause sedation and ataxia, and (5) they are unsafe in overdose
	The benzodiazepines such as diazepam (Valium), chlordiazepoxide (Librium), and flurazepam (Dalmane), among others, have very long half-lives and long-acting metabolites. The shorter acting forms such as lorazepam (Ativan), oxazepam (Serax), and temazepam (Restoril) are preferable because they do not seem to show changes in pharmacokinetics with aging. These drugs too should be used in very small doses for the minimum period possible. They have potential for addiction, although they are safer, and should not be given long term. All of these drugs may cause confusion and ataxia, with the adverse effects appearing to be age related (Thompson et al, 1983)
Narcotics, analgesics	These drugs should be used in smaller doses in the elderly to prevent sedation, confusion, and respiratory depression (Burks, 1982). Constipation may be a problem with these drugs

A drug history provides data for evaluating the person in terms of drug therapy. This includes information about the following:

Drug allergies
Past adverse effects from drugs
Current prescription medications
Current nonprescription medications
Home remedies
Noncurrent or occasionally used prescription and nonprescription drugs and home remedies
Social drug use (smoking and alcohol use)

SOURCES OF DRUG HISTORY INFORMATION

Drug histories are most complete if they come from several different sources. The primary source is the person who is taking the medication. Secondary sources include family members, primary care takers, and the person's medical record, doctor's orders, and pharmacy profile. An invaluable source of information is the medication containers. Home visits allow health care workers to gather information about how medications are stored, the condition of medication containers, numbers of non- prescription drugs and noncurrent medications on hand, as well as memory aids and medication-taking systems used by the person. A substitute for the home visit is to ask the person to bring in all of the medications that he or she is taking or storing for potential use, both prescribed and nonprescribed.

BASIC INFORMATION

Ask the patient to bring in ALL drugs they are taking, prescribed and over-the-counter.

All Drugs For all medications used or stored by the person you would want to know the following:

Name of the medication
Purpose of the medication—why it is prescribed, why the person is using it or keeping it
Dose of medication—are pills divided?
Schedule used by the person
Date when medication was started/prescribed
Does it help?
Where is it stored (if necessary)?
Is it taken with food, should it be?

TABLE 10–3 *Drugs Commonly Used by Elderly Persons and Clinically Significant Drug Interactions*

Drug	*Interacting Drugs*	*Potential Consequences*
Digoxin (Lanoxin)	K$^+$ wasting diuretics Furosemide (Lasix) Bumetanide (Bumex) Chlorthalidone (Hygroton) Metolazone (Diulo, Zaroxolyn) Hydrochlorothiazide and other thiazide diuretics	Increased risk of digitalis toxicity due to hypokalemia
	Thyroid hormones	When converting a hypothyroid person on digoxin to normal thyroid function, may need to increase dose of digoxin
	Quinidine (Quinaglute, Quinidex)	Increased digitalis effect; may need to decrease digoxin dose
	Verapamil (Isoptin, Calan)	Increased digoxin effect; may need to decrease digoxin dose
Beta blockers Propranolol (Inderal) Metoprolol (Lopressor)	Barbiturates	Decreased beta blocker effect
	Cimetidine (Tagamet)	Increased beta blocker effect; may cause bradycardia, hypotension
Both of above plus Atenolol (Tenormin) Nadolol (Corgard) Timolol (Blocadren) Pindolol (Visken)	Indomethacin (Indocin)	Decreased beta blocker effect in hypertension control
Clonidine (Catapres)	Tricyclic antidepressants	Decreased antihypertensive effectiveness
Guanethidine (Ismelin)	Tricyclic antidepressants	Decreased antihypertensive effectiveness
	Sympathomimetics: Epinephrine Ephedrine Phenylephrine Phenylpropanolamine	Same as tricyclic antidepressants
Prazosin (Minipress)	Beta blockers	Increased hypotensive effects of prazosin; can increase risk of syncope with initial dose of prazosin
Insulins	Beta blockers; less with metoprolol and atenolol	Increased risk of hypoglycemia; also blocks tachycardia as a sign of hypoglycemia
Sulfonylureas Chlorpropamide (Diabenese) Tolbutamide (Orinase)	Phenylbutazone (Butazolidin)	Increased risk of hypoglycemia
	Sulfonamides, e.g., sulfisoxazole (Gantrisin)	Increased risk of hypoglycemia
Theophylline Aminophylline	Beta blockers; less with metoprolol and atenolol	Decreased effectiveness of theophylline
	Phenytoin (Dilantin)	Decreased effectiveness of theophylline and phenytoin
	Cimetidine (Tagamet)	Increased effect; possible theophylline toxicity
	Liprofloxacin	
	Erythromycin	Same as cimetidine

TABLE 10–3   *(Continued)*

Drug	Interacting Drugs	Potential Consequences
Corticosteroids	Insulin and oral antidiabetic agents	Decreased effectiveness of hypoglycemic drugs secondary to steroid-induced increase in serum glucose; may need larger doses of hypoglycemic drugs
	Barbiturates	Decreased effectiveness of corticosteroids
	Phenytoin (Dilantin)	Same as barbiturates
	High-dose salicylates, e.g., aspirin	Decreased blood levels of salicylates When steroids are withdrawn from person on high-dose salicylates, the blood level may increase, with higher risk of salicylate toxicity
Warfarin (Coumadin)	Barbiturates	Decreased warfarin effect
	Glutethimide (Doriden)	Same as barbiturates
	Cimetidine (Tagamet) Disulfiram (Antabuse) Phenylbutazone (Butazolidin) Salicylates (aspirin)	Increased warfarin effect; possibility of bleeding
	Thyroid hormones	Hypothyroid patients require larger doses of warfarin. When a hypothyroid patient becomes euthyroid, the dose may need to be decreased

Current Prescription Medications   For prescribed medications that the person is currently taking, some additional information is needed. This includes the following:

Who prescribed it?
Specific information about how the drug is used:
  How many tablets, capsules, teaspoonfuls?
  What time(s) of day is the drug taken?
  Is it taken before, with, or after meals?
  Is it taken at the same time as other drugs?
  Have there been changes in the prescribed dosage? If so, why?
  Has the person experienced benefit from the drug?
  What are the adverse effects of the drug?
  Has the person experienced adverse effects from the drug?
  What should the person do if they occur?

Current Nonprescription Medication   All the questions asked about prescription drugs should be asked about nonprescription drugs, plus the following:

Is the person following the directions listed on the product?
Who recommended this medication?
For what reason is the person taking the medication? Does it help?

Medications Used Occasionally

How does the person know when the drug is needed?
How frequently is it used?
Does the person check to see if medication is up to date?
Does the person tell their physician when they take it?

Drug Allergies

What drug caused the reaction?
What was the reaction to the medication?
Have there been past adverse drug reactions that were not allergies?
When there have been allergic drug reactions, did the person receive that medication again? If so, did the same reaction occur?

What was done to correct the reaction? Did it work?

DRUG THERAPY EVALUATION

The goal of drug therapy evaluation is to bring all of the parts of medication-related health care together: the person's medical and nursing problem list as well as prescribed medication orders and information on the way the medications are actually being used.

This involves looking at each drug separately and asking the following questions:

What is the drug for?
Is it accomplishing the purpose for which it was prescribed?
Is it still needed?
Is the dose appropriate?
Could the drug or dosage be causing adverse effects?
If adverse effects are suspected, did they start soon after the drug was started or dosage was changed?
Are there interactions with other medications in the person's drug list?
If interactions are listed in drug references for some of the drugs, does the person appear to be experiencing the consequences of the drug interaction?
Did the symptoms start soon after an interacting drug was added to the regimen?
Has the person had allergies or past adverse reactions to the medication?
Is the indication for the medication listed on the person's problem list?
Is the person taking and receiving the medication complying with the dose, schedule, and duration of therapy?
Is the drug stored appropriately?

Drug therapy evaluation also involves looking at the overall medication regimen. Gather information about what has changed for the person, such as the following data:

Are there any recent medication changes? Why were they made?
Does the person have any new symptoms? Are they possible adverse drug effects?
Are chronic symptoms changing?
Is the person taking nonprescription medications, home remedies, or using social drugs?
Is there information that has not been reported to the prescriber, e.g., self-medication, social drug use, symptoms, or noncompliance?
What is the pattern of follow-up with health care providers?
Is cost or physical disability a barrier to safe medication taking?

GUIDELINES FOR DOSES

The goal of therapy is to maintain the older person on the fewest number of medications possible at the optimal doses to decrease the likelihood of noncompliance, adverse drug reactions, or drug interactions. Consider the purpose and need for each drug. Consider whether there will be additive adverse effects from taking several medications. Question the use of medications that exacerbate the person's disease states.

Elderly persons often require lower doses of medication. Initial doses should be small, and the person should be monitored closely or taught how to monitor himself. Dosages should not be increased on a frequent basis.

Elderly persons appear to be more sensitive to the effects of drugs that act on the central nervous system (Vestal and Dawson, 1984); therefore, doses of psychoactive medications should be routinely smaller than for younger people. Some physicians stop all medications for an older patient and slowly one by one add them back. In many instances the number of medications eventually needed is markedly decreased.

HELPING THE OLDER PERSON TO ACHIEVE SAFE MEDICATION-TAKING BEHAVIOR

Health care providers can be an important external resource to older persons in their efforts to take medications safely and effectively. Start with an assessment of the knowledge and strengths that the person already has; use these as a foundation for additional information or assistance.

Adequate knowledge is one key to effective management of a medication regimen. For each drug certain data are needed, as noted in the following list:

The name of the medication, both generic and brand name
The purpose of the medication, what it does, and the disease or condition for which it is prescribed

The color, size, and shape of the dosage form (e.g., tablet, capsule, liquid)

The route of administration (by mouth, inhalation, etc.)

The dosing schedule. Consider these factors:

The individual person's actual daily schedule (eating, sleeping, activities). Work with the person to develop a feasible schedule. Specify the times of day and associated meals or activities, e.g., "Take one tablet at 7 AM when you get up, one at noon with lunch, one at 5 PM with your dinner, and one at 10 PM when you go to bed." Do not assume the number of meals, time of meals, or hours of sleeping.

Can the medication be taken with meals or not? Should it be taken with food?

Can the frequency of dosing be decreased to improve compliance?

Can the medication be taken at the same time with other medications?

Are there any restrictions on alcohol consumption while the person is taking this medication?

If the drug is prescribed to be taken as needed, how often can it be taken? What signs or symptoms should be used to decide if the medication should or can be taken?

Indicate what to do if a dose is missed. Should the dose be skipped? Should two doses be taken at the same time?

Where the dosage is to be changed after a period of time, be specific about instructions, e.g., "Take one tablet each day for the next 3 days, then increase to two tablets per day" would be changed to "Take one tablet in the morning each day for 3 days, starting tomorrow, Tuesday, July 3rd, then increase to one tablet in the morning and one at night, starting Friday, July 6th."

Develop a system to help the patient remember to take medications. Are each day's pills put in a plastic bag and pinned to a calendar? Are medications on the table to remind the person when he eats or in the bathroom for h.s.?

Indicate the length of time the drug will be taken, i.e., for a short period to treat an acute infection or for a prolonged period for a chronic problem.

Indicate whether a new medication is intended to replace or is added to current medications.

Describe the adverse effects so that they are recognizable and explain what action to take.

Point out which symptoms need the attention of a health care worker and the degree of urgency in reporting them.

Identify any special precautions, such as "Do not take this medication at the same time or within 2 hours of taking antacids."

Give special instructions regarding storage if this is important. Does the medication need to be refrigerated? Should it always be left in the original container? Does this medication have an especially short shelf life?

Give instructions on how to refill the prescription. Are the number of refills indicated and if so where? This is particularly important for hospitalized patients going home.

Give instructions in writing and go over them orally with the patient. Encourage the person to call you if he or she has questions.

When and how should the person follow-up with the prescriber?

What is the procedure for disposing of non-current medications?

PRACTICAL GUIDELINES FOR PROVIDING DRUG INFORMATION

It can be seen that there is a large amount of information to be learned about each drug. Even persons who are alert and interested may have problems remembering all of the information at one hearing. Written instructions, particularly on critical information, are essential. These should be dated and signed to minimize confusion when various written messages are left by several health care providers.

When there is the possibility of several or ongoing contacts with the older person, information can be explained and reviewed in smaller parts. It is important to check on the person's recall and understanding about the medication regimen and to repeat the information when this is indicated. One strategy that has proven helpful is to ask the person to bring in all of the medications currently being taken when making any visit to the ambulatory care setting. This helps both the health care provider and the patient to make sure that they are discussing the same drug.

A useful rule is *do not assume*. Do not assume that the person understands merely because he or she does not ask questions. Do not assume medications are being taken correctly merely because you have explained the regimen carefully.

A change in the patient's condition physically or mentally should be considered a problem with a drug.

References and Other Readings

Abrass I. University of Washington School of Medicine conference. Aging and elderly—a review course of geriatric medicine. February 1988.

Adamson KA, Smith DL. Nonprescription drugs and the elderly patient. Can Pharm J 1978; 111:80.

American Pharmacy. F.D.A. proposes geriatric labeling. Am Pharm (NS) 1984; 24:14.

Ascione FJ, James M, Austin SJ, et al. Seniors and pharmacists: improving the dialogue. Am Pharm 1980; 20:30.

Barnes R, Raskind M. Strategies for diagnosing and treating agitation in the aging. Geriatrics 1980; 35:111.

Baum C, Kennedy DL, Forbes MP, et al. Drug utilization in the U.S.—1982. Fourth annual review. Division of Drug Experience, National Center for Drugs and Biologicals. Food and Drug Administration. DHHS, 1983.

Burks TF. Narcotic drugs: special considerations. In: Conrad KA, Bressler R, eds. Drug therapy for the elderly. St. Louis: CV Mosby, 1982.

Cooper JK, Love DW, Raffoul PR. Intentional prescription nonadherence (noncompliance) by the elderly. J Am Geriatr Soc 1982; 30:329.

Dyer CC, Oles KS, Davis SW. The role of the pharmacist in a geriatric nursing home: a literature review. Drug Intell Clin Pharmacy 1984; 18:428.

Eberhardt RC, Robinson LA. Clinical pharmacy involvement in a geriatric health clinic at a high-rise apartment center. J Am Geriatr Soc 1979; 27:514.

Evans MA, et al. Gastric emptying rate in the elderly: implications for drug therapy. J Am Geriatr Soc 1981; 27:201.

Friesen AJD. Adverse drug reactions in the geriatric client. In: Pagliaro LA, Pagliaro AM, eds. Pharmacological aspects of aging. St Louis: CV Mosby, 1983.

Geokas MC, Haverback BJ. The aging gastrointestinal tract. Am J Surg 1969; 117:881.

Gibaldi M. Biopharmaceutics and clinical pharmacokinetics. Philadelphia: Lea & Febiger, 1977.

Gomolin IH, Chapron DJ. Rational drug therapy for the aged. Comp Ther 1983; 9:17.

Gouveia WA, Miller RR. Drug interaction screening—a screen or a sieve? Am J Hosp Pharm 1978; 35:667.

Gral T, Young M. Measured versus estimated creatinine clearance in the elderly as an index of renal function. J Am Geriatr Soc 1980; 28:492.

Greenblatt DJ, Sellers EM, Shader RI. Drug disposition in old age. N Engl J Med 1982; 306:1081.

Hale WE, Marks RG, Stewart RB. Drug use in a geriatric population. J Am Geriatr Soc 1979; 27:374.

Hansten PD. Drug interactions. 4th ed. Philadelphia: Lea & Febiger, 1979.

Henney HR. Altered drug effects in the elderly. U.S. Pharmacist 1985; 10:41.

Hurwitz N, Wade OL. Intensive hospital monitoring of adverse reactions to drugs. Br Med J 1969; 1:531.

Jones J. Drugs and the elderly. In: Reichel W, ed. Clinical aspect of aging. 3rd ed. Baltimore: Williams & Wilkins, 1989.

Jue SG. Adverse drug reactions in the elderly. In: Vestal RE, ed. Drug treatment in the elderly. Boston: ADIS Health Science Press, 1984:29.

Knapp DA, Knapp DA. The elderly and non-prescribed medications. Contemporary Pharmacy Practice 1980; 3:85.

Knapp DA, Knapp DA, et al. Drug prescribing for ambulatory patients 85 years of age and older. J Am Geriatr Soc 1984; 32:138.

Lamy PP. Prescribing for the elderly. Littleton, MA: PSG Publishing Company, 1980.

Larrat EP. Patients' medication errors discovered by "brown bag" study. American Druggist 1990; 202:53.

Lely AH, Van Enger CHJ. Large-scale digitoxin intoxication. Br Med J 1970; 3:737.

Levy M, et al. Hospital admissions due to adverse drug reactions: a comparative study from Jerusalem and Berlin. Eur J Clin Pharmacol 1980; 17:25.

Lott RS, Hayton WL. Estimation of creatinine clearance from serum creatinine concentration—a review. Drug Intell Clin Pharm 1978; 12:140.

Mayersohn M. Drug disposition. In: Conrad KA, Bressler R, eds. Drug therapy for the elderly. St Louis: CV Mosby, 1982.

Mediphor. Drug interaction facts. St Louis: JB Lippincott, Facts and Comparisons Division, 1984.

Melmon KL, Morrelli HF. Drug reactions. In: Melmon KL, Morrelli HF, eds. Clinical pharmacology: basic principles of therapeutics. 2nd ed. New York: Macmillan, 1978.

Mitchard M. Drug disposition in the elderly. In: Crooks J, Stevenson IH, eds. Drugs and the elderly: perspectives in geriatric clinical pharmacology. Baltimore: University Park Press, 1979.

Morse ML. Drug utilization review: implications for patient compliance. U.S. Pharmacist Supplement, Rutgers Symposium, 1987.

Nananda, Col. MMP, Fande J, Kronholm P. Role of medication noncompliance and adverse drug reaction in hospitalization of the elderly. Arch Int Med 1990; 1:841.

Ostrom JR, et al. Medication usage in an elderly population. Medical Care 1985; 23:157.

Patrick M, Davignon D, Enloe C, Milburn P. Prescriptions for the high cost of drugs in nursing home geriatrics. J Geriatr Nurs 1991; 2:88.

Plein JB, Plein EM. Aging and drug therapy. In: Eisdorfer C, ed. Annual review of gerontology and geriatrics, Vol 2. New York: Springer Publishing, 1981.

Reidenberg MM. Drugs in the elderly. Bull NY Acad Med 1980; 56:703.

Robinson AF. Prescription medication practices of the elderly. Contemporary Pharmacy Practice 1980; 3:131.

Siegelman S. The coming wave of RX-To-OTC switches. American Druggist 1990; 202:41.

Simonson W. Medications and the elderly—a guide for promoting proper use. Rockville, MD: Aspen Systems, 1984.

Simonson W, Pratt CC. Assessing geriatric patients and their drug therapy regimens: evaluation using high-risk criteria. QRB 1981; 7:19.

Simpson T. New drugs for 1991. The Consultant Pharmacist 1991:103.

Sjoqvist F, Alvan G. Aging and drug disposition—metabolism. J Chron Dis 1983; 36:31.

Spokane Area Society of Hospital Pharmacists. Reduction of ADRs via an intervention network in institutionalized elderly patients. Research study in progress, 1991.

US Department of Health & Human Services. Healthy people 2000: national health prevention objectives. January 1991.

Vestal RE. Handbook on biology of aging. Schneider E, Rowe J, In: Drugs in elderly, 3rd edition. San Diego: Academic Press, 1990.

Vestal RE, Wood AJJ. Influence of age and smoking on drug kinetics in man: studies using model compounds. Clin Pharmacokinet 1980; 5:309.

Vestal RE, Dawson GW. Pharmacology and aging. In: Finch CE, Schneider EL, eds. Handbook of the biology of aging. 2nd ed. New York: Van Nostrand Reinhold, 1984.

Weintraub M. A different view of patient compliance in the elderly. In: Vestal RE, ed. Drug treatment of the elderly. Boston: ADIS Health Science Press, 1984.

Wilkinson GR. Influence of liver disease on pharmacokinetics. In: Evans WE, Schentag JJ, Jusco WJ, eds. Applied pharmacokinetics: principles of therapeutic drug monitoring. San Francisco: Applied Therapeutics, 1980.

Williamson J, Chopin JM. Adverse reactions to prescribed drugs in the elderly: a multicentre investigation. Age Ageing 1980; 9:73.

Zaske D, Hunter T. Polypharmacy and altered pharmacokinetics in the elderly. Today's Nursing Home, July 1985.

11
Oral Health and the Elderly

JAMES BENNETT   HOWARD CREAMER*

Perspectives

Advances in preventive medicine and dentistry are contributing significantly to the number of people living into later years of life with natural teeth and prosthetic or restorative stabilization of the mouth. The dental status of many active, responsible older individuals is that of the following:

Possess varying numbers of natural teeth restored with fillings or crowns, fixed bridge work, and even dental implants
Periodontal disease and dental decay being reasonably treated and contained by timely visits to the dentist
Being knowledgeable and skilled about oral self-care procedures

Theoretically, many adults can maintain their existing dental status for the rest of their lives, unless debilitating disease intervenes (Kiyak and Bennett, 1982).

The rapidly expanding population over 75 who are retaining more natural teeth is resulting in a change in dental practice among the elderly (Douglass and Furino, 1990; Matthiessen, 1986). There is a major difference between maintaining natural teeth, partial dentures, fixed bridges, and implants versus dealing with removable dentures.

Preventive dentistry's motto of "teeth for a lifetime" still begs the question of who will care for the mouth when the older, compromised individual can no longer maintain that responsibility. When older individuals become dependent and are cared for in acute or long-term care facilities, the nursing profession usually becomes the primary source of oral health maintenance. Therefore, it is appropriate to define nursing care of the mouth and to apply the same ethical and legal significance to dental care as to the prevention and care of decubiti, incontinence, and contractures. Dentists must also accept responsibility to provide basic dental services to this population in a manner consistent with the elderly person's medical and dental status and his desires for dental care (Saunders, 1990).

One irony in the current situation is that Medicare does not financially reimburse for dental care, even though dentists frequently treat extremely sick older patients for whom the mouth is the primary source of sepsis. It seems to be acceptable for fragile, institutionalized older people to suffer silent septic oral conditions that actually cause death. This chapter examines the working relationship nursing and dentistry can establish and describes standards of oral health for elderly patients.

Definition of Geriatric Dentistry

Geriatric dentistry is defined as the area of professional dental services that has the goal of at-

*Deceased

taining and stabilizing a reasonable level of oral health in older individuals, who may have significant physical, medical, emotional, and social deficits (Tryon, 1986; Bates and Adams, 1984). These patients are often under the care of medical and nursing professionals (Ettinger, 1989). Thus, geriatric dentistry involves frequent contact with primary physicians and nursing staff.

Normal Changes in Oral Structures

The mouth undergoes changes in the tissues as aging occurs as do bone, glands, nerves, muscle, connective tissues, and epithelia elsewhere in the body (Holm-Pederson and Loe, 1986). Therefore, in the mouth similar forms of atrophy, decreasing function, and loss of regenerative cellular units may be found. Teeth, being unique to the mouth, also undergo changes over time.

TEETH

The natural teeth that survive into later periods of life tend to be darker, with stress lines in the enamel that accumulate stains easily. The crown and root structure over the years suffer varying degrees of caries, abrasion, and erosion, depending on the nature of the diet, tooth-brushing habits, employment, environment, and the degree of grinding (bruxing) of the teeth. Sharp tooth edges that may lacerate the soft tissues are often produced by abrasion, tooth or filling fractures, and decay.

The pulp of the tooth usually lays down calcified tissue on the walls of the pulp chamber until there is only a fragment of tissue left in the tooth root canal (Fig. 11–1). This has significant implications for treatment. Given the reduced tooth sensitivity, fillings can sometimes be placed without anesthesia. If the crown of the tooth fractures as a result of trauma or caries, the nerve is often safe and may not require root canal therapy.

MUCOSA AND CONNECTIVE TISSUE

The mucosal tissue of the mouth changes with age. As the epithelium atrophies the normally pink mucosa and firm gingiva become thinner, smoother loosing elasticity and stippling. The connective tissue becomes more fibrous and less vascular. These soft tissues then become more friable and vulnerable to trauma and infections. They are also slower to heal (Rogers, 1989). Food selection and preparation should take into consideration the traumatic effect that coarse foods can have on aging mucosa.

The loss of periodontium over many years usually leaves root structure exposed to the environment and provides decreasing support for

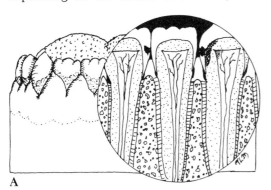
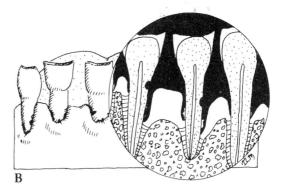

A   B

FIGURE 11–1 Diagrammatic contrast of the diseased dentition of a young person (A) with that of an older adult (B). A, the gingiva surrounds the crown (enamel) of the tooth and there are accumulations of dental plaque about the necks of the teeth. The teeth are close together, and dental caries (decay) is shown occurring in the enamel of the teeth. One carious lesion is shown involving the enamel and dentin and encroaching on the pulp. Early formation of calculus is occurring in several sulcular spaces. B, The gingiva, periodontal ligament, and bone have receded, leaving the tooth poorly supported. The enamel is markedly thinned owing to attrition and abrasion, and the pulp has filled in the inner chamber, leaving only a thin remnant of pulp in the root of the tooth. The teeth have separated as a result of periodontal disease. Such conditions tend to exacerbate disease because of increased stresses during eating and accumulations of bacteria and food debris in the interdental spaces, caries, and periodontal pockets. Note the marked change in the size of pulp, the anatomic features of the crown (enamel), and the relationship of tooth to supporting tissues in the two figures.

the teeth. This results in increasing mobility of teeth and root decay. Such changes have been used as a reasonable excuse for removal of such teeth even when the condition could be treated and the teeth maintained. Age-related changes in teeth and supporting structures compared with disease states are illustrated in Figure 11–1.

LOSS OF CHEWING EFFICIENCY

Chewing efficiency is also compromised with aging as a result of loss of tooth units, reduced muscle strength, increased tooth mobility, and obliteration of cusps on the chewing surfaces. Broad, flattened chewing surfaces do not incise food in the normal manner, and there is increased stress on the tooth. The biting force gradually decreases for those who retain their teeth. Those with dentures suffer additional losses of chewing power and end up with about one fifth the efficiency in food partitioning. This loss of chewing effectiveness may explain the decreased interest in meat and the "tea and toast syndrome." It certainly suggests that food should be selected and prepared to accommodate for the lost ability to chew food effectively.

LOSS OF ALVEOLAR BONE

Loss of alveolar bone also occurs. Periodontitis, removal of tooth units, and osteoporosis contribute to loss of alveolar bone. The result tends to be a loss of facial height, with the chin being closer to the nose. The loss of intermaxillary space may lead to problems in the temporomandibular joint and accentuate the commissures of the mouth. The latter condition is exacerbated when there is a concomitant vitamin deficiency, microbial infection, and/or chronic drooling.

CHANGES IN SALIVARY GLANDS

Recent studies in carefully defined elderly populations report no general reduction in salivary performance with aging (Merck Manual, 1990). Most age-related changes in salivary function can be attributed to systemic disorders or their treatment and drugs (Fox et al, 1985). Drugs that can decrease salivation include thiazide-type diuretics, tranquilizers such as promethazine, sympathomimetics (Actifed), parasympatholytics (hyoscyamine sulfate), antihistamines (Benadryl), antidepressants (both monoamine oxidase inhibitors and nonmonoamine oxidase inhibitors), decongestants (Trinalin), estrogens, and anorectics (amphetamines) (Baker et al, 1991).

Other Areas Affected by Age-related Oral Changes

Changes in one part of the body often have ramifications for other aspects of daily living. Changes in oral structure and functioning are no exception. They can affect body image, nutrition, and taking of medications.

BODY IMAGE

The emotional overlay associated with oral cavity dysfunction in the elderly is not easy to evaluate. There are many instances in which an older person will not eat or socialize while dentures are being repaired. Men in our practice tend to be less overtly sensitive about esthetics and are more likely to request that diseased teeth be removed. More edentulous men than women do not wear their dental prostheses and masticate food on toughened healthy gingiva and alveolar bone. Women tend to seek aesthetic restoration, and some wish to retain natural teeth.

COMMUNICATION

Teeth are essential for communicating with others. If dentures are removed during an acute phase of illness for diagnostic or surgical procedures, they should be returned to the patient as soon as it is safe to do so. Trying to speak without teeth while dentures are repaired is tiring for the person and represents significant loss of dignity. Teeth in a locked drawer are not useful.

NUTRITION

Nutrition may be a major key in the aging of oral tissues since there are such complex effects associated with chewing, tasting, sensing, and finally swallowing food. The systemic effects of food are well known; however, the local effects of quality and quantity of foods have been linked to oral health (Steen, 1986).

Nurses who care for the elderly need to be aware of the implications of oral age-related changes as these relate to diet. Nurses can alert the older person, particularly the denture wearer, to the need to consciously chew food longer because of the loss of chewing efficiency. They can gather data on usual eating patterns and cooking styles and recommend food preparation methods and food selections that accommodate for tissue vulnerability and lost chewing power. In general the nurse will be interested in (1) the person's chewing capability, (2) symptoms associated with decreased salivary flow that would suggest more frequent eating, drinking, or mouth rinsing, and (3) ability of the soft tissues to withstand the abrasion of coarse, hard foods.

DRUGS

Drugs are frequently associated with a variety of oral problems. A few common adverse drug–mouth interactions are offered here.

Some drugs act directly on oral hard and soft tissues. For example, aspirin, when held in the mouth for periods of time for a toothache, causes oral ulceration and decalcifies teeth.

Drugs that alter the immune system can significantly alter the oral environment. Often the mouth is the first area to reflect toxic levels of cytotoxic drugs. Before beginning chemotherapy, a thorough evaluation is done of the mouth and teeth.

Drugs can mask or partially inhibit oral disease processes so that the person is unaware of pathology or the progression of pathology. Antibiotics, analgesics, and steroids may have such effects.

Drugs that decrease salivary flow and exacerbate existing xerostomia (the complaint of oral dryness) were discussed earlier in the section on age-related changes in the salivary glands (Baker et al, 1991).

Progressive Oral Dysfunction Syndrome and Constellation Effect

One of the great frustrations for dentists treating elderly individuals is the rapid deterioration of teeth, gingiva, and periodontium that frequently occurs in a once well-maintained mouth. Surprising findings include lack of pain in the presence of gross destruction of teeth, increasing chewing dysfunction, loss of esthetics, and the person's obliviousness to the changed oral status. This has led to the development of two concepts: progressive oral dysfunction syndrome (PODS) and the constellation effect (Bennett and Creamer, 1984).

PROGRESSIVE ORAL DYSFUNCTION SYNDROME

The essential features of PODS include the following:

Uncontrolled presence of dental plaque for weeks or months

Rampant, painless decay of teeth, often involving exposed roots

Rapid loss of tooth crown from decay or breaking of the crown at the gingival margin

Extensive periodontal disease, especially in multirooted teeth

Significant loss of chewing efficiency, especially when opposing teeth are missing

Collapse of normal facial contours from tooth loss and loss of space between jawbones

Significant psychosocial effects with the changes in oral esthetics, loss of normal facial contours, and pervasive halitosis

Possible systemic sepsis, with or without fever

CONSTELLATION EFFECT CONCEPT

The concept of constellation effect describes the multiple factors and complex interactions that increase in scope and dimension with aging. These factors are related to the development of PODS and are illustrated in Figure 11–2.

FINANCIAL STATUS

Many older individuals have limited incomes. Most do not have dental insurance. Spending money on preventive maintenance or tooth problems that do not cause pain may have low priority. At times, a responsible relative may also assign less importance to dental health than to other health matters, particularly given the high cost of long-term care. The thought that the ailing older individual may not have a long life span may also result in neglect of dental health.

MEDICAL CONDITIONS

Concern over major health matters such as stroke, cardiac conditions, or cancer may distract the patient and others away from "silent" oral pathology.

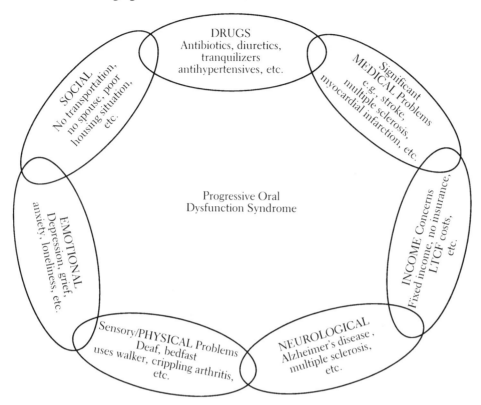

FIGURE 11–2   The constellation effect. Many factors are often associated with the development and progress of Progressive Oral Dysfunction syndrome.

NEUROLOGIC PATHOLOGY

Patients with dementias or cognitive impairments are often oblivious to their oral status. They can become fearful, suspicious, or threatened when attempts are made to brush the teeth or use other dental instruments. In addition, their motor skills are often impaired, making it difficult to engage in self-care.

PHARMACOLOGIC PRODUCTS

Older individuals who are taking tranquilizers or sedatives often seem detached from their oral pathology. Antibiotics and pain medications may mask significant oral diseases.

PHYSICAL STATUS

Many older individuals become increasingly frail or restricted in their flexibility and mobility and are no longer physically able to engage in effective oral hygiene.

EMOTIONAL STATUS

Emotional conditions such as depression, anxiety, grief, loneliness, apathy, and withdrawal can interfere with regular self-care of all kinds including the teeth and mouth.

SOCIAL STATUS

Many independent individuals whose physical capabilities are compromised seek to continue their oral self-care and refuse assistance from others. Older individuals with altered dental appearance through loss of teeth or broken dentures or chronic bad breath may decrease their social contacts and become more isolated.

The previously listed factors are important considerations for dentists and nurses as they seek to formulate reasonable plans for oral health maintenance and further dental care. Data on these factors are often not found in patients' clinical records, but are known to the observant nurse.

INTERCEPTIVE DENTAL CARE

Once the elderly person is more debilitated and PODS and the constellation effect reach significant proportions, dental therapies are modified to interceptive dental care. These are procedures that detect, interrupt, and contain disease processes that may significantly affect oral and systemic health. Examples of interceptive dental care include timely detection of oral cancer, treatment of abscessed teeth, and temporary stabilization of loose dentures. Within this definition of interceptive dental care is the implication that further dental care is desirable if and when the patient can tolerate such dental treatment. General dentists may hesitate to treat fragile elderly beyond palliative measures due to health risks posed by the patient's condition; these patients should be referred to geriatric dental specialists.

Factors Contributing to Oral Disease and Problems

Oral disease and problems in the elderly are usually multifactorial. Some of the major factors involved in oral pathology among the elderly include the following:

Microorganisms can cause dental decay, periodontal disease, and other inflammatory and infectious conditions of soft tissues and bone. The organisms can spread from the mouth to other areas of the body, particularly to grafts or prostheses such as artificial heart valves

Poor nutrition can lead to dental decay, decreased tissue resistance to infection, and trauma. In turn, oral pathology can result in inadequate quantitative and qualitative intake of nutrients

Trauma is associated with ill-fitting dentures, sharp edges to teeth, sharp metal and acrylic edges of prostheses, as well as improper use of cleaning devices

Soft tissue changes are associated with infection, inadequate nutrition, trauma, and premalignant or malignant pathology

It is estimated that 95% of these factors are within the scope of nursing practice to assess, monitor, and seek to prevent.

Common Oral Problems in the Elderly

DENTAL PLAQUE DISEASE

Caries and periodontitis are the major infectious diseases of the oral hard and soft tissues caused by parasitic microorganisms (Bennett and Creamer, 1984). These diseases are examples of multiple diseases, each caused by different sets of microorganisms in different people or even in different sites in the same person's mouth (Creamer, 1991). The microbial etiology is multifactorial.

The microorganisms involved are considered to be part of the normal oral flora, rather than classic pathogens found only in diseased individuals. The oral flora of an adult appears to consist of some 100 to 200 different kinds (taxa) of bacteria from a group of 300 known oral taxa. In spite of this complexity, the vast majority of significant oral infectious diseases are preventable.

The microbial masses that populate the surfaces of oral hard and soft tissues are the cause of decay, gingivitis, and periodontitis (damage to the alveolar bone that supports the tooth). The nature of the damage of the microorganisms living and replicating on tooth surfaces is illustrated in Figure 11–3.

Tissue invasion by the bacteria is a relatively late event, occurring after significant damage has resulted from the effects of various microbial products (e.g., acids, enzymes, toxins) that have been released by the surface plaques. These plaques grow naturally and soon come to have concentrations of bacteria found in feces (approximately 100 million bacteria per milligram wet weight). It is little wonder that oral malodors are associated with the heavily colonized, infected, and neglected mouth. What is surprising is that this area of the body can successfully withstand such insult for such long periods. The dental plaque disease cascade is illustrated in Figure 11–4.

The main points to be emphasized about dental plaque are the following:

Daily removal or inhibition of plaque by mechanical or chemical means will essentially control dental caries and periodontitis. Such control by the elderly adult is often difficult or impossible especially in deeper interdental areas.

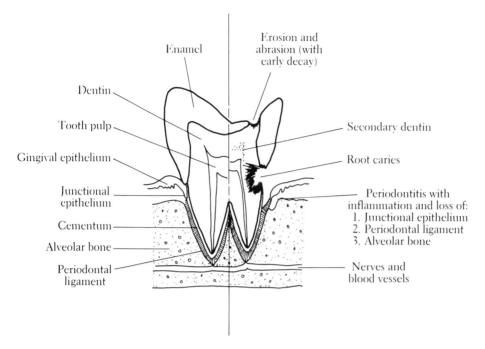

FIGURE 11-3 Diagrammatic scheme of a molar tooth contrasting a normal versus diseased area of crown and root. The disease process reflects the effect of dental plaque diseases (decay, gingivitis, and periodontitis) in which integrity of the gingival seal of epithelium is lost with subsequent root decay, loss of periodontal fibers, and loss of alveolar bone. The abraded and/or eroded enamel can be caused by such things as bruxism (tooth grinding) and acidic foods (e.g., citrus fruits).

Systemic bacteremia may occur whenever gingival and periodontal areas are manipulated (e.g., source of potential infection of damaged heart valves, prosthetic valves, or various implants).

PROBLEMS ASSOCIATED WITH DENTURES

Full and partial dentures will be important to elderly patients for many years to come, especially the denture units stabilized by dental implants. Several problems with dentures are regularly encountered by nurses. These include

Mixed-up or lost dentures. This can occur when dentures are lost down a toilet, left on food trays, or taken by another patient seeking a better denture fit. Denture marking kits are readily available.

Ill-fitting dentures. Soft and hard tissues change over time result in comfort and chewing efficiency. Regular dental examinations identify the problems early and are treatable.

Broken or poorly functioning dentures. Broken or worn out dentures increase the amount of energy and effort necessary to chew food. The sharp, broken edges of prostheses can lacerate soft tissue. Single teeth can be replaced on a denture and broken dentures can often be repaired. Poorly fitting dentures can be adjusted or relined to improve the fit.

Localized and generalized inflammatory problems. Inflammations often afflict denture-bearing tissues. Often they can be traced to poor oral or denture hygiene and a concomitant candidiasis infection.

Learning to live with dentures can present a variety of challenges to older persons. Even replacing old dentures with new ones can create difficulties. Most people make a smooth transition from natural teeth to dentures; however, some find it difficult and others impossible, and the treatments to resolve the problems vary widely. Older people may not know of options to dentures and wait until it is too late before seeking dental evaluation

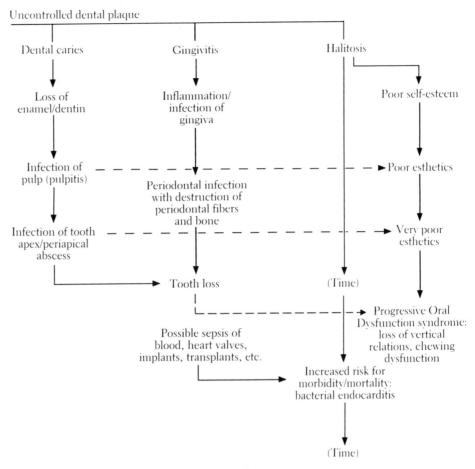

FIGURE 11–4 Dental plaque disease cascade.

when all that can be done is full-mouth extraction.

OTHER COMMON ORAL PROBLEMS IN THE ELDERLY POPULATION

The oral problems most commonly encountered in the elderly are listed in Table 11–1 together with the signs and symptoms of and comments about the condition or its treatment.

Nursing Management of the Older Person's Mouth

The major aspects of nursing responsibility for oral health include assessment of oral status, supervision of oral hygiene, and management of chronic oral problems such as dry mouth and cracked lips. Nurses should also be competent to carry out basic oral hygiene procedures if needed by the patient.

ORAL ASSESSMENT

There are two types of nursing assessment of the mouth: the initial or admission assessment and the ongoing assessment at timely intervals dictated by the patient's self-care ability, physical condition and disease, and the presence of chronic dental problems. Both subjective and objective data are needed. The goal is to achieve an oral "steady state" (Mulligan, 1984; Murray, 1989).

Nurses have two responsibilities in dealing with their findings. They should be recorded on the patient's clinical record. They should

(continued on p. 202)

TABLE 11–1 *Common Oral Problems (Clinical)*

Problem	Clinical Findings	Comments
Dental caries	Decay of enamel, dentin and/or roots (usually not painful)	May need pain medication if abscess present; antibiotics with acute infection
Fracture of crown	Tooth broken off at gingival margin	Sharp projections of enamel (or dentin) may perforate lip, tongue, cheek
Gingivitis	Gingiva red, swollen; bleeds easily with cleaning	Often not painful. May reflect changes in immune competency
Periodontitis	Deep red (to bluish) tissue; suppurative exudates from periopockets; mobile teeth (bone loss)	May develop abscess and fistula to gingiva
Abrasion (bruxism)	Marked loss of tooth chewing surface; flattened anatomic markings	May have significant loss of space between jawbone, e.g., collapse of facial features
Erosion	Cup-shaped loss of enamel and dentin; usually due to acidic or mechanically harsh foods	May occur on chewing surface or at the gingival margins
Xerostomia	Dry, leathery soft tissues; poor denture retention; much oral discomfort	May need fluids (water) available all the time; artificial saliva available
Keratoses	White, keratic buildup on soft tissues (may alternate with red, thickened epithelium)	May be a premalignant stage. Does not wipe off with cleaning
Snuff keratoses	Patchy keratoses and red, thickened areas	Usually in vestibule where snuff is held
Nicotine stomatitis	Soft and hard palate; keratotic buildup around inflamed minor salivary glands	May regress if smoking is stopped
Lichen planus	Lacy, white formations often bilateral on cheeks, tongue	Very common; cyclic in occurrence; may be premalignant
Lip keratoses	Usually thickening of tissues of lower lip	Often found in persons who spend much time in the sun
White, hairy leukoplakia	White, hairy projections on tongue, often lateral borders	May be one of earliest signs of aquired immunodeficiency syndrome
Candidiasis	White, patchy cords on a red tissue base	Colonies may be removed with a gauze sponge. May need antifungal therapy
Squamous cell carcinoma	Malignant change in surface epithelium of mucosa	Usually in the posterior areas of the mouth; biopsy required for diagnosis
Salivary gland enlargement	Parotid and submandibular glands most commonly enlarged may be due to increased gland size, blockage of ducts, neoplasm (benign and malignant)	
Ill-fitting prostheses	Atrophy and sore areas beneath dentures; loss of supportive alveolar bone	Temporary stabilization may be possible by packing cotton into denture base

Nursing Oral Assessment Guide (Allen System)

1. Ask the patient (and/or relatives) about
   a. Current and past dental problems
   b. Bleeding, swelling, areas of pain
   c. Loose and/or sharp teeth; loose, ill-fitting dentures
   d. "Bad" taste in the mouth; bad breath
   e. Ability to chew
2. Look at perioral areas including jawbone and neck for
   a. Firm or fluctuant swellings of lymph nodes, salivary glands, tissue spaces
   b. Areas painful to palpation
   c. Keratosis, tumors of lips and adjacent areas
3. Look into mouth using tongue blade and flashlight for
   a. Blood or pus exuding from about teeth (gums), fistulae, ulcers, etc.
   b. Uncontrolled accumulation of dental plaque about teeth, gums, and tongue; food accumulation in cheek vestibules and/or beneath tongue
   c. Full or partial dentures that are not being removed or cleaned
   d. Loose teeth
4. Enter oral findings into patient's chart
   a. Intake records should show presence of removable dentures
   b. Oral hygiene measures should be entered into patient's nursing care plan
5. Notify appropriate parties about oral status
   a. Patient's responsible parties must approve any dental procedures and cost
   b. Patient's physician must be alerted to significant dental problems and should approve dental procedures and any drug prescriptions
   c. Arrange for dental examination, coordinate dental care, plan routine, timely visits to (from) dental hygienist

Nursing–Dental Interactions

1. Can the nurse describe the general condition of the patient's mouth to the dental team?
2. Is the dental team provided with a complete and accurate medical history on the patient, especially allergies, presence of hip (or other) prosthesis, artificial heart valves, heart murmurs, organ transplants, and severe hormonal problems? Is antibiotic premedication required for invasive dental procedures?
3. Has the primary physician (of the patient) approved of dental procedures and drugs to be used on the patient?
4. Has the dental team made the appropriate chart notes in the correct areas, e.g., progress notes and doctor orders?
5. Does the patient need nursing while receiving dental care (at the dental office or at the care facility)? Will a sedative premedication allow the dental team to treat the patient more effectively?
6. Has the patient's responsible party approved the proposed oral health and dental procedures?
7. Are there patient factors (constellation effect) not easily detected in patients' chart that will assist the dental team in providing treatment or working with responsible parties?
8. Can the nursing, medical, and dental team agree on an acceptable oral status "steady state" (customized for each patient)?

also be reported to the dental team for appropriate treatment. See box on p. 201 for guidelines on nursing-dental interaction.

EQUIPMENT

Protective gloves, a face mask, a flashlight, and tongue blade are needed to undertake extraoral and intraoral examination. The tongue blade can be helpful in moving the tongue and cheek to one side to check for loose teeth or dentures (full or partial).

Guidelines for making an oral assessment are shown in the box on p. 201.

CLINICAL JUDGMENTS ASSOCIATED WITH ORAL ASSESSMENTS

Nurses need to be prepared to make some initial clinical judgments about the significance of their findings in order to seek appropriate treatment. Systemic problems are frequently reflected in the oral cavity. Some examples of problems that are manifested in the oral cavity include the following:

Drug-related iatrogenic stomatitis or generalized gingivitis

Chronic or acute malnutrition evidenced by thin atrophic oral mucosa and a smooth, reddened, painful tongue

Some specific deficiencies such as pernicious anemia

Changes in the immune system, frequently manifested in the mouth as a yeast infection (candidiasis)

Acute, suppurative periodontitis associated with cyclic neutropenia

Acute mucositis associated with cytotoxic chemotherapy

White hairy tongue or acute rampant periodontitis as an initial manifestation of acquired immunodeficiency syndrome or tumors secondary to the disease, e.g., Kaposi's sarcoma (Levine and Glick, 1991)

While oral findings may be indicators of the presence of systemic disease, conditions in the mouth also may be the cause of other pathology. Chronic suppurative periodontitis or chronic periapical infections (both often painless), may produce fever of unknown origin. Sooner or later these chronic infections may finally appear as swellings over the teeth (in the gums or jawbones), and fistulae may appear as purulent blebs or draining tracts in gingiva, palate, or even external skin. If the infections enter tissue spaces below or around the eye socket or mandible, the management problem becomes critical.

A fever of unknown origin in a nursing home resident was resolved by a nurse brushing a patient's teeth and gums very thoroughly the day before the dentist arrived to treat a "purulent, swollen, and painful mouth."

Clinical findings may indicate local pathology, requiring medical or dental intervention. Oral swellings may indicate infections, tumors, or blocked salivary glands. Tumors tend to be firm, painless, and involve the oral mucosa, lymph nodes, or salivary glands. Tumors of the minor salivary glands may occur in the oral mucosa, especially the palatal areas. An 86-year-old woman with left cheek swelling, but no pain or fever, had been tested extensively (including computed tomography) for a brain abscess. A 15-minute procedure in the dental office for localized periodontitis took care of the problem.

Since nurses are most closely involved with observation and care of the oral cavities of dependent elderly individuals, the observations they make and the clinical judgments they have the knowledge and experience to consider can make a significant contribution to the older person's well-being.

ORAL HYGIENE MANAGEMENT

Nurses should be able to provide effective oral hygiene when necessary and to supervise other nursing staff in these tasks. Inservice training of sufficient frequency to maintain awareness and skills is important even though state and federal regulations require infrequent reviews. It helps to have the dentist and hygienist conduct inservice sessions at least twice a year.

Oral hygiene management consists of five general elements:

Timely assessments as described in the previous section

Assistance with dental plaque control (Pader, 1988)

Access to the dental team as needed

Inclusion of oral hygiene measures in the nursing care plan (ideally these orders are written by the dentist/hygienist)

Documentation of findings and actions on the clinical record

MECHANICAL PLAQUE REMOVAL

Dental plaque should be removed from teeth, soft tissues, and dentures at least once a day, but better still twice a day. With older individuals who have had earlier radiation and chemotherapy for head and neck cancers, it is imperative to follow all the guidelines for mechanical, chemical, and nutritional control of dental plaque.

Dental plaque should be debrided by direct mechanical means. Equipment includes gloves, a glass of water, emesis basin and clean towel, moist 2 × 2 or 4 × 4 gauze sponges, appropriate type of toothbrush, tooth picks mounted on a handle, and interdental devices such as dental floss, yarn, interdental brushes, or gauze strips (Fig. 11–5).

Electric (battery-powered) toothbrushes can provide good mechanical cleaning; however, in institutional settings they tend to disappear rapidly. Toothbrushes may be modified for easier use by the patient as shown in Figure 11–6; however, patients with motor impairments are usually relatively ineffective in using them, so they may be most useful as a means of maintaining their dignity.

After gloving, gently scrub the teeth with the toothbrush using a scrubbing or vibrating motion. With very heavy plaque, several scrubbings are required in most areas of the mouth.

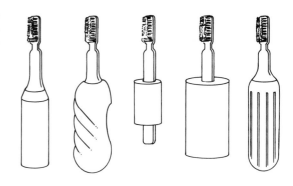

FIGURE 11–6 Modification of toothbrush and other handles for improved motor control in oral hygiene.

If the patient is uncooperative, stand behind and cradle the head with one arm, exerting downward pressure on the chin with the hand of the cradling arm; brush with the other hand as illustrated in Figure 11–7.

It may be necessary to assist patients in holding the mouth open, especially if they tend to bite. Mouth holding devices include several tongue blades taped together, a rolled-up wash-

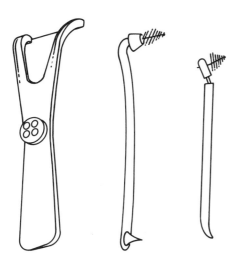

FIGURE 11–5 Interproximal cleaning devices. Dental floss, small brushes, rubber tips, and toothpicks are all useful; however, many elderly persons cannot use these instruments appropriately.

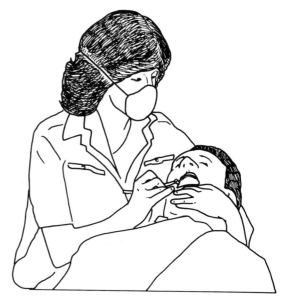

FIGURE 11–7 Cradling the patient's head for better control during oral hygiene.

cloth, or a mechanical mouth prop illustrated in Figure 11–8.

Water pics and glycerin cuvettes are also used for oral hygiene. They are inefficient plaque control measures.

CHEMICAL PLAQUE REMOVAL

Chemical plaque control using fluoride toothpaste and gel preparations has been very helpful in the management of dental plaque disease, particularly in dental caries. Daily use of the stronger fluoride gels is particularly recommended in patients at high risk for dental caries from radiation or iatrogenic drug effects.

Chlorhexadine mouth rinses have recently been introduced in the United States for treatment of gingivitis. The drug has a wide range of antibacterial and antifungal activity. Patients at high risk for chronic dental plaque disease may have to use the chlorhexadine preparation indefinitely, whereas it may be preferable to switch the patients to the fluoride toothpaste and rinses after 30 days of chlorhexadine oral use. Patients who cannot rinse and spit should have small amounts of chlorhexadine (or fluoride) preparation brushed onto the teeth and gingiva, using 2 × 2 sponges to remove excess fluids.

PLAQUE DISEASE CONTROL BY NUTRITION

The third major means of dental plaque disease control is appropriate nutrition. Desserts, candy, canned fruits, and certain oral drug preparations (e.g., oral nystatin) may have high sucrose content and can be devastating to natural teeth. Well-meaning relatives often provide candy or condiments (against dental advice), feeling it is the final pleasant experience for the older relative. Desserts are also served and used as rewards at many long-term care functions or at events older people attend.

MEDICATION THERAPY FOR GINGIVITIS AND PERIODONTITIS

The major antibiotic drugs are effective in gingivitis and periodontitis; however, systemic sensitivity and toxicity are significant possibilities. The tetracyclines are particularly good for the management of periodontal disease, especially if they can be adapted for local, intraoral use (Gabler and Creamer, 1991).

DENTURE MANAGEMENT

It is extremely important for nurses to assess the types of prosthetic devices present in any patient's mouth, especially removable appliances. This should be done on admission and recorded in the chart. Both the prostheses and the mouth need to be regularly cleaned. Failure to remove the prostheses for a protracted period can result in the need for painful surgical removal. Dentures are not necessary to sustain life; indeed the food in long-term care facilities usually does not require extensive chewing. At times it may be preferable to remove the dentures at meals and use them primarily for aesthetic effect.

Denture care involves the following:

Removal and cleaning at least once daily, but preferably after each meal

Cleaning with a denture brush and mild soap and water over a basin filled with water or one containing a towel (to avoid chipping or breakage)

Leaving them out of the mouth in clean water at night (some patients cannot tolerate leaving dentures out for prolonged periods)

Identifying each person's dentures with name or social security number

Seeking dental care regularly but especially to modify or replace ill-fitting dentures (plastic liners placed by the dental team can help for short periods of time). Ill-fitting dentures untreated over long periods may cause significant loss of denture-bearing tissue and bone or may damage abutment or natural teeth

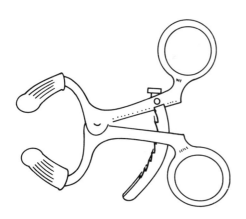

FIGURE 11–8   Mechanical mouth prop.

Nurse–Dental Team Interaction

Nurses tend to be the immediate, direct managers of health care for institutionalized or frail elderly who are living at home. Therefore, the older person's oral health can depend on effective relationships between the nursing caregivers and members of the dental team. Although the dentist must frequently consult with the patient's primary physician, the patient's nurse must be appraised of diagnosis and treatment plans. Conversely, it is important that the nurse appraise the dentist of oral findings that require further diagnosis or treatment. Nurses often have essential data related to the constellation effect.

In institutional settings a formal agreement delineating relationships and services of the dental team and the institution is highly desirable. A sample of such an agreement is found in Display 11–1.

The mouth is an important part of the admission assessment for each patient, and it must be cared for daily or more frequently for the prevention of illness, spread of disease, and physical discomfort and for esthetics and communication of the patient. The most common and significant oral health problems of the elderly, dental plaque disease and oral tumors, tend to be silent in their earlier stages. They can reach an advanced, destructive status before detection. Effective, knowledgeable nurses can make the difference in early detection and management of oral problems by working with the dentist. Basic expertise in the nursing care of the elderly should include both oral assessment and oral hygiene skills.

Standards of practice should include the following:

A complete oral assessment on admission and at predetermined intervals as dictated by the patient's medical and oral condition

Basic oral health management procedures, including use of emollients on dry, cracked, eroded, or ulcerated soft tissues, monitoring of fluid and food intake, performing or supervising oral hygiene measures, and implementing treatment prescribed by the dentist or physician

Supervision of nursing staff in oral hygiene tasks

Incorporation of appropriate oral hygiene or care measures as a part of the total nursing care plan

Dental care in both routine preventive and emergency situations

References and Other Readings

Baker KA, Levy SM, Chrischilles EA. Medications with dental significance: usage in a nursing home population. Spec Care Dent 1991; 11:20.

Bates JF, Adams D. Dental treatment of the elderly. Bristol, UK: Wright, 1984.

Bennett J, Creamer H. Oral disease. In: Cassel CK, Walsh JR, eds. Geriatric medicine, 2nd ed. New York: Springer-Verlag, 1984.

Creamer H. Adult periodontitis; biological and control. J Oregon Dent Assoc 1991; 36:60.

Dolan TA, Monopoli MP, Kaurich MJ, Rubenstein LZ. Geriatric grand rounds: oral diseases in older adults. J Am Geriatr Soc 1990; 38:1239.

Douglass CW, Furino A. Balancing dental requirements and supplies; epidemiologic and demographic evidence. J Am Dent Assoc 1990; 121:587.

Ettinger RL. Dental care and management of the aging dental patient. J Tenn Dent Assoc 1989; 69:10.

Fox P, Van der Ven P, Bonias B, et al. Xerostomia: evaluation of a symptom with increasing significance. J Am Dent Assoc 1985; 110:519.

Furino A, Douglass CW. Balancing dental service requirements and supplies; the economic evidence. J Am Dent Assoc 1990; 121:685.

Gabler WL, Creamer HR. Suppression of human neutrophil functions by tetracycline. I Periodont Res 1991; 26:52.

Geriatric Merck Manual. Rahway, NJ: Merck Sharp & Dohme Research Laboratory, 1990.

Holm-Pederson P, Loe H, eds. Geriatric dentistry. Copenhagen: Munksgaard, 1986.

Kiyak HA, Bennett J. Special problems of geriatric patients. In: Ingersoll B, ed. Behavior aspects in dentistry. New York: Appleton-Century-Crofts, 1982.

Levine RA, Glick W. Rapidly progressive periodontitis as an important clinical marker for HIV disease. Compendium 1991; 12:478.

Matthiessen PC. Demography—impact of an expanding population. In: Holm-Pederson P, Loe H, eds. Geriatric dentistry. Copenhagen: Munksgaard, 1986.

Mulligan R. Preventive care for the geriatric dental patient. J Calif Dent Assoc 1984; 12:21.

Murray JJ. The prevention of dental disease. Oxford University Press, 1989.

Pader M. Oral hygiene products and practice. New York: Marcel Dekker, 1988.

Rogers VC, Duvall DJ. Geriatric dentistry. In: Reichel W, ed. Clinical aspects of aging. 3rd ed. Baltimore: Williams & Wilkins, 1989:464 .

Saunders MJ. Challenges in managing the special geriatric patient. Texas Dent J 1990; 107:7.

Steen B. Nutrition in the elderly, implications for oral health care. In: Holm-Pederson, Loe H, eds. Geriatric dentistry. Copenhagen: Munksgaard, 1986.

Tryon A. Oral health and aging. Littleton, MA: PSG Publishers, 1986.

Display 11–1   Sample contract for dental services.

RETAINER AGREEMENT TO PROVIDE SERVICES

This Agreement is entered into this _____ day of _____, 199__, by and between ORAL HEALTH CARE GROUP, P.C., an Oregon Professional Corporation, dba Geriatric Dental Group (herein GDG), and _____ (herein Contractor).

RECITALS:

WHEREAS, Contractor operates a residential care facility and has need of certain services relating to the dental care of its residents; and WHEREAS, GDG is willing and able to undertake such care either at Contractor's facility or at its clinic at _____.

1. PROVISION OF SERVICES. GDG agrees to provide dental care to the residents of Contractor's facility, and to provide training and consultation to the staff of Contractor's facility, subject to the terms and conditions of this agreement.

2. RETAINER. Contractor agrees to pay GDG the sum of _____ upon execution of this Agreement, and a like sum each year thereafter on the anniversary date of this Agreement, provided, however, GDG reserves the right to increase the amount of the annual retainer by giving notice of a new sum at least thirty (30) days prior to the anniversary date of this Agreement.

3. TERM. This Agreement shall be effective as of the date first written above and shall continue for a twelve consecutive month period thereafter, unless terminated by virtue of some provision contained herein. This Agreement shall be renewed automatically for succeeding terms of one year unless either party, at least thirty (30) days prior to the expiration of any term, gives written notification of an intention not to renew the Agreement.

4. NOTIFICATION OF FINANCIALLY RESPONSIBLE PARTY. GDG agrees to notify the party who is financially responsible for each resident (herein Responsible Party) as to the availability of dental services. For each resident for whom services are to be provided, GDG agrees to obtain from the Responsible Party written agreement on the form attached to pay for an initial oral examination.

5. INITIAL ORAL EXAMINATION. Upon receipt of the written agreement as provided in paragraph 4, GDG shall send the original copy of the executed agreement to the Contractor. GDG and the Contractor shall mutually arrange for the initial oral examination. The examination shall take place at either Contractor's facility or the GDG clinic.

6. ROUTINE DENTAL TREATMENT. GDG shall advise the Responsible Party as to the results of the initial oral examination. If dental treatment is necessary, GDG shall obtain written authorization from the Responsible Party for such treatment. Routine dental treatment shall not take place until authorization has been received. Dental treatment shall take place at either Contractor's facility or the GDG clinic. If treatment occurs at Contractor's facility, there will be an additional charge for each patient to cover the dental team's travel expense.
   A. Travel expense will be determined by etc.
   B. Residents' Responsible Party will be notified of the travel expense when the written authorization is issued.

7. EMERGENCY DENTAL CARE. GDG agrees to provide emergency dental care for the residents of Contractor on a 24-hour on-call basis. Contractor shall obtain written authori-

---

Display 11–1   (Continued)

zation from the Responsible Party to pay for emergency dental care of all private pay residents. Such authorization is required to be given to GDG before treatment will be provided. Medicaid residents shall be transported to GDG clinic.

8. PATIENT BILLING. All dental treatment provided to residents of Contractor's facility shall be on a fee-for-service basis. GDG shall bill resident's Responsible Party directly, etc.

9. CLINIC SERVICES. When services are to be provided at the GDG clinic, an employee of Contractor shall accompany the resident to and from the clinic, and shall remain present at the clinic during the entire appointment. Contractor may substitute a member of the resident's family in place of the employee.

10. SCHEDULING. When scheduling routine dental treatment, GDG shall give Contractor notice at least forty-eight hours in advance.

11. TRANSPORTATION TO CLINIC. When services are to be provided at the GDG clinic Contractor is responsible for providing transportation for residents to and from the clinic.

12. PATIENT CONDITION. Contractor agrees to notify GDG as to changes in a resident's medical condition or changes in a resident's medication.

13. ANNUAL CHECK-UPS. GDG agrees to notify Contractor as to when annual oral examinations are due.

14. INSERVICE TRAINING. Contractor agrees to employ GDG to provide inservice training to Contractor's employees on the subject of proper dental care methods for residents at least once each twelve months. The fee for such training shall be at the rate of _____ per in-service.

15. CONSULTATIONS. GDG shall consult with Contractor's nursing staff about oral hygiene status of residents, and shall make specific recommendations about the oral hygiene care of residents, as needed.

16. COMMITMENT TO PROPER ORAL HYGIENE. By entering into this Agreement, Contractor acknowledges the importance of proper daily oral hygiene care to the health and well-being of its residents. Contractor agrees to provide appropriate nursing staff training and supervision to insure an optimal level of oral care within the facility.

17. TERMINATION. This Agreement shall be terminated upon etc.

18. PATIENT RECORDS. Upon termination of this Agreement, all patient records normally maintained by a party which are separate from the records normally maintained by the other party shall be the sole property of the party.

19. DOCTOR–PATIENT RELATIONSHIP. Contractor acknowledges that all residents of Contractor's facility have the right to receive dental treatment from the practitioner of their choice, that residents treated by GDG become patients of GDG, and that the doctor–patient relationship arising as a result of such treatment is not limited by the terms of this Agreement. Upon termination of this Agreement for any reason, GDG reserves the right to provide treatment to any of Contractor's residents who request such services.

20. NOTICES. Any notices shall be given in writing and transmitted by certified mail, postage prepaid, and shall be deemed given on the date postmarked etc.

Display 11-1 *(Continued)*

21. <u>ATTORNEY FEES</u>. In the event of arbitration or litigation respecting enforcement of any of the terms of this Agreement, it is agreed that the prevailing party shall be entitled to etc.

22. <u>ARBITRATION</u>. Except as otherwise provided, any controversy or claim arising out of or related to this Agreement shall be settled by arbitration in accordance with the rules etc.

23. <u>GOVERNING LAW</u>. This Agreement shall be governed etc.

24. <u>BINDING EFFECT</u>. This Agreement shall be binding upon the parties, their heirs, legal representatives, successors, and assigns.

25. <u>INTEGRATION</u>. This writing contains the entire Agreement of the parties and supercedes all prior negotiations or agreements either written or oral.

26. <u>HEADINGS</u>. All headings set forth in this Agreement are intended for convenience only and shall not control or affect the meaning, construction or effect of this Agreement or of any of the provisions hereof.

27. <u>CONSTRUCTION</u>. As used herein, the singular shall include the plural, etc.

IN WITNESS WHEREOF, the parties hereto have executed this Agreement in duplicate on the day and year first above written.

ORAL HEALTH CARE GROUP, P.C.
An Oregon Professional Corporation
dba Geriatric Dental Group

BY: _____
     President
CONTRACTOR:
Name: _____
BY: _____
     Title _____

12
Nutrition

JOAN M. KARKECK

BONNIE WORTHINGTON-ROBERTS

As recently as 1970, people over age 65 constituted less than 10% of our population and drew little attention politically or scientifically. Few studies on nutrition have been directed toward the elderly adult as a special segment of our population. Nutritional requirements of the elderly were thought to vary little from those of younger adults and people paid lip service to the importance of nutrition for the older person, with no particular support available in the scientific literature. The 1980s, however, brought about a revolutionary change in the demographics of age. Studies of nutritional requirements for older people proliferated, as have studies relating the consumption of more or less than usual intakes of nutrients to longevity and to the prevention of disease and deteriorating physiologic structure.

There are still few definitive studies of nutrition as it relates to the aging population, but there is at least a growing body of evidence to support the relationship between nutrition and healthful living in the elderly.

It is clear that food plays a variety of roles in the lives of individuals. Attention is given in this discussion to the diverse meanings of food in our society. Basic to the discussion of this topic, however, is the critical need for food and its constituent nutrients for support of life itself as well as for growth, tissue repair, and resist-ance to infection. The nutrients in foods are clearly vital to the support of basic biochemical and physiologic mechanisms in the human body; each individual must provide his body with its basic needs or suffer the consequences of suboptimal performance with advancing years.

Basic Nutrient Requirements of Older Adults

Before examining the specific nutritional needs of elderly persons, emphasis must be placed on the reality that individuals cannot be pooled or lumped into what is called the "old-age group." Clearly, this tendency makes for convenience in discussing the needs of older people, but common sense strongly supports the concept of increasing individuality with increasing age. As rough guidelines, however, for assessing nutritional needs of groups and for planning dietary programs for the elderly, the Recommended Dietary Allowances (RDAs) of the National Academy of Sciences serve a useful purpose (Table 12–1). It must be remembered, however, that the actual nutritional status of groups of healthy people or individuals must be judged on the basis of physical, bio-

208

TABLE 12–1 *National Research Council Recommended Dietary Allowances for Healthy People over 51 years (1989)*

	Men*	Women[†]
ENERGY		
Kilocalories (kcal/kg[‡])	30	30
Protein (g/day[§])	0.63	0.50
FAT-SOLUBLE VITAMINS		
Vitamin A (mg RE)	1000	800
Vitamin D (mg)	5	5
Vitamin E (mg)	10	8
Vitamin K (mg)	80	65
WATER-SOLUBLE VITAMINS		
Vitamin C (mg)	60	60
Thiamin (mg)	1.2	1.0
Riboflavin (mg)	1.4	1.2
Niacin (mgNE)	15	13
Vitamin B_6 (mg)	2.0	1.6
Folate (μg)	200	180
Vitamin B_{12} (μg)	2.0	2.0
MINERALS		
Calcium (mg)	800	800
Phosphorus (mg)	800	800
Magnesium (mg)	350	280
Iron (mg)	10	10
Zinc (mg)	15	12
Iodine (μg)	150	150
Selenium (μg)	70	55

*Based on reference man 77 kg, 173 cm in height.
[†]Based on reference woman 65 kg, 160 cm in height.
[‡]Based on recommended body weight.
[§]Based on biologic value of protein represented by usual American diet.
Reprinted with permission from Recommended Dietary Allowances, 10th edition, © 1989 by the National Academy of Sciences. Published by National Academy Press, Washington, D.C.

chemical, and clinical observation combined with observations of food or nutrient intake. If the RDAs are used as reference standards for interpreting records of food consumption, it should not be assumed that malnutrition will occur whenever the recommendations are not completely met. Conversely, it is important not to assume that nutritional adequacy is ensured by fulfilling the RDAs.

The concept of individuality has particular relevance for the aged. The overwhelming majority of elderly people have one or more chronic illnesses, such as atherosclerosis, digestive disorders, malabsorptive phenomena, rheumatologic disorders, osteoporosis, obesity, alcohol addiction, lack of teeth or poorly fitting dentures, and a whole host of other medical and psychologic problems. Certainly the aged person hardly represents the healthy reference man indicated in the RDAs. It is, therefore, a real challenge to health professionals not only to identify and manage the great variety of medical problems of the aged but also to determine and establish an appropriate nutritional program that will ensure individual nutrient adequacy, particularly in the face of these multifaceted problems. By no means does this imply that the RDAs should be disregarded but instead that they should serve as a guideline on which individual nutritional status is estimated and dietary recommendations are prescribed. In the final analysis, nutritional requirements (like most other needs) represent individual characteristics.

CALORIES

With increasing age, a gradual reduction in energy requirement takes place. Part of this reduction reflects the decrease in basal metabolism, resulting from the decline in functioning body cells. The cells that remain continue to demand the same nutritional support as cells from younger persons. In addition, a reduction in daily physical activity is commonly observed in the aging individual. This has been clearly documented in studies involving both men and women. Because of the decrease in physical activity with age, basal metabolism represents a higher proportion of the total energy needs of elderly persons than of young adults who are physically more active (Vaughan et al, 1991).

Because of the decrease in physical activity and basal metabolism with age, calorie intake should be reduced gradually as persons become older.

The Food and Nutrition Board of the National Academy of Sciences recommends that calorie allowances be reduced to reflect the 2% decrease in basal metabolic rate in each decade of adulthood and the reduction in activity levels for men and women over 51 years of age. They estimate the energy allowance for activity to decline 211 kcal/day for men and women over age 31 and 500 kcal/day for men and 400 kcal/day for women over 75 years. This results in a calorie recommendation for persons beyond 75 years reduced to 75% to 80% of that required for a young adult.

In practice, calorie needs of individuals may vary according to age, sex, basal metabolism, size, occupation, environment, hormonal balance, and physical activity patterns. Total calorie intake should be adjusted to a level that will prevent the patient from becoming overweight or underweight. Both problems are common among the aged, with overweight and obesity afflicting the greatest percentage.

The average body weight of men and women over 65 has been decreasing over the last two decades but NHANES II data indicate that 25% of black and white American men 65 to 74 are overweight when a body mass index (weight [kg]/height [cm²]) of 27.8 is used as an indicator. Thirty-six percent of white women 65 to 74 years are overweight (body mass index ≥ 27.3); but up to 60% of black women are overweight and apparently becoming more so (Fanelli and Woteki, 1989).

Body weight tends to increase throughout the adult years, peaking in the 50s for men and in the 70s for women and declining slowly thereafter.

This masks the continuing loss of lean body tissue and the accumulation of less metabolically active adipose tissue. The average man is expected to lose 50% of his lean body mass by age 70.

The degree to which this upward trend in percentage of body fat could be restrained by diet and exercise is not fully known. Studies of body composition in adults suggest that the proportion of body fat to body weight inevitably increases with age, but the rate of change can be slowed by exercise. It would be desirable to minimize this compositional change by attempting to maintain a desirable body weight for height throughout life.

The ideal weight range for older men and women is the subject of controversy. Andres et al (1985) suggest upward revision of height-weight tables for each decade after 25 years based on an analysis of the 1979 Body Build and Blood Pressure study. The data show the lowest curve of mortality to be at a body mass index between 27 and 28. Usually a body mass index of 25 is considered ideal. Analysis of NHANES II data support this conclusion (Tayback et al, 1990). Many reviewers still ob-

ject to the suggestion that weight should be allowed to increase with age (Willett et al, 1991); however, the 1990 US Department of Agriculture Dietary Guidelines for Americans adapted the table developed by Andres supporting the concept that rigorous adherence to lower weight standards might not be required. Both the widely used Metropolitan Life Weight ranges and the Andres table are presented in Table 12–2.

Both underweight and marked overweight

TABLE 12–2 *Comparison of Suggested Weight Range for Men and Women over 65*

Height (ft-in)	Metropolitan Life Tables*		Gerontology Research Center
	Men (lb)	Women (lb)	Men and Women (lb)
4-10	—	100–131	115–142
4-11	—	101–134	119–147
5-0	—	103–137	123–152
5-1	123–145	105–140	127–152
5-2	125–148	108–144	131–163
5-3	127–151	111–148	135–168
5-4	129–155	114–152	140–173
5-5	131–159	117–156	144–179
5-6	133–163	120–160	148–184
5-7	135–167	123–164	153–190
5-8	137–171	126–167	158–196
5-9	139–175	129–170	162–201
5-10	141–179	132–173	167–207
5-11	144–183	135–176	172–213
6-0	147–187	—	177–219
6-1	150–192	—	182–225
6-2	153–197	—	187–232
6-3	157–202	—	192–238
6-4	—	—	197–244

*Data in this table are for height without shoes and weight without clothes.
Reproduced with permission from Andres R, Elahi D, Tobin JD, et al. Impact of age on weight goals. Ann Intern Med 1985; 103:1030.

are associated with increased mortality and morbidity in this population, and both extremes should be avoided. An analysis of NHANES subjects followed for 8.7 years found little increased risk for moderate excess weight in men and women 65 to 74 years, but marked increased mortality in elder Americans in the lowest decile of body weight. These statistics were corrected for smoking and hypertension (Tayback et al, 1990).

Recently, several studies have indicated that the distribution of body fat with a concentration of adipose tissue in the upper trunkal area of the body carries greater risk than overweight for both young and elderly people for diabetes, hypertension, and coronary artery disease. Circumferences of waist to hip ratio in women and waist to upper thigh ratio in men appear to be relatively uninvasive and accurate measures of body fat distribution (Mueller et al, 1991).

There is general agreement that obesity in persons with hypertension and diabetes mellitus II is a risk factor that greatly increases morbidity and that weight loss may decrease both the clinical signs and consequence of these chronic conditions. Weight loss goals can be very moderate in these patients since even losses of 5 to 8 kg have been shown to decrease blood sugar and blood pressure levels in older subjects (Stamler et al, 1987).

Dietary counseling is essential for the older person who has laid down undesirable adipose tissue. Because activity generally is limited, the restriction of calories to bring about weight loss must be carefully planned so that the diet supplies adequate amounts of the essential nutrients. To achieve a loss of 1 lb of body fat per week, a reduction of daily intake of 500 calories is required. Restriction of dietary fat has the dual advantage of decreasing calorie intake and decreasing the serum lipid values, which is often a problem with these diseases. Moderate exercise may also assist in increasing expenditure of calories to a limited degree. Whatever program is devised, its success relates directly to the ease with which it can be adapted to the lifestyle and established food habits of the person in question.

The Health Assessment Nutrition Examination Study II (NHANES II) completed in 1980 shows a mean intake in kilocalories of 1295 in women and 1828 in men (Tables 12–3 and 12–4), far below the RDA. A significant percentage of the elderly over 75 years of age are at great risk for being markedly underweight and malnourished. These underweight elderly may require dietary counseling and well-planned support to increase their weight and nutritional status.

PROTEIN

Protein (and its constituent amino acids) is required by the body for synthesis of body proteins and other nitrogen-containing substances. Humans are unable to synthesize about ten of the amino acids, and these must be present in the diet for maintenance of life and health. Since proteins are vital structural and regulatory components of the body, it is not hard to understand that older people feel better and have fewer complications from acute and chronic illnesses when they ingest a diet adequate in protein content. Unfortunately, the self-selected diets of elderly individuals are sometimes deficient in this nutrient.

Although differences in opinion exist about the protein and amino acid requirements of the elderly, considerable evidence suggests that elderly persons use dietary proteins less effectively for protein synthesis and deposition of protein reserves. Studies by Young (1990) and others showed that healthy elderly people do not achieve nitrogen balance when they consume high quality protein at the level recommended by the RDA of 0.8 g/kg body weight. From these data, the minimum protein needs of older persons appear to increase slightly with advancing years.

Dietary protein derives from a number of food sources that basically can be classified as animal or vegetable materials. Animal protein foods, such as meat, fish, poultry, milk, eggs, and cheese, contain protein with a nice balance of essential amino acids and thus these protein sources are called *complete proteins*. Elderly people eat significantly less red meat, perhaps accounting for their less than adequate dietary intake. Vegetable proteins also are significant in the daily diet and largely derive from a variety of plant products such as wheat, corn, soybeans, and rice. Because the essential amino acid composition of these proteins is not as appropriate for the needs of humans as that of animal proteins, vegetables are said to contain protein that is partially complete or incomplete. It should be remembered, however, that combinations of vegetables that contain an amazingly well-balanced pattern of essential amino acids can be developed. Several good

TABLE 12–3   *Reported Intakes of Individuals Over 65 in the US Population: Preliminary Data from NHANES II, 1977–1978, for Women*

Nutrient	Mean Intake* + Standard Deviation		RDA	Percentile Distribution				
				5	25	50	75	95
Calories	1295	± 503	1600	607	972	1221	1570	2173
Protein (g)	51.18 ±	23	44	21	36	48	63	92
Carbohydrate (g)	158.47 ±	69		64	111	151	194	285
Fat (g)	50.21 ±	26		16	33	46	62	99
Calcium (mg)	541.9 ±	336	800	141	259	475	714	1156
Phosphorus (mg)	880.0 ±	417	800	350	594	823	1078	1573
Iron (mg)	10.23 ±	5.0	10	4.28	6.63	9.05	12.20	19.81
Sodium (mg)	1990	± 1086		678	1269	1818	2433	3891
Vitamin A (IU)	5486	± 8090	5000	832	1990	3376	6255	15,500
Niacin (mg)	14.44 ±	8.31	13	5.19	8.96	12.90	17.35	30.23
Thiamin (mg)	.99 ±	.76	1.0	.37	.63	.85	1.15	1.97
Riboflavin (mg)	1.36 ±	1.12	1.2	.42	.79	1.13	1.60	2.88
Vitamin C (mg)	105 ±	86	60	7	37	90	147	260

*Values usually rounded to the nearest tenth.

Abstracted from the preprint of NHANES II Preliminary Statistics, DHEW, 1982. Abrahams CS, Dresser CM: Dietary source data: United States, 1976–1980. Vital and Health Statistics Series 11, No. 231 DHHS. Publication No (PHS) 83–1681 Public Health Services, Washington, DC, 1983.

collections of recipes for such vegetarian dishes are available in most bookstores (Wasserman and Mangels, 1991; Robertson et al, 1979). Those elderly persons who maintain an enthusiasm for cooking might profit immensely from including some of these food combinations in their diets.

Not only is it necessary for the essential amino acids to be present in the diet, but they also must be available to the body tissues simultaneously and in proper proportions for utilization. This necessitates that some degree of regularity be established in presenting a balanced amino acid pattern to body tissues. The protein needs of most older people generally will be met if approximately 12% to 15% of the daily calorie intake is derived from protein. This need is easily met by the daily inclusion of two glasses of low fat milk and an average portion of meat or meat alternate in the diet. These along with the small amounts of protein found in other common foods will serve to meet daily needs. However, culture, personal preference, oral problems, and a variety of other factors may serve to make these recommendations useless; in such cases, other acceptable sources of dietary protein need to be identified and included in the diet on a regular basis.

CARBOHYDRATES

Under most conditions carbohydrates provide at least 50% of the total calorie content of the diet. Anywhere from 50% to 75% of total calories should come from this source, with 12% to 15% of the calories from protein and 10% to 40% of the calories from fat. Carbohydrates thus represent a very important source of energy for the body, and attempts to reduce carbohydrate intake drastically in an effort to lose weight are potentially harmful.

When dietary carbohydrates are drastically reduced, several things can happen. First, loss of tissue proteins (amino acids) occurs to make

TABLE 12–4 *Reported Intakes of Individuals Over 65 in the US Population: Preliminary Data from NHANES II, 1977–1978, for Men*

Nutrient	Mean Intake* + Standard Deviation		RDA	Percentile Distribution				
				5	25	50	75	95
Calories	1828 ±	753	2000	948	1529	1966	2554	3481
Protein (g)	73.29 ±	34	56	29	50	67	89	135
Carbohydrate (g)	203.0 ±	92		72	140	193	253	366
Fat (g)	75.10 ±	40		27	49	68	93	141
Calcium (mg)	698.0 ±	443	800	186	370	597	915	1564
Phosphorus (mg)	1197 ±	541	800	483	813	1119	1468	2275
Iron (mg)	14.09 ±	8.22	10	5.49	9.13	12.27	17.02	27.92
Sodium (mg)	2892 ±	1620		1047	1843	2577	3593	5603
Vitamin A (IU)	6572 ±	12,535	5000	976	2229	3914	7062	17,161
Niacin (mg)	19.93 ±	11.45	16	6.56	12.48	17.68	24.12	40.20
Thiamin (mg)	1.33 ±	.88	1.2	.47	.82	1.13	1.57	2.77
Riboflavin (mg)	1.84 ±	1.35	1.4	.57	1.07	1.56	2.25	3.95
Vitamin C (mg)	100 ±	87	60	5	33	79	140	271

*Values usually rounded to the nearest tenth.
Abstracted from the preprint of NHANES II Preliminary Statistics, DHEW, 1982. Abrahams CS, Dresser CM: Dietary source data: United States, 1976–1980. Vital and Health Statistics Series 11, No. 231 DHHS. Publication No (PHS) 83–1681 Public Health Services, Washington, DC, 1983.

up the calorie deficit if one exists and to maintain blood sugar concentration at appropriate levels. Second, mobilization of fat may occur, with a concomitant increase in blood cholesterol and triglycerides. Third, a significant loss of sodium and water through the kidneys may take place with the consequence of potential development of dehydration and renal damage. Even 10% of dietary calories from carbohydrate can overcome most of these problems. The human is known to exhibit a wide range of adaptability and thus no specific requirements for dietary carbohydrate have been defined.

Of significance, however, is the observation that some aged persons consume excessive amounts of *refined* carbohydrates because they usually are less expensive than other foods. Diets rich in refined carbohydrates not only may limit intake of other important nutrients but they also frequently contain excessive fat and calories. Complex carbohydrates are quali-

tatively much better in that the concentration of calories per unit of food is less, the content of other nutrients usually is higher, and the presence of fiber is probably vital to maintenance of the health of the gastrointestinal system.

With relation to fiber it is interesting to note that constipation may easily develop in individuals with a poor intake of dietary fiber. Constipation is known to occur in at least 25% of older patients and many reasons have been cited as potentially influential. Among the factors believed to be contributory are the following:

1. Lack of fiber in the diet to stimulate peristalsis
2. Abuse of laxatives
3. Decrease in fluid intake
4. Decrease in motor tone and motor function of the bowel
5. Lack of exercise
6. Blunting or loss of the defecation reflex as a consequence of neglect of the urge to defecate

7. Organic lesions such as poor dentition, anorectal lesions inducing spasm of the anal sphincter, tumors, and prolonged immobilization associated with fractures or paralysis
8. Medications such as sedatives or tranquilizers, antihypertensive and ganglionic blocking agents, narcotics, and calcium carbonate antacid

Poor dietary fiber intake accompanied by excessive laxative use is by far the circumstance of greatest significance; efforts to improve dietary composition and reduce laxative abuse should be aggressively made by all health professionals who care for older individuals in institutions or other community settings. Both soluble fiber (oat bran, pectin) and insoluble fiber (wheat bran and many vegetables) contribute to increased bulk and decreased transit time. Elderly people should be encouraged to consume a variety of whole grains, fruits, and vegetables and adequate fluids to encourage bowel health. Foods and beverages that aid in preventing constipation are summarized in Table 12–5.

FATS

The diet of the typical American is high in fat. Recent statistics indicate that almost 40% of the daily calorie intake is obtained from this source. This fat is derived largely from animal

---

TABLE 12–5 *Foods and Fluids That Aid in the Prevention and Management of Constipation*

Food with bulk (fiber)
    Vegetables (especially raw)
    Fruits (especially raw)
    Whole grain cereal products
    Bran (in moderation)
    Legumes
    Nuts

Prunes and prune juice

Water (at least 6 glasses per day)

Benefit is also achieved by regular meal patterns, regular time for elimination, sufficient rest and relaxation, and adequate exercise

---

sources but increasing use of vegetable oils in recent years is contributing to a slow change toward intake of less animal fat (saturated fat) and more vegetable fat (largely unsaturated fat). Fat is used by the body in various ways, serving as the vehicle for the absorption and distribution of fat-soluble vitamins A, D, E, and K, reducing the acid secretion and muscular activity of the stomach, and providing a vital energy source. Fats also increase the feeling of satiety, increase palatability of foods, and facilitate cooking. For these reasons, fats may be nutritionally, physiologically, and psychologically important to people.

A basic problem in our society is not one of fat deficiency but rather one of excessive fat consumption. Multitudes of research studies have indicated that high intake of dietary fat and cholesterol is directly correlated with incidence of atherosclerosis. In advanced industrialized societies the complications of atherosclerosis are the immediate cause of death for 50% of individuals. The lesion of atherosclerosis involves the formation of plaques in the inner lining of the arterial walls. Plaques contain several lipids and are rich in cholesterol and thus the lesions have long been associated with blood and dietary cholesterol. It is now well documented that deposition of cholesterol appears earlier and is more severe in those individuals whose blood cholesterol values are elevated. The level of blood cholesterol has been shown to depend on a variety of factors including genetic endowment, hormone interrelationships, exercise, and diet. A number of techniques have been used to lower serum cholesterol concentrations including drugs, exercise, and dietary change. An elevated serum cholesterol can be lowered by decreasing the total fat intake to less than 30% of calories from fat, eating less saturated fats and cholesterol, and substituting polyunsaturated vegetable fats for some animal fats.

Recent publication of the results of the Lipid Research Clinics' coronary primary preventional trials confirm that reducing serum cholesterol levels can reduce the incidence of coronary heart disease (Lipid Research Clinics Program, 1984). It is not clear, however, that altering serum cholesterol concentrations in the elderly would have such a beneficial result. Serum total cholesterol alone is not a useful predictor of coronary heart disease in people over 60. The relative ratios of total cholesterol of low density lipoproteins to high density lipoproteins appears much more predictive (Ben-fante and Reed, 1990).

Recent studies also suggest that the total fat in our diet may contribute substantially to the incidence of breast and colon cancer and to obesity. This information has caused critical evaluation of the amount of eggs, high-fat dairy products, and meats that should be in an optimal diet at any age. The consensus is that fewer than 30% of dietary calories should be derived from fat and that the fat that *is* consumed should contain a significant proportion of poly-unsaturated fatty acids.

Practically speaking, calories as well as fats can be reduced in a variety of ways. Substituting fish, poultry, and lean meat for other meats, rich dairy products, and eggs will contribute significantly to reduction in fat intake. (Maintenance in the diet of *low-fat* dairy products is sensible in the long run, however, because much nutritional value is obtained from the protein, riboflavin, calcium, and other nutrients that these foods contain.) The substitution of polyunsaturated margarines for butter and the use of vegetable oil instead of hydrogenated shortenings and standard salad dressings is also advisable. Avoidance of fatty desserts is particularly effective in reducing not only fat intake but sugar and calorie intake as well. There is no need for an individual to make these dietary changes overnight. This is very difficult for most people to accomplish; a much better approach to take is a gradual introduction of several new items into the diet each week as the fat-rich foods are gradually withdrawn or restricted in amounts.

It seems appropriate to insert a word of caution about working with people toward major dietary change. *Reasonable dietary changes for a man of 60 may not necessarily be right for a man of 90. If a person has done well for 90 years on a particular diet (high-fat or otherwise), there seems little reason for him to institute change at this point.* Diet therapy must be individualized. Recognition of the multitude of factors that influence eating patterns is basic to the planning and implementation of *any* special recommendations for dietary modification. There is concern that some elderly people concentrate so much on restriction of dietary fat and calories that they fail to eat a reasonable diet, lose excessive weight, and find less pleasure in eating. The skilled clinician finds a workable means of squeezing these restrictive adjustments into the existent dietary patterns of elderly patients.

VITAMINS

Vitamins are required by all humans throughout life, basically to allow for efficient operation of a variety of metabolic processes. Deficiency in one or more vitamins, consequently, impairs functionality of the biochemical processes that support physiologic activities. As a person grows older, the need for each of the vitamins remains, and the level of need is largely comparable to that of younger individuals. Unfortunately, the diets of many aged individuals are inadequate in terms of regular vitamin intake from natural sources.

Data from the NHANES I update conducted late in 1981 to 1982 (Murphy et al, 1989) indicate that, although many older persons are well nourished, a significant proportion are poorly nourished.

Fanelli and Woteki (1989) summarized the results of NHANES II dietary studies of older Americans. Vitamin A was rarely a problem except occasionally in institutionalized elderly patients; thiamin was more likely to be a problem. Several studies suggested that one third of the populations studied consumed less than the recommended intake of riboflavin, thiamin, and niacin, but it appeared not to be a problem clinically, though recent small studies indicate improved health in people with marginal thiamin intake supplemented with the vitamin. Intake of vitamin C has risen sharply, but the median intake of 55- to 74-year-old men and women with poverty level income was below the recommended allowance. Vitamin C intake in this population appears highly related to income and may well present risks for depressed immune responses.

Folate and vitamin D are considered nutrients likely to be deficient in the elderly. A follow-up evaluation of NHANES data found the mean intake of folate for men over 65 years was 281 μg ($= 36$) and 207 ($+ 29$) μg for women compared with the 400 μg recommended allowance (Subar et al, 1989). Folic acid status may be a significant problem for individuals over 65, resulting in increased anemias and would be of greater concern for the 3% to 10% of elderly people thought to be alcoholics. Folic acid supplements may be useful for some although dietary sources such as orange juice, bananas, green leafy vegetables, and beans will provide a balanced intake.

The recommendations concerning vitamin D and the elderly are subject to some contention (Gloth et al, 1991). It appears safe to say that vitamin D levels appear to decline with age, probably as the result of a combination of factors, including lack of sunlight exposure and poor nutritional intake (Webb et al, 1990). It is evident that conversion of 7-dehydrocholesterol in skin to vitamin D by sun exposure requires more time in the elderly (Machaughlin and Holick, 1985) and that institutionalized individuals are at increased risk for vitamin D deficiency and increased bone demineralization. Because bone diseases are so common in an elderly population and so highly related to vitamin D, special efforts should be made to provide for an adequate but not excessive vitamin D supply.

A number of drugs that may be used frequently by an elderly population affect vitamin status. Perhaps most evident is the effect of prolonged use of anticonvulsants on vitamin D and B_{12} status or antibacterial agents on vitamin K status. Patients on long-term anticonvulsant therapy now present with early osteoporosis (Roe, 1988). Vitamin K stores can be so severely deficient that a prolonged prothrombin time occurs, with the potential for excessive bleeding. When intestinal bacteria are eliminated as a source of vitamin K, food sources may be emphasized. Good food sources include alfalfa sprouts, dark green leafy vegetables such as spinach and kale, the cabbage family (especially cabbage and cauliflower), soybean oil, whole grain wheat, liver, eggs, and cheese. A number of antidepressants with anticholinergic actions can have profound effects on food intake, and thus on nutritional status, because they decrease saliva flow, peristalsis, and gastric acid secretion, thus decreasing gastrointestinal motility and causing difficulty with dry mouth, altered taste, slow gastric emptying, and constipation (Roe, 1988).

Nonspecific symptoms such as fatigue, weakness, and mild paralysis may result from prolonged inadequate vitamin intake. Both the poor and the elderly who have severely restricted their diets without a physician's advice may be especially prone to vitamin deficiencies. Additionally, individuals with chronic diseases are especially susceptible. A number of vague complaints of ill health, suboptimal performance, impaired resistance to infection, poor wound healing, and other qualities may improve by the elimination of vitamin deficit.

Functioning may be depressed by poor nutrition. (Tucker et al, 1990) evaluated nutritional status and cognitive function in elderly men and women and found a significant relationship between depressed nutritional status and the results of tests for abstract thinking ability and memory. Recent studies have focused on the relationship between low serum cobalamin levels and depressed cognition (Herbert, 1988). Martin et al (1992) suggest that there is a window in time during which altered cognition related to depressed cobalamin levels will respond to vitamin supplementation. Patients should be counseled regarding improving dietary intake of specific vitamins; if dietary improvement seems unlikely or long in coming, supplementation with appropriate, low-level multivitamin preparations including B_{12} is often desirable.

Unfortunately, there are surprisingly few well-controlled studies of the effects of vitamin supplementation on the health of the elderly. A well controlled, 2-year study of chronically ill, hospitalized elderly patients found that 95% showed some sign of nutritional deficiency and 90% had low serum levels of vitamin C and thiamin (Taylor, 1968). It was found that those patients receiving supplementary vitamin B complex and vitamin C showed highly significant improvement in physical and mental condition, although this improvement took up to 1 year. When the vitamins were discontinued, signs of deficiency reappeared in about 6 months in many of the subjects, even while they were provided the general hospital diet that was designed to be complete in all nutrients. More recent studies in the United States and Great Britain compared placebo with vitamin and/or mineral supplements, especially thiamin, vitamins A, C, and D and zinc and copper improved self-rated scores of well-being, increased several components of immune function, decreased wound healing time, and hospital length of stay (Lehmann, 1989).

Many older persons take vitamin supplements on their own initiative with the hope that improved health and vitality will develop. Several national studies indicate 30% to 55% of people over 65 use vitamin and mineral supplements, sometimes to such an extent that the costs impair their financial ability to buy food. Often physicians recommend vitamin supplements for patients of advanced age without any real knowledge about their nutritional status. Classic vitamin deficiency diseases (i.e., beriberi, pellagra, and scurvy) are infrequently seen in developed countries today, but subclinical deficiency is hard to prove or disprove. To suggest that vitamin deficiencies cause most debilitation states in the elderly is unscientific but to disregard the fact that they do cause some is naive.

Unfortunately, elderly individuals who choose to use vitamin supplements may not be the ones with deficient diets. Several surveys have been conducted to judge dietary adequacy of older persons who regularly took vitamin supplements. Not surprisingly, it was found in one study that half of the vitamin users were consuming a completely adequate diet. Of the respondents whose diets were poor (less than two thirds of the RDA), only one in four such people were using vitamin supplements that covered all of their vitamin shortages. Only two out of four persons were using preparations that provided some, but not all, of the nutrients in which their normal diets were deficient. One fourth of the people whose diets were rated as poor were using the wrong supplements, i.e., replacing none of the vitamins or minerals that their normal diet lacked (Levy and Schucker, 1987).

Some older people need to be warned not to depend exclusively on vitamin preparations to provide for all of their nutritional needs. A report from Florida indicates that some elderly persons spend as much as $70 dollars per month on dietary supplements. Most of these were with no prescription from a physician (Hale et al, 1982). Elderly people sometimes think that vitamin supplements take care of all nutritional problems or even all health problems. This certainly is not the case and such neglect of total individual requirements for maintenance of health most surely will lead to deterioration in nutritional status in some circumstances. Among elderly people who eat an ample diet, there is little evidence that supplementary protective vitamin therapy is required. Adequate medical and dietary histories and an awareness of the importance of nutritional status are required to ensure that the individual is ingesting a balanced regimen.

A rational approach, then, to the use of vitamin preparations by the elderly must take into account their special problems and needs. Realistically, a diet with less than 1200 calories, particularly if it is poorly planned, is likely to be deficient in some vitamins. Under such circumstances, supplementation with a low-level, *appropriate* vitamin preparation may be justified. Common sense must be used in the selection of a vitamin supplement. For example, if a regular source of vitamin C can be identified in the diet, there is likely no need to include this vitamin in the supplement. Similarly, if milk or milk products are consumed on a regular basis, additional amounts of vitamin D are unnecessary.

Consideration should always be given to the possible danger associated with the indiscriminate use of vitamin supplements. Available information suggests that water-soluble vitamins are generally nontoxic, even in large doses, since the body is believed to excrete excesses in the urine. Several cases have been reported, however, of adverse responses to large doses of vitamin C, niacin, vitamin B_6, and folic acid. The fat-soluble vitamins A and D have long been recognized as toxic in large amounts. Vitamins E and K may produce similar problems but only recently have case reports appeared in the scientific literature; complaints associated with vitamin E excess include nondescript diarrhea, nausea, discomfort, fatigue, and other nonspecific symptoms. Some trace elements in vitamin preparations may be toxic if the dosage is excessive and an additional problem might be the creation of significant vitamin imbalances by the use of single vitamin preparations. Without doubt the greatest danger in the use of vitamin supplements is failure to recognize and treat the underlying disease or social or psychologic problems that caused the deficiency state to begin with.

MINERALS

A number of minerals are required by the body to allow for normal operation of most chemical processes and adequate development of skeletal tissues. Most mineral elements are well distributed in food, with the exception of iron and calcium. These minerals are most frequently consumed in inadequate amounts by the elderly, and the incidence of iron deficiency anemia and skeletal problems is consequently high in this age group. Therefore, special attention must be paid to calcium and iron intake and ideally appropriate and acceptable food sources of these nutrients can be included in recommendations for dietary improvement.

CALCIUM

For millions of Americans over age 65, osteoporosis is a debilitating disease that reduces their mobility and independence (see the section on osteoporosis in Chapter 30). Bone loss occurs after age 35 regardless of sex, age, economics, or geographic location. The average rate of bone loss in men is about 0.3% of total mass per year and in women about 1% until the menopausal acceleration to 2% or more (Cumming, 1990).

The etiology of osteoporosis is multifactorial, but little doubt remains that the inadequate intake of calcium contributes to negative calcium balance (Cumming, 1990). Factors thought to increase net bone losses of calcium include the following:

Inadequate dietary intake: calcium, vitamin D
Excessive dietary intake of oxalates and to a lesser extent phosphorus, phytates, and protein
Lack of physical activity
Inheritance pattern: Northern European
Race: Caucasian, Asian
Habits: smoking, excess alcohol consumption, and possibly excess caffeine consumption

The NHANES II study (Fanelli and Woteki, 1989) found the average intake of calcium fell below the RDA for both men and women over 65 years. It was the least adequate nutrient intake for all ages. The mean intake for women over 65 years was less than 60% of the RDA (Table 12–3). Matkovic et al (1979) compared two rural populations in Yugoslavia in terms of lifelong calcium intakes of about 1000 and 500 mg/d. The population with higher calcium intakes had higher bone mass at all ages past 30 and those over 60 suffered lower fracture rates.

The summarized data from several studies of osteoporotic people found that they reported a lifelong history of lower calcium intake when compared with control subjects (Need et al, 1990). There is a growing weight of evidence supporting the need for adequate calcium intake throughout life, with special emphasis on the growing and consolidating years between ages 15 and 30. Recent work also emphasizes the 10 years following menopause for women when calcium balance cannot be maintained unless the calcium intake is 1500 mg daily or estrogen supplements are prescribed (Nordin et al, 1990).

Some factors appear to be protective of bone density premenopausally. Excess body weight is inversely related to the premenopausal and postmenopausal rate of bone loss. Several underweight/fat anorexic women and

excessive female exercisers have decreased bone density related to their body fat and circulating estrogen levels.

Calcium losses postmenopausally can be inhibited by increasing calcium intake or by estrogen supplementation. A number of other treatments and treatment combinations have been studied with varied success. Riggs and co-workers (1984) and Aloia and associates (1982) report the greatest success using estrogen, fluoride, and calcium to reduce fracture rates. Chestnut (1984) divides treatment plans into one for prevention of excess losses using calcium fluoride and vitamin D and one for restoration of mineral losses in which estrogen plus calcium, fluoride, and vitamin D are required. In his suggested treatment of postmenopausal osteoporosis, the woman would

- Consume adequate calcium, 1000 to 1500 mg/d
- Ensure an adequate supply of vitamin D (400 IU daily) plus sunlight exposure
- Take fluoride supplements for 1 to 2 years, especially in areas where water sources are low
- Exercise
- Take anabolic steroids or calcitonin (physician discretion)
- Receive estrogen/progestin 0.3 mg daily in a 3- to 4-week cycle (physician discretion)

Weight-bearing exercises such as daily walking are a component of both treatment programs. Exercise programs have been shown to decrease calcium losses and even increase secretion in those who have already suffered fractures (see box on p. 219).

Thus it may be said that the high incidence of osteoporosis found in the population over age 50 is related to long-term low calcium intake and decreased absorption. Although some people can adapt to relatively low calcium intake, there are others who continue to excrete large quantities of calcium in the urine in spite of low intake, indicating poor utilization in the body. Calcium balance tends to become negative with aging, and there are many patients with osteoporosis who are in negative calcium balance. This may relate in part to reduction in the ability of the intestine to absorb calcium, impairment in the ability of the renal tubules to reabsorb calcium, and decreased physical activity that may promote increased urinary excretion of calcium. Increasing the calcium intake,

Health Benefits of Exercise for Older People

Retention of lean body mass
 Increased requirements for kilocalories
 Increased strength and flexibility
 Decreased percentage of adipose tissue
 Increased glucose clearance

Retention of bone density
 Decreased frailness

Exposure to sunlight for vitamin D

Maintenance of normal bowel function

Prevention of depression

Maintenance of normal appetite

Decreased risk of some chronic diseases
 Noninsulin dependent diabetes mellitus
 Atherosclerotic heart disease
 Hypertension

if the total protein and other nutritional intake is adequate, usually will restore calcium balance. Measures to prevent osteoporosis are as follows:

- Consume adequate calcium 800 to 1000 mg daily. Postmenopausal women may need 1200 to 1500 mg each day
- Ensure an adequate but not excessive supply of vitamin D—400 IU per day and regular sunlight exposure
- Get some regular exercise (walking, racket sports, bike riding, dancing, etc.)
- Avoid excesses of caffeine and alcohol
- Do not smoke

Increasing the calcium content of the diet alone will not necessarily prevent or retard development of osteoporosis. More research in this area is required at the biochemical and developmental level in order that the specific relationship between diet and bone integrity can be clarified.

IRON

A number of nutrients are required for blood cell formation and deficiency of any of them can compromise synthetic activities, and thereby lead to the development of anemia. Iron deficiency is the most common problem, especially among individuals with low incomes or with chronic diseases. The usual case of iron deficiency is related to a combination of poor dietary iron intake plus chronic blood loss, and poor absorption or inadequate utilization of iron by the body.

While the average intake of iron reported by NHANES II for persons over age 65 meets the RDA, individual variations were great and subgroups of the population would be expected to have low values. Those people living on poverty incomes or those with unusually poor dietary habits would be at particular risk.

There is little direct evidence of widespread iron deficiency in the elderly. Although absorption apparently declines with age, requirements also decline for women postmenopausally and only inappropriate bleeding would cause significant losses. There are people who remain anemic from youth into later years and others who develop iron deficiency anemias due to blood loss.

Iron deficiency is characterized by hypochromic microcytic anemia with serum iron less than 50 μg/dL and iron binding capacity increased to levels of 450 to 650 μg/dL. Iron deficiency is most commonly diagnosed by the finding of low hemoglobin value in the blood and by reduction in the size of erythrocytes. When poor iron intake is found to be involved, dietary correction should be instituted whenever possible. Sufficient iron-containing foods such as fish, poultry, meats, legumes, and egg yolks should be incorporated into the diet on a regular basis. An adequate supply of vitamin C will help to ensure higher absorption. Sometimes iron supplementation may be needed on at least a temporary basis. Ferrous salts are the most readily absorbed source of iron, and ferrous sulfate, ferrous fumarate, or ferrous gluconate are usually regarded as appropriate in this respect. But they are not without problems. Lipschitz (1990) suggests that the anemia of chronic disease is very common in this population and is often misinterpreted as iron deficiency. Iron supplements are not effective in treating the anemia of chronic disease and may have unproductive negative side effects.

Although iron deficiency may be the most common diet-related cause of anemia in the elderly, deficiency of folic acid and vitamin B_{12} should also be recognized as important. Deficiency of these vitamins, singly or simultaneously, may lead to the development of macrocytic or megaloblastic anemia. The incidence of this type of anemia in the elderly is especially high as compared with its presence in younger segments of the population (Herbert, 1988).

SODIUM

Sodium is another mineral vital to maintenance of life in the human organism. It serves many functions as an ion in the fluid milieu of the body; one of its most significant roles is to assist in the regulation of fluid balance. The daily sodium requirement is unknown but a sufficient amount is easily obtained from almost any selected diet. More frequently, excessive amounts of sodium are consumed on a regular basis. The kidneys are helpful in dealing with this circumstance in that urinary excretion of sodium increases when diet excess occurs. It appears, however, that in some individuals who are genetically predisposed to hypertension, excessive sodium consumption may serve to contribute to the severity of their hypertensive disorder (Miller et al, 1987).

Excessive intake of sodium in relation to intake of potassium may, therefore, lead to the elevation of blood pressure in some individuals, especially among African-American and Asian people. Obesity and sedentary lifestyles are considered primary risk factors for all races, and moderate weight loss and exercise are considered keystones in prevention and treatment. Moderate sodium restriction is also useful as a treatment alone or in conjunction with antihypertensive medications (Stamler et al, 1987).

The pharmaceutical industry developed a series of diuretics including some that are extremely efficient in producing marked diuresis and also effective natriuresis. Chlorothiazide, furosemide, and ethacrynic acid are three such drugs that produce a sharp increase in excretion of both sodium and potassium. The availability of these drugs has been a major contribution to the management of essential hypertension and has largely eliminated the need for severe dietary restriction of sodium. Avoidance of excessive sodium intake, however, decreases potassium losses and the potential negative impact of hypokalemia and enhances the efficiency of most diuretics. Newer drugs used to treat hypertension, classed as beta blockers, promote sodium retention and may also be best used with a moderate sodium restriction. Foods with high to moderately high sodium composi-

tion are as follows. Added salt, however, is still the major source of sodium in most diets.

1. Processed, smoked, or cured meats and fish (ham, bacon, corned beef, cold cuts, frankfurters, sausage, tongue, salt pork, chipped beef)
2. Salted foods (potato chips, nuts, popcorn, crackers)
3. Meat extracts, bouillon cubes, and meat sauces
4. Vegetable salts and flakes (onion, garlic, or celery salt; celery and parsley flakes)
5. Prepared condiments, relishes, Worcestershire sauce, catsup, mustard, pickles, and olives
6. Sodium in various additive compounds (e.g., sodium benzoate, monosodium glutamate)
7. Breads and bakery products (unless prepared specially for low-sodium composition)
8. Shellfish (except oysters)
9. Prepared flours, cake and cookie mixes, baking powders, and baking soda
10. Some frozen dinners
11. Most canned meat and vegetable products unless specially prepared without salt

POTASSIUM

Potassium is the major cation in the intracellular fluid and a significant component of the extracellular fluid compartment as well. Potassium (along with sodium) is involved in the maintenance of normal water balance, osmotic equilibrium, and acid–base balance. It also acts with calcium in the regulation of neuromuscular activity. Any circumstance that significantly increases or decreases the level of potassium in the extracellular fluid may be regarded as indicative of serious disturbances in muscle biochemistry since change in the extracellular concentration of potassium occurs late in the process of potassium depletion.

Potassium deficiency is not likely to develop in healthy individuals under normal circumstances. Potassium is widely distributed in foods and the average intake is estimated to be 0.8 to 1.5 g per 1000 calories. An adequate intake of milk, meats, cereals, vegetables, and fruits will provide adequate potassium. Significant food sources of potassium are the following:

- Legumes
- Potatoes
- Whole grains

- Winter squash
- Leafy vegetables
- Milk and yogurt
- Meats

Certain fruits, such as the following, are potassium-rich foods:

- Bananas
- Dried prunes, apricots, dates, peaches
- Raisins
- Cantaloupe
- Citrus fruits

Excessive loss of extracellular fluid may result in potassium deficiency, especially in the elderly. The loss may be due to vomiting, diarrhea, excessive diuresis, prolonged malnutrition, or use of potassium-wasting diuretics. In these conditions, potassium from the intracellular fluid is transferred to the extracellular fluid. The serum potassium level is low and ionized potassium excretion is increased. In hypokalemia (low serum potassium), cardiac failure can result from depletion of ionized potassium in heart muscle. Prevention of potassium deficiency is of considerable importance in overall management of any patient with persistent gastrointestinal disorders, diuretic use (e.g., chlorothiazide, acetazolamide), or adrenocortical hormone therapy. Consumption of foods rich in potassium and a moderate sodium restriction should be recommended (unless contraindicated by accompanying problems) but in some cases, potassium supplementation of the diet will be required.

FLUID

Water or fluid is not often thought of as food but it probably is the most important single compound required by the body. Water is essential for maintaining an environment for all chemical reactions within the body and also is vital for the functioning of urinary excretory mechanisms and for prevention of constipation. So significant is water that it constitutes about two thirds of the weight of an adult; it also is present in all body secretions and is involved in regulation of body temperature. Although the body usually can survive for many weeks without food, death will occur in less than a week when an individual is totally deprived of water.

Consequently, enough fluids should be consumed on a daily basis to allow for normal 24-hour urine volume of about 1 to $1\frac{1}{2}$ quarts. The sensation of thirst will generally provoke intake of sufficient fluid, but elderly individuals, especially those with chronic illness, may lose this regulatory capacity. Both familial and cultural patterns may also serve to deemphasize the drinking of water. Health care providers should emphasize the importance of fluid sources and regular consumption to elderly patients.

In institutions where mealtime is regulated, the fluid needs of some individuals may not be met if much time elapses between dinner and breakfast. Dehydration may easily develop overnight, especially if dinner has been served early and breakfast served late. Therefore, it may be desirable to routinely provide an evening fluid snack, or at least water, to prevent the potential serious problem of water deficit.

Factors That Determine Nutritional Needs

To a large extent, the nutritional needs of the older adult are related to the problems of nutritional balance. Nutritional balance is not solely a matter of appropriate nutrient intake, but many other factors participate in altering the circumstance of nutritional equilibrium. Factors that serve to prevent achievement of balanced nutritional status include interference with food intake, modification of intestinal absorption, interference with storage and utilization, increase in urinary and fecal excretion, and change in nutrient requirements.

INTERFERENCE WITH FOOD INTAKE

Many factors in isolation or in combination with each other lead to reduction in food intake among the elderly. Since *low income* prevents the purchase of an adequate diet for some elderly persons, this factor may be of prime significance in limiting the available food supply in the home. However, the most common social factor interfering with appetite is the sense of loss and loneliness common in older individuals preparing and consuming meals alone. The risk for depressed nutritional status is highest among those elderly persons living alone and homebound and those dealing with the impact of recent changes such as the loss of a spouse or the family home (Davies, 1990). Additionally, however, *loss of teeth* and use of poor-fitting dentures along with age-related *loss of the senses of smell and taste* may have important effects on dietary intake. The sensory losses may render food monotonous, unattractive, and uninspiring. Oral problems may lead to the adaptation of a soft diet high in refined carbohydrate and low in protein. *Physical handicaps* may contribute to either primary or secondary loss of motivation by older persons in preparing meals, thus leading to the dependence on high-priced convenience foods or fad diets and ultimately the acceptance of a variety of dietary restrictions. In addition, certain *disorders of the esophagus* prevalent in the aged (such as spasm, cancer, or hiatal hernia) may retard the passage of food into the stomach. Such conditions may remain hidden to caretakers or attending health professionals until the individual progresses to the point of obvious deterioration in health.

As far as disorders of the oral cavity are concerned, these have frequently been considered a major factor in the poor eating habits of aged people. By age 60, about 45% of the people in the United States have lost all their teeth. Some studies, however, have indicated that satisfactory dentition was not necessarily required for maintaining good nutritional status as determined by height, weight, skinfold thickness, hemoglobin level, and other factors. Totally edentulous individuals are capable of gumming food surprisingly well and lack of teeth may not be a significant factor in compromising nutritional status. Probably more important than whether or not teeth or good dentures are present and used is the overall adequacy of the diet available to the individual. It has been observed that regardless of dentition, many older persons, particularly those in institutions, consume nutritionally important foods if given satisfactory opportunity to do so.

Alcoholism may also contribute to reduction in food intake in the aged. Recent psychiatric studies indicate that alcoholism may be common, particularly in metropolitan areas, but it is often denied by both older persons and their families. The high caloric value of alcohol tends to satiate the appetite, reduce food intake, and lead to deficiency of essential dietary components, particularly protein. In the past, a variety of vitamin deficiencies were quite common, especially involving the B complex vitamins; however, the frequency of obvious clinical manifestation of vitamin deficiency has decreased in recent years, probably owing to widespread availability of vitamin-enriched bakery products and improved preventive care by health professionals.

Depression also is common in the elderly and may lead to anorexia or complete refusal of food. The severe depressive states often respond to appropriate treatment and increased appetite. Treatment of anorexia in demented patients is even more difficult and often is unsuccessful under the best of circumstances. Depression may also be the result of impaired nutritional status, leading many physicians to suggest a trial of B complex vitamin supplement as a part of the treatment.

MODIFICATION OF INTESTINAL ABSORPTION

A variety of phenomena associated with the aging process may interfere with the absorption of nutrients from the intestine. Significant changes include atrophy of the salivary glands, with an accompanying loss of enzymes, gastric achlorhydria, a decrease in the production and delivery of digestive enzymes in the stomach, pancreas, and small intestine, and diminished production and release of bile from the liver and gallbladder. Some of these changes may be the result of normal aging, whereas others may relate to the presence of pathologic conditions.

Drugs may also affect food absorption and interact with nutrients in a variety of ways. Mineral oil, for example, is an effective laxative because it is not absorbed. Since it is not absorbed but is able to bind fat-soluble vitamins, these vitamins will be lost in the stool and fat-soluble vitamin deficiencies eventually develop. Additionally, numerous drugs are known to promote malabsorption as a result of their irritating or destructive effect on the intestinal mucosa or their interference with normal epithelial cell renewal. Other drugs alter the normal intestinal pH, decreasing absorption of pH-sensitive nutrients such as vitamin B_{12}, calcium, and iron. Hydrogen ion inhibitors are examples of such drugs.

INTERFERENCE WITH STORAGE AND UTILIZATION

Diminished storage and utilization of nutrients from food may occur with aging for several reasons. There may be a diminished or altered endocrine pattern, leading to impaired metabolism. With aging there may be a loss of cells involved in the utilization and storage of nutrients; there may also be loss of structural units that produce the enzymes required for these processes. Additionally, diminished efficiency of delivery by the vascular system may develop because of intrinsic changes within that system and because of the increase in fibrous tissue that accumulates in many organs; this latter condition may create a barrier between capillaries and the parenchymal cells of affected body tissues.

INCREASE IN URINARY AND FECAL EXCRETION

The aging process, in general, is not associated with significant increases in excretory losses from the body other than the possible passage through the large bowel of undigested food because of impaired digestion and absorption. There may develop in some older persons, however, a considerable loss of protein in the urine as a consequence of kidney disease. At the same time, there is also a loss of potassium and intracellular water with aging, but there is no evidence that this is related to increased excretion.

CHANGE IN NUTRIENT REQUIREMENTS

Most of the diet is used to provide energy for body functions. Energy-producing food constituents include carbohydrates, fats, and those proteins not needed for maintenance of structural and regulatory proteins of the body. The components of the diet required for maintenance and repair of structure and regulation of biochemical processes include nine or ten essential amino acids (constituents of proteins), several unsaturated fatty acids, vitamins, and minerals. During the aging process, the body's need for some of these nutrients changes in accord with changing physiologic activities, exercise patterns, and overall lifestyle. Conditions of nutritional deficiency or excess may develop if eating patterns are not adjusted to accommodate the change in body needs.

In addition to the normal changes in nutrient requirements related to advancing age, many diseases produce a hypermetabolic state that may create a dietary need in excess of intake. Fevers of any type, especially if prolonged, consume excess calories and produce tissue wasting and weight loss if dietary intake is not increased to cover the calorie require-

ment. Persistent fevers, even of a low-grade type, may produce the same result. The most common cause of emaciation or cachexia, however, is malignancy. Cancer causes tissue wasting that seems excessive in many circumstances for the increased metabolic activity that exists. This phenomenon may be due to preferential requirement by the tumor for particular amino acids that if found in short supply in the diet will be leached from available lean body stores.

The Significance of Food Beyond Its Nutrients

Fulfillment of the need for food is a significant concern in the management of patients at all stages of the life cycle. Beyond the basic role of food in providing for physical sustenance and growth, however, foods take on special meanings in the lives of most people. Eating is an important activity that serves to meet not only physiologic requirements but also to fulfill basic psychologic, sociologic, and emotional needs of individuals. Recognition of the significance of food and eating in the cultural patterns of aging persons is critical to the development of workable recommendations for improvement of health through modification of dietary practices.

Discussion of cultural patterns in relation to diet encompasses a variety of dimensions. For the practitioner who needs to understand fully what determines the behavioral patterns of people, it is particularly important to be consciously aware of ethnicity, regional or urban–rural cultures, socioeconomic status, and age-appropriate behavior.

ETHNIC FACTORS

Ethnicity includes those characteristics of behavior and habit that are part of national or ethnic custom. Ethnic patterns in food preference and use serve to consolidate group identity. Adherence to traditional patterns is particularly strong in connection with social and religious ritual. Culture defines those foods that are "good" and those that are not. Culture determines a group's perception of individual foods so that some highly nutritious food items may be considered good only as dog food and therefore totally unacceptable for human consumption.

Ethnic foods may be unsuitable for the aged only if they are medically contraindicated or if they consistently exclude necessary nutrients. The high fat diets of some Middle European cultures and the high starch diets of Southern Europeans are cases of dominance in the diet, but they are not necessarily inappropriate except as they may contribute to obesity. Soul foods of African-Americans also may contain excessive fats and a very low lean-protein content. Research on obesity, especially among women aged 55 to 70, indicates that ethnic diets contribute greatly to the persistence of weight problems.

It has been established by anthropologic studies, however, that indigenous foods and their manner of preparation and combination typically represent "good" nutritional balance for a particular native group. It is the imposition of alien food forms or preparation methods that most often subverts the inherent balance existent in a traditional diet of a group of people. Efforts to modify the diets of the various ethnic groups should be approached only by those with a detailed understanding of ethnic foods and the nutritional requirements of the population.

REGIONAL OR URBAN–RURAL CULTURES

There are traditional types of foods within the United States that are identified with certain areas of the country and that long-time residents of such areas associate with "home." For elderly persons, it is likely that the reintroduction of such foods in a social situation would have a positive reinforcement value. Presentation of foods from "down home" may encourage reminiscences, now considered a psychologic benefit in the aged's adjustment to the final stage of their life cycle. The exchange of memories may, in turn, facilitate the development of new interpersonal ventures, so necessary when old friends and many relatives have been lost.

SOCIOECONOMIC STATUS

Socioeconomic status is not strictly considered as "culture"; however, class often interacts in culture with, for example, rural origins of a mi-

grant group or ethnic group identity. The concept of a *culture of poverty* appears to have considerable practical reality as one observes and programs for those elderly who have lived their entire lives far below a minimum standard of living accepted as tolerable in this society. The class identification of certain foods may serve a detrimental function in the diet of poor people; status may be sought by selective purchase of high carbohydrate, processed foods thought to be preferred by the upper class.

AGE-APPROPRIATE BEHAVIOR

Of interest is the finding by social scientists that another culture factor in the behavior of older persons is the expectation held by the aged as to how they should act, i.e., what behaviors are appropriate or inappropriate to their chronologic level. These *shoulds* are reinforced by attitudes of younger adults so that a picture develops in the mind of young and old of appropriate *normal* behavior for old people in a particular culture. Age-appropriate behaviors relate especially to food choice and dietary habits since these are very often associated with the changed body image of the elderly. Older people, especially women, tend to be quite conscious about the internal and external states of their bodies and thus tend to develop protective attitudes in response to visible aging and body dysfunction. The dysfunctions or malfunctions may be real, imagined, or exaggerated. In any case, food selection and rejection is often justified by an appeal to the needs of the body. Areas of likely concern are related to digestion, constipation, tissue rejuvenation, blood, and muscle tone (fatigue).

The popularity of iron supplements among the elderly, for example, has been said to relate to the age-appropriate belief that high iron concentrations in the blood can reduce fatigue associated with aging. The reality that the fatigue of old age may mask (or be generated by) depression, cumulative social loss, or disease (none of which is affected by iron supplements) should create concern among health care professionals. Likewise, concern should also exist about the high use of pseudohealth foods among older persons. This recognized practice also suggests the widespread interest among the elderly for maintenance of body image through acceptable age-appropriate dietary behavior. Efforts should be made to counter myths about "bottled health" and "magic foods." The elderly person should be advised on how to spot a "quack."

Implications for Eating Habits of the Aged

Because of the multitude of roles that food plays in the lives of most people, feeding patterns and food preferences should be recognized as basic to happiness and survival. In particular, as far as the elderly are concerned, eating is remembering, eating is life-giving, and eating is relating.

EATING IS REMEMBERING

The aged person who uses "food for thought" as a means of gaining comfort in the present from reminiscence of the past is less concerned with the life-giving qualities of food and more concerned with the symbolic meanings of food. Eating habits that appear "unhealthful" to the nurse or nutritionist may be serving an important adaptive function for the aged person. Thus, there may be conflict between the primary nutritional goal and the aged person who is being served. The imposition of the health care professional's needs may, if not handled cautiously, undermine the intrapsychic needs of the person to be served. Although there is no easy solution to this conflict, it can be handled by a sensitive awareness of how particular eating habits play an adaptive function for the person. The older person can "have his cake and eat it too" if enough of the meaning of foods or particular detrimental routines to the individual are meshed into a more sensible nutritional regimen.

It may be more difficult, on the other hand, to introduce a beneficial food into a nutritional regimen when confronted with a lifetime of food aversions. Efforts to convince an aging person through a rational discussion that a new food might actually be rather tasty or indeed agree with him physically cannot help but conflict with persistent lifetime taboos and stereotypic attitudes. For example, the woman in her 70s with the common problem of constipation who says, "I don't eat cheese because it is constipating," is not about to be convinced that cheese is the obvious source of improved health. In her advanced age, such stereotypes form a convenient way of dealing with the

world, a world that seems manageable and comfortable by just such reassuring perceptions. The heroic task of introducing new foods into the diet of a younger person is made even more difficult in working with the aged.

EATING IS LIFEGIVING

When we are confronted with body deterioration, the primary function of food as bodily maintenance becomes increasingly important. Here, also, magical solutions that take the form of food as recuperative agents or as restoring youth are sometimes sought by the aged. In the extreme, this magic is seen in food faddism and in hoarding behaviors where having an immediate access to a particular food offers reassurance. Part of the institutionalization process has been seen to *depersonalize* the individual by restricting his free access to food. Some nursing homes and hospitals in the United States have instituted a 24-hour food availability system by providing refrigerators and cupboards for free snacking. Although psychologically of benefit, this type of program, if inadequately supervised, could lead to poor diet in the aged.

For the community-dwelling aged, an important aspect of the mechanism of food as reassurance may be shopping for and purchasing food in which the process of "gathering and storing" enhances feelings of life-maintenance. The more supportive an aged individual can be of his or her established food-related activities, the more likely that person is to maintain an optimistic outlook on his or her remaining life and a motivation to maintain health.

EATING IS RELATING

Securing, preparing, and consuming food are activities basic to family relationships. Most of the elderly in today's society have actively participated in home-based food activities and have enjoyed the mealtime as a period for family discussion. In most cases the wife has performed her maternal function of preparing and serving the food to her family; the husband typically has enjoyed the role of provider and consumer. Sex-role identification generally is well solidified so that when age-related losses reduce the opportunity for these activities, the corresponding identifications are weakened. Consequently, to facilitate the maintenance of these identifications, it may be necessary to find substitutes in the form of activities and persons that replace significant others. Where the elderly come together in senior centers, the opportunity for reestablishing and reaffirming their sex roles in food preparation and serving should be supported when possible by the practitioner. Similarly, in a home care program it may be easier to prepare all meals for the elderly widow who needs a special diet; this service, however, may be depriving her of the personal meanings inherent in food activities. Likewise, for persons who are unable to work for their food, effort should be made to locate an activity that might partially satisfy their needs.

Although maintenance of these food-related or meal-related activities is satisfying for most elderly people, several cross-cultural studies have shown that the need to maintain these activities is of less importance than the need to feel that one is comfortable and secure. Fulfilling the need for security may relate more to relationships with children than to spouse, especially if the spouse has died. Eating may thus become part of an intergenerational conflict where inadequate eating may function to arouse concern of a daughter, who may feel guilty about her caretaking relationship with a parent. The comment that "she doesn't eat enough to keep a bird alive" may reflect a generational conflict that must be handled if the elderly parent is to receive nutritional requirements. In a situation where the daughter is of an advanced age herself, especially if the mother is in her 70s or 80s, then inventive techniques geared toward the more elderly person may, by necessity, include therapeutic help for both.

Inadequate food intake as a plea for attention must be understood in the context of feelings of loneliness and of isolation and desolation. When faced with loneliness, food can become a solace, because it facilitates memories; on the other hand, the rejection of food may relate to a plea for immediate attention and caring. Often this plea is part of the paranoid behavior of the aged where the covert or unconscious message is, "If you really loved me you would care for me and make me well again." Whereas all efforts made to reduce these irrational feelings seem to be unsuccessful and all efforts to ameliorate the nutritional inadequacies appear to fail, the very contact between the provider and the elderly person may relieve feelings of loneliness and isolation.

Because of the multitudes of meanings that food has for aged individuals, part of the goal of any nutrition program for older people should be to keep them not only physically alive but also socially and psychologically active. This means that a good nutrition program for the aged includes more than the proper balance of nourishing food, even nourishing food adapted to the individual's past tastes, prejudices, and taboos. It includes at least some opportunity for the meaningful social involvement and some opportunity for individual planning and choice of both food and social involvement to suit varying personality types. Recent government-sponsored demonstration projects on the nutrition of the aged have paid careful attention to the multiple facets of the eating experience. Some of these programs and ideas are further discussed in the remainder of this chapter.

Assessing Dietary Patterns and Nutritional Status

The nutritional evaluation of the individual is as important as any other aspect of a thorough evaluation and consequently involves the acquisition of as much relevant information as possible. Effort should be made to identify significant factors known to adversely influence nutritional well-being. The evaluation must include a thorough physical examination, with special emphasis on those clinical signs that have been associated with malnutrition in humans. Unplanned weight loss is the most significant predictor of depressed nutritional status, leading to morbidity and mortality. It is important to track weight and to investigate causes of weight loss both in free-living and institutionalized patients. Also of particular importance are neurologic findings and examination of the skin, eyes, and oral cavity including the tongue, lips, gums, and teeth. In addition, selected and relevant biochemical data must be accumulated to confirm or extend the clinical judgment derived from the physical and nutritional evaluation. Particular attention must be given to the latent aspect of nutritional deficiency that frequently is present but extremely difficult to define in concrete observations.

Most circumstances of nutritional deficiency are complex in their development (Fig. 12-1). Primary nutritional deficiency disease may occur solely because of inadequate dietary

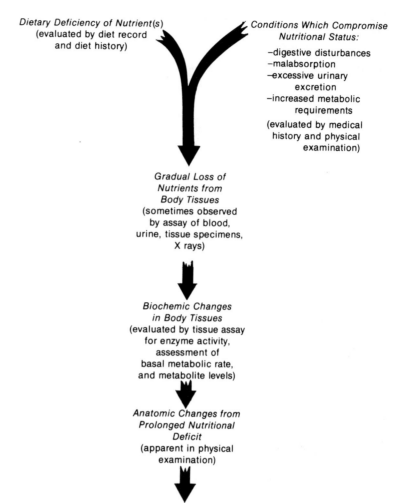

Dietary Deficiency of Nutrient(s)
(evaluated by diet record
and diet history)

Conditions Which Compromise
Nutritional Status:
–digestive disturbances
–malabsorption
–excessive urinary
    excretion
–increased metabolic
    requirements
(evaluated by medical
    history and physical
    examination)

Gradual Loss of
Nutrients from
Body Tissues
(sometimes observed
by assay of blood,
urine, tissue specimens,
X rays)

Biochemic Changes
in Body Tissues
(evaluated by tissue assay
for enzyme activity,
assessment of
basal metabolic rate,
and metabolite levels)

Anatomic Changes from
Prolonged Nutritional
Deficit
(apparent in physical
examination)

Death

FIGURE 12–1 Sequential steps in the development of malnutrition.

intake, but this is rare unless the poor diet persists for a long period. More commonly, especially in the elderly, such factors as malabsorption, decreased use of nutrients, increased excretion and destruction of nutrients, and increased nutritional requirements related to genetic or metabolic factors must be considered. The typical sequence of events in the development of clinical malnutrition is the initial desaturation of tissue content of various nutrients. Usually this is evidenced by biochemical alterations in blood, urine, and biopsy specimens. As tissue depletion proceeds, biochemical deficits may become increasingly manifest. It should be recognized, however, that these biochemical changes in the blood, like clear-cut observable clinical changes attributable to malnutrition, seldom develop in well-defined stages, but rather present in a series of gradua-

tions in which the duration of the deficit is most important. Clinical manifestations of nutritional deficiencies never appear as black or white problems, but more often present as a spectrum of irregularities appropriately assigned to the "gray zone" (Table 12–6). It has been suggested that the sequencing of events in the development of deficiencies may vary in elderly individuals, thus causing clinical changes before the expected biochemical changes. This suggests a more aggressive pursuit of a nutritional diagnosis.

If malnutrition continues long enough or if trauma or illness precipitate it, the classic anatomic and pathologic lesions or signs of deficiency disease become obvious. At this point of severe deprivation, complete responses to nutritional rehabilitation usually are slow. Clearly, it is important to diagnose malnutrition before

TABLE 12–6   *Clinical Syndromes Associated with Deficiencies of Specific Nutrients*

Calories: Underweight, underheight, weight loss, lethargy, anemia, edema, marasmus

Protein: As above, fatty liver, kwashiorkor

Fat: Dermatoses (essential fatty acid deficiency), deficiencies of the fat-soluble vitamins A, D, E, and K

Vitamin A: Follicular hyperkeratosis, night blindness, xerophthalmia, keratomalacia

Vitamin D: Tetany, osteomalacia

Vitamin E: Macrocytic anemia, altered immune responses

Vitamin K: Decreased plasma prothrombin activity with prolonged coagulation time and hemorrhages

Thiamin: Anorexia, beriberi, polyneuropathy, toxic amblyopia, heart disease, the ophthalmoplegia of Wernicke's syndrome

Riboflavin: Photophobia, corneal vascularization, angular stomatitis, glossitis, dermatitis

Niacin: Pellagra, dermatitis, glossitis, diarrhea, mental confusion and deterioration, encephalopathy

Pyridoxine: Anemia, polyneuropathy, seborrheic exzema

Pantothenic acid: Nutritional melalgia (burning feet syndrome)

Folic acid: Glossitis, macrocytic anemia, megaloblastic anemia of infancy, megaloblastic anemia in adults

Vitamin B_{12}: Glossitis, macrocytic anemia, peripheral neuropathy, combined system diseases (posterolateral column degeneration), mental changes and deterioration

Biotin: Seborrheic dermatitis

Choline: Unknown

Inositol: Unknown

Carnitine: Unknown

Ascorbic acid: Scurvy, scorbutic gums, subperiosteal hemorrhages, petechial hemorrhages, anemia, impaired wound healing

Iron: Anemia, achlorhydria, glossitis

Iodine: Simple goiter

Fluorine: Dental caries

Calcium: Osteomalacia, a role in the production of senile osteoporosis

Magnesium: Neuromuscular irritability, tetany

Potassium: Alkalosis, muscle weakness and paralysis, cardiac disturbances

Salt: Anorexia, nausea, vomiting, lassitude, asthenia, muscle cramps, circulatory collapse

Water: Thirst, dehydration, oliguria, mental changes progressing to coma

Zinc: Impaired wound healing, altered immune response

From Shils ME, Young VR. Modern nutrition in health and disease, 7th ed. Philadelphia: Lea & Febiger, 1988. Reprinted with permission.

the full-blown deficiency condition develops and to treat it aggressively to prevent the rapid and sometimes devastating decline often seen in hospitalized older patients (Morley, 1990). In view of recent Supreme Court rulings making withdrawal of nutrition support delivered enterally or parenterally more difficult, the decision to move to a "more heroic" feeding method should be considered carefully in the severely demented or very aged patient. The guidelines developed for withdrawal and withholding of treatment state that the difference between withholding and withdrawing treatment is not one of moral importance, but there is a widely recognized psychological distinction. The rights and opinions of the patient should be solicited early and should be considered along with the extent of discomfort and burden imposed by enteral and parenteral feeding (Meyers and Grodin, 1991) (see Chapter 4).

To summarize, the basic principles underlying the evaluation of nutritional status are not much different from those used in a general medical evaluation of a patient. The nutritional evaluation is based on (1) observing the general appearance of the individual, (2) obtaining a complete medical, personal, and social history, (3) recording an accurate diet history, either elaborate or concise, (4) completing a thorough physical examination, including measures of body weight and height, and (5) compiling pertinent laboratory data as they relate to suspected nutritional deficits.

As far as biochemical or laboratory data are concerned, several basic principles deserve attention in establishing guidelines for sensible lab work-ups. First, laboratory assays should be carefully selected to answer specific questions about the patient's nutritional status. Second, the laboratory work should provide substantiation of the clinical judgment or remove lingering doubt. Third, a number of do-it-yourself procedures may save time and costs for both patient and health care staff. A simple urinalysis, evaluation of a blood smear, and microscopic study of the stool for the presence of fat can be completed rather easily in an office or clinic. Fourth, the importance of appropriate timing of laboratory tests should be fully recognized. A fasting blood sample should be just that and assessment of vitamin level in the bloodstream or urine has no value if the therapeutic provision of vitamins has already begun. Last, at least two points should be established sequentially in a series of laboratory evaluations to determine the progress of the illness or the effects of therapy.

The American Academy of Family Physicians, The American Dietetic Association, and The National Council on the Aging, Inc. came together in a National Screening Initiative Consensus Conference in 1991 (White et al, 1992). They agreed that all health and social services professionals need to be aware of the importance of nutritional health and need to recognize the warning signs that identify people at nutritional risk. The Nutrition Screening Initiative published a checklist to be read by the lay public to determine a nutritional score and a two-level screening procedure. The level-one and level-two screens are designed to be administered by health or social services professionals to determine a category of nutritional risk—high or moderate—which will help with diagnosis and referral. Complete copies of the checklist, the level one and two screens, and the manual developed to explain their implementation can be obtained from the Nutrition Screening Initiative, 2626 Pennsylvania Ave. NW, Washington, DC 20037.

THE DIET HISTORY

The diet history may turn out to be the most important piece of information available in completing a routine evaluation of nutritional condition. Unfortunately, recording an accurate diet history is not always easy and usually requires considerable time and patience. One aspect of this procedure that may prove to be especially valuable as a screening mechanism is the listing of foods in major categories and determining the number of times per week that the patient consumes them. This process may easily identify the individual who tends to follow some fad diet, who restricts the diet to only several foods, who ingests significant amounts of "empty calories" such as alcohol and sugar, or who follows highly unusual dietary practices that exclude important foods or food groups. Generally speaking a balanced dietary regimen best fulfills daily needs, and such a dietary pattern should provide no more than 20% to 25% of daily calories from a single food. It is also important to inquire about eating habits and the distribution of meals, particularly the omission of certain meals, such as breakfast, and the type and frequency of snacks. Some people do not regard between-meal snacks as "food" and frequently do not report these as part of their daily diet. Obtaining this important information by careful questioning is important if accurate overall assessment of nutrient intake is to be secured.

Nutritional Status of the Elderly in Developed Societies

The results of a number of recent nutrition surveys support the concept that the diets of elderly individuals are often nutritionally adequate. Yet we also know that advanced age is a distinct risk factor for poor nutritional status. We can marry these two concepts by realizing that the population over age 65 is not homogeneous. Subgroups of the elderly are poorly nourished and require close attention. The findings of NHANES I and II and surveys from Australia and Europe support this concept (Wahlquest, 1990). For most people, calorie consumption declined with age; therefore, the intake of most nutrients declined with age. The *nutrient density* of their diet increased, however, so that as calories declined, the intake of other nutrients did not decline as rapidly. The elderly also ate food of higher nutritional quality and purchased more high-quality food for their food dollar.

NHANES II reported that mean intakes for

both men and women met the RDA for all nutrients except calcium and thiamin. Recent updates identify the mean intakes of people over 55 of folate and B$_{12}$ as insufficient to meet the RDAs. The ranges of nutrient intakes were very great, with those people at and below the 25th percentile failing to achieve recommended allowances for almost all nutrients. NHANES II data allowed a comparison of biochemical measures of nutritional status with reported nutrient intake. Biochemical evidence of decreased nutritional status occurred in 2% to 7% of the population over age 65, with increased evidence in African-American women and people with poverty incomes.

Numerous smaller studies have yielded information about institutionalized and free-living people. The study by Garry et al (1982) of a healthy middle-aged group of men and women over 60 and the study by McGandy et al (1986) of healthy free-living people in Boston both found values similar to NHANES II, with dietary calcium being the most deficient nutrient, but mean values for some other nutrients were also supplied in less than adequate amounts. They also found wide ranges, with more than 20% having significant deficits of vitamins B$_6$, D, and folate.

Several studies found that free-living populations fare better than the institutionalized, although frequently the deficits found are simply different. Patients admitted to acute care settings in the United States, France, and England have a high incidence of protein-calorie malnutrition, perhaps suggesting, at least in part, their reasons for admission (Mowe and Bohmer, 1991; Constans et al, 1992). Folic acid, vitamin C, and thiamin are deficit in 5% to 15% of older patients (Drinka, 1991).

Of those nutrients less studied in major surveys, zinc is one most frequently suggested to be in inadequate supply in diets of the elderly. Poor zinc nutrition is linked to common problems of the elderly: decreased taste acuity, decreased immune response, and decreased wound healing. Several small studies of zinc status suggest that older persons with inadequate intakes are at higher risk of poor zinc status. The adequate intake of zinc is difficult to maintain at low income levels, but available data are insufficient to determine the frequency of decreased zinc nutrition and its contributions to immune and wound healing deficits (Sandstead et al, 1982).

Efforts to Solve Nutritional Problems of the Elderly

Recognition of the serious problem of malnutrition among the elderly increased during the 1960s to the point where significant government involvement developed. The Department of Health, Education, and Welfare became increasingly involved in 1965 and, by 1973, under Title VII, now Title III-C, of the Older Americans Act, The Administration on Aging instituted The National Nutrition Program for the Elderly (National Clearing House on Aging, 1974).

The overriding goal of this massive undertaking was to provide inexpensive, nutritionally sound meals to older Americans. Additionally, however, the program was designed to reduce the isolation of older people by offering them an opportunity to participate in community activities that combine food and friendship. As the amended form of the Older Americans Act stated:

> Many older persons do not eat adequately because (1) they cannot afford to do so, (2) they lack the skills to select and prepare nourishing and well-balanced meals, (3) they have limited mobility which may impair their capacity to shop and cook for themselves, and (4) they have feelings of rejection and loneliness which obliterate the incentive necessary to prepare and eat a meal alone. These and other physiological, psychological, social and economic changes that occur with aging result in a pattern of living which causes malnutrition and further physical and mental deterioration.

To cope with this national problem of widespread concern, nutrition projects have been established throughout the country that provide at least one hot meal per day, 5 days a week, to older citizens (aged 60 and over) and their spouses (any age). Meals are prepared and served in group settings if at all possible. Meal sites include schools, churches, community centers, senior citizen centers, public housing, and other public and private facilities where other social services may also be available. Outreach programs to identify persons most in need of services (as well as transportation to meal sites) are also part of the program's responsibilities.

The nature and format of the individual programs now in existence depends on the composition and orientation of community personnel and resources. The aim of such assistance is to provide supplemental or enabling services to the older person who has the capabilities to function alone if this is desired. A typical group of elderly persons includes a wide range of individuals with a variety of needs; their physical and mental capabilities may not be the prime considerations. In such a group one might find the following: the older man who is widowed and has never prepared meals for himself, the person with a disabling illness that is not completely incapacitating but does cause pain in undertaking meal preparation activities, the person who always has had meals of his own "cultural derivation" and who is now faced with trying to maintain a special diet as a result of a disease condition or weight problem, and the individual in dilapidated housing whose cooking equipment is less than optimal and whose mental or physical state involves a safety hazard. A number of other examples could be cited. Some of these individuals may require other community services in the home such as public health nursing, nutrition services, and the home economics and related services of voluntary health, social, and civic agencies.

Area agencies on aging provide outreach services to help older persons to learn of community services available to them. It is true, however, that health care providers need to be aware of locally available services in order to make appropriate referrals.

Special facets of the federally supported nutrition demonstration-research projects are basic to the success that many of these projects have appreciated. Among the supplemental provisions are the following:

1. Auxiliary services such as transportation, dental care, and counseling on individual dietary requirements to make it possible for older people to use the services
2. Research projects to gain new knowledge on such matters as dietary needs and habits of older persons
3. Social settings designed for personal adjustment and adequacy of diet
4. Tools and appliances for food preparation, handling, and storage that older persons can use with greater safety and ease
5. Unit cost analyses of different systems for improving diets
6. Settings conducive to eating meals with others

7. Surplus or donated foods or food stamps from the USDA.

The nutrition projects currently funded under Titles III C-1 and C-2 Congregate Meals and Home Delivered Meal Programs began serving hot meals to the elderly in July 1973. Since then they have grown from 32 holdover projects from the research and demonstration days to over 1300 projects in operation in 1987. These projects comprise over 14,000 meal service sites staffed by over 30,000 paid staff and 195,976 volunteers. The nutrition program now serves over 220 million meals to Americans over 60 years of age (ADA Testimony, 1987).

Organization of the individual nutrition projects and administration of the federal funds are handled by the separate state agencies on aging unless another agency is designated by the Governor and approved by the Secretary of Health, Education and Welfare. This administering body makes grants to or contracts with public and nonprofit organizations for actual provision and delivery of the meals. Advisory assistance is available through the state agency to assist with consumer problems and overall planning for provision of high-quality nutrition services at the local level.

Most nutrition projects funded under this program primarily serve low income elderly persons and spouses who are determined to be in greatest need of nutrition services. Effort is made by the governing state body to see that awards are made to initiate projects to serve minority groups and individuals with limited English-speaking abilities within the state. Meal sites are required to be located in urban areas that have heavy concentrations of target-group elderly and in rural regions where high proportions of elderly eligibles reside.

Payment for meals obtained in the nutrition projects is not required and no one is turned away because of lack of funds. Participants *do* have the opportunity, however, to pay part of the cost of the meal if they wish. The project directors must establish either a range of contributions or a single flat sum as a suggested contribution by participants. Each participant determines for himself what he is able to contribute and collection of money is handled confidentially.

Title III C-2 of the Older Americans Act provides specifically for provision of home-delivered meals that can be delivered to home-bound elderly persons when appropriate or necessary. The demand for meals, either as hot complete meals or frozen (or freeze-dried) components, increased rapidly in the 1980s, with services increasing 10% to 12% annually. Although this type of arrangement does not provide an effective mechanism for socialization, the volunteer drivers are often a welcome contact with the outside world and home-delivered meals can help meet the ongoing nutritional needs of persons who otherwise would be inadequately nourished or forced to reside in an institution.

The aims of early portable meals programs were quite specific and were beautifully defined by Martin Keller and Charlotte Smith (Howell and Loeb, 1969). These authors state:

> The prevention of institutionalization is a basic aim in preventive medical and public health programs. In every community, there are people who can be helped to live successfully in their own homes by a number of simple services. Aside from the salutary benefits of relative independence, there is a distinct economic advantage (to the community) in the extension of such services.

The further point is made that the provision of such meals would prevent malnutrition and allow these persons to continue living at home. They are needed and

> ... aside from their virtue, such programs serve to elevate the level of the community action in the general area of the health of the aged and in chronic disease control. They can serve as a direct way into larger, more comprehensive programs.

The authors take great care in pointing out:

> ... that in the enthusiasm generated by (portable meals) programs, the fundamental aim may be, overlooked. *The object is to increase the independence of the recipient. Unless the activities are constantly reviewed with reference to this objective, the program may, instead, foster dependency.*

Portable meals are not designed for persons who can leave their homes and dine in restaurants, for those who can shop for food and prepare adequate meals for themselves, or for those who can obtain family or neighbor help in doing so. Their particular value may exist during periods of convalescence, especially when earlier hospital discharge is driven by prepayment systems such as the Diagnostic Related Groups System.

Specific portable meals programs have some common features, although there are variations in the administrative aspects based on local need and available resources. One survey indicated that 22 such services studied had the following characteristics:

1. A typical portable meals program is a community service, most often located in a metropolitan area.
2. The average number of persons served is approximately 20 to 40 per day, with the midday and evening meals being delivered 5 days a week, Monday through Friday.
3. The program has the professional assistance of a dietitian, nutritionist, or home economist.
4. The meals are prepared in an agency kitchen and modified diets are provided.
5. Various vehicles transport the meals to the recipient's home and a fee for service is charged according to the person's ability to pay.

Not so typical are efforts by some programs to offer extended services to the elderly homebound, including home-delivered groceries and home-delivered breakfasts.

A home-delivered meals program is only one part of a comprehensive approach to providing food to older persons in the community and must be viewed in this context. To be sure, it is a very important service and can be critical to survival for the person who needs it. It may be that the prevention of dependency requires that some recipients evolve from portable, home-delivery meals to counseling of family and neighbors in food preparation assistance, to neighborhood group meals, and to self-responsibility as the person's autonomy improves.

Educational and Consultative Services for the Elderly

All nutrition programs administered under the Older Americans Act are required to include an educational component. There is concern, however, for the effectiveness of this aspect of the program and the limited skills in communities for designing sound educational evaluation. The problem of appropriate teaching materials is a prime concern. There are many prepared written materials on nutrition and age, special diets, and other topics. They are often randomly distributed to older persons, even though they may not be tailored to this population or even readapted for special aged subgroups. These materials may be of better use in the training of aides than in reshaping the eating habits of the elderly directly.

Appropriate nutrition guidance for a given geriatric patient needs to be highly individualized—physical, psychologic, socioeconomic, and cultural factors must all be recognized as highly relevant. To provide the most effective counseling, the answers to a number of questions must be obtained. The following questions may prove helpful in the development of a more complete picture of the individual patient who needs advice:

1. What are the patient's physical limitations?
2. Is he able to plan for his food needs?
3. Does he know what his food needs are?
4. Is he physically able to shop for his food?
5. Does he have a convenient means of transportation?
6. Can he handle the food himself and get it back to his residence?
7. If he has special nutritional needs or limitations, is he able to read and understand labels on food packages?
8. Does he understand his condition and needs well enough to follow dietary directions?
9. If he cannot shop for food himself, what other options are open to him?
10. What are his housing arrangements?
11. Does he live alone or with others?
12. If he cannot take care of himself, will those with whom he lives take over this responsibility?
13. Are they capable of this responsibility? Are they willing to accept it?
14. What facilities are available for food storage, refrigeration, preparation, cleanup, and garbage disposal?
15. Is the patient able to use the facilities to prepare an adequate diet?
16. What kinds of utensils are available?
17. Have the utensils been rearranged to be within easy reach?
18. Is there a pleasant place to eat comfortably?
19. Are there enough dishes and tableware for attractiveness and sanitation?
20. Does the person have someone with whom he can eat?
21. What is the person's usual eating pattern?
22. Is there an eating pattern?
23. Are there foods that are disliked or do not agree with the patient?
24. Have any dietary limitations been prescribed?
25. What food items are eaten in a representative day (24-hour recall)?

This series of questions provides much information to the health care worker who needs to counsel the patient about nutrition. Using these data and knowledge of the nutritional needs of the elderly, the counselor can make reasonable suggestions in tune with the patient's physical condition, lifestyle, and unique circumstances (Davies and Knutson, 1991). A daily food guide, such as that seen in Table 12–7, may be useful in discussing diet with some individuals. Budgeting tips may also be very informative (see Getting the Most for Your Money on p. 235) as are many hints on encouraging good food intake for persons living alone (see Suggestions for People Eating Alone on p. 235). In some circumstances, however, the use of these materials may be awkward and other educational tools may serve the purpose more effectively. The health care providers are always on the lookout for well-designed nutrition education materials. The development of a repertoire of approaches and methods will serve the educator well in the real world where people are amazingly different in their response to specific educational experiences.

Teaching nutrition and consumerism to an elderly group is an exciting and rewarding experience if it is done properly with a thorough understanding of the audience before starting. The nutrition education experience must be based on the awareness that older persons come to the learning experience as voluntary participants, mature adults with a wealth of past experiences, special interests, training, and expertise, and not as young impressionable students. For this reason, they are ready to learn different things. In short, the adult learner will probably be most interested in knowledge that is immediately useful (Kieklighter, 1992).

If effective learning is to take place, the instructor must stimulate an interest in the subject of nutrition. Since learning depends on attention, retention, and recall, the instructor's greatest ally is the individual's desire to learn. Interest in the subject aids in the mental organization necessary for attention and retention. The first session is extremely important in get-

TABLE 12–7   *Daily Food Guide*

MILK, CHEESE, DAIRY DESSERTS—(2 OR MORE CUPS DAILY)

Leading source of calcium and riboflavin; excellent source of high-quality protein and vitamin A; lesser quantities of other nutrients

May be taken in many forms: fresh whole or skim, reconstituted dried whole or skim, evaporated, buttermilk, whole or skim cheese, ice milk or frozen yogurt

If calories or fat, or both, are restricted, skim milk fortified with vitamin A and B may be used

The calcium equivalent of 1 cup of milk is $1\frac{1}{3}$ oz cheddar cheese, 1 lb cream cheese, $\frac{3}{4}$ lb creamed cottage cheese, 8 oz yogurt; with restricted calories or fat, either skim or lowfat milk is the best source of calcium

MEAT, FISH, POULTRY, EGGS, DRY BEANS AND PEAS, NUTS—(2 OR MORE SERVINGS DAILY)

Meat, poultry, and fish are of particular value for high-quality protein and also provide iron, thiamin, riboflavin, and niacin; at least 1 serving daily

Eggs are a source of high-quality protein, iron, vitamin A, thiamin, riboflavin, and vitamin D; 3 to 4 servings weekly unless cholesterol is restricted

Nuts and dry beans and peas contain good protein, iron, and some B vitamins; protein value is enhanced if some animal protein is served with them

GRAIN PRODUCTS—(4 TO 5 OR MORE SERVINGS DAILY)

Provide significant quantities of iron, thiamin, riboflavin, and niacin if made with whole grain or restored or enriched with minerals and vitamins; include breads, cereals, noodles, macaroni, rice, and corn meal

VEGETABLES AND FRUITS—(AT LEAST 4 SERVINGS DAILY)

Should include at least 1 serving daily of fruit rich in vitamin C and at least 3 or 4 servings per week of vegetables rich in vitamin A value and folate

Fruits particularly rich in vitamin C are oranges, grapefruit, and tomatoes; the vitamin C equivalent of 1 orange is $\frac{1}{2}$ grapefriut, 4 oz orange or grapefruit juice, 10 oz tomato juice, $\frac{1}{2}$ medium-sized cantaloupe, $\frac{1}{2}$ to $\frac{3}{4}$ cup fresh strawberries, 1 cup shredded raw cabbage, $\frac{1}{2}$ cup broccoli, $\frac{3}{4}$ to 1 cup dark green leaves from kale, spinach, or brussel sprouts, or a small green pepper

Vegetables rich in vitamin A (dark green and deep yellow vegetables) also provide some riboflavin, iron, calcium; and folic acid, chard, collards, kale, spinach, carrots, yellow winter squash, pumpkin, sweet potatoes; broccoli; green peppers

Potatoes provide some of several minerals and vitamins, including iron, thiamin, riboflavin, and vitamin C and can be eaten every day

Other vegetables and fruits; 1 to 3 or more servings should be used daily to total at least 4 servings of fruits and vegetables per day

FATS AND OILS—(SOME BUTTER OR MARGARINE DAILY)

Butter and margarine are rich in vitamin A

All fats and oils are high in calories and should be used sparingly if calories are restricted

Many authorities recommend reduction of the total quantity of fat in the American diet, with an increase in the proportion of polyunsaturated fats and oils and a decrease in the proportion of saturated fats; in general, the use of fat as salad oil (especially corn, cottonseed, safflower, sesame, and soybean oils) and soft corn-oil margarines in preference to animal fats such as meat fat, cream, butter, and cheese, is encouraged

SUGARS AND SWEETS—(CAN BE USED SPARINGLY TO ADD FLAVOR)

Sugars, jellies, jams, syrups, molasses, honey, and candy essentially provide calories for energy

Getting the Most for Your Money

Plan ahead—that's the key

Shop with a list

Check newspapers for specials and coupons

Buy specials only if you can use them within their shelf lives

Generic brands may offer similar quality at lower prices

Buy large quantities of meat and divide into smaller serving sizes to freeze

Buy fresh fruits and vegetables at different stages of ripeness so they are ready when you are

Cook ahead. By making large casseroles and stews and freezing individual portions, you'll save time and money

Use eggs, skim milk powder, and beans to substitute for meat and add protein to meals

Adapted from Senior Sense for Healthy Eating. Washington State Dairy Council, Seattle, WA, 1982.

Suggestions for People Eating Alone

Set an attractive table—make meals an event

Eat by a window or any pleasant setting

Watch TV or listen to radio

Eat outdoors when weather allows

Treat yourself to a meal out every now and then

Invite guests often—a potluck or meal exchange is a good idea

Participate in Senior Nutrition Programs in your area. Call your area's agency on aging for locations

Adapted from A Guide for Food and Nutrition in Later Years, Society for Nutrition Education, Berkeley, CA, 1980.

ting off on the right foot. It should be carefully planned and given advance publicity. Large attractive posters may be placed in strategic places in the community or dining room of a program site so that everyone is aware of the upcoming event. The title of the nutrition class should not be too general or too dull. Many interesting presentations can be labeled with provocative titles that will help to attract the appropriate audience to the gathering.

The best ideas for discussion topics come from the elderly themselves. Clearly they are most responsive to information that meets their specific needs rather than abstract or generalized information not concretely related to their immediate concerns. As can be seen in Table 12-8, topics related to nutrition and health, cholesterol, and weight control were often indicated, with some degree of interest apparent for food labeling, storage, and preparation. Goldberg et al (1990) surveyed 459 members of the Massachusetts Chapter of the American Association of Retired People to determine nutrition-related issues they were most concerned about.

A significant percentage of the elderly

TABLE 12–8 *Concern about Selected Food and Nutrition Issues in an Elderly Population*

Topic	Percent Expressing Moderate to Great Concern
Additives, preservatives, and environmental contaminants	78.0
Food safety in the home	76.9
Weight control	71.1
Salt and hypertension	65.8
Sugar consumption	53.4
Serum cholesterol	46.6
Nutritional adequacy of their diet	35.8

No. = 459 AARP members aged 55 to 89 years.

TABLE 12–9 *Preferred Teaching Mode Reported by Older Adults*

Method	Percent Reporting Interest to High Interest (No. = 116)
Demonstration	57
In-person discussion	57
Literature	57
Lectures	41
Group discussion	37
Movies	38
Phone discussion	25
Cooking classes	25
Field trips	24

Adapted from Krinke UB: Nutrition information topic and format preferences of older adults. J Nutr Ed 1990; 20:292.

would place health issues before cost and taste in selecting food, although groups can be divided based on values reflecting preference for qualitative-pleasurable factors above all others and for largely economic factors above all others. Perhaps most salient to the issues of nutrition and the elderly is the fact that older Americans do change their diets and most frequently report making changes for health reasons.

Just how effective the final educational product happens to be relates directly to the enthusiasm, skill, sincerity, and creativity of the teacher. It takes more than just a list of relevant topics and an understanding of the subject matter to develop a program that is truly outstanding. There are absolutely no limits to designing an interesting presentation of nutrition information. Practice inevitably improves one's abilities and generally it also reduces the difficulty involved in the development of subsequent presentations. In a nutshell, a good teacher knows the audience and the subject matter well and uses creativity in the development of interesting, provocative, and relevant programs for the elderly.

Krinke (1990) conducted interviews with 116 free-living older adults to determine their interest in selected topics of interest for nutrition education programs and for their preferred pre-

sentation method. The subject preference does not seem to differ significantly from previous studies on this area. Unlike younger people, the elderly appear to prefer in-person discussion and demonstration rather than higher tech teaching methods (Table 12–9). It is interesting that these older adults considered magazine articles the most helpful source of food and nutrition information.

References and Other Readings

ADA testimony on the 1987 reauthorization of the Older Americans Act of 1965. J Am Diet Assoc 1987; 87:943.

Aloia JF, Zanzi I, Vaswani A, et al. Combination therapy for osteoporosis with estrogen, fluoride and calcium. J Am Geriatr Soc 1982; 30:492.

American Dietetic Association testimony on the 1987 reauthorization of the Older Americans Act of 1965. JADA 1987; 87:943.

Andres R, Elahi D, Tobin JD, et al. Impact of age on weight goals. Ann Intern Med 1985; 103:1030.

Axelson ML, Penfield MP. Food and nutrition related attitudes of elderly persons living alone. J Nutr Ed 1983; 15:23.

Benfante R, Reed D. Is elevated serum cholesterol level a risk factor for coronary heart disease in the elderly? JAMA 1990; 263:393.

Block G, Cox C, Madans J, et al. Vitamin supplement use by demographic characteristics. Am J Epidemiol 1988; 127:297.

Chestnut CH. Treatment of postmenopausal osteoporosis. Comp Ther 1984; 10:41.

Constans T, Bacq Y, Bréchot J-F, et al. Protein-energy malnutrition in elderly medical patients. J Am Geriatr Soc 1992; 40:263.

Cumming RG. Calcium intake and bone mass: a quantitative review of the evidence. Calcif Tissue Int 1990; 47:194.

Davies L. Socioeconomic psychological and education aspects of nutrition in old age. Age Aging 1990; 19:537.

Davies L, Knutson KC. Warning signs for malnutrition in the elderly J Am Diet Assoc 1991; 91: 1413.

Drinka PJ, Goodwin JS. Prevalence and consequences of vitamin deficiency in the nursing home. J Am Geriatr Soc 1991; 39:1008.

Fanelli MT, Woteki CE. Nutrient intakes and health status of older Americans: data from the NHANES II. Ann NY Acad Sci 1989; 561:94.

Garry P, Goodwin JC, Hunt WC, et al. Nutritional status of a healthy elderly population: dietary and supplemental intakes. Am J Clin Nutr 1982; 36:319.

Gloth FM, Tobin JD, Sherman SS, et al. Is the recommended daily allowance for vitamin D too low for the homebound elderly? J Am Geriatr Soc 1991; 39:137.

Goldberg JP, Gershoff SN, McGandy RM. Appropriate topics for nutrition education for the elderly. J Nutr Ed 1990; 22:303.

Hale WE, Stewart RB, Cerda JJ, et al. Use of nutritional supplements in the ambulatory elderly population. J Am Geriatr Soc 1982; 30:401.

Herbert V. Don't ignore low serum colbalamin (vitamin B_{12}) levels. Arch Intern Med 1988; 148:1705.

Howell SC, Loeb MB. Nutrition and aging: a monograph for practitioners. Gerontologist 1969; 9:1.

Kicklighter JR. Characteristics of older adult learners. J Am Diet Assoc 1991; 91:1418.

Krinke UB. Nutrition information topic and format preferences of older adults. J Nutr Ed 1990; 22:292.

Lehmann AB. Review: undernutrition in elderly people. Age Aging 1989; 18:339.

Levy AS, Schucker RE. Patterns of nutritional intake among dietary supplement users: attitudes and behavioral correlates. JADA 1987; 87:754.

Lipid Research Clinics Program. The Lipid Research Clinics Coronary prevention trial results. JAMA 1984; 251:351.

Lipschitz DA. The anemia of chronic diseases. J Am Geriatr Soc 1990; 38:1258.

Machaughlin J, Holick MF. Aging decreases the capacity of human skin to produce vitamin D_3. J Clin Invest 1985; 76:1536.

Martin DC, Francis J, Protetch J, et al. Time dependency of cognitive recovery with cobalamin replacement: report of a pilot study. J Am Geriatr Soc 1992; 40:168.

Matkovic V, Kostial K, Simonivoc I, et al. Bone status and fracture rates in two regions in Yugoslavia. Am J Clin Nutr 1979; 32:540.

McGandy RB, Russell RM, Hartz SC, et al. Nutritional status survey of health in noninstitutionalized elderly: energy and nutrient intakes from 3-day diet records and nutrient supplements. Nutr Res 1986; 6:785.

Meyers RM, Grodin MA. Decision making regarding the initiation of tube feeding in the severely demented elderly: a review. J Am Geriatr Soc 1991; 39:526.

Miller JZ, Weinberger MH, Christian JC, et al. Familial resemblance in the blood pressure response to sodium restriction. Am J Epidemiol 1987; 126:822.

Morley JE. Anorexia in older patients: its meaning and management. Geriatrics 1990; 45:59.

Mowé M, Bøhmer T. The prevalence of undiagnosed protein-calorie undernutrition in a population of hospitalized elderly patients. J Am Geriatr Soc 1991; 39:1089.

Mueller WH, Wear ML, Hanis CL, et al. Which measurement of body fat distribution is best suited for epidemiologic research? Am J Epidemiol 1991; 133:858.

Murphy SP, Everett DF, Dresser CM. Food group consumption reported by the elderly during NHANES I epidemiologic follow up study. J Nutr Educ 1989; 21:214.

National Center for Health Statistics: Health Assessment Nutrition Evaluation Studies, NHANES II Preliminary Statistics, DHEW, 1982.

National Clearing House on Aging: National Nutrition Program for the Elderly. Washington, DC, US DHEW, Office of Human Development, Admin on Aging, 1974.

National Research Council Recommended Dietary Allowances. 10th ed. Washington, DC, Food and Nutrition Board, National Academy of Sciences, 1989.

Need AG, Nordin BEC, Horowitz M, et al. Osteoporosis: new insights from bone densitometry. J Am Geriatr Assoc 1990; 38:1153.

Nordin BEC, Need AG, Chatterton BE, et al. The relative contributions of age and years since menopause to post-menopause bone loss. J Clin Endocrinol Metab 1990; 70:83.

Report of the Dietary Guidelines Committee on the Dietary Guidelines for Americans. USDA Human Nutrition Information Service, Washington, DC: US Printing Office, 1990.

Riggs BL, Seeman E, Hodgson SF, et al. Effect of the fluoride/calcium regimen on vertebral fracture occurrence in post-menopausal osteoporosis. N Engl J Med 1982; 306:446.

Robertson L, Flinders C, Godfrey B. Laurel's kitchen. Petaluma, CA: Nilgiri Press, 1979.

Roe D. Diet and drug interactions. New York: Van Nostrand Reinhold Publishing, 1988:89.

Sandstead HH, Henriksen LK, Greeger JL. Zinc nutrition in the elderly in relation to taste acuity, immune response and wound healing. Am J Clin Nutr 1982; 36:1046.

Stamler R, Stamler J, et al. Nutritional therapy for high blood pressure. JAMA 1987; 257:1484.

Subar AF, Block G, Jones LD. Dietary folate intake and food sources in the US population, NHANES II. Am J Clin Nutr 1989; 50:508.

Tayback M, Kumanyika S, Chee E. Body weight as a risk factor in the elderly. Arch Intern Med 1990; 150:1065.

Taylor GF. A clinical survey of elderly people from a nutritional standpoint. In: Exton-Smith AN, Scoll DL, eds. Vitamins in the elderly. Bristol, UK: John Wright and Sons, 1968, p. 51.

Tucker DM, Penland JC, Sandstead HH, et al. Nutrition status and brain function in aging. Am J Clin Nutr 1990; 52:93.

US Dept of Health and Human Services, Public Health Services. Healthy people 20: National health promotion and disease prevention objectives. Washington, DC: US Government Printing Office, Publication 017-0000474, 1991.

Vaughn L, Zurlo F, Ravussin E. Aging and energy expenditure. Am J Clin Nutr 1991; 53:827.

Wahlquest ML. Vitamins, nutrition and aging. In: Nutrition and aging. New York: Alan R. Liss, 1990:175.

Wasserman P, Mangels R. Simply vegan: quick vegetarian meals. Baltimore, MD: Vegetarian Resource Group, 1991.

Webb AR, Pilbeam C, Hanafin N, et al. An evaluation of the relative contribution of exposure to sunlight and diet to the circulating concentrations of 25-hydroxy vitamin D in an elderly nursing home population in Boston. Am J Clin Nutr 1990; 51:1075.

White JV, Dwyer JT, Posner BM, et al. Nutrition screening initiative: development and implementation of the public awareness checklist and screening tools. J Am Diet Assoc 1992; 92:163.

Willett WC, Stampfer M, Manson J, et al. New weight guidelines for Americans: justified or injudicious. Am J Clin Nutr 1991; 53:1102.

Young V. Amino acids and proteins in relation to the nutrition of elderly people. Age Aging 1990; 19:510.

13
Families of the Elderly

LEE-ELLEN COPSTEAD

At one time, the extended family—parents, grandparents, and children—lived under one roof and pooled their material and emotional resources to provide a nurturing environment from birth to death. Today there are forces that tend to separate different generations. Employment opportunities for women and increased mobility have often decreased the physically close family environment and at times have increased psychologic distances as well. However, research is showing that the stereotype of children not caring about their aging parents is invalid (Brody, 1985; Carnevali and Reiner, 1990). The strategies for maintaining contact and giving support are changing, but the caring remains.

Within the family network, there is an ongoing intergenerational transfer characteristic of reciprocal relationships. Often the financial and physical capacity of the older person is a key factor in the pattern of these exchanges. With declines in health status, activities of daily living, and functional capacities, older people may not only require greater levels of support, but may find it increasingly difficult to reciprocate. Little is known about that period in late adulthood in which intergenerational exchanges become redefined as caregiving. There is clearly a continuum of caregiving from the beginning phases of a caring career to the full-time commitment documented among the caregivers of severely impaired elderly. Several demographic, social, and epidemiologic trends

have converged to make caring for the impaired elderly problematic.

Today's medical advances have resulted in an increased life span, and social patterns are resulting in the birth of healthy babies to women in their mid-30s and older. Thus, nurses increasingly encounter both middle-aged children at the peak of their own generativity as well as elderly children, born when their parents were very young, who are facing the demands of caring for sometimes frail, aged parents.

In addition, the current pattern of divorce and single parent households with associated financial strains has resulted in the return of children to their parents' homes. This produces three- and even four-generational households where the care of the very young and the very old creates severe stresses. Researchers have only recently begun to investigate yet another problematic issue: the multiple role responsibilities faced by the substantial number of Americans who serve as informal caregivers for noninstitutionalized disabled older persons and also hold full-time or part-time jobs (Steuve and O'Donnell, 1989). Another family constellation in which problems in daily living may arise is one in which an age mate—spouse, sibling, or companion—is the primary care giver to an ill, dependent, aged person.

These groups of adults are at high risk for developing problems in daily living associated with meeting their own needs and those of the

239

dependent, aged person. The nurse is in a position to identify risk factors and intervene so that these primary care givers receive the support they need in order to care for those who depend on them. The well-being of the ailing elderly depends on the well-being of their care givers.

High-risk Areas in Daily Living Associated with Being Primary Caregiver to the Ailing Elderly

Basically the difficulties in daily living for primary caregivers for the elderly with long-term illnesses arise from the *unremitting needs* of the elderly person for supervision and assistance. These needs are defined by both the caregiver and the dependent person and those definitions may not coincide. The depletion of physical, emotional, and financial resources is also a major dimension in managing daily living as a care giver to a dependent elderly person.

Examples of problems associated with continuous care giving include the following:

The inevitable advance planning for an appropriate substitute caregiver who is acceptable to the patient whenever there is any need to leave home

Impairment in personal and social activities such as time for oneself, time to visit friends, or privacy

The tension of not knowing what is going to happen with the elderly person in a given day (e.g., incontinence, falls, wandering, mood changes, setting fires, pulling out a catheter, not eating, developing infections, or other complications)

The tension created when the older person cannot tolerate *any* variation in schedule or environment and becomes distressed if changes occur in meals, bathing, location of objects, and so forth

The worry of how long the situation will continue and whether changes in status will require hospitalization or placement in a nursing home

The need to devote major portions of funds to the care and potential needs of the patient to the point where others can be seriously deprived

The long-term nature of the care and the complexity of technologic demands placed on the primary caregiver create problems in daily living. These include care of the elderly person with complex equipment such as hyperalimentation devices, ostomy care, chemotherapy and narcotic pumps, catheters (suprapubic and urethral), respirators—the list could go on. These demands add to the other stresses of daily living.

Interpersonal tensions between the primary caregiver and (1) the dependent elderly person and (2) other family members can generate additional stresses in daily living. Examples of situations that arise out of competing, continuing demands on a primary caregiver include the following:

Differences in perceptions of what is needed, such as the dependent person wanting more help or contact than is either feasible or actually required, or the caregiver giving more help or structure than the older person wants

Giving of time or resources to the older person to the deprivation of younger persons, spouses, and self

Work-related changes as a result of caregiving, such as using vacation time, making personal calls, taking a day off, too tired to work, or leaving work early

Guilt arising when the caregiver is unable to meet his own expectations of what is needed in giving care to the older person

Conflict between the expectations or values of self and others, e.g., institutionalization for the older person versus retaining them in noninstitutional settings

Often a combination of these problems impacts on the daily living of a primary care giver, whether that person is the adult child caring for parents or a sibling or spouse. Nursing diagnosis will identify and address issues in these major areas.

FACTORS INCREASING THE RISK OF PROBLEMS IN DAILY LIVING

Not all primary caregivers experience difficulties in their daily living associated with providing care to the elderly dependent relatives in their families. There are factors that should alert the nurse to anticipate higher risk of problems.

INADEQUATE INCOME

Families with moderate income often have inadequate financial resources and are at risk in managing the demands of the older patient over time. Money can purchase respite care (when this is available), services, transportation, supplies, equipment, and a comfortable environment. Even when insurance is available, third party payers tend not to cover long-term illness and home care, medications, supplies, and equipment. Low-income families may be quite sophisticated in learning to locate and mobilize the resources in the system, but this is not always so. There also are some levels of financial and people resources for those with lowest incomes. Those families that are middle class have great needs for help in managing dependent, ill parents and spouses. It is an area of high priority for nursing assessment.

LACK OF COMMUNITY RESOURCES

Many communities, particularly small towns and rural areas, lack support systems for families caring for older persons with long-term disabilities. They may not have respite care beds, day-care centers, chore services, home health care, visiting nurse services, long-term care facilities, or even persons who could be hired to come in and assist. This places increased burdens on family members, who must struggle with minimal support.

ENVIRONMENTAL BARRIERS

Housing and transportation that present physical barriers create risks for managing daily living when there are disabilities in the elderly. Such barriers include stairs into the house or within it, lack of bedroom and bathroom on one floor, and lack of heating or cooling equipment. Cars or public transportation that the person is physically unable to use constitute another major barrier. Lack of a phone creates a limitation for living alone. Lack of personal safety because of the kind of people in the neighborhood is another environmental hazard.

FAILING HEALTH

A potent risk factor in both the need for care and the capacity to provide care is the functional health status of the patient and the caregiver (Gaynor, 1990). The greatest risk occurs when both the patient and the caregiver are elderly or in poor health, e.g., the 85-year-old husband caring for the disabled 83-year-old wife, or the arthritic 70-year-old daughter trying to care for the 90-year-old arthritic mother.

Dementia or other psychologic and behavioral problems tend to create greater difficulties than physical problems. Families seem to have a greater capacity to deal with even major physical disabilities and the associated technology than to manage behavioral problems (see Chapters 18 and 19 for examples).

DEVELOPMENTAL DISSONANCE

When the caregiver feels "out of step" with respect to peers, there is a potential for anxiety and strain. Neugarten and Hagestad (1976) conclude from research that ". . . the age norm system . . . also creates an ordered predictable life course, it creates timetables, it sets boundaries for acceptable behavior at successive life stages." Few people are prepared to become caregivers of a dementia victim. Caregivers receive almost no socialization for this role before they enter it and little support once they take it on. Further, as they see their peers enjoying life, they may feel the stress of developmental dissonance—"why aren't *my* later years filled with enjoyment too?" Statements like, "Why is this happening to me?" "I feel like I am missing out on life" or "I expected that things would be different at this point in my life" reflect the feeling of burden. The burden of caregiving is also related to moral development (Klein, 1989).

SUBSTANCE ABUSE

Substance abuse, such as alcohol or other drug abuse, in either the caregiver or the patient will increase the difficulties in managing daily living. In cases in which the caregiver abuses substances, physical abuse or neglect of the patient may be evident. If the aged person abuses substances, increased physical and mental debilitation result. Neglect from caregivers over the long-term may occur.

PREVIOUS FAMILY RELATIONSHIPS

When previous relationships between the caregiver and the patient have been positive, there is less likely to be unwillingness to provide care at this stage. However, when the caregiver has not been satisfied with the relationship or when there was frank abuse as a child or by a spouse, there may be understandable reluctance to expend the tremendous amounts of physical and emotional energy required to maintain the well-being of the older dependent person.

LENGTH OF TIME CAREGIVING SERVICES MUST BE PROVIDED

Research suggests that providing assistance to an older person over an extended period undermines the elder–helper relationship (Stoller and Pugliesi, 1989). Initially, the caregiver may be able to retain friendships and activities outside the immediate caring relationship. Later, as the older person's needs escalate and the caregiver experiences increasingly heavy demands and conflict between caring and other responsibilities, social isolation may occur. Eventually, the caregiver may become devoted entirely to the task of caring. Extended caregiving without relief has been linked to physical and mental health problems for the helper (Gaynor, 1990).

TIMES OF GREATER RISK

Problems in the care of the older person tend to be exacerbated at particular times of the day, week, or year. Nights are often a problem as the older person confuses the hours of the day, gets up, wanders about, turns on the stove or water, and places himself or the environment at risk. This can create sleep deprivation in the caregiver and rapidly reduce the stamina for caregiving. Weekends tend to be a time for younger, working care providers to gain some respite from the demands of the work world and have more time for home and children or grandchildren; yet these are also the times of greater loneliness for the older person. Vacations and holidays create conflicting demands. On vacations when there is the need for the family to be away, there is the problem of finding another caregiver or else failing in the other family members' expectations of what should be done. On holidays, often older persons could well participate, but they may lack the stamina to be surrounded by larger numbers of people and different generations. Again there is the conflict of meeting the older persons' needs and those of other family members.

DYNAMICS

The problems in daily living created for families of aging, dependent persons arise from several sources and are shaped by the associated relationships and factors. Major role changes are accompanied by role ambiguity and confusion. The former role relationships of parent–child, spouse–spouse, sibling, or independent companion are altered by the changing health status and capabilities of the patient (Carnevali and Reiner, 1990). A caregiver may argue with a spouse or other family members over how to manage the care receiver's needs. Caregivers may feel unappreciated and neglected by others. The inability or perceived inability of caregivers to meet the basic needs of the older person can result in frustration, guilt, anger, and resentment—even as the older person requires love and a sense of belonging. The physical fatigue associated with the caregiving activities and supervision, often on a round-the-clock basis, can deplete the resources for staying on top of the situation. Caregivers may also have to limit the time and energy that they invest in relationships or in their jobs. All these factors are interwoven to add to the complexity in daily living for families of ailing, dependent elderly.

Cultural norms shape role expectations for intergenerational and intragenerational attitudes and behaviors of family members at all ages. When nurses deal with families from cultures different from their own, it is wise to become informed about the cultural values and expectations that are having influence on family responses and activities.

SIGNS AND SYMPTOMS

Families of dependent elderly who are becoming ineffective in managing daily living with the additional responsibilities manifest signs and symptoms of their difficulties. Frequently, they are unable to identify the problems specifically enough to find solutions. They may also feel unable to ask for those resources that would restore some balance in their lives. Nurses who are aware of the risk situations and who have potential for contact with these families are in a position to look for the signs and symptoms that indicate a need for outside assistance.

EARLY SIGNS AND SYMPTOMS IN THE CAREGIVER

Even in the early stages of difficulties in managing daily living with primary care responsibilities there are signs and symptoms in the caregiver. They include multiple complaints about the situation, signs of anxiety, growing depersonalization of the older person, and fatigue.

Multiple Complaints   One may hear such statements as:

> "I just don't know what to do. Mother's care has been so demanding lately, I'm just worn to a frazzle. She never gives me a moment's peace. She's never satisfied. Nothing seems to be going right, no matter what I do."

Anxiety   The complaining statements may be accompanied by signs of anxiety such as:

Agitated pacing
Strident voice
Poor eye contact
Wringing hands
Short attention span
Inability to focus on any one problem area

Growing Depersonalization   One may see signs and symptoms that the family members are distancing themselves and seeing the older family member as less of a person. Symptoms of the depersonalization may take the form of statements such as:

> "There's no point in trying to talk to Dad; he doesn't understand what we're saying anyway."

Signs of depersonalization include the following:

Talking in front of the older person as though he were not present
Performing duties of care in an impersonal, detached manner, without talking to the person during the care
Failure to observe modesty

Fatigue   Fatigue may be diagnosed both by what the caregiver says and by accompanying signs. Nurses may hear comments such as:

> "In the last 6 months, Mother has slept poorly and so have I."

> "Dad gets up and wanders about many nights. He turns on the stove, runs water without checking to see if the drain is open—I just never know what to expect, so I have to sleep with one ear listening for him."

> "I just don't seem to have any pep these days."

> "I've had the flu twice this winter."

Signs of fatigue include irritability, stooped posture, dark shadows under the eyes, a pinched drawn expression on the face, and frequent sighing.

EARLY SIGNS AND SYMPTOMS IN THE AGED PERSON

The older person may also give evidence of the stresses in family dynamics associated with his care. These signs and symptoms fall into the same categories of multiple complaints, anxiety, and fatigue. One may hear complaints such as:

> "I'm just too upset to even think about getting stronger and relying less on my daughter. Everytime I ask for ANYTHING she gets mad. She won't even talk to me anymore. She just ignores me. She won't make my grandson turn the radio down—it gets so noisy, I can't even think straight. I just don't know what to do. . . ."

Such statements may be accompanied by the signs of anxiety as noted earlier in the caregiver section.

Fatigue may be alluded to in statements such as:

> "At night I just can't sleep. I lie awake for hours on end. The harder I try to fall asleep, the worse it gets. I wake up more tired than I was before going to bed."

The observable signs of fatigue are the same as noted in the earlier section on fatigue in the caregiver.

LATE SIGNS AND SYMPTOMS IN THE CARE GIVER

Without support, the imbalance between the requirements of daily living and the resources to meet them tends to worsen over time. Problems are compounded when assistance is either refused or is not available. Late signs and symptoms in the caregiver include depression (Drinka et al, 1987), open hostility and avoidance, and evidence of misappropriation of the older person's funds or property.

Depression   The caregiver's depression may be noted in complaints of insomnia characterized by early morning wakefulness, weight changes, sadness, brooding, fatigue inappropriate to activity, inability to concentrate, loss of interest in formerly pleasurable activities, headaches (particularly in the occipital region), feeling worse in the morning, being "shut down" in terms of activities and decision making, and flat affect.

Open Hostility   Overt hostility may be seen in verbal behavior and, in severe situations, in the abuse of the elderly person. One may hear angry comments such as, "I've HAD it! I can't sleep, can't take time to eat; I can't even make my own decisions. I'm fed up. . . ."

Avoidance or Distancing When the older person becomes a patient or resident in an institutional setting, avoidance may take the form of failure to visit or call as well as reluctance to participate in discharge planning. On an interpersonal level the communication between caregiver and older person may become either more formal or more superficial and routine or sparse.

Misappropriation of Financial Resources Those who make inquiries about the financial resources or property management of the elderly person may receive vague, noncommittal responses from the caregiver who is managing them. Further investigation may show bills unpaid and bank accounts depleted.

LATE SIGNS AND SYMPTOMS IN THE OLDER PERSON

In the aged person the late signs and symptoms of disintegration of the relationships with the caregiver can be seen in fear, indications of personal neglect or physical abuse, withdrawal, confusion, depression, and open hostility.

Fear One might observe the fear of asking for needed care in such comments as:

> "My son and daughter-in-law leave me alone for hours and I can't get to the bathroom without help. That's why I don't dare drink much water. My daughter-in-law yells at me if I do happen to wet the bed, but sometimes I just can't hold it."

> "My son hasn't picked up my ear medicine and I've been out of it for the past 3 days."

Signs of fear may include seeing:

the aged person shy away from the touch of the caregiver
abrupt cessation of conversation on the arrival of the caregiver
an alarmed facial expression at the caregiver's approach
furtive glances in the caregiver's direction
unusual passivity
ingratiating behavior

Personal Neglect or Physical Abuse Signs and symptoms of neglect or abuse are readily available to the nurse who knows what they are. Subjective data may include reports of long periods of isolation, such as being made to stay alone in a bedroom, or expressions of concern that the older person's money is being used for the caregiver's personal gain.

Signs of neglect and abuse include body odor, clothing consistently soiled or in poor repair, long dirty fingernails, and neglected feet with long nails and buildup of corns and calluses. Physical abuse can be inferred from the presence of fingerprint bruises on the upper arms or bruises on the inner thighs or other areas not explained by injury.

Withdrawal The unhappiness and powerlessness of the older person in his relationships to caregivers may be seen in withdrawal. One may observe the older person curling into the fetal position more often, initiating no spontaneous conversation, replying to questions in monosyllables, sitting or lying with eyes closed, or making poor eye contact.

Cognitive Changes One may note regression in cognitive capabilities, with increased impairment of short-term memory, decreased ability to think abstractly or make logical decisions, and even failure to recall basic personal information, e.g., age, address, birthdate (see Chapter 16 for additional signs and symptoms of cognitive changes).

Depression The older person may exhibit signs and symptoms of depression (see Chapters 17 and 19 for discussions of depression in the aged).

Open Hostility Because of compromised physical status and dependency, open hostility in the older person will most often be seen in verbal behavior. One may hear angry statements such as:

> "I'll never forgive my daughter-in-law. She went to work and now she doesn't bring me my dinner. She has no right to do this to me. Who does she think she is? I've got my rights too, you know. . . ."

When an older member in a family constellation requires ongoing care, assistance, and supervision, there is a high risk of changes in family dynamics and possible maladaptive responses. The previously mentioned signs and symptoms, taken together, should suggest diagnoses in the area of maladaptive responses and a need for external assistance.

PROGNOSIS

The prognosis for families of the elderly is based on risk factors, such as adequacy of personal support that satisfies needs and keeps the personal well-springs of the caregivers reasonably full. Poor prognosis is associated with poor health in the caregiver, low economic resources, inadequate housing, dementia or other psychiatric problems, and prolonged, demanding needs for care. It is also associated with past history of abuse of the caregiver, lack of trust between caregiver and patient, negative cultural values (e.g., lack of valuing of the elderly), and the inability either to identify the need for help or to accept it. Care demands that extend to 2 to 4 years increase the stress on the caregiver (Gaynor, 1990).

Good prognosis for effective management of daily living in families of dependent, ailing elderly persons is associated with having reasonably good health, an adequate income, strong family ties and affection among various elements of the family, positive views on aging, ego strength, and mutual respect and adequate available outside support services.

COMPLICATIONS

When families do not manage effectively in their daily living to include care of the elderly member, complications can occur for both the caregivers and family members and the older person. There can be physical or mental breakdowns in either party. Financial resources may be depleted. An unnecessary or premature downward trajectory in the older person's health may take place, with premature institutionalization. Suicide is another possibility.

Nursing Management

ASSESSMENT OF THE FAMILY SITUATION

In order to maintain or restore effective management of daily living in a family involved in care of a dependent elderly person, an accurate initial assessment of the patterns of daily living,

the demands affecting both caregivers and the older person, and the available internal and external resources for managing the requirements of daily living and the deficits that are present. Alerting all the participants—caregivers and older person—to the risks inherent in the situation and some options for preventing, minimizing, or delaying dysfunction is an important function for the nurse.

As with assessment of patients, it is important in a family assessment to work at the family's pace, address their agenda first, allow sufficient time for them to share their perception of the situation, and maintain a neutral objective data collection attitude, withholding one's personal values and judgments of the situation.

Areas of assessment include:

Perception of the primary problem areas—What are they? How did they occur? How long has the problem(s) existed?

Problem-solving strategies attempted—What have they tried? What has worked? What do they think would resolve or relieve the problem?

Goals—What goals do they have for the older person? for themselves?

Strengths—What internal and external resources are available to address the situation?

Needed assistance—What additional external resources do they feel are needed and usable? What barriers to needed resources do they see?

Patterns of daily living—What are the usual or preferred patterns of daily living for care giver and the older person as these are relevant to the presenting situation? What is the nature of the home environment as this is relative to the functional status of the older person?

When data in the above areas have been organized, nursing diagnoses can be generated that, in turn, form the basis for the plan of nursing management. The nurse and family can work together to develop realistic goals and negotiate the activities that each will implement. Early intervention is, of course, the ideal; however, nurses most frequently become involved when the situation has developed to the point where intervention is critical to patient and family well-being.

MANAGEMENT OF EMOTIONAL RESPONSES TO DEMANDS OF CAREGIVING

When the demands on primary caregivers and other family members are seen to exceed their resources and disrupt their daily living, emotional responses normally occur. These responses may include feelings of helplessness, hopelessness, and frustration, resulting in turn in anger accompanied by guilt feelings. Other emotional responses may be those of sadness or depression. The caregivers may feel neglected insofar as their own needs (including recognition or appreciation) are perennially forgotten.

The nurse has a role in helping the family members to:

1. Recognize and accept their own emotional responses to the presenting situation
2. Accept these responses as normal and legitimate

In the same way, the changes in lifelong role relationships may need professional attention. The nurse can suggest that the person who is experiencing discomfort in altered role relationships:

1. Specifically identify the changes that have occurred or are occurring
2. Note the reactions that these changes are generating in each party
3. Identify the reason or basis for the changes that have occurred or are occurring

Beyond this the nurse can propose some options for action to gain a sense of control over the situation. These include:

1. Negotiations to acknowledge and establish new expectations for the relationships between the parties
2. Where this is not feasible, identification of the areas of change, the basis for the changes, and the *acceptable options* the caregiver has in adapting to the changes

The nurse who notes that the emotional tone of a family member seems out of proportion to the existing situation needs to recognize that the individual may be responding to feelings dating back to earlier experiences and relationships. It may be important to verify this history as a basis for assisting the people involved to understand and possibly alter their current behavior.

RELIEF FROM UNRELENTING RESPONSIBILITY

Many problems in families' care of the dependent elderly person can be relieved by *planned, predictable* periods of respite (Bader, 1985). With physical care problems (treatment, equipment), it may be possible to contact the physician and obtain home health care nursing services, e.g., Visiting Nurse Service for physical care and private home health care agencies for broader care services including physical care, chore services, laundry, food preparation, light housework, and grocery shopping.

Other options include locating individuals—homemakers, retired persons, and high school or college students—to provide elements of care for periods of time, e.g., nights, evenings, weekends, or a couple of hours in the afternoon. Some churches or social groups could provide the names of people who may be available for several hours to stay with a person. The nurse, however, needs to ensure that the family member needing respite gets out of the house or at least leaves the presence of the patient in order to benefit from this respite. It may take time to establish the trust needed for this to occur, but it should not be taken for granted that the caregiver will experience respite merely because another support person is available—follow-up is needed.

FORMAL RESPITE CARE

Dependent elderly can be *admitted* to formal respite care. It is not often readily available at present and it can be expensive. It is one alternative and may become more accessible in the future in the United States, as it is in Scandinavia, for example. (For more information on respite resources, see Chapter 6.)

DAY-CARE CENTERS

Both private and community day-care centers are increasingly available. One needs to be assured that the services available will cover the needs of the older person.

MOBILIZATION OF NECESSARY COMMUNITY RESOURCES

Restoration or maintenance of balance in a family may require an interdisciplinary team. One member of that team must be identified as

Available Community Resources

AT THE LOCAL LEVEL

Senior citizen centers

Day-care centers

Food/nutrition programs
  Nutritional senior health services
  Delivered meals on wheels

Case management: Elderly services information and assistance

Legal services

Medical services
  Healthline for available physician
  Health screening
  Glaucoma screening

Dental services

Chore services

Social services

Department of Social and Health Services

Transportation

Home health care

Minor home repair

Energy assistance program
Community mental health center

Various kinds of information may be obtained by writing to the following national organizations. In addition, services of the various national agencies are usually available at the local level.

American Association of Diabetes Educators
500 N Michigan Ave, Suite 1400
Chicago, IL 60611

American Association of Retired Persons
1909 K St, NW
Washington, DC 20049

American Cancer Society
1599 Clifton Rd
Atlanta, GA 30329

American Diabetes Association
  National Service Center
PO Box 25757
1600 Duke St
Alexandria, VA 22313

American Heart Association
7320 Greenville Ave
Dallas, TX 75231

American Lung Association
1740 Broadway
New York, NY 10019

American Parkinson Disease Association
1600 John St, Suite 417
New York, NY 10038

Architectural and Transportation Barriers
  Compliance Board
1111 18th Street, NW, Suite 501
Washington, DC 20036

Arthritis Foundation
1314 Spring St, NW
Atlanta, GA 30309

Centers for Disease Control
1600 Clifton Rd, NE
Atlanta, GA 30333

(Continued)

Available Community Resources *(Continued)*

Leukemia Society of America
733 Third Ave
New York, NY 10017

Mental Health Materials Center
9 Willow Circle
Bronxville, NY 10708

National Alzheimers Association
70 East Lake St.
Chicago, IL 60601

National Association for Visually
   Handicapped
22 W 21st St
New York, NY 10010

National Council on the Aging
600 Maryland Ave, SW
West Wing, Suite 100
Washington, DC 20024

National Easter Seal Society
70 E Lake St
Chicago, IL 60601

National Epilepsy League
6 N Michigan Ave
Chicago, IL 60602

National Information Center for Children
   and Youth with Handicaps
Box 1492
Washington, DC 20013

National Jewish Center for Immunology
   and Respiratory Medicine
1400 Jackson St
Denver, CO 80206

National Kidney Foundation
2 Park Ave
New York, NY 10003

National Mental Health Association
1021 Prince St
Alexandria, VA 22314

National Multiple Sclerosis Society
205 E 42nd St
New York, NY 10017

Stroke Club International
805 12th St
Galveston, TX 77550

United Ostomy Association
36 Executive Park, Suite 120
Irvine, CA 92714

---

the coordinator responsible for the case management. This individual has the following responsibilities:

Conducts case conferences
Keeps team members informed about the care plan
Conducts ongoing evaluation and update of the care plan
Coordinates services

The nurse plays a vital role in linking families with needed or desired community resources. See box on p. 247 for a list of resources that may be available in the community.

EVALUATION

Response to intervention (or nonintervention) may be evaluated in terms of abatement or continuation of manifestations. When caregivers or family members begin to report being happier, having more enjoyable encounters with the older person, being busier and being able to get more done and concentrate more easily, then improvement is being made. Family members and the older person may have fewer complaints about each other. They may report sleeping better, eating better, being less tired, or having fewer headaches. They may make fewer demands on the health care system and be less intense in reporting their symptoms.

Both the caregiver and the person receiving the care may voice actual satisfaction with the living arrangements or plan of care. Financial arrangements are more adequate and improvements in the living environment, such as less crowding, may bring greater comfort. Usable and acceptable outside support services have been identified and mobilized.

In the event of the institutionalization or death of the older person, the family members are able to find satisfaction and effective living with the situation.

Long-term care and family dynamics tend to change even when there seems to be stability. It becomes important to listen for subtle cues and to anticipate changes where the intervention needs to change, or where support needs to be offered.

References and Other Readings

Azarnoff RS, Sharlach AE. Eldercare: the sandwich generation's coming of age. Personnel Journal 1988; 67:60.

Bader J. Respite care: temporary relief for caregivers. Health needs of women as they age. Binghamton, NY: Haworth Press, 1985.

Brody EM. Parent care as a normative family stress. Gerontologist 1985; 25:19.

Brody EM, Kleban MH, Johnsen PT, et al. Work status and parent care: a comparison of four groups of women. Gerontologist 1987; 27:201.

Brody EM, Johnsen PT, Fulcomers MC, Lang AM. Women's changing roles and help to elderly parents: attitudes of three generations of women. J Geront 1983; 38:597.

Cantor MH. Strain among caregivers: a study of experience in the United States. Gerontologist 1983; 23:597.

Carnevali D, Reiner A. The cancer experience: nursing diagnosis and management. Philadelphia: JB Lippincott, 1990 pp. 19–27, 88–103, 265.

Cook-Degan RM. Dealing with the impact of dementia. Business and Health 1986; 3:26.

Drinka TJ, Smith JK, Drinka PJ. Correlates of depression and burden for informal caregivers of patients in a geriatrics referral clinic. Geriatr Soc 1987; 35:522.

Families and chronic illness. University of Washington Symposium, Seattle, WA, 1990.

Gaynor SE. The long haul: The effects of home care on caregivers. Image: J Nurs Schol 1990; 22:208.

Gilhooly ML. The impact of caregiving on caregivers: factors associated with the psychological well-being of people supporting a dementing relative in the community. Br J Med Psychol 1984; 57:35.

Gilleard CJ. Problems posed for supporting relatives of geriatric and psychogeriatric day patients. Acta Psychiatr Scand 1984; 70:198.

Goldstein V, Regnery G, Wellin E. Caretaker role fatigue. Nurs Outlook 1981; 29:24.

Houlihan JP. Families caring for frail and demented elderly: a review of selected findings. Fam Sys Med 1987; 5:344.

Klein S. Caregiver burden and moral development. Image: J Nurs Schol 1989; 21:94.

Neugarten BL, Hagestad GO. Age and the life course. In: Binstock RH, Shanas E, eds. Handbook of aging and the social sciences. New York: Van Nostrand Reinhold, 1976.

Poulshock SW, Deimling GT. Families caring for elders in residence. J Gerontol 1984; 39:230.

Reece D, Walz T, Hageboeck H. International care providers of non-institutionalized frail elderly: characteristics and consequences. J Geront Soc Work 1983; 5:21.

Rivers C, Barnett R, Baruch G. Beyond sugar and spice: how women grow, learn and thrive. New York: Putnam, 1979.

Scharlach AE. Role strain in mother-daughter relationships in later life. Gerontologist 1987; 27:627.

Soldo B, Myllyluoma J. Caregivers who live with dependent elderly. Gerontologist 1983; 23:607.

Steuve A, O'Donnell L. Interacting between women and their elderly parents. Res Aging 1989; 11:331.

Stoller EP. Parent caregiving by adult children. J Marr Fam 1983; 45:851.

Stoller EP, Pugliesi K. The transition to the caregiving role. Res Aging 1989; 11:312.

Stone RS, Cafferata GL, Sangl J. Caregivers of the frail elderly: a national profile. Gerontologist 1987; 27:616.

14
Managing Daily Living with Diminishing Resources and Losses

CAROLYN ENLOE

As individuals in our society enter the seventh to tenth decades of their lives, environmental changes and challenges to health continue to occur, as they have throughout their lifetimes. A major difference, however, is a reduction in the adaptive ability to meet the stressors incumbent to change. In the *old–old* (over age 75), this results in a narrower range in homeostasis, one which is readily compromised in the presence of physical illness, limitations or disability as well as cumulative losses of internal and external resources, social roles and relationships. Any of these phenomena represent a psychophysiologic assault to the steady state of the individual. Physiologic assaults, for example, anemia or pneumonia, stress the internal environment of the elderly person. Psychologic events of either a positive (e.g., anticipating a trip) or negative character (e.g., bereavement) can trigger physiologic events. Both physical and psychologic states threaten the balance and well-being of the individual. Balance can be restored if:

The body is not stressed too vigorously, too profoundly, or too repeatedly over time; and
The intervals between assaults are long enough to meet the elderly person's requirement for longer time to return to a baseline state.

As the elderly person begins to look at quality of life and engage in the developmental tasks of the later years, the rate of change in re-

sources may seem to accelerate. Integrating either losses or diminishing resources into an adjusted lifestyle is the major task of the elderly "survivor." Individualized goals at this time of life fairly universally revolve around the following issues (Comfort, 1976):

Maintaining dignity
Managing one's financial affairs
Obtaining proper health care
Engaging in useful activity

Impediments to a rich and satisfying old age include the following:

Physical transformation or disability
Alterations in social roles and unmet expectations
Loss of an optimal state of health
Diminution of external resources

Losses in any one of the above areas usually can be handled well by an elderly person. When losses occur in multiple areas or become cumulative and profound, intervention by a health care provider is necessary to assist the person to regain a previous level of coping or to manage an acceptable level of functioning.

Mrs. A is an 80-year-old retiree who raised three children as a single parent in the late 1930s when this was not the norm. She built her own home 15 years ago, maintained an acreage garden, and lives a preferred lifestyle during this time with a long-term roommate who is her major support system. Family members are attentive but separated by distance and habit. In the past year her roommate had a successful hip replacement. Mrs. A cared for her during the convalescence despite her own extensive arthritis. This depleted her endurance. As a result she discontinued her gardening and lifelong self-employment and hobby of making pottery. She sold the garden equipment and gave away the potter's wheel to a friend.

Two months ago these roommates went on a month-long automobile trip, even though they worried about the costs. During the trip, Mrs. A developed a series of painful mouth ulcers. Just after their return, Mrs. A's grandchild was killed in an accident.

With the onslaught of stressors, she experienced insomnia, loss of appetite (together with worry about not eating properly), increased joint pain, decreased energy, and intense feelings of loss. She turned to self-medication, taking meprobromate 800 mg nightly in addition to the usual anti-inflammatory drugs and the prescribed antibiotics for the mouth ulcers. Her previous experience had been relief of symptoms with medication; it did not occur this time. Now, feeling increasingly unorganized, fragmented, and anxious, she sought consultation with a visiting nurse.

In the assessment of Mrs. A it was important to recognize that in earlier life she had dealt successfully with the majority of the problems that she was now experiencing. This time both the number and intensity of her losses and the global diminishing of her normal resources created a crisis that she could not handle alone. The case points out the interrelationships between diminishing resources, losses, and the well-being of an individual whose usual efficient coping has been overwhelmed by circumstances. Without intervention, the prognosis for this woman would have been negative, because the cycle of events and her responses were in a downhill spiral. Together, a decision was reached to consult a geropsychiatrist.

Normal age changes most often are manifested in the form of physical changes that alter the individual's capacity to meet the requirements and expectations in daily living; modifications gradually or suddenly ensue. Still, about 85% of the over-65 population learn to adapt to diminishing resources and losses and continue to live "independently" in the community. These individuals are able to look at options and select activities and environments that meet their own value systems and maintain their currently desired roles and activities.

The impact of any *loss* is best analyzed by defining the direction of its impact on the total status of the person. This involves the following:

The person's definition of loss
The person's concern regarding potential losses
Objective data indicating loss or risk of loss
The significance of the loss to the person
The areas of daily living and lifestyle that are being affected by the loss and the nature of the effect
The person's responses in coping with losses, both past and present

The value the person attaches to the area within which the loss occurs will determine in part the intensity of the deprivation experienced. It will be a factor in the response to nursing intervention.

Response to Losses

Elderly people, like younger persons, need to work through perceived problems to a resolution. The stages of loss resolution have been identified as shock, denial, anger/guilt, depression, understanding, and finally acceptance. These stages precede any restitution that is possible. Individuals will vary in their involvement with these stages—not all will go through each stage, nor will they necessarily occur in the sequence mentioned here. However, normal response to any significant loss regardless of magnitude is grief. This is manifested individually in behaviors that indicate emotional suffering. With the elderly, the sadness, depression, or guilt caused by grief are often translated into physical symptoms of dysfunction. These may include immobilization, insomnia, loss of appetite, or intensification of preexisting illness. It may even present with a broad nonspecific syndrome of "failure to thrive."

Normal grieving should resolve in a period of months. Unresolved grieving of a year or more in duration suggests the need for help from a mental health specialist. The extreme reaction of depression leading to suicide is not common, but must always be considered in unresolved grieving situations.

At the other extreme, normal grieving should not be avoided or abnormally foreshortened. Well-meaning friends and even professionals may seek to help by "cheering up" the grieving person. This may only result in delayed grieving or other problems.

Areas for Diminished Resources and Losses in Later Years

PHYSICAL LOSSES

DIMINISHED FUNCTIONAL CAPACITY

Many of the diminishing internal resources in the elderly are based on normal biologic age-related changes (see Chapter 8). The capacity to tolerate the effects of medications is narrowed so that the therapeutic dosages may come perilously close to toxic doses. (In Chapter 10 the relationship between medications and aging is discussed.) As a result of biologic changes, the individual experiences alterations in associated functional capabilities for managing daily living. The requirements of everyday life must be managed with decreased flexibility, agility, balance, strength, endurance, and sensual acuity. When alterations become great enough, adaptations are needed in the strategies for meeting the requirements of daily living and often in elements in the environment for that daily living.

DIMINISHED RESISTANCE TO DISEASE

Increased vulnerability to pathology and trauma is another facet of diminishing psycho-physiologic resources. This in turn can create a sense of greater vulnerability and associated loss of confidence in moving about in society.

LOSS OF BEAUTY OF FACE AND BODY

Another physical change occurs that is not so much in function but in appearance. Inevitably the older person lives in a body with more wrinkles and sagging tissues, skin discolorations, and thinning, graying, or whitening hair. For those who have valued beauty of face and body, this loss can create great discomfort—almost a sense of disbelief except when one gazes in the mirror. The young image that lives inside is an alien to the aging outside.

DEATH

Death may be defined as the ultimate loss. Some elderly persons, however, see it as a welcome alternative rather than a loss; in fact, it may be wistfully wished for if not actively sought. This is a major difference between the old-old and those who are younger. The elderly more often see death as a natural summation of life. Indeed it may be seen as a preferred state to feared alternatives such as outliving children, becoming cognitively impaired, becoming dependent on family, being involved in a catastrophic illness that depletes an estate carefully built for future generations, or placement in a nursing home.

Some elderly people actively seek death in overt or covert suicide. These attempts to die are often successful and are more likely to succeed in the over-75 age group. Although only about 12% of the population in the United States is classified as elderly, 25% of all suicides occur in this group. The group at greatest risk is white males. Added risk factors for this group include depression, alcoholism, bereavement (in the first year), new knowledge of expectation of death from another cause, and living alone. The means chosen is most often guns or explosives (Barnes, 1981). These demographics and statistics relate only to the overt suicides; undoubtedly there are many others who by their behavior engage in a gradual covert suicide.

It is possible to gather information about suicidal thoughts in the elderly. One may talk about whether they (Wolanin and Phillips, 1981):

Think about dying and under what circumstances they imagine it

Have ever considered taking their own life and the strategy and timing of the effort

Actually have developed a plan for ending their lives should living become not worthwhile

PSYCHOSOCIAL LOSSES

LOSS OF FIRST-CLASS CITIZENSHIP

One of the major losses common to the aged is the curse of being ejected from the adult majority. Some elderly persons have never experienced being a member of a minority before;

others now experience a double minority status. The elderly recognize this change in status as they experience being patronized, tolerated, ignored, or treated in a "special" way. Membership in the adult majority is associated with work and being able to make an accepted contribution. Often with age comes "demeaning idleness" (Comfort, 1976). One is not useful, and is therefore not called on to contribute. One carries no weight. It is as if the elderly person is told to "run away and play," until death "calls them to bed" (Comfort, 1976). Comfort (1976) proposed that many older people are in fact young people who live in old bodies.

LOSS OF DIVERSION OPTIONS

With reduced mobility, visual and hearing deficits, and decreased finances may come a diminution in the kinds of activities that one may use to occupy the hours of the day. The options of the elderly person narrow, depending on the losses in other areas, e.g., vision for reading or handiwork; hearing for radio, television, or being part of groups; and with reduced mobility, appropriate transportation for visiting events and places.

ECONOMIC LOSSES

As one grows older economic losses occur for many persons, some of them severe. Reduced finances result in an inability to purchase needed goods and services. There is a decline in the use of support services that require a fee-for-service. This can include such basic factors as heating and cooling of the home, health care, telephone, and transportation. For some it may even mean loss of housing and inadequate food.

PERSONAL NETWORK ALTERATIONS

Attrition of personal support systems occurs through deaths of age-mates and children as well as changes in family structure. Family structure is altered by the mobility of family members and the multiplication of relationships associated with divorce and remarriage. Greater employment of middle-aged women, the primary care givers of the past, also alters the personal external resources of the elderly (see Chapter 13 on the families and caretakers of the elderly).

ROLE CHANGES

Elderly people face role adjustments and changes. Those who have had spouses or housemates face moving into the role of the single older person. The provider–giver role may be changed to the dependent–receiver role. Parent-child roles may be reversed to dependent parent-dominant child roles. The losses of some roles and assimilation of others can be stressful and demanding.

RISK FACTORS

Many elderly manage daily living effectively and with a degree of satisfaction well into their eighth and ninth decades. A small minority, approximately 5%, have physical and health changes that severely impede activities of daily living as related to independent living. This population is most often dysfunctional in areas of physical endurance and disability. Less often there are cognitive deficits. The smallest segment of this group may have global loss in all areas.

Several factors increase the risk of failure to manage daily living effectively in the face of diminishing resources. Some concern the nature of the losses and others the nature of available support systems. Losses are not likely to be effectively managed when they

Occur in multiple areas concurrently

Occur singly, but in too rapid a succession to allow time to regain balance from one loss before another occurs

Are too profound to allow the individual to compensate for them or accommodate them

Those whose external resources are inadequate to support them in the face of diminished resources are the persons who are single—those who have not married or who have been widowed (Shanas, 1979). Those who are widowed face the highest risk within the first 2 months of bereavement when physical symptoms tend to be exacerbated.

SIGNS AND SYMPTOMS

The effectiveness in management of daily living with diminishing resources and losses can be observed both in the comments of the elderly (and those around them) and in their observable status and that of their environments. The nurse should particularly observe for changes when there have been increases in the risk factors.

The data base should include the following:

Antecedent preferred lifestyle and functional ability

Past experiences and current expectations in the high-risk areas

Status of balance between requirements and resources for managing daily living

Areas of strength to be maintained

Areas of existing deficits or dysfunctions, or those the person is at risk for

Perceived options

Acceptable external resources and support systems

SUBJECTIVE DATA

The elderly may not be comfortable with direct verbal expression of feelings or acknowledgment of failing performance. There is a general tendency to adhere to a cultural sense of what is proper and improper to reveal of one's personal life (Malatesta and Kalmak, 1984). Genuine denial of diminishing function also may result in muted or *disguised* patterns of communicating actual status. These factors suggest the need to listen carefully and also to adapt data-gathering strategies that take into account the potential reluctance for disclosure. Being perceptive of data that reveal strengths and giving feedback about them may also allow the person to share areas in which strengths are lacking.

The reporting of concerns over losses or concern for potential or imminent losses may be overt. An example is the individual with failing eyesight who is worried about his driver's license renewal test. On the other hand, a loss may be alluded to only in an indirect and obscure manner: "I used to be so active in my garden." "I can't keep up the house the way I did—sad to see it go downhill, but. . . ." "I was head of the fire brigade in this town, during the early years." "I once was able to give the children and grandchildren nice things at Christmas; now I don't even bother with a tree." Some of the losses that are most personally devastating or demoralizing, however, may be the most difficult to share. Given the sensitive nature of data in these areas, the nurse will want to maintain the person's dignity, support strengths, build trust, and move at the elderly person's pace (unless it is a crisis situation). Where confronting a loss is too painful because

the person's resources are inadequate at the time, the nurse will need both patience and sensitivity.

Gathering basic information on the nature of the person's typical days can give the nurse a great deal of data in a nonthreatening format. The person is asked to describe a daily schedule on an hourly basis, as shown in the box on p. 255.

This information can then be supplemented by following up on high-risk areas, e.g., the interrupted sleep pattern and daily naps, and daily bathing and the risk of dry skin. A more extensive data base on diet could be achieved by asking for a daily diary of food intake for 3 days. Other areas would be that of medications being taken, and knowledge of them and their effects. Areas of strength appear to be mobility and daily exercise plus the ability to manage the instrumental functions of daily living. The failure to mention social contacts (other than the phone call to his daughter) and the amount of time spent watching TV and napping may suggest boredom or social isolation. Further exploration is indicated here. The nonthreatening description of a typical day can be a springboard for moving into areas of ambitions, goals, frustrations, and plans for the months ahead. In subsequent contacts, as trust and the relationship evolve, subtle cues will become easier to recognize and sharing may become easier for the client.

OBJECTIVE DATA

Objective data to validate information derived from the subjective data and to suggest unrecognized areas of loss can be obtained from the medical data base, from functional assessment, and from observation of the elderly person and his environment. Systematic assessment of the individual's functional strengths and weaknesses in relationship to the requirements of daily living is a crucial foundation for development of management strategies. Additional objective data can be obtained about the presence and status of the older person's personal support network, i.e., availability of family, transportation, housing, and so forth. In some circumstances a home visit is invaluable to observe directly the demands that the home situation makes on the functional abilities of the person and to observe how they are being managed.

One should note the richness or barrenness of the sensory environment, the contrast be-

Analysis of a Typical Day's Activity

AM

6	Rises and performs ablutions
7–7:30	Fixes breakfast and eats, e.g., cold cereal and coffee
7:30–8	Gets dressed and calls daughter "to touch base"
8–9	Sits in chair and watches TV game shows
9–10	Completes chores for the day (e.g., pays bills, writes letters, makes shopping list)
10–11:30	Reads morning newspaper and takes a nap
11:30–12:30	Prepares and eats lunch (canned soup, sandwich, and milk)

PM

12:30–2:30	Takes a walk to the store or around the neighborhood
2:30–4	Watches TV
3–5	"Rests," usually on the couch
5–6:30	Fixes dinner (TV dinners, canned or frozen entrées, bread, and coffee), eats while watching TV news, and then cleans up the kitchen
6:30–8:00	Sets up medications for the next day. Takes bath and gets ready for bed. Putters around
8:00	Goes to bed, "tosses and turns"
10:00	Goes to sleep, but sleeps fitfully. Up two or three times to go to bathroom
4 AM	Wakens, stays in bed thinking, sometimes falls asleep again

tween beauty and form in old photographs and present appearance, the roles the individual occupies (or lack of them), and the condition of the immediate environment, activity, mobility, cognitive ability, and finances. All of these circumstances yield concrete data to help determine loss and response to it, if assessed in the context of the individual's earlier life to determine whether a loss in truth exists and what its nature is.

PROGNOSIS

Prognosis is based on the frequency and intensity of losses and their cumulative effect, when new significant losses occur before restitution and adjustment have been accomplished for earlier ones. In addition to the incidence of losses, prognosis is related to resources and past coping styles. Prognosis is improved if at least two of the following three resources are available:

1. Ongoing capacity for making friends and maintaining relationships
2. Financial status seen as adequate by the person
3. Physical status viewed as "healthy" or positive by the individual

Successful aging, including coping with losses, is related to retaining some sense of control—feeling able to "make do" rather than being victimized by events or fate (Wagnild and Young, 1990). Careful assessment of just *how much* adaptive change is being required and the resources that are available is essential in predicting prognosis.

COMPLICATIONS

Complications associated with diminishing resources are associated with failures in crisis management when appropriate help is not received in a timely fashion and major unnecessary losses occur. Exacerbated illnesses, deteriorating environment, and a downward spiraling in managing daily living can occur when gradually occurring resource losses are not managed effectively.

When bereavement occurs, nurses must be alert to the possibility that a great deal of the person's energy is invested in mourning, with little available for carrying out the tasks of daily living. Anorexia, insomnia, severely restricted activities in daily living, and sensory deprivation can occur.

Treating chronic illness is not seen as the most rewarding enterprise. Many professionals are reluctant to get involved with the elderly. This is especially true among those professionals who cannot overcome their "rescue fantasies," i.e., those who tend to avoid patients they cannot cure because they regard both the patients and themselves as failures if a cure is not established. Mutual discouragement can be hard to avoid and may result in spiraling complaints or "shopping" for miracles. Nurses and the elderly persons they serve need to seek contentment with small increments of improvement and gain or even stability or small losses. Comfort instead of cure may be the goal.

PREVENTION AND MANAGEMENT

PREVENTION

Most diminishing resources are a part of the aging process, so that perhaps the only bulwark that can be erected against disintegration is a persistent effort to develop constructive ways of dealing with losses. *Denial* or *making do* is seen frequently among the aged, and for some these serve as an effective defense.

Reminiscing is another mechanism for avoiding or minimizing a present that is painful or empty from losses. It is a recalling of time when one had more self-worth and greater capabilities, and when life was more rewarding and pleasant. It was reported that elderly persons who were discharged from hospitals in New York who engaged in reminiscing tended to survive longer with fewer readmissions than those who focused on a bleak present and uncertain future.

Nurses can engage with elderly persons by fostering reminiscing as well as giving recognition for earlier achievements. Recognizing reminiscing for its therapeutic value should enable nurses to participate genuinely in the ac-

tivity and seek to gain the maximum positive effects from its use.

Planning ahead in terms of organizing an environment and determining goals and options compatible with normal diminution in functional capacity may make transitions and adjustments more comfortable and efficient. The anticipation of risk situations and creation of preset plans for their management also can contribute to greater peace of mind.

Obviously, engaging in a lifestyle that enhances health and good functioning in a safe environment is one way of delaying or preventing some losses.

MANAGEMENT

Effective nursing treatment to enable the elderly to manage daily living with diminishing resources needs to be based on precise diagnoses. There is need to identify the specific areas of daily living that are being affected, the dysfunction or inadequate resources that are creating the difficulty, the cause of the problem (may be in the daily living itself, the dysfunction, the absent external resources, or the environment), and possibly the person's response (if this too is dysfunctional). An example might be as follows:

> Inadequate knowledge and skills in shopping and cooking and inexperience with eating only refined carbohydrate and coffee, avitaminosis, confusion, and weight care.

This would result in nursing interventions different from another diagnosis:

> Lack of funds for food and inability to negotiate for food stamps and supplementary Social Security, leading to 3 days without eating.

Beyond being based on a precise diagnosis, treatment needs to incorporate documented strengths and underused potential or resources.

Since the management of daily living for more than 90% of the elderly is under their own control, any treatment plan, in order to be successful and acceptable, is a negotiated, jointly determined set of goals and activities. The role and participation of all parties is agreed on. Where cognitive deficits are involved, adjustments in participation and control are required.

Specific nursing interventions associated

with particular functional deficits are dealt with in the daily living sections in Parts Four and Five of this book.

EVALUATION

As with the resolution of interpersonal losses, so too with intrapersonal loss one must depend on observation of what people who experience losses are able to say and do. Alertness to the ebbing of sadness and reawakening of interest and involvement is critical to these developments that must be encouraged and supported. Activity patterns in general, but especially those connected with the activities of daily living, and reinvolvement in the lives of others are probably the most reliable indices of loss-coping behavior. Even people who may be unable to verbalize feelings of devastation or discouragement can begin to engage in behavior that reflects the regaining of a firmer grasp on their bootstraps. As they begin to experience this control, some people can be openly verbal about an increase in feelings of well-being. It is helpful to give reassurance that it is normal to have setbacks in progress. Resources in the community for the support of older people are one of the most significant consequence of recent social policy and planning. Professionals should be well informed of these developments and encourage older people to take full advantage of the emerging fact that our society no longer tolerates the abandonment and neglect of our older citizens.

Future Perspectives on Long-term Care for the Elderly with Diminishing Resources

It has been estimated that one out of four older persons will be admitted to a nursing home within their lifetime for varying periods of time (Fuchs, 1984). This rate may be increased to one in two with the advent of prospective payment for acute care.

When a previously independent elderly person is admitted to a long-term care facility, assessment of previous level of functioning as well as current disabilities is imperative. This group is at high risk of continued institutionalization unless the nurse is actively involved in assessment of the individual for discharge planning. These individuals may be involved in

potentially transitional states of diminished resources that can be compounded by the loss of hope related to the new dependent lifestyle of institutionalization.

National Policy and Geriatric Health Care

Nowhere are the elderly more at risk for potential risk of external resources than in the current controversy over planning for use of health care resources. "Cost-effectiveness" and "bottom line" are the slogans of the day. Costs and outcomes of treatment or programs are being quantified in these terms. One health planner has devised a "human capital" approach. This is a rationale wherein the projective lifetime earnings are calculated from average earnings by periods within the life span of adults. Using this index, a 30- to 34-year-old adult is valued at $205,062; a 60- to 64-year-old at $45,169, and an 80- to 84-year-old person at $2,820. Using such a value system, it is easy to see that the support of health care resources would become another major deficit in the other predictable diminishing resources of old age, and would result in a systematic devaluation of health care for the elderly (Avorn, 1984).

Nurses interested in providing appropriate therapy in managing daily living for the elderly with diminishing resources have twofold directions and obligations for their efforts. The first is to provide the kind of sound, sensitive, *direct nursing care* that will promote person-defined quality of life. The second is to engage in the political processes necessary to influence national values, policies, and thus appropriate resources for the elderly.

References and Other Readings

American Nurses' Association. Nursing: a social policy statement. Kansas City, ANA, 1980.

Anderson F. Retirement can damage your health. Nursing Mirror 1984; 158:42.

Avorn J. Benefit and cost analysis in geriatric care: turning age discrimination into health policy. N Engl J Med 1984; 310:1295.

Barnes R, Kieth R, Raskin M. Depression in older persons: diagnosis and management. West J Med 1981;135:463.

Beck SH. Retirement preparation programs: differentials in opportunity and use. J Gerontol 1984; 39:596.

Berkman LF. The assessment of social networks and social support in the elderly. J Am Geriatr Soc 1983; 31:743.

Butler RN, Lewis IM. Aging and mental health: positive psychological and biomedical approaches. New York: CV Mosby, 1982.

Comfort A. Practice of geriatric psychology. New York: Elsevier, 1980.

Comfort A. A good age. New York: Crown Publishers, 1976.

Fuchs V. "Though much is taken": reflections on aging, health and medical care. Milbank Mem Fund Q 1984; 62:143.

George LK, Fillenbaum GG, Palmore E. Sex differences in the antecedents and consequences of retirement. J Gerontol 1984; 39:365.

Kahn RL. Productive behavior: assessment, determinants, and effects. J Am Geriatr Soc 1983; 31:750.

Kane RL, Ouslander JG, Abrass AB. Essentials of clinical geriatrics. New York: McGraw-Hill, 1984, p. 50.

Linn MW, Linn BS. Self-evaluation of life function (SELF) scale: a short comprehensive self report of health for elderly adults. J Gerontol 1984; 39:603.

Malatesta CZ, Kalmak M. Emotional experience in younger and older adults. J Gerontol 1984; 39:301.

Markides KS, Vernon SW. Aging, sex-role orientation and adjustment: a three-generation study of Mexican Americans. J Gerontol 1984; 39:586.

Palmore EG, Fillenbaum GG, George LK. Consequences of retirement. J Gerontol 1984; 39:109.

Shanas E. The family as a social support system in old age. Gerontologist 1979; 19:169.

Somers AR. Why not try preventing illness as a way of controlling Medicare costs? N Engl J Med 1984; 311:853.

Thompson LW, et al. Effects of bereavement on self perceptions of physical health in elderly widows and widowers. J Gerontol 1984; 39:309.

Wagnild A, Young HM. Resilience among older women. Image: J Nurs Schol 1990; 4:252.

Wolanin MO, Phillips LRF. Confusion: prevention and care. St. Louis: CV Mosby, 1981.

PART FOUR

Neurologic and Behavioral Problems in the Elderly

Neurologic and behavioral problems of the elderly are the focus for Part Four. Normal age-related cognitive changes are covered in Chapter 15. Abnormal changes associated with delirium and dementia are discussed in Chapter 16. Other psychiatric problems as they are manifested and treated in the elderly are considered in Chapter 17. All three chapters are written by a geropsychiatrist.

The remainder of this section focuses on nursing, addressing the problems in daily living associated with the dysfunctions and demands of Alzheimer's disease (Chapter 18), and other behavioral problems (Chapter 19). The reader will find that some behavioral problems considered in Chapter 18, such as agitation and restlessness, are applicable to other conditions, so refer to both Chapters 18 and 19 regarding behavioral problems. A gerontological nurse specialist, practicing in a large mental hospital, has written these chapters. The two chapters on parkinsonism and stroke were written by a clinical specialist who works daily with these patients and their families.

15
Cognitive Changes of Normal Aging

ROBERT WILLS

There are few significant changes that predictably occur in normal aging (Comfort, 1979; Bortz, 1982). This is good news to the young and middle-aged members of our society, but no news to millions of older persons who lead full and intellectually satisfying lives. In 1990 George Burns and Bob Hope turned 95 and 85, respectively. Both continue to perform with remarkable vigor. Ronald Reagan, who completed his second term as our oldest president, continues to lecture and teach as an octogenarian. In the following discussion, changes in neuroanatomy are addressed, followed by known changes in cognitive function.

Neuroanatomic Changes of Normal Aging

GROSS STRUCTURAL CHANGES IN THE BRAIN WITH AGING

The brain undergoes measurable reductions in size and weight with aging. Structure, once lost, cannot be replaced because of the postmitotic nature of nerve cells. Shrinkage of the brain tissue is most prominent in the frontal halves of the cerebral hemispheres, with less loss in the posterior halves, brain stem, and cerebellum. There is associated progressive enlargement of the ventricles (Rossman, 1986). Computerized axial tomography has shown sig-

nificant brain atrophy starting at 50 years. Atrophy relates better to age than to dementia, while enlargement of the ventricles seems to be better correlated with dementia (Ford and Winter, 1981).

MICROSCOPIC BRAIN CHANGES WITH AGING

LOSS OF NEURONS

Microscopic studies show progressive loss of neurons beginning, surprisingly, in the 20s. By age 90, approximately 30% of cerebral neurons are lost (Brody, 1955). Of more clinical consequence, some areas of the brain seem to lose neurons at a higher rate than others. The focal loss of cells in the substantia nigra that results in Parkinson's disease is an example.

INTERCELLULAR CHANGES

Intercellular changes include the progressive appearance of neurofibrillary tangles and senile plaques, which, when present to a marked degree, are characteristic of senile dementia of the Alzheimer's type. Tangles and plaques represent different changes in aging neurons. Although they are both increased in frequency after age 60, they are not related directly to each other in terms of intensity and distribution (Dayan and Lewis, 1985). In general, there is still little known about the relationship of neuronal degeneration and loss of cognitive function and behaviors.

Cognitive Changes of Normal Aging

Changes in cognitive function are included within the neuropsychiatric parameters of consciousness, attention, language, memory, constructional ability, and higher cognitive function (Albert, 1981, 1984; Granacher, 1981; Strub and Black, 1977; Taylor et al, 1980). These same functional areas form the basis of clinical testing discussed in the mental status examination in Chapter 16. The clinical examples used here to clarify cognitive functions may be incorporated with the standard tests included in the discussion of the dementias.

CONSCIOUSNESS

Evaluation of consciousness is really an evaluation of alertness, the ability to be aware of and respond to external and internal stimuli. It is a function of complex interactions between the arousal center in the brain stem and higher cortical function. No impairment in this fundamental brain function occurs in normal aging.

Consciousness is tested by observation of response to verbal and touch stimuli and is stated in terms of four levels:

Alert: Fully awake, able to interact with the examiner
Lethargic: Unable to stay awake without stimulation and unable to sustain attention. Lethargic persons are not "with you," giving the impression of lack of interest and dullness
Stuporous: Responds to aggressive stimulation with no meaningful recognition or cooperation
Coma: Unable to be aroused with any vigorous stimulation

Lethargy is the usual level of consciousness in delirium and is sometimes confused with the more chronic changes of dementia. Patients with decreased levels of consciousness cannot be accurately assessed for the other functional parameters.

ATTENTION

Attention describes the ability to maintain concentration adequately enough to remain task oriented. Although alertness is necessary for attention, the opposite is not true. A simple test of attention is digit span. Normal older persons are able to easily repeat four random digits and usually six to eight digits.

The ability to maintain attention over a longer period of time can be evaluated by reading a series of random letters containing a target letter to be identified by the patient with a tap of the finger (Strub and Black, 1977). Abnormal responses include errors of omission as well as incorrect tapping with nontarget letters.

Although elderly persons are able to attend accurately to single tasks, more complex tasks involving divided attention demonstrate age-dependent impairment. This has practical implications for the person in a managerial or executive position who may interpret this natural change as a sign of dementia. Along with reassurance, guidance may be given in simplifying or reorganizing job requirements (Albert, 1984). Older persons need to be encouraged to set up tasks in a serial format and not attempt to work at several tasks in parallel. Successful completion of each task increases confidence and may actually accelerate the number of completed tasks over time.

LANGUAGE

Healthy older individuals demonstrate changes in naming objects and individuals (Albert, 1984). This is not solely a function of memory; amnesic persons with severe memory impairment are able to name objects successfully. Although generally ascribed to old age, naming problems begin to be experienced in middle age, with a common example being the inability to name friends of many years when making introductions. The inability to name an object is separated from the intact ability to describe its use or function in detail. In addition, the name may be readily available at other times.

Impaired naming can be assessed by confrontational testing using items such as a watch, pen, ring, body parts, and so on (Strub and Black, 1977). The recognition of abnormal responses is based on clinical experience and a knowledge of the person's educational level and experience. Specific problems with language, e.g., aphasia, are common in disease and their testing is useful in localizing brain pathology.

MEMORY

Memory is a complex process involving several steps. Sensory input obtained through sight, smell, sound, or touch is received and registered (Strub and Black, 1977; La Rue, 1982). This input is transferred to short-term or immediate memory while the person consciously focuses on the information. A further step involves storage of input in a more permanent form, resulting in long-term or remote memory. The final step is retrieval or recovery of the stored information.

It is clear that problems affecting alertness, attention, and language can prevent the registering of new information.

Information deemed critical to relationships, work, or survival is more apt to be permanently encoded. Performance anxiety also impairs retrieval of stored information. This phenomenon can be experienced by any reader asked to retrieve particular information at test time.

For testing purposes memory is divided into *immediate, recent,* and *remote memory.* Recent memory is a rather nebulous term in contrast with the other and really refers to the learning of recently received data, e.g., the day's new events, what was eaten for breakfast, the date, and so forth. Because deficits in new learning are the most sensitive indicators of early cognitive loss, most formal tests of memory focus on this period. Immediate memory is adequately tested by digit recall. Remote memory is tested by historical data such as the names of presidents, dates of wars, and similar kinds of information. More personal data include birth date, names of schools attended, jobs held, and so on, but requires verification that is not always readily available.

Although normal persons begin to demonstrate mild memory loss in their mid-years, it is more often described in the 60s and 70s. Neuropsychiatric testing may demonstrate losses of approximately 30% without accompanying evidence of cortical disease. A significant improvement can be shown with the use of memory aids, coupled with relaxation training. This suggests that what is found on testing is not true memory loss (Yesavage, 1984). As previously discussed, complaints of memory loss

may actually evolve from a misperception due to problems of divided attention and naming. The term *benign forgetfulness* encompasses this type of apparent loss of memory. Immediate and remote memory appear little affected in normal aging. The habit of some elderly persons to control conversation with comfortable old material may be an attempt to avoid the embarrassment of not holding new material on the tips of their tongues. This behavior should not be interpreted as demonstrating the confabulating behavior of dementia without further inquiry.

CONSTRUCTIONAL ABILITY

The ability to accurately draw figures on command or copy simple one- and two-dimensional shapes or figures is well maintained in the elderly. This exercise demands complex, integrated skills of perception, cortical function, and motor ability and is particularly sensitive to bilateral cortical dysfunction. Demonstrating dysfunction in constructional ability offers a simple sensitive tool to evaluate early diffuse cortical disease (Thal, 1982).

HIGHER COGNITIVE FUNCTION

That the majority of elderly persons live active independent lives affirms their ability to assimilate, process, and successfully use information. This is particularly important in a complex urban culture that demands high levels of performance to supply most of the basic needs, e.g., paying utility bills, shopping at the supermarket, repairing the automobile, and getting health needs met. Nevertheless, there are measurable changes in the speed of learning new material and the performance of complex tasks.

Higher cognitive function is evaluated by testing for the fund of basic knowledge, ability to use acquired knowledge, social skills, judgment, and abstract thinking. Interpretation of responses should consider the person's educational level, past occupations, and life experiences.

NEUROPSYCHIATRIC TESTING

Until recently there has been minimal interest in geriatric neuropsychiatry; the elderly have been given tests standardized for younger persons (Raskin and Jarvik, 1979). In addition, their specific physical and emotional needs have not been addressed, e.g., easy fatigue, hearing and sight deficits, need for additional instruction and time, and fear of being judged incompetent. Medical and psychiatric disease or unrecognized drug toxicity may create responses ascribed to chronic brain dysfunction. Because of potential problems in testing, all results should be carefully compared with the clinical data. This is particularly important with tests that are timed or required rapid movement. No doubt the future will provide excellent age-standardized tests that will be useful in diagnosis and therapy. However, these are not presently available.

Normal aging is characterized by minimal cognitive deterioration. The aged show some slowing of learning and respond less well to a complex presentation of new tasks. Naming is decreased. Recent memory is mildly impaired, in part because of inattention and inadequate registration.

References and Other Readings

Albert MS. Geriatric neuropsychology. J Consult Clin Psychol 1981; 49:835.

Albert MS. Assessment of cognitive function in the elderly. Psychosomatics 1984; 25:310.

Bortz WM. Disuse and aging. JAMA 1982; 248:1203.

Brody H. Organization of the cerebral cortex: a study of aging in human cerebral cortex. J Comp Neurol 1955; 102:511.

Comfort A. The myth of senility. Postgrad Med 1979; 65:130.

Dayan A, Lewis P. The central nervous systems—neuropathology of aging. In: Brocklehurst J, ed. Textbook of geriatric medicine and gerontology. 3rd ed. New York: Churchhill Livingstone, 1985, p 274.

Ford C, Winter J. Computerized axial tomograms and dementia in elderly patients. J Gerontol 1981; 36:164.

Granacher RP. The neurologic examination in geriatric psychiatry. Psychosomatics 1981; 22:485.

Hultsh D, Dixon R. Learning and memory. In: Birren J, Schaie KW, ed. Handbook of psychology of aging. 3rd ed. San Diego: Academic Press, 1990, p 259.

La Rue A. Memory loss and aging: distinguishing dementia from benign senescent forgetfulness and depressive pseudodementia. Psychiatr Clin North Am 1982; 5:89.

Raskin A, Jarvik LF. Psychiatric symptoms and cognitive loss in the elderly: evaluation and assessment techniques. Washington, DC: Hemisphere Publishing Corp, 1979.

Rossman I. The aging brain. In: Clinical geriatrics. 3rd ed. Philadelphia: JB Lippincott, 1986, p 17.

Strub RL, Black FW. The mental status examination in neurology. Philadelphia: FA Davis, 1977.

Taylor MA, Abrams R, Faber R et al. Cognitive tasks in the mental status examination. J Nerv Ment Dis 1980; 168:167.

Thal LJ. Diagnosing and treating dementia. Drug Therapy—Hosp 1982; 7:51.

Yesavage JA. Relaxation and memory training in 39 elderly patients. Am J Psychiatr 1984; 141:778.

16
Delirium and Dementia

ROBERT WILLS

Disorders involving diffuse impairment of brain function are common in the elderly, particularly in relation to chronic illness and drug therapy. Until recently, many terms were interchangeably used to describe these clinical syndromes. In 1987, the American Psychiatric Association revised the third edition of its *Diagnostic and Statistical Manual of Mental Disorders* (DSM-III-R). These diagnostic criteria are used in the following discussions of specific disorders.[*]

Delirium

Delirium is a descriptive word meaning literally "off the track." It is a common condition, particularly in the hospital setting, and is most often a manifestation of serious, systemic disease or an abnormal response to treatment. Altered consciousness, the inability to sustain attention, and a fluctuating clinical course are important distinguishing features.

INCIDENCE

Estimates of prevalence vary, but one third to one half of hospitalized elderly patients become delirious at some time during their hospi-

talization (Lipowski, 1983). No data are available on outpatients, but personal experience suggests a significant incidence in the medically ill who are taking multiple medications.

ETIOLOGIC FACTORS

The elderly seem particularly disposed to symptoms of delirium. Table 16–1 presents a partial list of conditions causing delirium. Drug intoxication is emphasized because of the high percentage of elderly persons taking multiple drugs and the increased sensitivity of the brain to many prescription and over-the-counter medications (Table 16–2). Most psychotropic medications, which include antipsychotics, antidepressants, tranquilizers, and sedatives, can cause delirium. Alcohol alone or in combination with other drugs causes symptoms of delirium and should be considered in both outpatient and inpatient settings. Unfortunately patient and family denial make this diagnosis difficult. Failure to consider alcohol abuse or lack of persistence in pursuing the diagnosis leads to diagnostic confusion and failure of all therapies (see discussion of alcoholism in Chapter 17).

Other factors include premorbid dementia, reactions to hospitalization, the nature of treatments or procedures (e.g., bypass surgery), general anesthesia, and unfamiliarity with medical personnel. Many situations and conditions

[*]DSM-IV will be published in 1994 according to the American Psychiatric Association.

(continued on p. 268)

TABLE 16–1 *Disorders Causing Delirium in the Aged*

Disorder	Examples
CENTRAL NERVOUS SYSTEM	
Neoplasm	Primary intracranial neoplasm, metastatic neoplasm—bronchogenic carcinoma, breast carcinoma
Cerebrovascular disease	Arteriosclerosis, cerebral infarction, subarachnoid hemorrhage, transient ischemic attacks, hypertensive encephalopathy, vasculitis (lupus), cranial arteritis, disseminated intravascular coagulation
Infection	Neurosyphilis, brain abscess, tuberculosis, meningoencephalitis (bacterial, viral, fungal), septic emboli (subacute bacterial endocarditis)
Head trauma	Chronic subdural hematoma, extradural hematoma, cerebral contusion, concussion
Ictal and postictal states	Idiopathic seizures, space-occupying lesion, post-traumatic lesions, electroconvulsive therapy
CARDIOVASCULAR DISEASE	
Decreased cardiac output	Congestive heart failure, cardiac arrhythmias, aortic stenosis, myocardial infarction
Hypotension	Orthostatic hypotension, vasovagal syncope, hypovolemia
METABOLIC DISORDERS	
Hypoxemia	Respiratory insufficiency, anemia, carbon monoxide poisoning
Electrolyte disturbance	Kidney disease, adrenal disease, diabetes mellitus, diuretics, edematous states, syndrome of inappropriate secretion of antidiuretic hormone, dehydration, starvation
Acidosis	Diabetes mellitus, kidney disease, pulmonary disease, chronic diarrhea
Alkalosis	Hyperadrenocorticism, pulmonary disease, psychogenic hyperventilation
Hepatic disease	Acute hepatic failure, cirrhosis, chronic portahepatic encephalopathy
Uremia	Chronic glomerulonephritis, chronic pyelonephritis, acute renal failure, obstructive uropathy
Endocrinopathies	Hypothyroidism, thyrotoxicosis, "apathetic" hyperthyroidism, hypoglycemia, hyperglycemia, hypoparathyroidism, hypoadrenocorticism, hyperadrenocorticism
Deficiency states	Hypovitaminosis—thiamine, nicotinic acid, vitamin B_{12}, folate deficiency, iron deficiency
OTHER DISORDERS	
Trauma	Burns, surgery, multiple injuries, fractures (fat embolism)
Sensory deprivation	Cataracts, glaucoma, otosclerosis, darkness ("sundown syndrome")
Exogenous toxins	Medications, alcohol, withdrawal syndromes, heavy metals, solvents, insecticides, pesticides, carbon monoxide
Temperature regulation	Exposure and accidental hypothermia, heat stroke, febrile illnesses

From Liston EH. Delirium in the aged. Psychiatr Clin North Am 1982; 5:49; with permission.

TABLE 16–2 *Common Medications Causing Delirium in the Aged*

Disorder	Medication	Common Examples
Cardiovascular conditions	Antiarrhythmics	Procainamide, propranolol, quinidine
	Antihypertensives	Clonidine, methyldopa, reserpine
	Cardiac glycosides	Digitalis
	Coronary vasodilators	Nitrates
Gastrointestinal conditions	Antidiarrheals	Atropine, belladonna, homatropine, hyoscyamine, scopolamine
	Antinauseants	Cyclizine, homatropine–barbiturate preparations, phenothiazines
	Antispasmodics	Methanthelene, propantheline
Musculoskeletal conditions	Anti-inflammatory agents	Corticosteroids, indomethacin, phenylbutazone, salicylates
	Muscle relaxants	Carisoprodol, diazepam
Neurologic-psychiatric conditions	Anticonvulsants	Barbiturates, carbamazepine, diazepam, phenytoin
	Antiparkinsonism agents	Amantadine, benztropine, levodopa, trihexyphenidyl
	Hypnotics and sedatives	Barbiturates, belladonna alkaloids, bromides, chloral hydrate, ethchlorvynol, glutethimide
	Psychotropics	Benzodiazepines, hydroxyzines, lithium salts, meprobamate, monoamine oxidase inhibitors, neuroleptics, tricyclic antidepressants
Respiratory-allergic conditions	Antihistamines	Brompheniramine, chlorpheniramine, cyproheptadine, diphenhydramine, tripelennamine
	Antitussives	Opiates, synthetic narcotics
	Decongestants and expectorants	Phenylephrine, phenylpropanolamine, potassium preparations
Miscellaneous conditions	Analgesics	Dextropropoxyphene, opiates, phenacetin, salicylates, synthetic narcotics
	Anesthetics	Lidocaine, methohexital, methoxyflurane
	Antidiabetic agents	Insulin, oral hypoglycemics
	Antineoplastics	Corticosteroids, mitomycin, procarbazine
	Antituberculosis agents	Isoniazid, rifampin

From Liston EH. Delirium in the aged. Psychiatr Clin North Am 1982; 5:49; with permission.

common to the elderly can cause delirium in the outpatient setting. Nutritional deficiencies, hypothermia, undiagnosed medical illness, head trauma, cardiovascular and pulmonary disease, metabolic imbalance, and drug toxicity are potentially important factors.

CLINICAL COURSE

The onset of delirium is usually abrupt—hours to days—and the course is usually less than 1 week. Common exceptions would include delirium associated with medical conditions known to have insidious onsets, e.g., hypothyroidism.

Characteristically there is global impairment, with rapid fluctuations in specific cognitive functions over time, i.e., problems in orientation, attention, consciousness, or memory may dominate the clinical picture at any moment. Patients may show inappropriate changes in mood such as demonstrating anger, fear, apathy, or irritability that is unrelated to the clinical situation. Perceptual disturbances include frightening visual hallucinations and illusions. Psychomotor disturbance is common, with extremes of motor activity occurring through the day. Sleep–wake cycles are disrupted, with accentuation of confusion during the night. The latter is a more severe form of "sundowning" activity observable in less impaired elderly persons during hospitalization. *Full recovery depends on accurate, rapid diagnosis and aggressive early treatment.* Delay in either may cause irreversible cortical damage and dementia.

DIAGNOSIS

Table 16–3 presents the major criteria for diagnosis of delirium. Delirium is a clinical diagnosis that is not difficult to determine if the premorbid state of health is known. Unfortunately the elderly are assumed to have some degree of cognitive dysfunction as a part of normal aging, increasing staff tolerance for abnormal behavior in the hospital setting. Subtle confusion and inattention are often recognized but ignored as expected behavior. Furthermore, medical specialization itself places the elderly at risk, particularly in the hospital setting. Major treatment decisions are increasingly made by hospital staff who have never seen the patient before admission. The patient's premorbid condition needs to be verified with their regular providers. Information from friends or relatives may be less reliable as they tend to overes-

TABLE 16–3 *Diagnostic Criteria of Delirium*

1. Reduced ability to maintain attention to external stimuli (e.g., questions must be repeated because attention wanders) and to appropriately shift attention to new external stimuli (e.g., perseverates answer to a previous question)

2. Disorganized thinking, as indicated by rambling, irrelevant, or incoherent speech

3. At least two of the following:
   a. reduced level of consciousness, e.g., difficulty keeping awake during examination
   b. perceptual disturbances: misinterpretations, illusions, or hallucinations
   c. disturbance of sleep–wake cycle with insomnia or daytime sleepiness
   d. increased or decreased psychomotor activity
   e. disorientation to time, place, or person
   f. memory impairment, e.g., inability to learn new material, such as the names of several unrelated objects, after 5 minutes, or to remember past events, such as history of current episode of illness

4. Clinical features develop over a short period of time (usually hours to days) and tend to fluctuate over the course of a day

5. Either a or b:
   a. evidence from the history, physical examination, or laboratory tests of a specific organic factor (or factors) judged to be etiologically related to the disturbance
   b. in the absence of such evidence, an etiologic organic factor can be presumed if the disturbance cannot be accounted for by any nonorganic mental disorder, e.g., manic episode accounting for agitation and sleep disturbance

From Diagnostic and Statistical Manual of Mental Disorders (DSM-III-R), Third Edition, Revised. Washington, DC: American Psychiatric Association, 1987, pp. 77–78; with permission.

timate the patient's prehospital function through denial. Procrastination in evaluating early symptoms is common, resulting in higher risk of harm to the patient.

The diagnosis of delirium should always be immediately followed by a careful review of the clinical course of the primary disease, with emphasis on metabolic abnormalities and drug toxicity. Often several factors are found to be operative, and all members of the treatment team can play important diagnostic roles.

DIFFERENTIAL DIAGNOSIS

The previous discussion has emphasized the problem of mistaking delirium for dementia. This diagnostic confusion should be short-lived because the rapidly changing nature of delirium is in marked contrast to the more stable, slowly progressive dementia (Table 16–4). Premorbid information is extremely helpful. Finally, it is not unusual to have both conditions present, with the dementia heightening the susceptibility to delirium.

TREATMENT

If the clinical situation allows, all drugs should be withdrawn for at least a few days. It is often surprising how many medications can be reduced in dosage or discontinued without a significant change in the patient's physiologic status. A partial explanation lies in the tendency to add new drugs without removing old ones.

Specific therapy obviously hinges on aggressive and successful therapy of the primary medical or surgical problem. In addition, general measures directed at correction of anemia, nutritional deficiencies, electrolyte imbalance, and dehydration should be rapidly undertaken.

Nursing care involves frequent neurologic assessment, protection of the patient, and maneuvers directed at maintaining orientation. Physical restraint is occasionally needed, but carries the usual risks of superficial trauma, more agitation, and occasional musculoskeletal injury.

Psychotropic medication should be considered when confusion is protracted, physical maneuvers fail to adequately protect the patient or staff, or when insomnia is a major factor delaying recovery. Neuroleptics is the major

TABLE 16–4 *Differential Diagnosis of Delirium and Dementia*

Feature	Delirium	Dementia
Onset	Rapid, often at night	Usually insidious
Duration	Hours to weeks	Months to years
Course	Fluctuates over 24 hours; worse at night; lucid intervals	Relatively stable
Awareness	Always impaired	Usually normal
Alertness	Reduced or increased; tends to fluctuate	Usually normal
Orientation	Always impaired, at least for time; tendency to mistake unfamiliar for familiar place or person	May be intact; tendency to confabulate
Memory	Recent and immediate impaired; fund of knowledge intact if dementia is absent	Recent and remote impaired; some loss of common knowledge
Thinking	Slow or accelerated; may be dream-like	Poor in abstraction, impoverished
Perception	Often misperceptions, especially visual	Misperceptions often absent
Sleep–wake cycle	Always disrupted; often drowsiness during the day, insomnia at night	Fragmented sleep
Physical illness or drug toxicity	Usually present	Often absent, especially in primary degenerative dementia

From Lipowski ZJ. Transient cognitive disorders in the elderly. Am J Psychiatry 1983; 140:1432; with permission.

class of drugs used. Haloperidol is frequently used because of its high potency and lack of anticholinergic effects. It is given intramuscularly or orally and doses of 0.5 to 2 mg every 2 to 4 hours are well tolerated. Higher doses will add to the sedative effect but will not shorten the course of the delirium. Common side effects include extrapyramidal symptoms resembling Parkinson's disease. Benzodiazepines can also be effective. They, like the neuroleptics, can produce paradoxical worsening of the delirium. Therapeutic goals include a reduction in confusion and agitation with associated improvement in sleep.

PROGNOSIS

Most delirium improves with removal of the noxious agent or treatment of the underlying disease. Late diagnosis and incomplete treatment increase the potential for slow recovery. Permanent brain damage can occur.

Dementia

Dementia, like delirium, is an ancient term taken from the Latin and means literally "out of one's mind." The dementias are actually a group of diseases sharing a gradual onset, global decline in intellectual capacity and performance, and progressive social incapacitation. They are *never* a normal consequence of aging (Comfort, 1979). Regardless of etiology there will eventually be a diffuse and permanent loss of neurons involving all areas of the brain.

PREVALENCE

Dementia is common, afflicting 4% in the 65 to 75 age group and 25% over age 80. With 12% of the population of the United States presently over age 65 and with an anticipated doubling of this percentage by the year 2030, the problem of dementia looms as a significant personal and public health problem.

DEFINITION

At the present time, there is no single accepted manner of grouping the dementias. One useful method divides them into primary and secondary disorders (Table 16–5). Primary dementias have in common a progressive, unremitting course, obscure etiology, irreversibility, and ab-

TABLE 16–5 *Primary and Secondary Dementias*

Primary Dementias	Secondary Dementias
Primary degenerative dementia (Alzheimer's type)	Normal pressure hydrocephalus
Multi-infarct dementia	Parkinson's dementia
Pick's disease	Drug-induced dementia
Huntington's disease	Pseudodementia
Creutzfeldt-Jakob disease	Metabolic disorders Other neurologic disorders

sent or inconsistent response to therapy. Secondary dementias show an identifiable etiology and some measure of reversibility. Regardless of the etiology, all dementias share general diagnostic features described in Table 16–6. These are discussed in detail in the following sections on specific disorders of dementia.

PRIMARY DEGENERATIVE DEMENTIA

DESCRIPTION

Primary degenerative dementia (PDD) is more commonly known as Alzheimer's disease, being named for the pathologist who first described the characteristic brain pathology in 1907. Both presenile and senile dementia are included in this diagnosis because they demonstrate similar pathology. Approximately 50% of patients presenting with dementia have PDD. (Wilcock, 1989). Another 25% show mixed PDD and multi-infarct dementia (MID). Women are affected twice as often as men, and the incidence in both sexes increases with age.

ETIOLOGIC FACTORS

Although the etiology is unknown, specific biochemical and pathologic changes have provided a foundation for ongoing research (Shalat, 1989). The characteristic pathology includes neurofibrillar tangles, neuritic plaques, and granulovascular degeneration. The origin of these findings is not known. Neuritic plaques and neurofibrillar tangles are also seen in Down's syndrome and scrapie viral disease

TABLE 16–6 *Diagnostic Criteria of Dementia*

1. Demonstrable evidence of impairment in short- and long-term memory. Impairment in short-term memory (inability to learn new information) may be indicated by inability to remember three objects after 5 minutes. Long-term memory impairment (inability to remember information that was known in the past) may be indicated by inability to remember past personal information (e.g., what happened yesterday, birthplace, occupation) or facts of common knowledge (e.g., past presidents, well-known dates)

2. At least one of the following:
   a. impairment in abstract thinking, as indicated by inability to find similarities and differences between related words, difficulty in defining words and concepts, and other similar tasks
   b. impaired judgment, as indicated by inability to make reasonable plans to deal with interpersonal, family, and job-related problems and issues
   c. other disturbances of higher cortical function, such as aphasia (disorder of language), apraxia (inability to carry out motor activities despite intact comprehension and motor function), agnosia (failure to recognize or identify objects despite intact sensory function), and "constructional difficulty" (e.g., inability to copy three-dimensional figures, assemble blocks, or arrange sticks in specific designs)
   d. personality change, i.e., alteration or accentuation of premorbid traits

3. The disturbance in 1 and 2 significantly interferes with work or usual social activities or relationships with others

4. Not occurring exclusively during the course of delirium

5. Either a or b:
   a. there is evidence from the history, physical examination, or laboratory tests of a specific organic factor (or factors) judged to be etiologically related to the disturbance
   b. in the absence of such evidence, an etiologic organic factor can be presumed if the disturbance cannot be accounted for by any nonorganic mental disorder, e.g., major depression accounting for cognitive impairment

From Diagnostic and Statistical Manual of Mental Disorders (DSM-III-R), Third Edition, Revised. Washington, DC: American Psychiatric Association, 1987, pp. 78–79; with permission.

of sheep. Neurofibrillar tangles are seen in Parkinson's disease. Similar changes occur with normal aging, but to a markedly lesser degree.

The typical histologic appearance of PDD associated with viral particles in animal diseases has suggested a slow virus as the etiologic agent. Unfortunately, no virus has been cultured from human brain tissue (Heston and White, 1983). The finding of increased amyloid has pointed toward an immunologic cause, and research in this area is active. The finding of increased aluminum in the brains of patients with PDD has directed research toward a toxic etiology (Allen et al, 1979).

Biochemical abnormalities have been known for two decades (Thal, 1983; Goodnick and Gershon, 1984). Choline acetyltransferase, the enzyme active in the synthesis of acetylcholine, is decreased. The importance of cholinergic involvement in memory function has also been extensively studied. Unfortunately, attempts at increasing brain choline levels have not been successful in reversing the course of PDD (Goodnick and Gershon, 1984). More recently, attention has been focused on deficits of serotonin and its principal metabolite, 5-hydroxyindoleacetic acid, in the frontal and temporal cortex. Although the functional significance is presently unclear, serotonin is known to play an important role in such complex and diverse processes as memory, sleep, mood regulation, appetite, anxiety, and aggression (Lawlor, 1990).

Genetic factors are also important, but there is not a simple model that explains how the disease appears in specific families. The risk to siblings up to the age of 75 is about 7%. Children may have about the same percentage risk, but this is not known because families have not been studied long enough for children to grow up and be affected (Heston and White, 1983).

CLINICAL FEATURES

The onset of symptoms in PDD is insidious. Although global involvement characterizes the later stages of the disease, initial findings may suggest a more specific diagnosis. An example is the person who is referred for psychiatric evaluation because of lability of mood. Impaired memory is first suspected by friends and relatives or health care personnel. Patients may never spontaneously seek help because they are embarrassed about or unable to appreciate their gradual deterioration. The ability to confabulate with old, well-rehearsed stories and the retention of good social skills obscure early memory deficits. Family and friends may delay diagnosis through the process of denial and rationalization.

Initial impairment involves recent memory. Immediate recall and remote memory are affected later. Cognitive changes in PDD occur in a continuum with normal aging and can be divided into fairly distinct stages (Reisberg, 1986). Because of the complexity of modern life, memory deficits and disorientation often evolve around losing objects and getting lost in new surroundings. On the other hand, patients may be able to drive across a busy city if the route is familiar, only to forget the purpose of their visit while there and the substance of the visit on returning home.

Suspiciousness and paranoia are often associated with early loss of orientation, somewhat analogous to the response of persons losing their hearing, i.e., life that is heard unclearly may be experienced as threatening. Confusion may be first evident at night, with associated insomnia, wandering, irritability, and combativeness, known as the sundown syndrome. Changes in personality are seldom for the better and are perceived as negative or hostile. This further isolates the patient because social support is withdrawn. Perceptual problems include hallucinations and illusions. In later stages patients show reduced motor activity, become mute and apathetic, and lose control over urine and stool. Death often occurs from aspiration or infection.

COURSE AND PROGNOSIS

PDD is a progressive unremitting disease with a highly variable course. Prognosis is worse if the disease begins early in life. Average life span is approximately 6 to 8 years, with reports of some persons living 15 to 20 years (Heston and White, 1983). Unfortunately many of these years are personally and socially unproductive.

MULTI-INFARCT DEMENTIA

DESCRIPTION

Until recently almost all dementia was thought to be due to arteriosclerosis, e.g., senile brain disease. This misconception probably arose because many older persons have evidence of arteriosclerosis in other organs. Even when ath-

erosclerosis is present in cerebral vessels, it is the occurrence of multiple small infarcts, not cerebral ischemia, that causes deterioration in brain function. When infarcts have softened 50 to 100 mL of brain tissue, dementia becomes clinically apparent (Hachinski et al, 1974; Roth, 1978).

INCIDENCE

Approximately 15% of dementia is secondary to MID, with 25% mixed MID and PDD.

CLINICAL FEATURES

MID may not be distinguished from PDD unless the longitudinal course is known. Stepwise deterioration is a common feature in contrast to the smoothly progressive course of PDD. Each small infarct is followed by a partial recovery and plateau. Associated neurologic deficits also help to identify the natural progression. Although these specific features may be helpful, they are usually subtle and the clinical picture is one of progressive, global involvement showing the signs and symptoms discussed with PDD.

COURSE AND PROGNOSIS

MID is less predictable in its course than PDD. Functional plateaus may last for many months. Diagnosis and treatment of hypertension may retard its progress but not the basic disease process of multiple small infarcts. When associated with PDD, the course is generally more rapid.

HUNTINGTON'S DISEASE

An autosomal dominant pattern of inheritance, early cognitive disturbance (usually before age 45), and abnormal involuntary movements describe Huntington's disease. Fortunately it is an uncommon disease and represents less than 5% of dementias. It is untreatable and premature death is the rule.

PICK'S DISEASE

Pick's disease is a rare hereditary disease of the fifth and sixth decades affecting frontal lobe function before the occurrence of global deterioration. Frontal lobe symptoms include apathy, emotional lability, and social inappropriateness. This distinction is seldom appreciated clinically, and differentiation from the more common PDD is usually impossible. Post-mortem findings are distinctive, with the so-called Pick's bodies present but not the characteristic neurofibrillary tangles, senile plaques, or granulovacuolar degeneration of Alzheimer's disease.

CREUTZFELDT-JAKOB DISEASE

Creutzfeldt-Jakob disease is rare and rapidly fatal, with mental deterioration, sleep disturbance, weight loss, and neurologic symptoms. A slow virus is the suspected cause. Human-to-human transmission has been reported. No treatment is available.

SECONDARY DEMENTIAS

Secondary dementias have a specific organic basis that is often reversible. *Early diagnosis is essential.* Collectively they account for 15% to 20% of the dementias. It is their diagnosis and treatment that is the chief stimulus for a thorough work-up of dementia.

DEPRESSIVE PSEUDODEMENTIA

In 1961, Kiloh described findings of apparent cognitive loss in a group of psychiatric patients with multiple diagnoses. Because there was no evidence of progressive global loss of function the condition was called pseudodementia. More recently the term has been reserved to describe elderly depressed persons with dementia-like symptoms.

Approximately one third of all secondary dementias are related to depression. Table 16–7 lists the clinical features of pseudodementia and true dementia. Persons with depressive pseudodementia demonstrate a significant mood disorder, with better acquisition and recall of new information and minimal disorientation. They make feeble "don't know" attempts when questioned and can be irritable and uncooperative during a mental status examination. Persons with dementia more commonly demonstrate perseveration or confabulation in attempts to cover up their deficits. Even when the diagnostic evaluation has included neurologic examinations and appropriate laboratory studies have been done, up to 30% of persons thought to be demented were found on subsequent evaluations to be misclassified (Ron et al, 1979). It is obvious from these studies that longitudinal assessment may be the best diagnostic tool in some cases.

To further complicate the evaluation there are a significant number of persons with early dementia who are depressed. Depression is more unusual in the severely demented because the cognitive rationale underlying depression is complex and unavailable to their subconscious.

Diagnosis may be assisted by a trial of antidepressant medication (Plotkin and Small, 1984). A significant improvement in mood should occur in 60% to 70% of the depressed group and in 20% to 30% of the mixed depressed-demented individuals. Suspected pseudodementia is one situation in which a clinical drug trial may always be indicated. Even when early dementia is clearly evident, subtle depression may be missed. Improvement in depression will significantly improve function, allowing improved management of the residual dementia.

NORMAL PRESSURE HYDROCEPHALUS

The classic triad of dementia, gait disturbance, and urinary incontinence are diagnostic features of normal pressure hydrocephalus (NPH). Approximately one fourth of persons with a secondary dementia have NPH. No specific obstruction to cerebrospinal fluid circulation occurs; hence there is no elevation of pressure. One type of NPH follows injury to the brain with impaired absorption of cerebrospinal fluid from the surface of the brain. A second type appears to be idiopathic. A history of head injury or encephalitis favors the former and is an important distinction because treatment with a shunt has been more effective in the injury type than in the idiopathic type.

INTRACRANIAL MASS LESIONS

Tumors and subdural hematomas are potentially treatable conditions that may present early in their course as cognitive deficits with minimal neurologic disability. Mood changes with emotional lability or depression may further obscure the etiology. A history of head injury and more rapid progression with eventual appearance of focal neurologic deficits lead to neurologic evaluation and diagnosis. Early consideration of this diagnosis, particularly after subdural hematoma, can result in dramatic im-

TABLE 16–7 *Clinical Features of Pseudodementia and True Dementia*

	Pseudodementia	Dementia
Duration of symptoms before physician consulted	Short	Long
Onset can be dated with some precision	Usual	Unusual
Family aware of dysfunction and severity	Usual	Variable* (rare in early stages, usual in late stages)
Rapid progression of symptoms	Usual	Unusual
History of prior psychopathology	Usual	Unusual
Patient's complaints of cognitive loss	Emphasized	Variable* (minimized in late stages)
Patient's description of cognitive loss	Detailed	Vague
Patient's disability	Emphasized	Variable* (concealed in late stages)
Patient's valuation of accomplishments	Minimized	Variable*
Patient's efforts in attempting to perform tasks	Small	Great
Patient's efforts to cope with dysfunction	Minimal	Maximal
Patient's emotional reaction	Great distress	Variable* (unconcerned in late stages)
Patient's affect	Depressed	Labile, blunted, or depressed
Loss of social skills	Early	Late
Behavior congruent with severity of cognitive loss	Unusual	Usual
Attention and concentration	Often good	Often poor
"Don't know" answers	Usual	Unusual
"Near miss" answers	Unusual	Variable* (usual in late stages)
Memory loss for recent versus remote events	About equal	Greater
Specific memory gaps ("patchy memory loss")	Usual	Unusual
Performance on tasks of similar difficulty	Variable	Consistent

*Wells lists the characteristics of the later stages of dementia. These manifestations, however, can be variable early in the course of dementia and are helpful in the differential diagnosis only if they are in the direction seen in later stages of dementia.
From Small GW, Liston EH, Jarvik LF: Diagnosis and treatment of dementia in the aged. West J Med 1981; 135:469; with permission; and adapted from Wells CE: The differential diagnosis of psychiatric disorders in the elderly. In: Cole JO, Barrett JE, eds. Psychopathology in the aged. New York: Raven Press, 1980.

provement and restoration of cognitive and motor skills.

METABOLIC, NUTRITION, TOXIC DISORDERS, AND INFECTIONS

Many conditions and diseases are included in this broad category, as indicated in Table 16–1. Delirium may occur early, but with less clouding of consciousness. If the noxious agent is not removed or the metabolic or nutritional prob-

lem continues unaltered, a progressive, global loss in cognitive function follows. An example is the progressive memory loss seen clinically in Korsakoff's syndrome, a disease of thiamine depletion found in alcoholics. Early in the disease they may experience a delirium secondary to encephalopathy (Wernicke's encephalopathy).

Diagnosis The goal of *diagnostic evaluation* is not to make a diagnosis of dementia. In the majority of cases the diagnosis of cognitive im-

TABLE 16–8 *The Mental Status Questionnaire for Evaluation of Brain Dysfunction in the Aged*

Questions	Interpretation of Answer	
	Total Incorrect Answers*	Estimate of Degree of Brain Dysfunction
1. Where are you now? (name and kind of place)	0–2 incorrect	None or mild
2. Where is this place? (address)	3–8 incorrect	Moderate
3. What month is it?	9–10 incorrect	Severe
4. What year is it?		
5. What day of the month is it? (Correct if within 2 days)		
6. Hold are you? (age in years)		
7. What month were you born?		
8. What year were you born?/When were you born?		
9. Who is President of the United States?		
10. Who was President before him?		

Questions 3, 4, 5 bracketed together: What is the date?

*Includes unanswered questions.
Adapted from Liston EH. Delirium in the aged. Psychiatr Clin North Am 1982; 5:49; with permission.

pairment is obvious. The work-up must be thorough enough to define with reasonable certainty that a treatable (secondary) dementia is not present (Eisdorfer and Cohen, 1978; Raskin and Jarvik, 1979). This is important to emphasize because many early dementias are not being aggressively evaluated. Ageism and ignorance about dementia may be factors. The widespread promotion of Alzheimer's disease, although important, may be supporting a false impression that all dementia is Alzheimer's disease, and this disease is presently untreatable.

A careful history and physical examination including past history and old medical records may establish the onset and course of the illness. Diseases known to be associated with dementia may also be detected. A family history of dementia only weakly supports a diagnosis of primary dementia and should not be allowed to interrupt the evaluation. Careful evaluation of diet and the adequacy of living arrangements should be supplemented by home visits when feasible. Medication history and present medications may also need to be evaluated in the home. The tendency for elderly persons to use multiple medications, both prescription and over-the-counter agents, and to trade medications is well known. An alcohol history is important but is often minimized or avoided altogether. The physical examination should place special emphasis on detecting specific neurologic deficits.

The mental status examination (MSE) is used to determine the severity and course of the disease (Wells, 1978). The basic examination is used in both neurologic and psychiatric evaluations. It is not generally useful in determining the etiology of neurologic disease, but is the basis for diagnosis of psychiatric disorders. In this discussion the focus is on the cognitive aspects of the MSE. In Chapter 18 the behavioral and affective components are considered in more detail.

The MSE includes statements about the person's environment and personal appearance. The person's behavior and relationship to the examiner and the process of examination are recorded. Observation of speech production and pattern are noted. Thought content includes statements about delusions, hallucina-

TABLE 16–9   *Mini-mental State Examination*

Maximum Score	Score	
		Orientation
5	( )	What is the (year) (season) (date) (day) (month)?
5	( )	Where are we (state) (county) (town) (hospital) (floor)?
		Registration
3	( )	Name 3 objects: 1 second to say each. Then ask the patient all 3 after you have said them. Give 1 point for each correct answer. Then repeat them until he learns all 3. Count trials and record. (trials _____)
		Attention and Calculation
5	( )	Serial 7's (begin with 100 and count backwards by 7). 1 point for each correct answer. Stop after 5 answers. Alternatively spell "world" backwards.
		Recall
3	( )	Ask for the 3 objects repeated above. Give 1 point for each correct answer.
		Language
9	( )	Name a pencil, and watch (2 points)
		Repeat the following: "No ifs, ands, or buts." (1 point)
		Follow a 3-stage command: "Take a paper in your right hand, fold it in half, and put it on the floor." (3 points)
		Read and obey the following: Close your eyes (1 point)
		Write a sentence (1 point)
		Copy design (1 Point)
30	_____	Total score
		Assess level of consciousness along a continuum:

Alert	Drowsy	Stupor	Coma

From Folstein MF, Folstein SE, McHugh PR. "Mini-mental state": a practical method of grading the cognitive state of patients for the clinician. J Psychiatr Res 1975; 12:189; with permission.

tions, illusions, and suicide. Observations and statements about mood are recorded. Cognitive testing completes the MSE and focuses on the evaluation of functions previously discussed under normal aging, e.g., consciousness, attention, language, memory, constructional ability, and higher cognitive function. Two widely used tests are described. They are simple to memorize and use and they form a basis for neuropsychiatric referral when they are abnormal.

As previously discussed, it is important to observe for problems of consciousness and attention; deficits in either will prevent accurate testing of the other functions. Patience and flexibility are also important during the initial evaluation, beginning naturally with references to activities of daily living, such as what was eaten for breakfast, and if in the home names of persons in pictures on the tables and walls. Goldfarb and other workers have developed a simple 10-point test that is widely used as a rapid screening test of orientation and memory when evaluating both delirium and dementia

(Table 16–8). With modifications the test can be used both with inpatients and outpatients.

More specific tests of memory as well as constructional ability and cognitive function are contained in the Mini-Mental State examination developed by Folstein and coworkers (1975). Normal persons score 25 points and above. Persons with dementia usually score fewer than 20 points, with many scoring fewer than 10 points. Both tests are useful in initial evaluation and for following the course of dementia and response to intervention (Table 16–9).

Laboratory studies are listed in Table 16–10. Most are routine and included in standard screening profiles. When a specific diagnosis is suspected or an obvious medical condition exists, the laboratory work-up should reflect those problems.

Computed tomography is the single most useful diagnostic study (Heston and White, 1983; Eisenberg, 1978). It is safe and noninvasive. Some treatable dementias such as NPH, subdural hematoma, and tumors can be specifically diagnosed by this test. PDD (Alzheimer's type) can be strongly suspected if ventricular dilatation and diffuse cortical atrophy are found. A normal CT scan, however, does not exclude the diagnosis of dementia, and mild cortical atrophy may be seen in normal elderly persons.

TREATMENT OF DEMENTIAS

The primary dementias are defined as irreversible diseases without specific therapies. Although this continues to be true, intensive investigation is presently focused on halting or reversing known biochemical abnormalities. Goodnick and Gershon (1984) reviewed the chemotherapy of cognitive disorders.

Of more immediate importance is the need for education and support of patients and their families (Rabins et al, 1982). Because of the chronic nature of dementia, families and friends willing to join in giving care need continuous information and mutual support. See Chapters 18 and 19 for specific nursing care strategies. Medical therapy should support the maintenance of good general health, with special attention to detection and treatment of infections, skin breakdown, nutritional deficiencies, insomnia, and mood disorders (Maletta, 1990).

Insomnia can be managed with small doses

**Table 16–10   *Laboratory Work-up for Dementing Illnesses* **

ALL PATIENTS

Urinalysis

VDRL *and* FTA

Chemical survey (e.g., SMA-20)

CBC, erythrocyte sedimentation rate

Serum vitamin B_{12}, RBC, folate levels

Thyroid function tests (e.g., T_4, RT_3U, T_3, etc.)

Computed tomography

Electrocardiography, chest radiography

Pap smear, stool for occult blood

COMMON ADDITIONAL STUDIES *(As Indicated)*

Electroencephalogram

Lumbar puncture

Lumbar cisternogram (only for normal pressure hydrocephalus)

Psychological testing

Other laboratory tools that may be indicated are bone scan, mammography, ABGs, and arteriography.

---

*After completion of the history and physical examination. From O'Daniel R, Lippman S, Patel P. Depressive pseudodementia. Psychiatr Ann 1981; 11:357; with permission.

---

of short-acting benzodiazepines, e.g., flurazepam, 15 mg, or triazolam, 0.125 to 0.25 mg. These compounds do not accumulate with chronic use, although they may lose their effectiveness if used nightly for extended periods and, in addition, anterograde amnesia may occur.

Chronic anxiety, if functionally disabling, may respond to benzodiazepines with a longer half-life such as lorazepam, 0.25 to 0.50 mg twice a day. Nonbenzodiazepines, including antidepressants, neuroleptics, and antihistamines, have been used for anxiety with some success but have significant side effects. Buspirone in doses of 5 to 10 mg three times a day has the advantage of moderate effectiveness in chronic anxiety without the side effects of sedation or amnesia and no potential for abuse (Maletta, 1990).

Depression, particularly when recognized

early in the disease, can be successfully treated with standard therapies, using general criteria of selection and dosage for the elderly.

Confusion, agitation, paranoia, and perceptual problems respond to neuroleptic medication in relatively small doses, e.g., 0.5 to 2 mg of haloperidol per day (see Chapter 18). Trazodone, 25 to 50 mg twice a day, and buspirone, 5 to 10 mg three times a day, may also be effective.

The secondary dementias are treated by interrupting the disease or condition responsible for the cognitive deterioration. This may include specific treatment of an underlying disease, e.g., thyroid replacement for myxedema, antidepressants for pseudodementia, improvement of metabolic and nutritional disorders, and removing noxious agents, including medications. Unfortunately, full reversal of the cognitive dysfunction is unusual and supportive measures may be needed, as with the primary dementias.

References and Other Readings

American Psychiatric Association. Diagnostic and statistical manual of mental disorders—revised. Washington, DC: APA, 1987.

Arieff, Allen I, Armstrong D et al. Dementia, renal failure, and brain aluminum. Ann Intern Med 1979; 90:741.

Comfort A. The myth of senility. Postgrad Med 1979; 65:130.

Eisdorfer C, Cohen D. Cognitively impaired elderly: differential diagnosis. In: Storandt M, Siegler I, Elias M, eds. The clinical psychology of aging. New York: Plenum Publishing, 1978.

Eisenberg L. Computer tomography: a critical assessment. Drug Therapy—Hosp 1978; 3:21.

Folstein MF, Folstein SE, McHugh PR. Mini-mental state: a practical method of grading the cognitive state of patients for the clinician. J Psychiatr Res 1975; 12:189.

Goodnick P, Gershon S. Chemotherapy of cognitive disorders in geriatric subjects. J Clin Psychiatry 1984; 45:196.

Hachinski VC, Lassen NA, Marshall J. Multi-infarct dementia: a cause of mental deterioration in the elderly. Lancet 1974; 2:207.

Heston L, White J. Dementia: a practical guide to Alzheimer's disease and related illnesses. New York: WH Freeman, 1983.

Jenike MA. Alzheimer's disease: what the practicing physician needs to know. J Geriatr Psychiatr Neurol 1988; 1:37.

Jenike MA. Geriatric psychiatry and psychopharmacology. Chicago: Year-Book Medical Publisher, 1989.

Kiloh LG. Pseudo-dementia. Acta Psychiatr Scand 1961; 37:336.

Lawlor B. Seritonin and Alzheimer's disease. Psych Ann 1990; 20:567.

Lipowski ZJ. Transient cognitive disorders (delirium, acute confusional states) in the elderly. Am J Psychiatry 1983; 140:1426.

Liston EH. Delirium in the aged. Psychiatr Clin North Am 1982; 5:49.

Maletta G. Pharmacologic treatment and management of the aggressive demented patient. Psych Ann 1990; 20:446.

O'Daniel R, Lippman S, Patel P. Depressive pseudodementia. Psychiatr Ann 1981; 11:43.

Plotkin DA, Small GW. Pseudodementia: an approach to treatment. Drug Ther 1984; 14:52c.

Rabins PV, Mace NL, Lucas MJ. The impact of dementia on the family. JAMA 1982; 248:333.

Raskin A, Jarvik LF: Psychiatric symptoms and cognitive loss in the elderly: evaluation and assessment techniques. Washington, DC: Hemisphere Publishing Corp, 1979.

Reisberg B. Dementia: a systematic approach to identifying reversible causes. Geriatrics 1986; 41:30.

Ron MA, Toone BK, Garralda ME, Lishman WA. Diagnostic accuracy in presenile dementia. Br J Psychiatry 1979; 134:161.

Roth M. Epidemiological studies. In: Katzman R, Terry RD, Beck KL, eds. Alzheimer's disease: senile dementia and related disorders of aging, vol 7. New York: Raven Press, 1978.

Shalat S. Risk factors for Alzheimer's disease: fact or theory? Geriatric Medicine Today 1989; 8:26.

Thal LJ. Neurotransmitters and receptors in neurologic disease. Res and Staff Physician 1983; 29:43.

Wells, CE. Chronic brain disease: an overview. Am J Psychiatry 1978; 135:1.

Wilcock G. Update on Alzheimers's disease. Geriatric Medicine Today, 1989; 8:23.

17
Psychiatric Problems of the Elderly

ROBERT WILLS

Psychopathology represents a serious problem to the elderly. Approximately 15% to 20% of individuals aged 65 and over demonstrate functional psychiatric disorders (Jarvik, 1982). This translates into 4 or 5 million potential patients. If one adds persons with dementia, up to 25% of the elderly population may, at some time, be in need of neuropsychiatric evaluation and treatment. Unfortunately the elderly are underserved by psychiatry, representing only 3% to 5% of visits to psychiatrists' offices and community mental health clinics while accounting for 12% of the population (Gurland and Cross, 1982). Many who might benefit from care remain hidden in the community. Their problem may not be recognized; or they or their families resist evaluation. Many are victims of the same problems being actively publicized in the past few years. Physical and sexual abuse, inadequate parenting, divorce, poverty, alcoholism, and drug abuse have been active ingredients of mental illness for centuries.

Many elderly with obvious neuropsychiatric problems lie ill in hospitals and long-term care settings. As many as 65% of elderly persons with psychiatric disorders have significant medical disease. The psychiatric disorder is interpreted as an inevitable consequence of the primary medical disorder. ("I'd be depressed if I had chronic arthritis, wouldn't you?") Depression or other psychiatric disorders should never be considered just a normal response to other disease. If specific therapy is to be initiated, it is critical that the psychiatric symptoms are recognized as distinct from those of medical and surgical disorders. One of the objectives of this chapter is to better equip clinicians to make a presumptive diagnosis of psychiatric disease, even when associated with significant medical or surgical disease.

The following sections focus on commonly encountered psychiatric disorders. Diagnostic criteria from the recently revised *Diagnostic and Statistical Manual* (DSM-III-R), of the American Psychiatric Association is used as a framework for discussion where applicable. In psychiatry, unlike modern medicine and surgery, the clinical criteria provide the major evidence for diagnosis. This is analogous to the practice of medicine in Galen's time and provides a unique interpersonal diagnostic experience unencumbered by gadgets and blood tests. Although we discuss some attempts to bring the laboratory to the psychiatric couch, they have practical usefulness in only a small number of cases.

Major Depressive Disorder

DESCRIPTION

Depression is the most commonly encountered psychiatric disorder. Few escape its mood and if a depressed or dysthymic mood were its only symptom, most persons—young and old—

would lay claim to experiencing it on a frequent basis. In addition to mood, persons with a major depression must describe associated cognitive and physical dysfunction. This distinction is statistically as well as clinically important (Hendrie and Crossett, 1990). When the full triad of dysthymia, cognitive deficits, and physical complaints is present, approximately 5% to 10% of elderly persons will be diagnosed as having major depression. If only mood is considered, 15% to 20% will admit to sadness, feeling blue, or depression.

ETIOLOGY

Modern theories of depression have concentrated on disorders of neurochemical regulation of mood in specific brain structures known to be involved in this control, e.g., the limbic system. Derangement or reduction in neurotransmitters, including serotonin, dopamine, and epinephrine, would logically result in impaired neuronal conduction and clinically evident depression. This theory has been supported by the known actions of antidepressant medications. Their ability to improve depression seems linked to their ability to increase neurotransmitter levels by reducing their chemical degradation. They may also act to increase the sensitivity of postsynaptic neurotransmitter receptors. In what appears to be a paradox, levels of monoamine oxidase (MAO), an enzyme responsible for degradation of norepinephrine, are increased in the elderly (Lehman, 1982). This could result in less available neurotransmitter, leaving the elderly vulnerable to depression. Even though many questions remain to be explored, the biochemical basis of depression is firm.

What is less clear is the relation of life events to the genesis of depression. Former theories of depression focused on the life experiences of patients: how many losses had occurred, at what age, and with what meaning. Depression was felt to be the result of introjected ambivalent feelings about the lost object that were thought to contain hateful as well as loving aspects. When these feelings were unable to be openly expressed they were turned inward against the self, with resulting symptoms of depression.

In addition to specific losses, modern persons are afflicted with stresses coming from many sources. The pace of society, job tensions, family and personal problems, and continuous change create a potentially unstable environment. To form a consistent theory we would have to know whether and how loss and stress created the biochemical changes that initiate the clinical picture of depression. At present this information is not known. In fact, the association of life events and depression, even in younger persons, appears weak. Many persons develop depression with minimal loss or stress, whereas many others face remarkably intense stress without developing major depression.

The situation at older age may be different. A general reduction in physical ability coupled with specific deficits in neurotransmitter levels may in some way reduce the threshold for depression when the individual is faced with recurrent and serious adverse life events (Wilkie et al, 1982). Retirement, inadequate income, loss of friends, and loneliness may progressively deplete "psychic energy," resulting in depression. Chronic illness, chronic psychiatric disorders, alcohol and drug addiction, and previous episodes of depression may also lower the depression threshold.

The past 100 years have produced many theories of depression that have led naturally to various psychotherapies. Because of the recent biochemical emphasis, most psychotherapy is now combined with medication.

CLINICAL FEATURES

Table 17–1 outlines the clinical diagnostic criteria for major depressive disorder. As noted in the introduction, depressed mood is not in itself an adequate symptom on which to base the diagnosis. To further complicate matters, the mood may not even be the dominant symptom. In some Far Eastern cultures there is no specific term to describe the mood, and depression is diagnosed from cognitive and physical symptoms as manifested by withdrawal, loss of work, and somatic preoccupation. Many elderly persons have an analogous resistance to naming their problem "depression." Past experience and cultural bias suggest that depression is weakness and admission of this weakness is a humiliating experience. Confrontation with statements like, "You seem depressed," often is countered with strong denial and retreat from the diagnostic encounter. In this situation it is more fruitful to move to a discussion of daily living activities, hopefully to focus on the cognitive and physical symptoms of depression.

TABLE 17–1   *Diagnostic Criteria for Major Depressive Disorder*

1. At least five of the following symptoms, have been present during the same 2-week period and represent a change from previous functioning; at least one of the symptoms is either (1) depressed mood, or (2) loss of interest or pleasure. (Do not include symptoms that are clearly due to a physical condition, mood-incongruent delusions or hallucinations, incoherence, or marked loosening of associations)
   a. depressed mood (or can be irritable mood in children and adolescents) most of the day, nearly every day, as indicated either by subjective account or observation by others
   b. markedly diminished interest or pleasure in all, or almost all, activities most of the day, nearly every day (as indicated either by subjective account or observation by others of apathy most of the time)
   c. significant weight loss or weight gain when not dieting (e.g., more than 5% of body weight in a month), or decrease or increase in appetite nearly every day (in children, consider failure to make expected weight gains)
   d. insomnia or hypersomnia nearly every day
   e. psychomotor agitation or retardation nearly every day (observable by others, not merely subjective feelings of restlessness or being slowed down)
   f. fatigue or loss of energy nearly every day
   g. feelings of worthlessness or excessive or inappropriate guilt (which may be delusional) nearly every day (not merely self-reproach or guilt about being sick)
   h. diminished ability to think or concentrate, or indecisiveness, nearly every day (either by subjective account or as observed by others)
   i. recurrent thoughts of death (not just fear of dying), recurrent suicidal ideation without a specific plan, or a suicide attempt or a specific plan for committing suicide

2. a. It cannot be established that an organic factor initiated and maintained the disturbance
   b. The disturbance is not a normal reaction to the death of a loved one (uncomplicated bereavement)

   Note: Morbid preoccupation with worthlessness, suicidal ideation, marked functional impairment or psychomotor retardation, or prolonged duration suggest bereavement complicated by major depression

3. At no time during the disturbance have there been delusions or hallucinations for as long as 2 weeks in the absence of prominent mood symptoms (i.e., before the mood symptoms developed or after they have remitted)

4. Not superimposed on schizophrenia, schizophreniform disorder, delusional disorder, or psychotic disorder NOS

From Diagnostic and Statistical Manual of Mental Disorders (DSM-III-R), Third Edition, Revised. Washington, DC: American Psychiatric Association, 1987, pp. 222–223; with permission.

Sleep and appetite are easily identified areas of concern. Whereas younger persons often experience increased hours of sleep and overeating, the elderly person experiencing an initial depression commonly describes severe problems in getting to sleep or early morning awakening. Occasionally these symptoms progress to nights of almost total insomnia. The emergence of confusion and frank psychosis may be as much secondary to sleep deprivation as to the depression and the picture is one of a cyclic worsening of the person's physical and emotional status. Poor appetite with significant weight loss is a common presenting complaint and may lead to a sidetracking of medical workup for occult disease. When no organic diagnosis is made, weeks or months of fruitless dietary advice and manipulation may follow. The depression is overlooked because the depressed mood is interpreted to be secondary to anorexia, nausea, or lower bowel complaints. The gastrointestinal tract is the organ most often included in the somatic ruminations of elderly depressed persons. Of the two thirds presenting with somatic complaints, 50% are focused on the stomach and bowel, with the remainder divided between neurologic and cardiovascular problems. Because many elderly depressed persons also have medical disease, it is not uncommon to encounter confusion around mind–body issues.

Agitation is common and may be manifested

by increased rate and volume of speech, irritability, obsessive rumination or perseveration, and increased motor activities, e.g., pacing, gesturing, and so on. Agitation seems to be naturally associated with insomnia and poor appetite. Other persons are slowed down and retarded in speech and movement. Marked latency is characterized by long pauses between apparent thought and action. Questions may appear to go unanswered unless sufficient time is allowed for answering. The simplest tasks may take hours to accomplish. Health care providers who are used to aggressive action do not do well with either agitated or retarded persons because neither seem able to effectively manage their problems. Monitoring one's countertransference (how the clinician reacts to the client) can be diagnostically helpful. Many elderly persons who irritate us with their poor response to our efforts may be depressed, not just noncompliant.

Anhedonia, or the loss of pleasure, in hobbies, reading, travel, and so forth, is common and may be of major concern to family and friends because of the progressive isolation. The person becomes "homebound" and unable to show interest in, or initiate action toward, previously enjoyed activities. Spouses, family members, and friends become upset and angry because their own goals and interests are frustrated. Depressed persons not only isolate themselves, but are rejected by others because of their obstinate spirit.

Although *guilt* is experienced by many elderly depressed persons, statements suggesting low self-esteem may be more common, e.g., "I don't feel guilty. I'm just not able to change anything in my life." Limited social and financial resources, health problems, and personality disorders contribute to feelings of low self-esteem and a distorted view of the future. If guilt is prominent, it tends to lock the person into the past. Present events are interpreted in relation to perceived past mistakes and any thought of the future is filled with hopeless despair.

Cognitive deficits are apparent to the elderly depressed person (see the section Depressive Pseudodementia in Chapter 16). Problems of *concentration and recent memory* are most often noted, but unlike true dementia, past and immediate memory also seem impaired. The person appears bored or irritable and is quick to reply "I don't know" to test questions directed at memory. This behavior contrasts with the denial and confabulation that characterize dementia.

Suicidal ideation must always be taken seriously particularly in the elderly, white, widowed man with a chronic incapacitating disease or cancer. The incidence of suicide is highest in this group, being seven times more frequent than in women of the same age. Alcoholism and isolation are also more frequent in this high-risk group. All depressed persons should be specifically questioned about suicide intent. Previously stated concerns about discussing suicide, e.g., "If we talk about it, they may start considering suicide," have no basis in fact. Suicide results from a distorted view of life in which all sense of control has been lost. Discussion can provide an opportunity to reorganize a concept of reality within a framework of empathetic support.

When paranoid delusions and hallucinations are present, there may be initial confusion with schizophrenia or paraphrenia. *Perceptual distortions* associated with depression are mood-congruent, that is, of the same emotional tone as the depression itself. For example, statements like, "God is punishing me for my past sin," or "I know my husband is going to divorce me because I failed as a wife" are common. Depressed persons do not describe the bizarre distortions common in psychotic disorders.

CLINICAL COURSE

The onset of depression may be insidious. Elderly persons, particularly those living alone, may experience progressive functional loss and, believing they have a physical illness, take to bed. Friends and relatives may become alarmed when the person begins to miss usually enjoyed activities or stops eating. Avoidance behavior, isolation, and confusion give a false impression of early dementia, further delaying evaluation and treatment. As with many diseases, the full clinical course is seldom observed. Interruption with medication or electroconvulsant therapy leads to significant improvement in the majority of cases, shortening the course and reducing suffering. In approximately 10% to 15% of cases all therapeutic efforts may fail. Physical debility, withdrawal from society, institutionalization, and premature death occur. Suicide, as previously discussed, terminates the illness in a tragically high number of cases.

DIAGNOSIS

Table 17–1 described both the clinical and diagnostic features of major depression. When the depressed mood is prominent and other symptoms are aggressively pursued, the diagnosis is usually not difficult. When the person is a poor historian or has a medical illness, the distinctive diagnostic features may be blurred. A careful history and complete physical examination are an essential part of any diagnosis of depression. Mental status examinations and rating scales (Yesavage et al, 1983) are sometimes used (Zung, 1965).

To help with this dilemma, recent efforts have been made to find biologic markers specific for depression. One of these, nonsuppressible elevations of cortisol, has lead to the use of the standard dexamethasone suppression test (DST) (Gold et al, 1981; Roy et al, 1984). This test uses an 11 PM dose of dexamethasone 1 mg and 8 AM and 4 PM blood levels of cortisol. The normal biologic response to high-potency synthetic steroid is to shut down the pituitary and lower the blood level of naturally produced cortisol. The elevated cortisol of depressed patients cannot be suppressed. The initial impression was that the DST test was specific (90%) for major depression, but was insensitive, missing approximately 50% of the obvious cases. More recently the specificity has been questioned, with high levels of nonsuppressive cortisol found in elderly persons with dementia (Roy et al, 1984). This finding squelched the initial enthusiastic statements that the DST is useful in differentiating between depression, pseudodementia, and dementia. Depressed persons also show reduced thyroid-stimulating hormone (TSH) response to thyrotropin-releasing hormone (TRH) (Gold et al, 1981; Roy et al, 1984). When the DST and TRH are combined, the diagnostic confidence is high for confirming the diagnosis of major depression. No doubt, future research will provide additional biologic tests that will be both sensitive and specific (Roy et al, 1984).

DIFFERENTIAL DIAGNOSIS

Depressed mood may occur as a reaction to many adverse events. The elderly experience multiple losses including retirement, the death of friends, chronic illness, and inadequate finances. If the depressed mood is not associated with cognitive or physical complaints, the diagnosis should be Adjustment Disorder with depressed mood.

This diagnosis describes

1. A maladaptive reaction to an identifiable psychological stressor, occurring within 3 months of the onset of the stressor
2. The maladaptive nature of the reaction is indicated by impairment in social or job functions and/or symptoms that are in excess of a normal and expected reaction to the stressor
3. The assumption that the disturbance will eventually remit after the stressor ceases
4. The symptoms as not being those of another diagnosis

Adjustment Disorder does not include the diagnosis Uncomplicated Bereavement, which is not considered a psychiatric disorder. Prolonged bereavement with progressive appearance of cognitive and physical symptoms should always suggest the insidious onset of Major Depressive Disorder with its attendant need for aggressive therapy.

Persons should be carefully questioned about prescription and over-the-counter medications since their side effects may include severe lowering of the mood as well as cognitive and physical symptoms indistinguishable from those of depression (Table 17–2). A careful review of systems may reveal subtle evidence of disease capable of causing depression, as listed in Table 17–3.

TREATMENT

Since the 1930s depression has been effectively treated with electroconvulsive therapy (ECT). Although strong opinions have been expressed against ECT, it remains a useful therapy particularly in the medically ill elderly person who is suicidal. The major arguments against ECT have dealt with physical injury and memory loss (Frith et al, 1983). The dangers of musculoskeletal injury and aspiration have been minimized by intubation, brief general anesthesia, and muscle relaxation. Unilateral application of electrodes has reduced the transient memory deficits noted after ECT. Even when therapy is bilateral, memory is regained within 6 months. Past impressions of severe memory loss were, at least in part, due to unrecognized premorbid dementia. Relief of the depressive symptoms with ECT allowed the memory deficits to be-

TABLE 17–2   *Drugs Frequently Associated with Depressive Reactions as Adverse Effects*

Class Name	Generic Name	Trade Name
Antihypertensives	Reserpine	Serpasil, Sandril
	Methyldopa	Aldomet
	Propranolol hydrochloride	Inderal
	Guanethidine sulfate	Ismelin sulfate
	Hydralazine hydrochloride	Apresoline
	Clonidine hydrochloride	Catapres
Antiparkinsonian agents	Levodopa	Dopar, Larodopa
	Levodopa, carbidopa	Sinemet
	Amantadine hydrochloride	Symmetrel
Hormones	Estrogen	Evex, Menest, Premarin
	Progesterone	Lipo-Lutin, Provera
Corticosteroids	Cortisone acetate	Cortone acetate
Antituberculosis	Cycloserine	Seromycin
Antineoplastic	Vincristine sulfate	Oncovin
	Vinblastine sulfate	Velban

Adapted from Klerman G, Hirschfeld R. Treatment of depression in the elderly. Geriatrics 1979; 34:51; with permission.

come manifest. As with any therapy, the risk-to-benefit ratio must be considered. In patients over age 75 confusion, falls, and cardiorespiratory complications occur with increasing frequency and are related to a higher incidence of medical disease and number of medications (Burke et al, 1987). In recent years ECT has been most often reserved for those who fail a course of antidepressant medication.

The major medications include tricyclics and tetracyclics, MAO inhibitors, and recently developed nontricyclics. Table 17–4 describes common side effects of the presently available drugs. Most of these drugs are prescribed to be taken in a single dose. This is a significant help in ensuring compliance. Special care must be taken when choosing the initial dose. Elderly persons with diminished liver function may need one third to one half the usual adult dose. An associated problem is determining how high to push the dose. The end point is usually taken as the appearance of side effects. Until the recent development of safer drugs, there was a narrow margin of safety between the therapeutic and toxic doses. Table 17–5 describes symptoms that suggest a need to reduce dosage. The anticholinergic effects are usually the earliest to appear and include reduced salivation, constipation, urinary retention, and toxic delirium (Hall et al, 1981). The elderly seem more susceptible to these effects because of a general reduction in autonomic tone.

Cardiac side effects are minimal when tricyclic antidepressants are used carefully with frequent evaluations (Davidson and Wenger, 1982). Severe arrhythmias and death occur with overdose, particularly with the older drugs such as amitriptyline. Newer drugs such as fluoxetine, bupropion, and trazodone appear less cardiotoxic even after significant overdose ingestion (Branconnier and Cole, 1981; Kulig et al, 1982; Gerner et al, 1980). In addition, fluoxetine and bupropion cause minimal sedation and orthostatic hypotension, which are significant side effects of the tricyclic antidepressants.

Alprazolam, a benzodiazepine, has been used effectively in treating depression with associated marked anxiety (Feighner, 1983; Feighner et al, 1983). It is unique in the respect

TABLE 17-3   *Medical Causes of Depression*

Deficiency States
  Pellagra
  Pernicious anemia
  Wernicke's encephalopathy

Drugs and Medication
  Alcohol
  Amphetamines
  Antihypertensive agents
    Clonidine
    Diuretics—hypokalemia*
      or hyponatremia*
    Guanethidine
    Methyldopa
    Propranolol
    Reserpine
  Birth control pills
  Cimetidine
  Digitalis
  Disulfiram
  Sedatives
    Barbiturates
    Benzodiazepines
  Steroids/ACTH

Endocrine Disorders
  Acromegaly
  Adrenal
    Addison's disease*
    Cushing's disease
  Hyper- and hypoparathyroidism*
  Hyper- and hypothyroidism
  Insulinoma
  Pheochromocytoma
  Pituitary

Infections
  Encephalitis
  Fungal
  Meningitis
  Neurosyphilis
  Tuberculosis

Malignant Disease
  Metastases
    Breast
    GI
    Lung
    Pancreas
    Prostate
  Remote effect: pancreas

Metabolic Disorders
  Electrolyte imbalance
    Hypokalemia
    Hyponatremia
  Hepatic encephalopathy
  Hypo-oxygenation
    Cerebral arteriosclerosis
    Chronic bronchitis
    Congestive heart failure*
    Emphysema
    Myocardial infarction*
    Paroxysmal dysrhythmias
    Pneumonia*
    Severe anemia*
  Uremia*

Neurologic Disorders
  Alzheimer's disease
  Amyotrophic lateral sclerosis
  Creutzfeldt-Jakob disease
  Huntington's chorea
  Multiple sclerosis
  Myasthenia gravis
  Normal-pressure hydrocephalus
  Parkinson's disease
  Pick's disease
  Wilson's disease

Trauma
  Postconcussion

*Acute life-threatening disorders.
From Jenike MA. Depressed in the E.R. Emerg Med 1984; 16:102; with permission.

that other benzodiazepines reduce anxiety but have little effect on depression. Doses of 0.5 to 1 mg four times a day are effective. Alprazolam must be given in divided doses because of its intermediate half-life of approximately 12 to 14 hours. The divided dose may complicate treatment by requiring a higher level of compliance.

MAO inhibitors are effective in the elderly and have the advantage of low anticholinergic side effects and cardiotoxicity (Gerner, 1984). Dietary restriction of foods containing tyramine must accompany the use of these drugs. Tyramine is a building block in the metabolic pathway of norepinephrine. MAO normally metabolizes norepinephrine. Inhibiting MAO allows a sudden buildup of catecholamines and the potential for a hypertensive crisis if tyra-

TABLE 17–4 *Relative Side Effects Profile of Common Antidepressant Medications**

Generic Name	Reference Trade Name	Side Effects†					Antidepressant Potency Relative to Amitriptyline
		Sedation	Orthostatic Hypotension	Anti-cholinergic	Cardiac Conduction Toxicity	Miscella-neous‡	
TRICYCLICS							
Tertiary							
Amitriptyline	Elavil	+++	+++	+++	++		1:1
Imipramine	Tofranil	++	+++	++	++		1:1
Trimipramine	Surmontil	+++	++	++	++		1:1
Clomipramine	Anafranil	+++	++	+++	+		1:1
Doxepin	Sinequan	+++	+++	++	++		1:1
Secondary							
Nortriptyline	Pamelor	+	+	+	+		2:1
Protriptyline	Vivactyl	0	++	+++	+	1	5:1
Desipramine	Norpramin	+	+	+	+		1:1
NONTRICYCLICS							
Amoxapine	Asendin	+	++	+	+	2,3	1:1
Maprotiline	Ludiomil	+	++	+	++	2	1:1
Trazodone	Desyrel	+++	+	0	0/++	4,5	$\frac{1}{2}$:1
Fluoxetine	Prozac	0	0	0	0	1,4,6	—
Bupropion	Wellbutrin	0	0	+	0	1,2,4,6	—
MONOAMINE OXIDASE INHIBITORS							
Isocarboxazid	Marplan	+	++	++	0		—
Phenelzine	Nardil	+	+++	+	0		—
Tranyl-cypromine	Parnate	0	+	0	0		—

*Symbols: 0, virtually absent; +, relatively mild; ++, relatively moderate; +++, prominent.
†Relative side effect and potency values according to Peterson. HW Psychoactive Medication Pocket Guide 1989. San Francisco: Langley Porter Psychiatric Institute, 1989.
‡Miscellaneous notes: 1, excitation; 2, greater seizure threshold lowering effect relative to other antidepressants; 3, extrapyramidal syndromes; 4, not lethal with overdose; 5, priapism as rare effect in men; 6, nausea.
From Martin R: Geriatric psychopharmacology: present and future. Psych Ann 1990; 20:686; with permission.

mine is ingested. Restricted foods when taking MAO inhibitors include the following:

Old cheese
Beer
Chocolate
Red wines
Pickled herring

Compliance may be difficult because the list contains several "favorite foods." Nevertheless many elderly persons are quite capable of strict adherence to these dietary restrictions, greatly benefiting from the MAO inhibitors (Small and Jarvik, 1982). Frequently there is a need to try different drugs to get maximal therapeutic benefit, and each drug should be used long enough to give it an adequate trial.

Psychotherapy includes cognitive, behavioral, supportive, and analytical approaches (Cohen, 1984). The choice of therapy and its ul-

TABLE 17–5   *A Summary of Tricyclic and Tetracyclic Antidepressant Adverse Effects* *

ANTICHOLINERGIC

Blurred vision (common; narrow-angle glaucoma may worsen)

Dry mouth (common)

Constipation (common)

Urinary retention (occasional)

Increased or decreased sweating (infrequent)

Sinus tachycardia (common)

Speech blockage, mental clouding (occasional); confusion, delirium (rare)

CARDIOVASCULAR

Postural hypotension, dizziness (occasional)

Hypertension (rare)

Sinus tachycardia (common, anticholinergic effect)

Premature atrial or ventricular beats (infrequent)

Antiarrhythmic effect, myocardial depression (additive with antiarrhythmic drugs)

Pedal edema (occasional; may worsen congestive heart failure)

ECG (ST-segment depression, T wave flattened or inverted, QRS prolongation)

NEUROLOGIC

Central anticholinergic effects as above (varies considerably with different drugs)

Drowsiness (varies considerably with different drugs)

Muscle tremors, twitches, jitteriness (occasional)

Extrapyramidal symptoms (rare)

Paresthesias, fatigue, weakness, ataxia (infrequent)

Seizures (with overdose or in patient with known seizure disorder)

Hallucinations, delusions, activation of schizophrenic or manic psychosis

GASTROINTESTINAL

Constipation (common, anticholinergic effect)

Nausea, vomiting, heartburn (infrequent)

ALLERGIC

Rash (rare; but somewhat more frequent with maprotiline [Ludiomil])

*Adverse effects may decrease or disappear with use of lower dosage or divided dosage regimen, or by changing to a different antidepressant.
From Bernstein J. New pharmacologic approaches to depression. Drug Ther—Hosp 1981; 6:66; with permission.

timate success depend on the training and interpersonal orientation of the therapist. Psychotherapy of major depression is usually combined with medication. The latter therapy provides an important adjunct by improving concentration, lessening fatigue and anhedonia, and improving sleep and appetite. This improvement may be crucial in allowing a patient to get on with the process of psychotherapy.

Schizophrenia and Paraphrenia

DESCRIPTION

Schizophrenia is a disorder that includes the following:

* Severe perceptual distortions including bizarre delusions and auditory and visual hallucinations

* Inappropriate speech and behavior
* Deterioration in social, school, or job functions
* Duration of at least 6 months

Elderly schizophrenics can resemble those with dementia. Many of these persons, previously in state institutions, are in need of continuous, intensive community support. Unfortunately they are also victims of crime and neglect, and in some cities, a tragically underserved or forgotten group.

Elderly persons with late onset psychotic symptoms are diagnosed as paraphrenic (Raskind et al, 1979). Although not included in DSM-III-R, paraphrenia enjoys popularity with geriatric mental health workers and is widely understood to describe a syndrome of mixed paranoid delusions, auditory and/or visual hallucinations, and bizarre thinking. Orientation and memory remain intact. The onset is usually rapid, with no premorbid medical or psychiatric disorder consistently identified. Some persons demonstrate brief confusion, and fear and agitation are common.

PREVALENCE

The prevalence of schizophrenia is approximately 1% of the entire population. Because of the diagnostic confusion related to the diagnosis of psychotic disorders in the elderly, no data on prevalence exist for this population.

ETIOLOGY

The etiology of schizophrenia and paraphrenia is unknown. Onset may appear to follow periods of intense stress, but, as in depression, this may be fortuitous. Many consider schizophrenia to have a genetic basis, with specific neurochemical alterations. This relationship is less apparent in paraphrenia.

TREATMENT

Neither disorder completely responds to current therapies. The treatment is usually directed at the functional incapacity. Initial therapy may involve immediate hospitalization if social support is absent or inadequate. Hospitalization in a psychiatric setting provides stability and safety while a long-term therapeutic plan is formulated. It also provides a monitored environment for the initiation of drug therapy. If the person has adequate social support it is possible to offer treatment on an ambulatory care basis.

Unless there is a specific contraindication, therapy usually includes medication with an antipsychotic drug. These are classified as neuroleptic medications. Dosage is so variable that few dependable guidelines can be offered. Most elderly persons are begun on relatively low doses, such as haloperidol 1 to 5 mg daily. Long-acting intramuscular preparations such as fluphenazine decanoate given in dosages of 6.25 to 25 mg (0.25 to 1 mL) every 3 to 6 weeks may significantly help with patient compliance (Raskind et al, 1979). This may be critical in those who show marked paranoia. Success in these individuals may be more dependent on early engagement maneuvers designed to lessen suspiciousness. Patience and gentleness, with a nonpressuring attitude may, in time, break through this resistance.

Although neuroleptic drugs are usually well tolerated, care must be taken in monitoring the sedative and hypotensive effects to prevent falls. Parkinson-like symptoms are occasionally seen and usually controlled with antiparkinson drugs such as Cogentin (benztropine mesylate) 1 to 2 mg daily. Tardive dyskinesia, a troublesome and often irreversible movement disorder, is not uncommon, particularly in elderly women. Intermittent withdrawal or reduced dosage may allow the treatment to continue.

Paranoid Disorders

DESCRIPTION

Psychiatrists recognize paranoia as both a symptom of several disorders and as a specific disorder. Paranoia related to paraphrenia and schizophrenia, depression, and personality disorders are discussed with the primary disorder. Table 17–6 describes the DSM-III-R criteria for Paranoid Disorder. This is a disabling disease, whether experienced in youth or advanced age. Both age groups use projection as the primary defense mechanism. Projection is an unconscious defense mechanism in which a person attributes to others the ideas, thoughts, feelings, and impulses that are part of his inner perceptions, but that are unacceptable to him. By externalizing whatever is unacceptable, the person deals with it as a situation apart from himself. Delusions are often focused on elaborate plots that the individual feels have been hatched to his disadvantage. Because the thoughts and feelings are unacceptable it is not surprising that they include subjects or material that society finds difficult to handle, e.g., sexual, religious, and criminal activities. Ideas of reference, i.e., the idea that personal messages are being received through the radio or TV, are common. Those whose delusions are threatening to them appear anxious or frightened. Others seem curious or even detached as if the delusion were usual or expected. Some delusions are experienced as comforting (e.g., the return of an old lover), and produce a mood of anticipation. Regardless of the content of the delusion and the associated mood, there is minimal disorientation, confusion, and loosening of associations. This is in contrast to schizophrenia or paraphrenia. In fact, unless the delusion is confessed during an interview, patients

TABLE 17–6 *Diagnostic Criteria for Paranoid Disorder*

PARANOID DISORDER

1. Nonbizarre delusion(s) (i.e., involving situations that occur in real life, such as being followed, poisoned, infected, loved at a distance, having a disease, being deceived by one's spouse or lover) of at least 1 month's duration

2. Auditory or visual hallucinations, if present, are not prominent

3. Apart from the delusion(s) or its ramifications, behavior is not obviously odd or bizarre

4. If a major depressive or manic syndrome has been present during the delusional disturbance, the total duration of all episodes of the mood syndrome has been brief relative to the total duration of the delusional disturbance

5. Has never met criterion for schizophrenia, and it cannot be established than an organic factor initiated and maintained the disturbance

Specify type: The following types are based on the predominant delusional theme. If no single delusional theme predominates, specify as **unspecified type**

EROTOMANIC TYPE

Delusional Disorder in which the predominant theme of the delusion(s) is that a person, usually of higher status, is in love with the subject

GRANDIOSE TYPE

Delusional Disorder in which the predominant theme of the delusion(s) is one of inflated worth, power, knowledge, identity, or special relationship to a deity or famous person

JEALOUS TYPE

Delusional Disorder in which the predominant theme of the delusion(s) is that one's sexual partner is unfaithful

PERSECUTORY TYPE

Delusional Disorder in which the predominant theme of the delusion(s) is that one (or someone to whom one is close) is being malevolently treated in some way. People with this type of delusional disorder may repeatedly take their complaints of being mistreated to legal authorities

SOMATIC TYPE

Delusional Disorder in which the predominant theme of the delusion(s) is that the person has some physical defect, disorder, or disease

UNSPECIFIED TYPE

Delusional Disorder that does not fit any of the previous categories, e.g., persecutory and grandiose themes without a predominance of either; delusions of reference without malevolent content

From Diagnostic and Statistical Manual of Mental Disorders (DSM-III-R), Third Edition, Revised. Washington, DC: American Psychiatric Association, 1987, pp. 202–203; with permission.

may present as socially appropriate, or at worst, somewhat eccentric. Women are paranoid more often than men. *There is also a strong association of paranoia with hearing loss.* It is logical that if information is distorted or only partially communicated, the hard of hearing will feel left out and misinformed. Suspiciousness becomes paranoia as suspected slights, insults, or plots become projected against the speakers. Blind persons do not demonstrate this phenomenon because often the problem seems to be one of communication.

TREATMENT

Treatment of Paranoid Disorder with neuroleptic medication has not been very successful. As previously discussed, the paranoid person thoroughly believes the delusion, seeing little need to take a drug to treat it. There is minimal confusion or loosening of associations, two symptoms that respond most dramatically to these medications. Psychotherapy has limited usefulness for the same reason. For talk therapy to be helpful the person must see a need to change.

Maintaining social contact is assisted by explaining the nature of paranoia to the person's family and friends, or to residents in the nursing home or the senior housing complex. Family and friends invariably feel rejected and others may be frightened of the behavior. Typical examples of situations that family members face include the spouse accused of adultery and grown children suffering verbal abuse because of a suspicion that they are altering the patient's will or stealing his property. Relief from guilt and a renewed desire to participate in a care plan often follow explanation of the problem as a disease and not a relational issue.

Paranoia is occasionally an early symptom of dementia. Because dementia interferes with the ability to formulate and retain information necessary to function in a complex society, it is not surprising that persons experiencing early cognitive loss begin to see the world as a threatening place. Unlike paranoid schizophrenia, paraphrenia, and paranoid disorder, the paranoia of early cognitive loss is more responsive to treatment. These individuals seem less convinced of the reality of their delusions and, when provided with a safe structured environment, are more willing to put them aside. In addition, low-dose medication, such as haloperidol, 0.5 to 2 mg, may be very effective. As the dementia progresses, paranoia becomes less a problem. The ability to formulate complex delusions is lost with cortical atrophy. Medication needs thus may lessen.

Personality Styles and Disorders

However personality may be defined, it forms the interface in all human transaction. Although the developmental aspects of personality are beyond the framework of the present discussion, it is clear that an individual's own style of interaction is present since early age. The ingredients of each personality style are a mix of positive and negative attributes. Whereas some styles rise to conquer adversity, many do not. Negative attributes may dominate a person's response to stress. Medical illness, personal losses, financial setbacks, isolation, and restriction of opportunity may cause maladaptive responses. Neuropsychiatric disorders by themselves or in addition to these stressors may lead to impaired coping strategies and the emergence of self-defeating patterns of behavior. A common example is the increased word production of some elderly who are attempting to cover up early memory loss. Friends and relatives are "driven crazy" by this defensive behavior and the very outcome the elderly are attempting to avoid eventually occurs—they are isolated and ignored.

OBSESSIVE-COMPULSIVE STYLE

Persons with obsessive-compulsive styles are common in Western culture. In fact, the modern caricature of a scientist, university professor, or computer type is the obsessive-compulsive personality. Although obsessive-compulsive behavior can be useful in helping to organize a very complex world, it is often experienced by others as inflexible. The obsessive-compulsive person is also intolerant of others' plans and purposes. This trait may be so strong as to have a moral flavor of rightness. This is the "I should" or "I need to" drive toward an imagined but always unattainable perfection. The initial impression of this quality is of great personal control. With continued observation, however, it is clear that the drive actually is in control of the person. The inflexibility, the moral imperatives, the pressure toward perfection, and the sense of being driven to accomplish are qualities that poorly serve the aging person. At a time when there is a greater need for the social skills of tolerance, flexibility, and personal warmth, the obsessive-compulsive individual manifests rigid stereotypic concepts and actions. These are persons who are imprisoned by minutiae while missing the real freedom of thoughts and actions. A common example is seen in the elderly person's preoccupation with maintaining a large bank account while claiming that he has insufficient funds to take a brief trip. The moral obligation to have money "for a rainy day" and the driving experience of maintaining the money, often counted down to the last penny, can prevent experiencing with any satisfaction the spending of money. Some of these people may become collectors, accumulating a house full of papers and junk that they seem incapable of discarding. Needed health care, clothing, and food may be sacrificed.

Paranoid thinking may occur and reach psychotic proportions, i.e., the obsessive person's preoccupation with the minute details of life may become the paranoid's search for the hidden clue spelling disaster. The defense mechanism of projection sees others as dangerous and attacking. Effective intervention is prevented and they may, e.g., not only refuse to spend money for necessary things, but will ask, "Why are you interested in helping me anyway?" If mild dementia is added to this scenario, what emerges is a situation where needed help is vigorously and repeatedly refused.

DEPENDENT STYLES

Dependent personality styles seek comfort and acceptance from others, but paradoxically they are fearful of developing genuinely warm and close relationships with others. This process involves significant problems of self-esteem. A typical example is the person who is always baking cookies for the group, but is never available to go on social outings. Closeness, which demands maturity and trust, is experienced as an unaccepted threat. The need for closeness is denied and defended against by the person's nonavailability. The ego may be salvaged by a statement such as, "You know how important it is that I finish knitting this sweater for my granddaughter." There is a precarious balance of needs with utilization of energy to maintain the defensive rationalizations.

As persons age, they become less able to shore up their defenses. The dependent person becomes actually more in need of others and less able to distance himself by rationalization or activity. Loneliness and isolation may lead to depression and anxiety as needs go unmet. These dependent elderly may resist attempts at making them independent and, at the same time, seem ambivalent about group-living experiences. Offering a private room with opportunities to be with others in a day room setting or cafeteria may fill the needs of wanting to be near others while maintaining a safe distance to avoid the anxiety generated by the closeness it-

self. The elderly person who quietly accepts the presence of others without direct participation may be demonstrating this paradoxical behavior without rationalization. This behavior should not be interpreted as the isolation of depression.

Dependent individuals often seem to reject advice from caregivers because their real need for affirmation "Do you love me?" is confused with their excuse for attention, the medical complaint (Groves, 1978). Care must be taken to provide the necessary interpersonal structure to meet both their physical and emotional needs while preventing caregiver burnout.

PERSONALITY DISORDERS

When compared with personality styles, personality disorders are more maladaptive or socially harmful. Persons with personality disorders are spared anxiety by a more rigid defense of the ego. Most are not seen in office psychiatry or mental health clinics. They are either oblivious to the adverse effect of their personalities on others' lives or have accepted their disorder as unchangeable.

ANTISOCIAL PERSONALITY DISORDER

Although mainly a problem of young and middle-aged men, Antisocial Disorder continues into old age. Over 80% of prison inmates carry this diagnosis. As the elderly increase in the general population, they will also increase in the country's prisons. However, as with other felons, they will spend most of their lives in the community. They are chronic users and abusers of the social welfare and health care systems, working hard for all they can get through guile and intimidation. In addition, there are many persons with antisocial disorder who are slick enough to spend little if any time in prison. Even though they may cause suffering in others, these people seldom feel compelled to seek treatment. When they do, it may be because they are facing divorce proceedings, driving while intoxicated citations (DWIs), or business problems.

Antisocial behavior begins in the early teen years with delinquent behavior and extends into mid-life manifesting itself by poor work effort, irresponsible parenting, legal problems, poor interpersonal relationships, impulsivity, and disregard for truth. Although successful in their early years even criminals experience ageism and may not be highly regarded by their colleagues. Many are disabled from chronic drug and alcohol abuse.

Treatment efforts are characteristically unsuccessful, with therapists soon caught up in the patient's antisocial behavior. These individuals generally only feel discomfort when they are discovered and threatened with punishment. Guilt is not experienced and desire to change is not sincerely in evidence. Structure, sometimes prison, is the only treatment available and is usually applied in defense of society's better interests.

Education and support for the family may be helpful in allowing them to disengage from the more destructive elements of the relationship. Setting limits and boundaries should lead to more helpful and less painful family interactions.

PARANOID PERSONALITY DISORDER

Persons with this disorder are identified by their tonic state of hypervigilance. They are intense, serious individuals who are always on the lookout for the "hidden clue." They are mistrustful and suspicious, searching every word and action for evidence that others are taking advantage of them. Unlike the Paranoid Disorder, they do not describe well-defined and intricately constructed delusions. They tend to be "loners," driving others from their company by their defensive projection. As with the other disorders that show symptoms of paranoia, therapeutic engagement is very difficult. These persons resist social activities and frustrate efforts to improve their "support systems." Giving them assistance in obtaining basic needs and supporting their attempts to deal with government and social agencies may be all the therapy that is practical or necessary. Their autonomy and privacy must be respected at all times. Medication is not helpful unless symptoms of psychosis or depression appear. When medications are prescribed, they are seldom taken.

Alcohol Abuse and Dependence

Few other disorders of the elderly so immediately invoke emotions associated with ageism and therapeutic nihilism as alcohol abuse and dependence. Several factors combine to severely limit treatment and community interest in providing effective programs for treatment of alcoholism. These include the following:

Confusion about the definition and etiology of alcoholism

Family and society ambivalence about limiting the "few enjoyments remaining in old age"

Broadly held views that this disorder is untreatable

An example is found in the author's own community where one of the nation's highest incidence of alcoholism is combined with a rare involuntary commitment to detoxification programs. In addition to the high number of identified alcoholics, we have personal observations from residents of retirement communities describing week-long "happy hours." Unless the recent trend among younger persons to reduce alcohol consumption continues, we can expect to see the alcohol problem in the older population worsen.

DESCRIPTION

The American Psychiatric Association's current definitions of alcohol abuse and dependence combine common behaviors associated with pathologic use and anticipated functional impairment (Table 17–7) (American Psychiatric Association, 1987). The more chronic state of dependence includes the physiologic changes leading to tolerance and withdrawal. These diagnostic classifications wisely avoid etiologic factors. Although included in a discussion of psychiatric problems of the elderly, several other disciplines are concerned with alcoholism, including the social sciences, medicine, and genetics (Miller and Chappel, 1991; Dinwiddie and Cloninger, 1991). Over one third of alcoholics have a positive family history. In addition, our society powerfully indoctrinates children and young persons about the beneficial effects of alcohol.

Elderly alcoholics often have associated problems, including poor health, loneliness, associated psychiatric problems, and continuous losses. Although the majority of elderly alcoholics have problems before age 60, approximately one third develop serious problems late in life, perhaps related to these stresses. The prevalence of alcoholism in the elderly is not accurately known. Reported incidence ranges from 2% to 10%, depending on the group studied.

TABLE 17–7 Diagnostic Criteria for Alcohol Dependence and Abuse

ALCOHOL DEPENDENCE

1. At least three of the following:
   a. Alcohol often taken in larger amounts or over a longer period than the person intended
   b. Persistent desire or one or more unsuccessful efforts to cut down or control alcohol use
   c. A great deal of time spent in activities necessary to get alcohol, use alcohol, or recover from its effects
   d. Frequent intoxication or withdrawal symptoms when expected to fulfill major role obligations at work, school, or home
   e. Important social, occupational, or recreational activities given up or reduced because of alcohol use
   f. Continued alcohol use despite knowledge of having a persistent or recurrent social, psychological, or physical problem that is caused or exacerbated by the use of alcohol
   g. Marked tolerance: need for markedly increased amounts of alcohol in order to achieve intoxication or desired effect with continued use of the same amount
   h. Characteristic withdrawal symptoms
   i. Alcohol often taken to relieve or avoid withdrawal symptoms
2. Some symptoms of the disturbance have persisted for at least 1 month, or have occurred repeatedly over a longer period of time

ALCOHOL ABUSE

1. A maladaptive pattern of alcohol abuse indicated by at least one of the following:
   a. Continued use despite knowledge of having a persistent or recurrent social, occupational, psychological, or physical problem that is caused or exacerbated by use of alcohol
   b. Recurrent use in situations in which use is physically hazardous
2. Some symptoms of the disturbance have persisted for at least 1 month, or have occurred repeatedly over a longer period of time
3. Never met the criteria for alcohol dependence

CLINICAL FEATURES

The typical signs and symptoms of alcoholism are well described in standard medical and nursing texts and are qualitatively similar in both young and old. The nature of the aging process itself creates special problems. Impairment in alcohol kinetics and increased vulnerability of organ systems prolongs the effect of alcohol and creates greater morbidity. The toxic effects of alcohol on the older brain causes symptoms and behaviors that are often diagnosed as depression, anxiety, or dementia. Attempts to treat these conditions with psychotropic drugs further depress brain function, delay diagnosis, and prolong recovery, causing increased morbidity from confusion, unsteadiness, and falls.

Dementia, with severe recent memory loss, may be a direct result of alcohol and may rapidly become irreversible. Alcohol can also worsen existing dysfunctional personality disorders, causing further isolation and alienation from family and friends. Denial is a major defense mechanism used by both patient and family. It is often combined with the justification, "Why deny me (them) a few of life's pleasures?" This denial and justification forms the rationalization that evades diagnosis and fuels the continued drinking. Alcohol's toxic effects on specific organs such as the liver, coupled with the patient's refusal to admit to excessive consumption leads to fruitless work-ups and misdiagnosis.

DIAGNOSIS

Diagnostic criteria are presented in Table 17–7. Unlike most other diagnostic situations, the major obstacle faced is not the correctness of the diagnosis, but the remarkable resistance shown by patient and family to data collection. Screening instruments, such as the CAGE questionnaire and the Michigan Alcohol Screening Test, must complement the diagnostic criteria and offer the interviewer a helpful, open-ended approach. The CAGE questions are

Have you ever felt that you should cut down on your drinking?

Have people annoyed you by criticizing your drinking?

Have you ever felt bad or guilty about your drinking?

Have you ever had a drink first thing in the morning to steady your nerves or get rid of a hangover (eye-opener)?

Two or more positive responses are associated with a sensitivity and a specificity of over 80% (Mayfield et al, 1974).

In nonalcohol-related medical and surgical conditions, alcohol abuse or dependency should be suspected when the patient shows inadequate or unexpected responses to therapy and noncompliance with medications and follow-up. Rapidly changing brain function suggesting delirium or early dementia may also suggest the diagnosis.

Because alcoholics always live in a dysfunctional family system, family members may show enabling or codependent behaviors. Home visits can be especially helpful in revealing direct evidence of alcohol use and in evaluating the family or social system supporting the behavior.

When the diagnosis is suspected, great care must be taken to initially avoid getting into arguments with the patient or the family. We may believe that the evidence is airtight, but the office or hospital is not a court of law, and patients and family are ready with defenses perfected over the years. Accusations and premature confrontation stiffens denial and justifies changing caregivers in the patient's mind. Initial engagement strategies must focus on acceptance of the patient as a person who may have an alcohol problem. In the patient presenting with a medical complication, an explanation that the cause seems "related to a toxin" may get both patient and family to focus on the possibility of alcohol playing a role, without blaming the patient for "causing" his or her disorder. The author uses the simple axiom, "If it's a problem, it's a problem." The approach avoids arguing definitions of alcoholism and so forth. A brief trial of abstinence may be accepted as reasonable and will allow all parties to evaluate the effect on target organ function. Demonstrating an improvement in central nervous system function to a skeptical family, with the potential of reduced care needs may help align them with the caregivers. Equally as important, it will demonstrate how difficult it is to stop the abuse, even briefly.

TREATMENT

Research and practical experience have consistently demonstrated the superiority of self-help programs patterned after the 12-step program of Alcoholics Anonymous. Inpatient abstinence programs using several treatment approaches have seen increasing use when community-based programs have failed. Patients more likely to need inpatient treatment have a history of long heavy use, previous treatment failures, associated medical problems, and brain dysfunction. Long-term success depends on continued participation in outpatient programs. In addition, problems of loneliness and isolation must be addressed. Depression and anxiety may have to be aggressively treated if they do not resolve with abstinence, otherwise alcohol will be resumed to self-treat the uncomfortable mood.

Family and friends must be involved in education and support groups to modify their denial patterns. In many cases, particularly the home-bound elder, they are the main suppliers of alcohol. Even if the patient will not cooperate with treatment, shutting off the supply will cause a significant improvement. Unfortunately, this can be very threatening to the family or friends, who may fear rejection.

Nihilism must be confronted with the reality that many older alcoholics can be helped. This is seen most often in the "late-onset" group, but may also occur in the longtime abuser.

References and Other Readings

American Psychiatric Association. Diagnostic and statistical manual of mental disorders—revised. Washington, DC: APA, 1987.

Bernstein J. New pharmacologic approaches to depression. Drug Therapy—Hosp 1981; 6:66.

Branconnier R, Cole J. Effects of acute administration of trazodone and amitriptyline on cognition, cardiovascular function, and salivation in the normal geriatric subject. J Clin Psychopharmacol 1981; 1(6 suppl):82S.

Burke W, et al. The safety of ECT in geriatric psychiatry. J Am Geriatr Soc 1987; 35:516.

Cohen GD. Psychotherapy of the elderly. Psychosomatics 1984; 24:455.

Davidson J, Wenger T. Using antidepressants in patients with cardiovascular disease. Drug Therapy—Hosp 1982; 7:89.

Dinwiddie SH, Cloninger CR. Family and adoption studies in alcoholism and drug addiction. Psych Ann 1991; 21:206.

Feighner JP. Open label study of alprazolam in severely depressed inpatients. J Clin Psychiatry 1983; 44:332.

Feighner JP, et al. Comparison of alprazolam, imipramine, and placebo in the treatment of depression. JAMA 1983; 249:3057.

Frith CD, et al. Effects of ECT and depression on

various aspects of memory. Br J Psychiatry 1983; 138:142.

Gerner RH. Antidepressant selection in the elderly. Psychosomatics 1984; 25:528.

Gerner RH, et al. Treatment of geriatric depression with trazodone, imipramine and placebo: a double-blind study. J Clin Psychiatry 1980; 41:216.

Gold MS, et al. Diagnosis of depression in the 1980s. JAMA 1981; 245:1562.

Griest J, Griest T. Antidepressant treatment. Baltimore: Williams & Wilkins, 1979.

Groves J. Taking care of the hateful patient. N Engl J Med 1978; 298:883.

Gurland BJ, Cross PS. Epidemiology of psychopathology in old age: some implications for clinical services. Psychiatr Clin North Am 1982; 5:11.

Hall RC, Feinsilver DL, Holt RE. Anticholinergic differential diagnosis and management. Psychosomatics 1981; 22:581.

Hendrie H, Crossett J. An overview of depression in the elderly. Psych Ann 1990; 20:64.

Jarvik LF. Aging and psychiatry. Psychiatr Clin North Am 1982; 5:5.

Jenike MA. Geriatric psychiatry and psychopharmacology. St. Louis: Year-Book Medical Publishers, 1989.

Klerman G, Hirschfeld R. Treatment of depression in the elderly. Geriatrics 1979; 34:51.

Kulig K, et al. Amoxapine overdose. JAMA 1982; 248:1092.

Lehman HE. Affective disorders in the aged. Psychiatr Clin North Am 1982; 5:27.

Martin R. Geriatric psychopharmacology: present and future. Psych Ann 1990; 20:682.

Mayfield D, McLeod G, Hall P. The CAGE questionnaire: validation of a new alcoholism screening instrument. Am J Psychiatry 1974; 131:1121.

Merck manual of geriatrics. Merck, Sharp & Dohme Research Laboratories, 1990.

Miller NS, Chapple JN. History of the disease concept. Psych Ann 1991; 21:196.

Raskind M, Alvarez C, Herlin S. Fluphenazine enanthate in the outpatient treatment of late paraphrenia. J Am Geriatr Soc 1979; 27:459.

Roy A, Pickar D, Paul S. Biologic tests in depression. Psychosomatics 1984; 25:443.

Small GW, Jarvik L. Depression in the aged, a commentary. Psychiatr Clin North Am 1982; 5:45.

Wilkie F, Eisdorfer C, Staub J. Stress and psychopathology in the aged. Psychiatr Clin North Am 1982; 5:131.

Yesavage JA, Brink TL, Rose TL et al. Development and validation of a depression screening scale: A preliminary report. J Psych Res 1983; 17:37.

Zung WWK. A self-rating depression scale. Arch Gen Psych 1965; 12:63.

18
Daily Living with Alzheimer's Disease

LYNDA CRANDALL

Nursing Management of Alzheimer's Disease

Alzheimer's disease (AD) is a type of dementia. The term *dementia* means "deprived of the mind." A diagnosis of AD means a progressive deterioration in memory, intellect, and personality. In functional terms, AD is the global impairment of higher cortical functions, including memory, the capacity to solve the problems of day-to-day living, the performance of learned perceptual and motor skills, the correct use of social skills, and control of emotional reactions in the absence of gross clouding of consciousness (U'ren, 1984). In emotional terms AD is a devastating illness for the patients and for their relatives. There is no available cure at this time. AD progressively destroys a lifetime of learning and skills, affecting the person in a manner more dramatic than any other chronic disorder. In fact, of all the chronic disorders, none is feared more than the loss of cognition and with it the essence of personhood.

Despite the neural devastation and the incurable nature of AD there is still much that can be done to make life better for the patient and the family. Incurability does not mean untreatability. Unfortunately, there continues to be an attitude of fatalism and pessimism toward the treatment and care of those persons. One can rarely afford to be pessimistic. With the current advances in biomedical research

and the individuality of each case, it is appropriate to be optimistic and positive, while realistically providing nursing assessment and process at all stages. Nurses have a tradition of maintaining the quality of life for persons for whom cure and treatment are not available (Buckwalter, 1986). Within this tradition day-to-day function can be improved at whatever stage of the disease the victim is found to be. Nursing comprehensively assists afflicted individuals to live safely, comfortably, and fully. Comprehensive care, however, reaches further than maintenance of health and safety. It calls for attention to helping relatives and caregivers to cope with the emotional and behavioral problems that often accompany this illness. One of the greatest challenges nurses face is that of capturing and preserving each victim's uniqueness since AD causes the loss of that which makes the victim unique. Nurses work toward blending the past and present to preserve the unique self. AD patients are helped by the fundamental nursing philosophy of caring about and skillfully caring for these individuals and their families. The outcome can be very rewarding.

PROGRESSION OF ALZHEIMER'S DISEASE

The course of deterioration has been outlined in phases or stages in which symptoms and behaviors are grouped for the purpose of roughly

296

Stages or Phases of Dementia of the Alzheimer's Type

Phase I   Prediagnosis (forgetful, early confusional)
        Forgetful of names, events, phone numbers
        Lost in familiar surroundings
        Difficulty telling time
        Difficulty making decisions
        Lack of spontaneity
        Easily angered, irritable
        Aware of losses
        May express concern

Phase II   During and after diagnosis (late confusional, early dementia)
        Word-finding problems
        Reverts to earlier language
        Difficulty following story line
        Abstract thought impaired, planning, problem solving
        Forgets routine tasks, hygiene
        Loses items and claims stolen
        Complains of neglect
        Distractible, decreased attention span
        Refuses help with activities of daily living
        Decreased ability to handle finances
        Overt anxiety
        Uses denial to cope
        Restless, impatient
        Social skills may remain

Phase III Early to middle dementia
        Gait changes, small steps, halting
        Increased rigidity
        Intolerance to cold
        Bowel and bladder incontinence
        Decreased ability to read, do math (dysgraphia, dyscalculi)
        Decreased ability to understand and express language (aphasia)
        Decreased ability in purposeful movement (apraxia)
        Decreased ability to recognize objects (agnosia)
        Perseveration
        Wandering
        Hyperorality
        Immodesty
        Swallowing problems
        Actively resists help with activities of daily living
        Affect flat
        Paranoia
        Agitation
        Hallucinations and delusions
        Violent behavior

(Continued)

Stages of Phases of Dementia of the Alzheimer's Type *(Continued)*

Phase IV   Late dementia
                  Seizures
                  Myoclonic jerking
                  Severe loss of body weight
                  Slowed movements
                  Automaticisms, lip smacking
                  Indifference to food
                  Little response to stimuli
                  Loss of verbal abilities
                  Use of agitation to communicate

gauging where the person is in the progression (see boxes on pp. 297 and 298). This information is helpful in planning care, setting goals and expectations, and relating the current level of capacity observed in an individual with the symptom groupings. Tracking the person's changes can be useful in determining the rate of deterioration over time as well as evaluating unexpected developments in physical health or behavior.

While the course of AD is progressive, the stages or phases of deterioration can be used

Reisberg Scale

STAGE	LEVEL OF FUNCTIONING
1	No decrement
2	Subjective deficit in word finding
3	Deficits in demanding employment settings
4	Assistance required in complex tasks
5	Assistance required in choosing proper clothing
6a	Assistance required in putting on clothing
6b	Assistance required in bathing properly
6c	Assistance required with the mechanics of toileting
6d	Urinary incontinence
6e	Fecal incontinence
7a	Speech ability limited to approximately a half dozen intelligible words
7b	Intelligible vocabulary limited to a single word
7c	Ambulatory ability lost
7d	Ability to sit up lost
7e	Ability to smile lost
7f	Consciousness lost

From Reisberg B, Ferris SH, Franssen E. An ordinal functional assessment tool for Alzheimer's type dementia. Hosp Community Psychiatry 1985; 36:593; with permission.

only as guideposts of function and capacity to assist in caregiving and anticipation of the next stage. The clinical presentation of any one phase rarely includes only the features listed within that phase. Rather, symptoms and behaviors often overlap phases. New deficits or behaviors should always be assessed for other potential causes before concluding that they are part of a deteriorating course. Many factors can contribute to loss of functional capacity or behavioral changes, such as physical health of the patient, the patient's reduced capacity to cope or problem solve, and changes in the environment. Reciprocally maintenance or improvement of functional performance can also be multifactorial. When deficits are noted, the nurse must focus attention toward identifying the potential underlying cause or causes of the new behavior, symptom, or deficit. For example, referring to the Reisberg scale, the loss of ambulation in a person currently assessed to be at stage 5 would indicate a need for additional assessment and work-up of that loss as a development separate from the AD process. Likewise, the onset of urinary incontinence in a person currently determined by other clinical indicators to be at stage 4 cannot be assumed to be a further deterioration before adequate evaluation has ruled out other potential causes.

The progressive global deterioration of someone with this illness is accompanied by an ever changing functional capacity of the afflicted individual. Not only does function progressively decline, it also can fluctuate so that performance and ability may be uneven and unpredictable from one day to the next. The person who yesterday could independently put his shirt on, but today cannot, may be viewed as "uncooperative" or "resistive." The person may in fact have truly forgotten the skill or the steps necessary to accomplish that task. The loss may be temporary or permanent. Often such a presentation is interpreted by the caregiver as willful behavior and may engender frustration or anger. Likewise there may be days when the afflicted person experiences "windows" of insight or clarity in which memory and cognitive and emotional functions seem improved. This too can be confusing to caregivers because it complicates performance expectations. As abilities and capacities vary from day to day, expectations of caregivers must likewise be fluid. It is best to assume the individual is working at maximum capacity at all times.

TREATMENT

The idea of treatment for persons with AD is relatively new. For a long time there were no known formal interventions or therapies to treat or manage this disease. Reality orientation was introduced in the late 1950s at the Veteran's Administration Hospital in Topeka, Kansas as the first method to treat memory loss and confusion. Caregivers attempted to stimulate and reorient the confused person by repeatedly verbally orienting him to time and place and putting him in a situation where he met and competed with others. The goal was to force him out of his isolation and back into his environment. Gradually it became apparent that reality orientation was most helpful for mildly confused persons, but could actually increase the distress and restlessness in the moderately or severely confused persons. In recent years there has been growing interest and research in environmental manipulation, communication, behavioral programming, management of behavior problems, caregiver support, etc., revealing that knowledge, understanding, and skillful intervention can produce positive results (see box on p. 300). Nurses must join with members of other disciplines in order to develop integrated services toward the goal of continuity of care throughout the changing clinical course. The ultimate goal is that the victim's function be maximized while maintaining quality of life of both the patient and his family (Buckwalter, 1986). Education and attitude preparation directed toward caregivers, both professional and lay, can serve to minimize the risk that inappropriate or incomplete care and treatment will occur. Education should focus on understanding the disease process, the stages and deficits commonly observed in the person, as well as skill building in communication, approach, space, and environment, strategies in routine establishment, and activities of daily living simplification. Even the expert and practiced caregiver would do well to review basic principles from time to time.

COMMUNICATION

After the survival needs, the need to communicate is one of the most important in the hierarchy of human needs. Self-esteem is largely based on meaningful communication on a verbal and nonverbal level (Wolanin, 1981). Making ourselves and our needs known and under-

---

Shells

By Phyllis S. Yingling

One day while walking on the beach, I found a fragment of what must have been a magnificent conch shell . . . a remnant of a masterpiece, an exquisite shard. I tried to imagine the part as the whole when it was at its best, before it was broken by the churning sea . . . and Time. The shell must have been an elegant ectoskeleton, a prime example of its species. Now, all that remained was a chunk of pink and white shell, its scalloped edge chipped and scratched. Its complex shape, intricate design, and brilliant colors had vanished as the crashing surf took its toll. I thought of my mother, a victim of Alzheimer's disease for the past five years. At 78, wheelchair bound, unable to walk or speak coherently, she resides in the nursing wing of a retirement home. In recent years she has become an exquisite shard of the magnificent person she once was, before she was broken by degenerative disease . . . and Time. She is the remnant of a masterpiece.

Those of us who knew and loved her in her prime still see her as the loving mother, warm-hearted wife, and fun-loving sister she used to be. We know her as the gifted teacher, the outstanding church and community leader, the confidante and friend, the lover of laughter and music, the wearer of beautiful hats that she was for most of her years. We love her all the more for the change in herself that she has had to endure.

Those of you who know her now see only the shell of a once-vital person, a lovely fragment of a magnificent individual. As caregivers for the elderly, it must be difficult to imagine the people you work with as the young people they once were. As you feed them, walk with them, change their clothes, endure angry outbursts, bathe them, and tuck them in at night, please know that families and friends . . . and the individuals themselves . . . are grateful when you show respect and kindness, and handle them as gently as a once-exquisite shell.

Phyllis Yingling resides in Baltimore. From J Gerontol Nurs 1985; 2:44; with permission.

---

standing messages given to us are fundamental to satisfactory interpersonal interaction. Since both the receptive and expressive dimensions of communication are impaired in persons with AD, the focus of intervention should be on full use of current capacity. The caregiver can preserve capacity and enhance the person's ability to send and to interpret messages.

The concept of agenda behavior introduced by Radar et al (1985) has great value in communicating with the chronically confused person. Agenda behavior has its roots in the basic premise that all behavior has meaning. With AD, communication is expressed through behavior to a larger extent than it is through the spoken word. Hence the patient's agenda must be understood. In the context of the confused person's world, behaviors may or may not be related to current reality. Additionally, the patient's agenda (i.e., behavior, emotion, or need) often are in conflict with the caregiver's agenda or needs, which adds stress to both the caregiver and the patient. Recognition of the patient's reality and acceptance of it are the first steps to closing the gap. The next step is developing a sense of sympathy and using appropriate communication skills. The fundamental principles of these communications skills are (1) acknowledging and accepting the agenda nonjudgmentally and (2) allowing the patient to follow or play out his or her agenda. This can be facilitated through both nonverbal and verbal interaction.

There is no question that effective communication is the key to quality care. There are several principles to be drawn from communicating with older persons that are particularly cogent when interacting with an AD patient.

1. Treat them with the same respect you would treat anyone
2. Allow independence and equal participation in interaction. Do not attempt to "protect" them by answering or choosing for them
3. Assess for sensory deficits and make appropriate adjustments (e.g., vision and hearing impairments)
4. Maintain the flexibility to alter your approach and planned intervention if indicated after assessing a situation
5. Maintain slow, gentle movement around the patient with AD. Walk unhurriedly and calmly with slow body movements, including hand and arm gestures, as these persons are sensitive to affect and movement and are at high risk for misinterpretation or may mirror fast-paced movement or harsh tones, resulting in overstimulation and anxiousness
6. Be reminded that *how* we say *what* we say can "make or break" the communication
7. Ensure that verbal and nonverbal messages are congruent
8. Situate yourself at eye level with the individual you are communicating with or lower than they are

See box on pp. 302–303 for specific communication guidelines.

ENVIRONMENT

Physical, emotional, and social surroundings can enhance or further confuse the daily function and coping capacity of all of us, but environment plays a particularly relevant role for persons with dementia. The Alzheimer patient is keenly sensitive and reactive to the climate around him. As capacities decline the stationary physical surroundings and more fluid psychosocial surroundings take on a greater role in splinting or supporting maintenance of comfort and function. Environments designed and adapted to the special needs of these persons will serve to not only maintain but also to heighten function. Likewise environments that are not designed to the particular needs of the person will minimize functional capacity. The environment can be manipulated to the level of the person with AD rather than requiring him to adapt to the environment.

PHYSICAL ENVIRONMENT

There are a number of important concepts to be included in the planning of the physical environment housing a person with AD. *Consistency* and *simplicity* are fundamental principles. Additional considerations are

- Furniture arrangements should remain unchanged
- A large face clock and calendar should be within easy view
- Bright primary colors are easily seen
- Toilet seats painted bright yellow can increase security and identification
- Reflective tape around the doorway to the bathroom may increase visability at night
- Walkways and halls should be clutter free and easily negotiable
- Colored pathways on the floor made with paint or cloth tape may assist the wanderer to find his way or serve as a diversion for a wanderer or pacer
- Signs identifying rooms such as the bedroom or bathroom can be helpful. The lettering should be bold print block letters. White letters on a black background are easily read
- When the written word is no longer understood, simple pictures may be useful room identifiers (e.g., of a bed, toilet, refrigerator)
- Pictures that are individualized to special interests of the person, e.g., flowers, dogs, cats, even a sheet of colored construction paper placed on bedroom doors, may assist the person to recognize his or her room more easily
- Decor should be simple. Busy wallpaper designs, detailed paintings, and numerous wallhangings or other decorations should be avoided
- In institutional settings efforts should be made to simulate a home-like environment to the extent possible, including furniture, dishes, photos, paintings, afghans, and pillows
- Attention should be given to appropriate lighting; bright lighting should be provided for activities that require it and subdued lighting can be used to create a calming atmosphere. Night lights can increase orientation and a sense of control at night
- Maintain floor waxes without glare to decrease the risk of falls or agitation related to

(*continued on p. 304*)

Guidelines for Communicating with Confused Persons

DELIVERING A MESSAGE

Approach	Use slow gentle movements
	Arms at side, hands open. Respect the person's need or preference for personal space
	Get at eye level to him
Getting the person's attention	Say the person's name. Use his formal name or the name he prefers. Avoid calling him "honey" or "dear" unless given permission by him to do so
	Establish eye contact using soft eyes. Be aware that on rare occasions direct eye contact can be threatening
	It can be helpful to touch his shoulder or arm to draw attention to you. Use discretion when touching
Delivering the message	Use short words, simple sentences. It may be necessary to use nouns and verbs only
	Use a friendly, calm tone of voice. Speak slowly, softly, and clearly
	Use concrete, direct wording. Abstract or hypothetical examples or explanations are easily misunderstood
	Use positive terms, "do" rather than "do not," e.g., "Please put your hands in your lap" rather than "Please stop pounding on the table"
	Use "please" and "thank you" where appropriate
	Make only one step requests at a time
	Allow time for him to process the request and respond to it before assuming he cannot or will not
	If he does not respond, repeat the question, comment, or request verbatim, i.e., do not try to rephrase
	To maintain his attention throughout the interaction it is helpful to say his name repeatedly and reestablish eye contact
	When there is more than one caregiver only one should deliver the verbal direction and under no circumstances should the caregivers carry on a conversation excluding the patient
	If he walks away as you are speaking pay attention to this nonverbal message and reapproach later. Avoid stopping him or trying to get in front of him. Sometimes walking along side and slightly ahead of him while delivering your message is effective

RECEIVING A MESSAGE

There are only two fundamental parts to receiving a communication. The first is to listen to what is said and the second is to respond to what is said. In the case of the patient with AD enhanced listening is required and projection as to the meaning behind the words is necessary as messages are often not the literal meaning of the words.

Guidelines for Communicating with Confused Persons *(Continued)*

Active Listening

Use all senses and watch the person closely while listening and feeling the environment and tone around him

Maintain eye contact and demonstrate an interest in his message. Lean toward him and nod as you listen. Be aware that lack of eye contact is a message and that the eyes alone can relate a great deal about thoughts and feelings

Every request should be attended to. Ignoring a request will ferment frustration and anger. Focus on the words he says as well as possible emotions or feeling behind the words, e.g., the woman saying she needs to go home to cook dinner for her children, may be expressing her need to feel useful or needed; the person who insists his daughter will be coming to pick him up, may be feeling lonely

Responding

Use the skills mentioned under getting attention and delivering messages

When the verbal message is unclear, try to pick out and repeat key words or phrases in an effort to trigger the patient's memory or ability to supplement or clarify the message. Using his vocabulary adds to his sense of effectiveness, letting him know he has been heard and encouraging him to continue talking

Restate his message as you understand it and ask if your interpretation is accurate, e.g., "Do you need to go to the bathroom?" "Do you want to call your daughter?"

Never say you understand if you do not. It is better to say honestly that you are trying to understand but have not understood yet

Try responding to the feeling you may have identified while listening to his message, e.g., "Did you cook dinner every night for the children? That is a big responsibility. What foods were favorites in your family?" "Tell me about your daughter"

More specifically, try overtly identifying out loud the emotion you think he may be feeling, e.g., "You seem sad. Are you?" or "It sounds like you are angry. Is that what you are feeling?"

If after repeated attempts the message meaning still cannot be uncovered and the patient is becoming anxious, it can sometimes be helpful to make a general statement such as "I'll take care of it" or "I'll work on it for you." This type of response frequently results in a sigh of relief from the patient. However, do not make promises or commitments you cannot or have no intention of following through with overstimulation or reduced visual acuity produced by the glare

- Attempt to create a sense of control for the patient with AD by avoiding rooms or spaces that are very large and empty as well as spaces that are small and cluttered with furnishings or people

SOCIAL AND EMOTIONAL ENVIRONMENT

Components particularly essential to the ideal social and emotional environment are flexibility and adaptability on the part of the caregiver. Nurses are in a position to assist in establishing and maintaining a relaxed climate, as well as to assess when shifts in approach and behavior are required. Similarly, the nurse maintains surveillance over the behavior of others and assesses the impact on the patient and then teaches the skills necessary to establish the model milieu as well as how to alter it when indicated.

Of all physical and psychological caregiving skills, there is none that yields greater influence than that of a positive, optimistic attitude and outlook on the part of the nurse and other caregivers. Optimism is a skill to be learned and nutured for growth. In its most dynamic state optimism can be felt as an aura around the nurse, creating a "can do" atmosphere for the patient with AD, the relatives, and the nurse herself. It increases the strength necessary to live with and effectively manage this illness and can make the differences between excellent and satisfactory care. The following additional considerations may positively influence the psychosocial environment.

Maintain the same caregivers whenever possible
Maintain a routine and schedule
When deviations or changes are necessary, the person should be informed of this and reminded of the change as needed
Activities should be paced slowly and offered frequently but not forced

SPECIAL ALZHEIMER UNITS

With increasing popularity and frequency, long-term care facilities have designed special units for their residents with AD. The special units vary tremendously in terms of their guiding philosophy, environmental design, and therapeutic approach (Ohta and Ohta, 1988). Debate exists about the efficacy of such units, supported on the one side by those who believe the units provide consistency and better care

through a smaller environment and the same staff, who are more knowledgeable about specific care. Those who oppose this model maintain that separation from the general population may accelerate deterioration by removing the person from the more normal and active environment of the rest of the facility and from more functional peers and role models. Whether in or out of a special unit, particular environmental features are desirable for the person with AD for functional maintenance and growth. It is theoretically easier for caregivers to learn the principles of care for a single diagnostic category and to learn specific care plans for a select group of persons, such as would be found in a special unit. Routine and consistency are easier to maintain when caregivers are the same. Whatever the physical setting, the environment and its delivery must be consistent.

DAY TO DAY

We cannot know what it feels like to experience the thoughts and emotions of someone with AD. It must be a bewildering, threatening, frightening, and depressing experience for the person who is affected, especially in the early stages before insight is lost. The realization that one cannot make sense out of normal experiences and cannot cope with situations that previously were handled with ease surely provokes severe apprehension and insecurity (U'Ren, 1984). Patients respond differently and may experience different levels of distress and problems. The impact of the same symptom picture or problems varies from family to family based on their interpretation, skill, and support structure. The better "armed" the caregivers are the greater the opportunity for success for the patient.

There are several principles to consider in designing the daily routine for the patient with AD. Two key components are *consistency* and *predictability*. Optimally, caregivers and routines, including meal time, exercise time, rising time, bed time, etc., are unchanged from day to day. The earlier in the disease process that the routine is established and repeated, the easier it is for the person to follow it. It may also reduce potential anxiety later.

The patient with AD relies on the skills that have become rote such as dressing, bathing, and social graces. Learning new skills becomes increasingly more difficult. Caregivers should use skills the person already possesses and adapt these to routine activities of daily living needs rather than attempting to teach new methods of accomplishing tasks. Repetition is helpful, along with frequent and clear cues. It is helpful to assume a matter of fact tone, quietly acknowledging accomplishments. All people like to be recognized for accomplishments, but oversolicitation or overpraise can be embarrassing or humiliating.

ACTIVITIES

An important concept in activity and daily planning concerns the need for balance in work, play, and rest. While leaving the patient with AD to independently plan and carry out activities is generally not appropriate, neither is it beneficial to plan and fill the day so tightly that in the long term it contributes to or is the sole cause of stress. Patients vary in their abilities and interests and both must be attended to. The following principles may serve as guidelines in designing activity:

1. The activity must be enjoyable to the individual and have meaning for him
2. The activity that focuses on or brings out old roles is often favored
3. The activity period should last only as long as it is pleasurable. Hour-long sittings may be overwhelming
4. Activity groups should be small, including from three to five persons, depending on the individuals and the activity
5. Patience on the part of the caregiver is necessary
6. Avoid placing demands on the person. Focus on accomplishments. Do not illustrate his deficits
7. When group activities are scheduled, do not change the schedule or routine of the group process
8. Activity groups should follow a structure similar to a social group. The activity itself should be fairly simple
9. The caregiver should define a goal of enjoying the activity herself as well

EXCESS DISABILITY

"Excess disability is the discrepancy that exists when a person's functional incapacity is greater than is warranted by actual impairment" (Brody et al, 1971). While there is evidence and demonstration of progressive deterioration in capacity and function in patients with AD, the added factor of unrecognized or untreated co-existing medical illness or unskilled or negative attitude in caregivers may well result in a greater disability than was originally present in the person. Physical health must be monitored daily. Persons with dementia are at high risk for suffering unrecognized acute medical illness or complications of chronic conditions due to reduced awareness and communication skills. Environmental assessments done throughout the day with timely adjustments can serve to improve function as well. When caregivers deliver routine care unskillfully or intervene with problems unskillfully, the result can be disastrous. The resulting disorganization, confusion, and distress is not only the cumulative product of both the patient and the caregiver not coping well, but is frequently further magnified through the spiraling effect of the patient mirroring frustration and disorganization presented by the caregiver. This additional stress can be conceptualized as adding fuel to an already out of control fire. Excess disability that caregivers project onto the patient can be prevented.

PROGRESSIVELY LOWERED STRESS THRESHOLD

Setting realistic expectations and problem solving requires an understanding of the relationship between progressive cognitive loss and the response to stress. Hal and Buckwalter (1987) designed a visual model of the incongruence between progressive functional decline and the incline in frustration tolerance. This is helpful in teaching coping and problem-solving skills to caregivers.

Progressively lowered stress threshold refers to the fact that persons with dementia experience increased frustration due to planning deficits, intolerance of multiple stimulus, and increased fatigue from processing information about their environment. The sequelae is a lowered tolerance for stress, often made worse by inappropriate or nontherapeutic response from caregivers (i.e., excess disability). When this already lowered threshold for stress is exceeded, the result is anxious behavior, which if not curtailed moves on to dysfunctional behavior. The goal of planning daily care is to focus attention on those times throughout the day when the person is approaching the stress threshold and intervene at that point to bring the patient back to baseline before he passes through the anxious behavior and into dysfunctional behavior. Appropriate interventions include the gamet of any and all strategies and principles that are customized to that individual in the care plan (Figures 18–1 to 18–4).

FAMILY SUPPORT

AD has been described by caregivers and families as "the long good-bye." The patient seems lost and gone long before physical death and yet daily care must continue. Families and caregivers are known as the hidden victims as they strive to maintain some semblance of life continuity during the many difficult hours, days, and months of caregiving. The physical, emotional, and spiritual strength required of all caregivers is phenomenal. While only a small percentage of victims are cared for in institutions, the majority are at home with family. It is imperative that the nursing discipline give attention to the needs of these caregivers both in the home and in institutional settings. Many communities offer support groups, respite care, day care, etc.

GUARDIANSHIP

At some point in this illness the competence of the person becomes an issue. The question of competence should never entirely exclude the person from decision making. The true essence

of adulthood is found in making decisions and being respected for the choices one makes. Competency refers to the ability to understand, reason, consider potential outcomes, and make decisions. Persons not competent to make complex legal decisions, drive a care, or even protect themselves from cold weather in the winter still maintain capacity to (1) have input into decision making and (2) make choices and decisions in other dimensions. For example, someone unable to make a totally informed decision with regard to determining medical treatment may still be able to demonstrate in some way his preferences.

There is debate over protecting the patient through guardianship on the one hand and preserving autonomy and dignity through no guardianship on the other. However, the focus should be shifted from whether a guardian should be appointed or not, to appropriate selection and education of the guardian so that he can indeed substitute judgment based on what the patient would likely have done for himself in the same situation.

The presence of one or even several of the deficits of AD does not mean total disability. The person who does not know the date or where he is may still be quite capable of finding his way around the house and finding or selecting clothing. Often there is a tendency to take

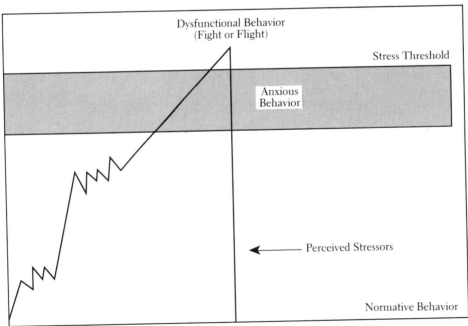

FIGURE 18–1   Stress threshold in normal individuals. (From Hall GR. Care of the patient with Alzheimer's disease living at home. Nurs Clin North Am 1988; 23:34; with permission.)

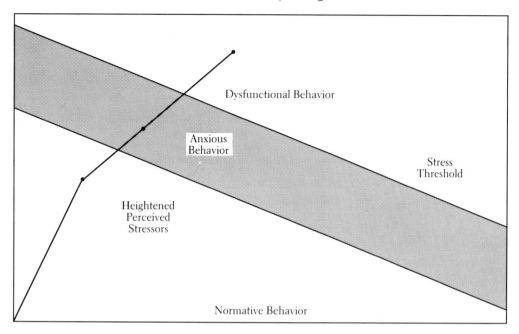

FIGURE 18–2   Progressively lowered stress threshold in adults with progressive degeneration of the cerebral cortex (Alzheimer's disease and related disorders). (From Hall GR. Care of the patient with Alzheimer's disease living at home. Nurs Clin North Am 1988; 23:35; with permission.)

over decision making for these persons too soon. It is particularly true for persons who are in the middle stages when dilemmas are presented to caregivers. The caregiver can expand the patient's functional capacity in the early stages by providing supplemental information, assisting him to identify pros and cons, and in more advance stages by supplying several choices from which the person can select his preference. At that point a guardian may be needed to assume responsibility for legal or more complex issues and the person can retain control over the issues of importance to him.

Behavioral Problems Associated with Dementia

Five common behaviors of patients with AD follow. In Chapter 19 daily living with other behavior problems are discussed including agita-

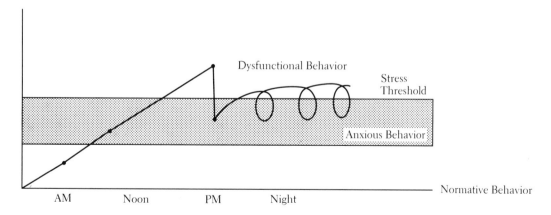

FIGURE 18–3   A typical day for an adult with a dementing illness in an unstructured care program. (From Hall GR. Care of the patient with Alzheimer's disease living at home. Nurs Clin North Am 1988; 23:38; with permission.)

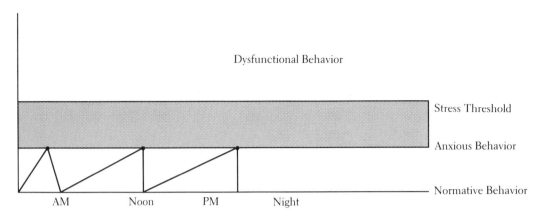

FIGURE 18–4   Planned activity levels for the adult with dementing illness. (From Hall GR. Care of the patient with Alzheimer's disease living at home. Nurs Clin North Am 1988; 23:41; with permission.)

tion, restlessness, aggressiveness, hostility, calls for attention, and suspicion.

DAILY LIVING WITH WANDERING

Wandering is a behavior associated most often with chronic confusion. It can occur within the immediate living environment or in the neighborhood on foot, in a wheelchair, or in an automobile. Some wanderers have a fixed destination in mind, whereas others wander aimlessly without a plan. Management in all cases is complicated, requiring time, energy, and a thoughtful balancing of caregiver needs versus wanderer needs.

RISK FACTORS

Wandering can pose significant safety considerations and disrupt the management of daily living. Perhaps the greatest risk the wanderer faces is institutionalization at the point when the family believes he is no longer safe. Even this measure is often unsatisfactory as not all long-term care facilities are secure settings or can guarantee the measure of safety that families often demand. This creates a risk of potential eviction from the institutional setting. Other risks include the following:

The risk of getting lost in inclement weather or a fall or other injury while wandering
The wanderer being subject to sedating medication or physical restraint with their associated adverse effects when other measures are ineffective

Emotional burdens of fatigue, frustration, fear, and worry by family and caregivers, with the ongoing efforts of management

PROGNOSTIC VARIABLES

Management of wandering is largely dependent on the caregiver's understanding of the behavior and skill in intervening. A greater success rate will be observed in cases where the caregiver is flexible and creative in finding interventions that not only produce a safe environment but attend to the emotional needs of the wanderer as well. Where comfort and control are engendered less disruption of daily living will occur.

TREATMENT

The nursing goal in management of this problem is to provide a safe environment and prevent injury. While there is no single cause there is likewise no single solution. While it does pose management questions, wandering may also be interpreted as a coping strategy and should therefore not be viewed negatively. Intervention should be pointed toward facilitating this coping or redirecting it. Behavioral interventions include the following:

1. Therapeutic communication skills (see Chapter 19)
2. Reality orientation is helpful to the mildly confused or delirious person but not generally effective for more confused persons. It might be tried, but if the wanderer be-

comes more upset or insistent abandon this approach

3. Tune in to exercise needs. Persons who by history have been physically active especially need to continue this activity
4. Activity programs and projects provide many benefits, including diversion from the wandering, an outlet for energy, a purpose, and an opportunity to touch and talk with others
5. Wanderers should wear identification bracelets with their name, address, phone number, and the words "memory impaired" on them
6. Be aware of providing rest periods for those who do not think to do so for themselves
7. Check feet daily on persons who walk all day
8. Work with the environment to change or create cues to assist the wanderer to develop walking patterns within safe areas (e.g., stop signs, colored tape paths on the floor, dutch doors). It is known that wanderers are drawn to or spend more time at points of interest, stimulation, or potential reinforcement
9. Provide cue cards for the wanderer to carry in his pocket that will guide him or whoever may find him as to who to call
10. Establish a quiet hour or time during the day when noise, movement, lighting, etc. is reduced to minimize confusion and assist the wanderer to calm and maintain his best coping
11. Long-term care facilities may find security door systems helpful
12. Long-term care facilities should have a procedure for responding to the report that someone is missing. Home caregivers should also have a protocol in mind with emergency numbers and a current photograph available

NIGHTTIME WANDERING

1. Recall that some sleep disturbance may be an unavoidable consequence of aging
2. Allow the confused person in long-term care facilities where there are night staff available to be up at night if awake. The focus of care should be on safety
3. Night lights may decrease disorientation and the desire to get up
4. Limit caffeine after 6 PM
5. Urinals or commodes at the bedside will facilitate problem solving when the wanderer wakes up at night needing to void. Alterna-

tively, reflector tape around the bathroom door and painting the toilet seat a bright parking-lot yellow will guide the confused person

6. Integrate the person's past sleep pattern and habits into the current routine
7. Experiment with naps or rest periods. It is not necessarily the case that every person who takes a nap will not sleep well at night or that those who do not nap will sleep well. Daytime behavior and needs must be weighed in the equation as well. The best routine for an individual will be found through trials with various schedules

DAILY LIVING WITH YELLING OR CALLING OUT

This behavior may include moaning, yelling, or calling out recognizable words, names, or messages or sounds that are not recognizable and is generally quite disruptive. Some yelling is intermittent and other yelling goes on continuously. Yelling may be viewed as a manifestation of some unmet need that is most often exhibited by persons suffering with chronic confusion. Frequently these persons are unable when questioned to identify why they are yelling. It then becomes a trial and error mystery for the caregiver to solve. In other cases yelling may occur as a manipulative or controlling gesture. Patients who moan may not even be aware that they are doing it. Calling attention to it may help to stop it.

RISK FACTORS

Risks for the older person who yells include the following:

Potential retaliation from others he shares a living environment with
Not having others take him seriously when he does need something
Social isolation as peers, family, and caregivers become frustrated and tired of listening to the yelling

PROGNOSTIC VARIABLES

Yelling is one of the most difficult problems to manage. The prognosis is better in cases where there is an identifiable and treatable physical or psychological etiology, and the caregiver is patient, flexible, and tolerant.

TREATMENT

Reduction of this behavior requires patience and consistency by all who are in contact with the person. Psychoactive medication does not alter behavior, rather it may sedate the person, who continues the yelling albeit more groggily. The following suggestions may prove helpful:

1. Attempt to identify why the person is yelling and meet the need to the degree possible
2. Experiment with diversional activity, as boredom may be part or all of the etiology. Customize the activity to the person's interest and skill level (e.g., earphones and a small radio or tape player is a useful tool)
3. Offer the person snacks in an attempt to discern if hunger is causing the yelling. Alternatively, offer ice chips or sugarless candy for him to suck on to divert attention from yelling
4. Regular rest or nap periods may reduce fatigue
5. Change position of the chair or bed-bound person
6. Gentle touch, hugs, or massage may relax an anxious or fearful person. Try encircling the person with your arms and rock with him close to you
7. A trial of an analgesic for pain administered as needed and routinely may decrease pain in some persons too confused to be able to articulate

DAILY LIVING WITH PILFERING AND HOARDING BEHAVIORS

This behavior may include going through drawers, closets, bags, etc., sometimes disrupting the order of things and other times moving things from one place to another or collecting and carrying things with them. It can be exasperating to family, caregivers, or other residents in long-term care settings who must watch the older person or their own possessions. Persons exhibiting pilfering behavior are most often those with chronic confusion who are looking for something, real or imagined. Other times it is the result of boredom or restlessness.

RISK FACTORS

Social isolation
Physical or verbal retribution from others whose things have been taken or disrupted

Emotional distress, which continues for the person who is desperately looking for something and cannot find it

PROGNOSTIC VARIABLES

Once again the response of the person who is pilfering and hoarding will to a large degree depend on how he is approached and what skill the caregiver has to attend to this person's need or "agenda."

TREATMENT

The following interventions may be of assistance in discovering why this behavior is occurring and identifying ways to rechannel or reduce it:

1. Diversionary activities are a beneficial method of distracting the person from the course of action. Activity that involves keeping the hands busy are best because the person is then not free to go through things or pick things up. Some examples include pushing a broom or dust mop, carrying specific things for the caregiver, pushing an empty wheelchair or one carrying laundry, clothing, etc., folding laundry, sanding blocks of wood, etc.
2. Short, frequent interactions by caregivers will serve both to monitor the patient's whereabouts and activity as well as to give the patient attention and regular cuing as to what he or she should be doing
3. In redirecting behavior the verbal cues should be given in a "please do" format rather than a "please stop" format. In other words, give direction as to what you would specifically like the patient to do. Telling the patient to stop doing something, even when done politely and gently, still does not give him or her the needed guidance as to what to do instead
4. Provide a box of interesting and varied things for the person to sort through, empty out, arrange, and rearrange. This will satisfy the need to look for something or collect things. A box of assorted pieces of PVC piping to be put together and taken apart does not require fitting one specific piece to another and thereby offers the person success in whichever way he or she fits them

References and Other Readings

Baldwin VA. Community management of Alzheimer's disease. Nurs Clin North Am 1988; 23:47.

Beck D, Heacock P. Nursing interventions for patients with Alzheimer's disease. Nurs Clin North Am 1988; 23:95.

Beisgen BA. Life enhancing activities for mentally impaired elders: a practical guide. New York: Springer Publishing, 1989.

Bergener M, ed. Psychogeriatrics: an international handbook. New York: Springer Publishing, 1987.

Brody E, Kleban M, Lawton MP, Silverman H. Excess disabilities of mentally impaired aged: impact of individualized treatment. Gerontologist 1971; 2:124.

Buckwalter KC, Abrams IL, Neundorfer MM. Alzheimer's disease. Involving nursing in the development and implementation of health care for patients and families. Nurs Clin North Am 1988; 23:1.

Calkins MP. Design for dementia. Owings Mills, MD: National Health Publishing, 1988.

Cherry DL, Rafkin MJ. Adapting day care to the needs of adults with dementia. Gerontologist 1988; 28:116.

Chocon JO, Potter JF. Age-related changes in human memory: normal and abnormal. Geriatrics 1988; 43:43.

Cohen D, Eisdorfer C. The loss of self. New York: NAL Penjuin Inc., 1986.

Cohen-Mansfield J. Agitated behaviors in the elderly. Preliminary results in the cognitively deteriorated. J Am Geriatr Soc 1986; 34:722.

Cox KG. Milieu therapy. Geriatr Nurs 1985; 6:152.

Crane Macdonald K. Occupational therapy approaches to treatment of dementia patients. Phys Occu Ther Geriatr 1986; 4:61.

Evans LK, Strumpt NE. Tying down the elderly. J Am Geriatr Soc 1989; 37:65.

Freidman R, Tappan R. The effects of planned walking on communication in Alzheimer's disease. J Am Geriatr Soc 1991; 39:650.

Galasko D, Corey-Bloom J, Thal L. Monitoring progression in Alzheimer's disease. J Am Geriatr Soc 1991; 39:932.

Given CW, Collins CE, Given BA. Sources of stress among families caring for relatives with Alzheimer's disease. Nurs Clin North Am 1988; 23:69.

Gwyther LP. Care of Alzheimer's patients: a manual for nursing home staff. American Health Care Association and the Alzheimer's Disease and Related Disorders Association, 1985.

Hall GR. Care of the patient with Alzheimer's disease living at home. Nurs Clin North Am 1988; 23:31.

Hall FR, Buckwalter KC. Progressively lowered stress threshold: a conceptual model for care of adults with Alzheimer's disease. Arch Psychiat Nurs 1987; 1:399.

Hamdy RC, Turnbull JM, Norman LD, Lancaster MM. Alzheimer's disease. A handbook for caregivers. St. Louis: C.V. Mosby, 1990.

Harvis KA, Rabins PV. Dementia: helping family caregivers cope. J Psychosocial Nurs 1989; 27:8.

Jenske M. In: Geriatric psychiatry and psychopharmacology. Alzheimer's disease and other dementias. Chicago: Year Book Medical Publishers, 1989, p 127.

Katzman R, Jackson JE. Alzheimer's disease: basis and clinical advances. J Am Geriatr Soc 1991; 39:516.

Lee VK. Language changes and Alzheimer's disease: a literature review. J Gerontol Nurs 1991; 17:16.

Maas M. Management of patients with Alzheimer's disease in long-term care facilities. Nurs Clin North Am 1988; 23:57.

Mace NL. Principles of activities for persons with dementia. Phys Occu Ther Geriatr 1987; 5:13.

Mace NL, Rabins PV. The 36-hour day (2nd ed.). Baltimore: The Johns Hopkins University Press, 1991.

Martin RL. Update on dementia of the Alzheimer type. Hosp Community Psychiatry 1989; 40:593.

Mitchell-Pedersen L, Edmund L, Fingerote E, Powell C. Lets untie the elderly. Quarterly 1985; 10.

Namazi KH, Rosner TT, Calkins MP. Visual barriers to prevent ambulatory Alzheimer's patients from exiting through an emergency door. Gerontologist 1989; 29:699.

Nolen N. Activity programming for withdrawn, confused residents. Act Adapt Aging 1987; 9:45.

Ohta RJ, Ohta BM. Special units for Alzheimer's disease patients: a critical look. Gerontologist 1988; 28:803.

Phelps Stevenson J. Family stress related to home care of Alzheimer's disease patients and implications for support. J Neuroscience Nurs 1990; 22:179.

Rader J, Doan J, Schwab M. How to decrease wandering, a form of agenda behavior. Geriatr Nurs 1985; 6:196.

Reifler FV, Larson E. Excess disability in demented elderly outpatients: the rule of halves. J Am Geriatr Soc 1988; 36:82.

Reifler BV, Larson E, Teri L, Poulsen M. Dementia of the Alzheimer's type and depression. J Am Geriatr Soc 1986; 34:855.

Reisberg B, Ferris SH, Franssen E. An ordinal functional assessment tool for Alzheimer's type dementia. Hosp Community Psychiatry 1985; 36:593.

Roberts BL, Algase DL. Victims of Alzheimer's disease and the environment. Nurs Clin North Am 1988; 23:83.

Roper JM, Shapira J, Chang BL. Agitation in the demented patient: a framework for management. J Gerontol Nurs 1991; 17:17.

Schafer SC. Modifying the environment. Geriatr Nurs 1985; 3:157.

Schwab M, Rader J, Doan J. Relieving the anxiety and fear in dementia. J Gerontol Nurs 1985; 11:8.

Scott RR, Bramble KJ, Goodyear N. How knowledge and labeling of dementia affect nurses' expectations. J Gerontol Nurs 1991; 17:21.

Shulman MD, Mandel E. Communication training of relatives and friends of institutionalized elderly persons. Gerontologist 1988; 28:797.

Sloane P, Mathers L. Dementia units in long term care. Baltimore: Johns Hopkins University Press, 1991.

Spencer B, White L. Understanding difficult behaviors. Ypsilanti, MI: Geriatric Education Center of Michigan, 1991.

Steele C, Rovner B, Chase GA, Folstein M. Psychiatric symptoms and nursing home placement of patients with Alzheimer's disease. Am J Psychiatry 1990; 147:1049.

Taylor JA, Ray WA. Managing behavior problems in nursing home residents. A manual for nursing home staff. Nashville, TN: Department of Preventative Medicine, Vanderbilt University of Medicine, 1990.

Teri L. Managing and understanding behavior problems in Alzheimer's disease and related disorders. Northwest Geriatric Education Center, University of Washington, HL-23, Seattle, WA. Videotape Training Series for Caregivers of Patients with Alzheimer's Disease and Related Disorders.

U'Ren R. Organic disorders. In: Cassel CK, Walsh JR, ed. Geriatric medicine. 2nd ed. New York: Springer-Verlag, 1984, p 553.

Wolanin MO, Fraelich Phillips LR. Confusion. St Louis: C.V. Mosby, 1981.

Zarit SH, Orr NK, Zarit JM. The hidden victims of Alzheimer's disease. New York: New York University Press, 1988.

Zgola JM. Doing things. A guide to programming activities for persons with Alzheimer's disease and related disorders. Baltimore: Johns Hopkins University Press, 1987.

19
Daily Living with Behavioral Problems

LYNDA CRANDALL

All people experience periods of agitation and restlessness, hostility and aggression, social withdrawal, and forgetfulness or confusion. These responses and behaviors can create difficulties in daily living at any age. But to the elderly who are at higher risk for a variety of reasons, these behaviors can be not only disruptive but life-threatening. They can interfere with essential elements of daily living such as sleeping, eating, drinking, eliminating, and being mobile. Long-term consequences can include malnutrition, electrolyte imbalance, urinary tract infections, and other pathology that may contribute in turn to further central nervous system dysfunction. Some behaviors can endanger other persons and threaten the security of the older person's living environment, and most behavior problems interfere with the emotional comfort and quality of life of the older individual and his family or caregivers.

Although changes in physical status tend to be more obvious, behavioral and cognitive dysfunctioning have a powerful impact on the social, interpersonal, and physical character of daily living. With the aged there are risks of overlooking changes or of attributing the observed signs and symptoms to normal aging rather than to other factors that can be equally potent in creating mental and behavioral problems. Other significant factors include pathophysiology, drugs (prescription or nonprescrip-

tion), malnutrition, change in the environment, and other life changes such as changes in roles.

Families of elderly persons with behavioral problems also need to be included in the nurse's assessment, diagnoses, treatment plans, and evaluations. The ability of the family members, spouse, or companion to adapt to or work with behavioral problems in the older family member can be hampered by their own lack of understanding of what is happening. This lack of information is an area for nursing diagnosis and treatment. Nursing expertise in proposing and mobilizing additional support systems can often make a difference in the quality of life for the family and older person alike. Both nurses and families need to know when it is timely to seek additional professional help and to know how to communicate about the patient's status with enough precision and confidence that others can understand the situation and provide appropriate consultation and care.

Daily Living with Behavioral Problems in General

RISK FACTORS

Factors that predict the likelihood of problematic behaviors reoccurring or continuing as an element in daily living include the following:

Previous history of a particular problematic behavior exhibited by an individual

The likelihood that the events triggering the behavior will recur

The rewarding nature of the reinforcement that the behavior has received

The pathology that may be underlying the behavior: progressive dementia, depression, strokes, schizophrenia, etc.

Exhaustion in the primary caregiver

COMPLICATIONS

Whereas individual behavior problems may follow different sequelae involving unique complications, there are also a number of complications and risks that may overlap from problem to problem. Most behavior problems tend to be more disabling when accompanied by confusion and memory loss. When behavior problems in daily living are not effectively managed, the resulting complications for the older adult may include:

Physical   Trauma, exhaustion, dehydration, ill effects from any undiagnosed organic or mental problem, sleep deprivation, increased risk of verbal or physical retaliation by peers or caregivers, immobility from physical restraints, and oversedation or other adverse effects from improperly used psychoactive medication

Emotional   Anxiety, sensory overload, fear, and sadness

Social   Social isolation, alienation and distancing from family and others, with increased risk of loneliness and loss of support, getting lost, institutionalization, establishment of a reputation that then sets negative expectations and interactions in subsequent encounters, not only with those who have experienced it, but also those who learn of it, and restrictions on physical or social activity

PROGNOSTIC VARIABLES

Daily living is likely to be compromised in an ongoing manner in the presence of behavior problems when the caregiver or those around the person:

Do not understand the phenomenon

Do not recognize and take seriously the physical or mental changes that may be occurring and thus fail to seek professional help

Cannot tolerate the behavior

Have no workable strategies for dealing with the situations

Are themselves disabled or somewhat depressed so that their own moods are exacerbated or they are physically unable to take on the added responsibilities of the person's care

The outcome is also impacted negatively when the older person:

Lacks insight about the problem

Chooses not to participate or cooperate with the problem solving process

For whatever reason is noncompliant with the treatment regime

The potential for effective management of daily living in individuals burdened with behavioral problems depends in part on two interrelated factors:

1. Accurate nursing diagnosis as to the cause of the problem
2. The attitude, outlook, and level of information and skill of the family or caregiver

NURSING INTERVENTION

Just as nurses must be knowledgeable in the signs and symptoms of physical health problems and skillful in their assessment and treatment, so must nurses be prepared to intervene in the assessment and management of behavior problems. Nursing intervention includes components directed toward both the older individual as well as the family or caregiver. This includes a working knowledge of treatment options and proficiency in designing intervention strategies appropriate to helping older persons and their families to manage everyday living that is complicated by behavior problems. Impressions and recommendations for managing daily living need to be communicated in a usable manner to families and primary caregivers. Nursing treatment involves helping the older person to:

Stay safe, minimizing the intensity, emotional discomfort, and potential injury related to the problematic behavior

Gain insight into the impact of the behavior on himself and others

Expand coping abilities and problem solving skills for managing his behavior and daily living as it relates to the behavior

Modify the behavior to more appropriate, socially acceptable, or safer levels

Nursing treatment involves helping the family and caregivers to

Understand the nature of the phenomena they are living with

Develop feasible plans for managing daily living for both the impaired elderly person and the caregiver, given the circumstances

SUPPORTING THE PRIMARY CAREGIVER

The companions, family, or staff of long-term care facilities caring for persons with behavior problems face real demands on their energy, stamina, and patience. Often the caregivers are agemates whose own health status is compromised. Exhaustion is common due to the constant disruption of usual activities, sleep deprivation, the worry or constant tension of having the older person always about, or the need for constant vigilance in many circumstances. If the nursing assessment and diagnoses are made in a timely fashion, then intervention to alter the patterns of behavior can be put into place before family or caregivers are so tired or frustrated that they have no energy or desire to work with the behaviors.

When chronic confusion is part of the clinical picture, adult day care is one modality that can provide relief for both the older person and the harassed caregiver. The older person can benefit from the structured daily living environment staffed with skilled personnel while his caregiver has time for work, rest, and recreation. Another strategy is the addition of home health aides to assist with activities of daily living that may be too demanding for the primary caregiver alone. Having someone to share the burdens of difficult caregiving can reduce the emotional and physical strain of long-term caregiving and dealing with difficult behavior. Support groups can bolster waning spirits and offer solutions to the caregiver.

PREVENTION

A primary focus of holistic health care is prevention. Nurses must expand the scope of prevention to include the realm of behavior problems. The axiom "prevention before intervention" should function as the guiding principle to be integrated in all treatment and care planning related to behavior problems. Prevention of the unwanted behavior also results in prevention of the associated complications in daily living. Nurses are obligated to become adept with prevention skills in concept as well as practice so they can teach the same to families and caregivers.

ASSESSMENT

Toward the fundamental goal of prevention, ongoing assessments of the mental, physical, and emotional presentations and changes in elderly persons are imperative. When problem behaviors surface, a comprehensive reassessment must precede diagnosis whether by the nurse or by the family with nursing support. Symptoms must never be treated before an assessment of the total clinical picture is done to determine the underlying cause. As medical problems are uncovered they are treated accordingly. The following steps and questions should be included in an initial assessment when problem behaviors arise:

1. Define behaviors specifically
2. Review medications
3. Onset: (a) Acute or chronic? (b) Precipitating event?
4. Any environmental or life changes recently?
5. Are there any accompanying physical changes?
6. Physical examination
7. Laboratory tests

Three interrelated aspects that give direction to the nurse's assessment include the precise nature of the problem, how it is identified, and who identifies it. One family or caregiver may describe a particular behavior as unmanageable and a crisis while the same behavior for another family or caregiving team is not viewed as problematic at all. Generally, problem behaviors are reported by the caregiver who has a vested interest in modifying the behavior. The perception or interpretation of the behavior is directly related to ownership; to whom does the problem belong? Ownership is critically related to determining intervention for modification or resolution of the problem (e.g., wandering through other resident's rooms and belongings in a long-term care facility may be problematic to the other residents but not to the wanderer; the frequent yelling by an older person may be more problematic for the caregiver than it is for the yeller). Ownership is often shared as in the previous examples where there are definite potential negative impacts for the older person as well as for the caregivers and peers.

The fact that a behavior has been identified as "deviant" or "problematic" does not necessarily indicate a need for intervention. It is the impact that the behavior has on the older individual and/or the family or caregivers that determines both the need for and the level of intervention required.

Nurses must understand the dynamics of the basic phenomena as well as the older person's particular situation and that of the family or caregiving team. Regardless of the presenting behaviors and symptomatology, the same thoughtful, thorough process is required in each case. This involves exercising critical thinking and problem solving skills. A general problem solving model that closely parallels the nursing process can be a functional tool (Fig. 19–1).

PROBLEM IDENTIFICATION

The most critical step in the problem solving process is that of accurate and specific identification of the target behavior or problem. Target behaviors must be described explicitly. Terms such as "worked up," "agitation," or "dither" are not very helpful because they are so vague. Labeling or categorizing behaviors before assessment should be avoided because this often leads to misidentification and/or time lost in pursuit of answers for the real problems. The objective of defining the problem is to set the stage for goal setting and treatment planning.

A fundamental premise is that the presenting behavior is rarely the primary problem. Most often the behaviors are symptoms of the real problem (i.e., the way the problem manifests itself). For example, wandering is a symptom of a primary problem that may be confusion, boredom, or an emotionally driven need to get some place. Similarly, combativeness is a symptom of the basic problem that may be pain, misinterpretation of caregiver intent, paranoid delusions. Some deviant behaviors in aged persons are protective defenses against perceived problems in their daily living. If the older person's perception of reality changes, communication and behavior may be altered. Such changes in long-standing patterns can confuse, threaten, and alienate family members and support figures. The result is to further reduce the older person's external resources at a time when they can ill afford to lose them.

Interpretation of the behavior is not always apparent and often requires a fair amount of detective work, particularly when the person suffers from cognitive impairment. In many cases a tedious process of empirical trial and error interventions using one's "best guess" is required to derive the etiology. *Determining what the behavior means* generally leads to the heart of the real problem. Directing attention toward reducing the problem or target behavior without understanding *why* it is occurring may do little to alter the behavior and may in fact exacerbate the problem or create new ones. However, there is frequently a strong desire by caregivers to find a quick solution to the visible behavior and thus a tendency exists to rush through this most important step of problem identification. The dangerous practice of trying to treat surface behaviors creates significant risks for both the older person and his caregiver.

Often several problem behaviors present concurrently. Not all can be addressed at the same time. It is necessary to prioritize the behaviors, weighing their impact on both the older individual and those persons around him in order to select which one or two problems should be addressed first.

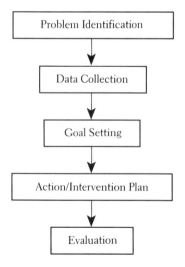

FIGURE 19–1   Problem solving model.

DATA COLLECTION

Once the problem behavior has been identified and described, the investigative process is initiated to determine other relevant information. Having a current, accurate objective data base is crucial to maintaining valid diagnoses.

A balanced approach to caregiving dictates that significant energy be put toward identifying the older person's strengths before attention is focused on deficits and problem behaviors. Questions to family members and significant others can yield invaluable information about the person's strengths, preferences, and routines. The families' perceptions of the specific target behavior, time of onset, triggers, associated factors or patterns, and interventions that to date have and have not been helpful will assist the nurse in rounding out the data base. Frequency of behavior and patterns of occurrence are particularly crucial pieces of information. Caregivers may overcount or exaggerate behaviors that are particularly annoying or

frustrating. This is only one of a number of reasons why it is helpful to write the behavior on paper to follow it and more accurately analyze it. A behavior management flow sheet, designed by Radar and Harvath (1990) (Fig. 19–2) is an especially useful tool for this purpose and can be easily incorporated into most caregiving settings and schedules. The observer notes the occurrence and intensity of a behavior through the use of a graded number system set up for that particular problem and individual. After 7 to 10 days a baseline for most behaviors can be analyzed as to frequency, patterns, associated factors (e.g., absence of or increases in the behavior at certain times of the day or when particular staff are on duty). Antecedent conditions (those conditions that precede the behavior) and consequences of the behavior can more readily be pinpointed. Caregivers are often surprised to see the emergence of patterns that were not evident before record keeping.

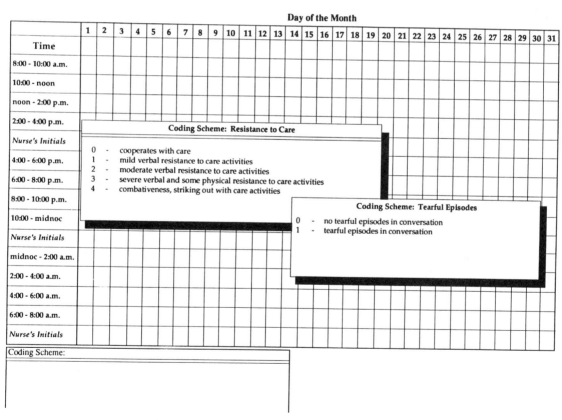

FIGURE 19–2 Behavior monitoring chart and coding examples. (From Rader J, Harvath R. Benedictine Institute for Long Term Care, Mt. Angel, OR 97362. © January 1990.)

GOAL SETTING

The primary rule in goal setting is that the goals be realistic. It is almost never realistic to expect to completely extinguish a problem behavior. Rather the caregiver should work toward modifying the behavior to a safe or tolerable level. Goals are most helpful when stated in positive rather than negative terms (e.g., Mr. Jones will participate in morning care, rather than Mr. Jones will not strike out during morning care). Finally, the treatment team must be able to gauge success so the goal must be stated in terms conducive to measurement (e.g., Mr. Jones will do morning care at least 5 days per week by January). Recall that only specific behaviors can be measured (e.g., "agitated" "worked up" cannot be objectively evaluated).

ACTION PLAN

Specific intervention strategies should use the person's identified strengths, known likes and dislikes, as well as interventions that by history have been helpful. Basic prevention and behavioral management principles form the backbone of the plan. Interventions that have been effective in similar cases may be tried. A measure of creativity in intervention design is frequently necessary as there are generally no management protocols addressing some of the most difficult behavior problems in daily living. Creative thinking is a skill that requires practice and openness to new ideas and possibilities. New and better ways of intervening should always be pursued. A current successful method of intervention never justifies not looking further as a better idea may be discovered.

EVALUATION

Evaluation reveals the effectiveness of the methods tried as shown primarily through decreased frequency of the target behavior and perhaps an increase in more appropriate or desirable behaviors. Once again the need for specific target behavior descriptions is highlighted. The behavior management flow sheet is useful in this process by providing an objective reflection of behavior frequency after interventions are initiated. While the subjective impressions of the family or caregiver are helpful and frequently accurate, access to the definitive data is more beneficial in determining whether the current interventions should be continued.

Daily Living with Agitation and Restlessness

Agitation and restlessness are two of the most pressing behavioral problems that create difficulties in managing everyday living. Both are nonspecific terms used frequently to describe one behavior or a cluster of behaviors (e.g., wandering, pacing, insomnia, handwringing, picking, inability to sit still, crying, etc.). Most commonly these signs are associated with anxiousness, an overall sense of unrest, or uneasiness. Mild agitation and restlessness may be behavioral patterns of a lifetime that become exacerbated as the person grows older and is more restricted in desired activities. These behaviors can occur episodically or seemingly continuously and the intensity may fluctuate. They can range from a moderate discomfort to a severely disabling force in daily living. The heightened activity frequently encroaches on the person's diurnal cycle, throwing sleep and activity periods out of synchrony with previously established household patterns.

Agitation generally refers to a more intense behavioral response than restlessness, but neither term is in and of itself very helpful in pinpointing what is going on with an individual or what to do about it. Specific description of the behaviors is much more useful. These nondescript signs of agitation and restlessness are often a tip-off that further investigation is needed. If neglected, the result is often a progression into distinct behavioral concerns such as wandering or combativeness.

The agitated or restless person can be quite well physically and appear mentally intact on initial observation. However, dementia and major depression are frequent underlying causes of severe and disabling agitation and restlessness.

RISK FACTORS

Agitation and restlessness tend to be more complicated when accompanied by chronic confusion. Deterioration and exacerbation of the symptoms are more likely to occur:

1. During periods of fatigue
2. During early evening hours for those with altered diurnal cycle ("sundowners")
3. When infections are present
4. With unameliorated chronic pain
5. When polymedicines are routinely used or

following ingestion of certain medications (Table 19–1)

6. When alcohol is used or withdrawn
7. With inexperienced caregivers
8. When confined to a restricted space devoid of familiar objects
9. When subjected to rapid routine or environmental changes
10. When physical restraints are used
11. When there is a lack of use of glasses or hearing aids to overcome sensory deficits

PROGNOSTIC VARIABLES

If the nursing assessment and diagnosis are made in a timely fashion, then intervention to attend to unmet needs and to harness the restless energy into constructive activity and alter

---

TABLE 19–1 *Some Commonly Used Drugs That May Cause Behavioral Symptoms*

ANALGESICS

Indomethacin (Indocin)	Confusion, depression, mania, paranoia, auditory and visual hallucinations, anxiety
Pentazocine (Talwin)	Depression, disorientation, paranoia, hallucinations

ANTICHOLINERGICS

Trihexyphenidyl (Artane), benztropine maleate (Cogentin), antidepressants	Confusion, delirium, disorientation, auditory and visual hallucinations, paranoia

ANTICONVULSANTS

Phenytoin (Dilantin), primidone (Mysoline)	Confusion, depression, paranoia, tactile and visual hallucinations, agitation, aggression, delirium

CARDIOVASCULAR DRUGS

Digitalis	Confusion, depression, delusions, visual hallucinations, belligerence
Propranolol (Inderal)	Confusion, depression, visual hallucinations
Methyldopa	Depression, hallucinations, paranoia

CORTICOSTEROIDS

Prednisone, cortisone	Confusion, depression, mania, paranoia, auditory and visual hallucinations

GASTROINTESTINAL DRUGS

Cimetidine	Confusion, depression, disorientation, paranoia, auditory and visual hallucinations, delirium

RESPIRATORY DRUGS

Ephedrine	Hallucinations, paranoia
Theophylline, aminophylline	Agitation, insomnia

MINOR TRANQUILIZERS

Diazepam (Valium), chlordiazepoxide hydrochloride (Librium)	Depression, excitement, rage, hallucinations

BARBITURATES

Phenobarbital	Depression, excitement, hyperactivity, visual hallucinations

the patterns of behavior can be put into place before the problem becomes less responsive to intervention. Concurrently effective management of the agitation and restlessness can also result in maintaining function or even gaining skills in daily living.

TREATMENT

Nursing treatment plans have various goals, which include the following:

1. Reducing the associated emotional distress
2. Harnessing the energy in ways that are constructive for the older person and acceptable to the caregivers
3. Maintaining nutrition and elimination
4. Arranging for adequate sleep and rest
5. Providing for a safe environment

HARNESSING ENERGY

The restless energy of these individuals (particularly their busy hands) can be channeled into *meaningful* activities that fall within their attention span, interests, and skills. They can fold laundry, dry silverware, help make beds, set the table, stir foods, mend, knit, crochet, hook or braid rugs, pull weeds in the garden, and go for walks.

MAINTAINING ADEQUATE NUTRITION AND ELIMINATION

Persons with agitation and restlessness burn up a lot of calories, yet these individuals often are unable to sit long enough to eat a full meal. One option is to provide nutritious finger foods such as sandwiches made with the essential nutrients, protein, and fiber, fresh fruits, and nutritious beverages. A second option is to serve small meals five to six times daily.

Bowel elimination is another high-risk area in daily living. Individuals with agitation and restlessness may not remember whether they have had a bowel movement, yet they may answer yes if asked. As a result, fecal impactions are common. Morning elimination is a helpful pattern to establish and bowel training should be provided to achieve this goal. Urinary incontinence may not be a problem if routine toileting is established (see Chapter 29 on urinary problems).

ARRANGING FOR ADEQUATE SLEEP AND REST

With rest patterns, as with activity, past patterns should serve as the guide to planning. The older person who has never napped in the daytime may only become more tense and anxious if he is scheduled to nap in the afternoon. Catnapping in a recliner in front of the TV may serve as well. Further, too much sleep in the daytime may result in greater nighttime wakefulness and activity. Fatigue levels need to be evaluated regularly. Finally, the strategies for gaining needed physical rest must be tailored to the individual's lifestyle, i.e., too much novelty in a treatment can have the insidious effect of increasing the level of anxiety and restlessness as the person tries to cope with the new elements in daily living.

EVALUATION

Response to nursing intervention can be evaluated in terms of reduced frequency or intensity of agitated or restless behaviors, improved record of patient safety, stability of weight, absence of fecal impactions or urinary problems, and evidence of a more satisfying quality of life for caregivers.

Daily Living with Aggressiveness, Hostility, and Combativeness

Aggressive or combative behavior is a complex problem occurring for numerous reasons and presenting in a variety of manners and intensities. It occurs at all levels of care and calls for sophisticated and creative problem solving skills. Combative, aggressive behavior or the fear of such behavior is poorly tolerated by families and staff of care facilities. This behavior affects literally every sphere of the older person's life. It can be manifested:

Verbally—(e.g., yelling, name calling, threats, swearing)
Physically—(e.g., hitting, biting, scratching, pushing, etc.)
Sexually—(e.g., exposing oneself or masturbating in public, touching or hitting caregivers on the breasts, or genitals)

At times intentional and at other times unintentional, aggressive behavior can be directed toward the self or toward other persons or objects. There is no way to predict in a foolproof manner if, when, or how aggression will occur. A history of aggressive behavior is the best indicator that it may be repeated. Current observations of behavior with the individual's history can increase the accuracy of foretelling the risk that this behavior may occur again. While such a process is helpful, the caregiver must constantly guard against the destructive sequelae that may result when labels (e.g., trouble maker, bully, fighter) of past behavior are brought to the present. It is wise to be prepared mentally and physically in planning care for persons with this problem, but it is imperative that the nurse offer each person an open nonjudgmental attitude that reflects not only genuine caring but an optimism as well that he will behave appropriately. This same attitude should be shown to persons who chronically demonstrate aggressive behavior.

ETIOLOGIES

The following five categories outline the range of possible etiologies associated with aggressive, hostile behavior in older adults:

1. Fear, misinterpretation, or inability to cope in delirium (acute confusional state) secondary to cerebral failure in acute medical or surgical conditions. Examples of such conditions are drug toxicity, pneumonia, postoperative states, metabolic derangement, and fecal impaction.
2. Fear, misinterpretation, or inability to cope in dementia (chronic confusional state) secondary to cerebral failure in chronic conditions such as Alzheimer's disease or multi-infarct dementia. This may occur in persons with known dementia or in cases of previously unrecognized and slowly developing dementia.
3. Delusions, hallucinations, fear, irritability, etc. in known psychiatric illness. Examples are chronic schizophrenia, paraphrenia, bipolar illness, major depression, or anxiety states. It is important to note that persons with psychiatric illness are no more dangerous than persons without such diagnoses. It is listed as an etiology due to the psychiatric symptom influence on some person's behavior.
4. Distress, frustration, or anxiety secondary to age-related losses, changes, and declining health. It is easy to understand these re-

sponses and increasing potential for aggression and hostility when older persons discover that society not only no longer needs or accepts them but merely tolerates, patronizes, or ignores them.
5. Intentional and chronic use of aggression as a lifelong coping and problem solving strategy. The person who resorted to aggression at ages 25, 35, and 45 will likely maintain the aggressive approaches when they are 75 and 85 years old.

Other risk factors include the following:

Sharing living space with persons who have similar sensory deficits as the patient

Acute or unresolved discomfort or pain related to unmet physical needs

Inappropriate action or behavior by an unskilled caregiver

Frustration at the perception that others are preventing the person from accomplishing something he wants to do

Times of higher risk may occur when families come to visit or when they leave, or in times of increased fatigue

PREVENTION

It is better to prevent an aggressive incident than to have to intervene during or after one has occurred. Prevention of overt aggression requires an understanding of the dynamics of the phenomenon.

PRINCIPLES AND STRATEGIES OF PREVENTION

1. Maintain a positive, optimistic attitude and outlook. Of all strategies for prevention and intervention none carries a greater influence or has a more lasting impact than the demeanor of the caregiver. At the very least, attitude presentation should be neutral.
2. Perform regular reviews of the health and circumstances of the older person to identify and reverse problems before a crisis arises. This review should include correction of hearing and vision deficits.
3. Keep medication use to a minimum.
4. Stroke frequently with physical touch and verbal recognition. Persons whose recognition needs are not met may resort to disruptive behavior to secure the attention they desire.

5. Assist the older person to maintain control in his life by increasing choices by involving him in decision making. Limited choices may have to be offered at first.
6. Maintain awareness of importance of social and environmental consistency—particularly important for the confused person. The goal is creating predictability, security, and stimulation without overstimulation in a stable, easily read environment:

   Establish a reasonably fixed daily routine
   Reduce apprehensions by reassuring, answering questions, orienting frequently, providing time frames, and posting schedules
   Provide reality orientation cues (e.g., clock, calendar, current magazines, newspaper)
   Keep furniture in the same arrangement
   Keep clutter to a minimum

7. Conduct daily, and as needed, environmental inspections:

   Assess and adjust lighting. Intense lighting, flickering lights, and reflective glaring surfaces can provoke aggressive acts. Likewise, inadequate lighting can trigger a similar response
   Adjust the noise level (television, radio, talking). Soft music can be quite calming
   Adjust crowded areas to reduce stimulation
   Reduce excessive movement and activity
   Ensure room temperature is within the comfort zone for the older person; offer sweaters when indicated

8. Maintain a working knowledge of therapeutic communication skills (refer to Chapter 18 for specific communication skills to be used with confused persons).
9. Record and maintain an awareness of individual triggers, escalation patterns, and cycles as well as known effective interventions. It is helpful to have identified two or three interventions discerned to be effective in deescalating the behavior once it has been triggered.
10. Anticipate times of confusion (i.e., change in schedule or environmental change, sleep deprivation, physical illness, etc.) and make adjustments in expectations.
11. Schedule routine exercise periods for both the older adult and the caregiver to increase tolerance to stress and better equip them to manage stress.

CRISIS CYCLE

The crisis cycle is a useful model to assist caregivers in both the assessment and intervention phases of problem solving with hostile, aggressive and combative behavior. It provides a visual depiction of the behaviors as they increase and decrease in intensity and can guide the caregiver in deciding which intervention to use depending on where the person is assessed to be in the cycle at any given point. Refer to Figure 19–3.

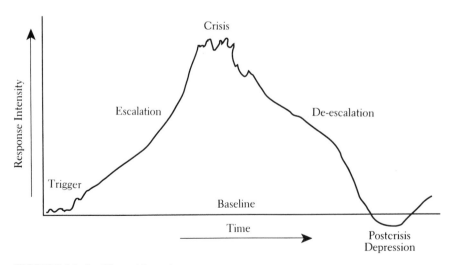

FIGURE 19–3   The crisis cycle.

TRIGGER

When individuals exceed their tolerance for stress they are said to have been triggered and the crisis cycle is started. Triggers can be internal (e.g., pain, constipation, hallucination) or external (e.g., hot day, demanding caregiver, invasion into personal space). Knowing what tends to provoke or trigger a person are key elements in planning care. This information should be documented and accessible to all caregivers.

ESCALATION

Escalation is generally manifested through increasing levels of activity. Alternatively, reduction of activity in an otherwise outgoing active person may signal escalation in that person. Changes from normal behavior are the tip-off that a closer look is indicated. Constant reference and comparison must be made to the person's baseline or normal behavior. The time from escalation to crisis may vary from minutes to days or weeks. Evidence that energy is building toward a critical level in a person may include the following:

Increasing agitation and irritability
Increasing impulsivity
Disturbed thought processes and perceptions
Anger disproportionate to events or mistrust
    and suspicion
Misinterpretation of sensory stimuli
Misinterpretation of the behavior of others

Specific behaviors may include

Crying (tears)
Widened eyes
Increased volume of voice
Increased rate of speech
Increased psychomotor behavior (pacing, picking, grabbing, hair twisting)
Frowning
Shaking or trembling

INTERVENTION

Early Intervention   The primary goal of early intervention is to assist the individuals to return to their baseline behaviors, thereby averting a crisis. Be alert for subtle cues. Apparently mild mannered people are capable of hostile acts. The guiding principle to follow is that the least intrusive and restrictive interventions should be tried first. Only if they are ineffective should more restrictive measures be considered. Therefore, nonphysical behavioral interventions are implemented initially. Medication and physical intervention (e.g., restraint) are considered more restrictive. Intervention strategies to be used during early escalation include the following:

1. Decrease environmental stimulation (e.g., turn television or radio down or off, turn heat up or down, check lighting, noise level).
2. Touch (i.e., hand holding, an arm around the shoulder or massage) when done with discretion can demonstrate caring, reduce tension, and lead to increased control for him.
3. Offer a diversional activity (e.g., rocking in a rocking chair or walking offers a physical outlet), reading, board games, snack, warm bath. This is a prime opportunity to use the interventions known by history to be calming to the person. It is not helpful to provide a pillow or punching bag so that the person can release anger; this perpetuates the anger rather than dissipating it.
4. Keep him talking, as this is an effective method to distract him from abusive thoughts. Talking and assaulting at the same time are generally not compatible.
5. One to one communication. (See box on p. 324.)
6. Medication may be used after behavioral interventions have been unsuccessfully tried but before a crisis develops. PRN medications are used to prevent a crisis from occurring or to minimize its intensity and duration if it does occur. In most situations it is not beneficial to medicate a person who is in the middle of an aggressive act or has already completed it. The natural course of the crisis cycle will be to deescalate and return to his baseline level, which can generally be facilitated through behavioral methods.

Continued Escalation and Later Intervention   Generally, hostile aggressive persons see themselves as helpless and powerless victims. They feel unable to act effectively. The situation becomes intolerable and aggressive behavior is seen as the only solution. When escalation continues as evidenced as exaggerated behaviors and louder, more specific verbal threats (e.g., "I'm going to hit you" and "I can't

Communication Techniques for Use During Escalation

1. Use a calm, quiet tone of voice and a calm manner. Behave in ways that model and support the person's ability to remain calm, cooperative, and in control supports his worth and self-esteem. The caregiver sets the tone and can change the direction of an escalation through modeling.

2. Maintain eye contact with "soft eyes."

3. Call the person by name. Repeat the name often (using the name he prefers) throughout the conversation at the beginning or end of sentences. This will help to maintain his attention.

4. Talk at eye level (e.g., sit down if the person is seated, stand if he is standing).

5. If the person is standing, use an oblique or side stance posture as it is safer should the person kick or strike out and may be less threatening to the person than a toe to toe posture.

6. Use active listening. Effective listening is a deceptively simple intervention that can make or break an interaction. Do not busy yourself with other tasks. Recognize the value of anger as an emotion and avoid equating it with aggression. Allowing verbal and emotional expression of anger can prevent a physical display of it. Try to determine whether there is a feeling that the person's viewpoint or feelings are being ignored and if this is causing discomfort.

7. Ask what is causing the tension you observe. If the person is unable to identify the cause immediately, anxiety may climb if pushed to come up with a reason.

8. Ask the person for clarification. Ask for specific examples: "What do you mean? I'm not clear." You may think you understand a complaint or a behavior. If in doubt, make sure. Paraphrasing can be helpful, e.g., "Are you saying you feel angry when John tells you what to do rather than asks you what you want to do?"

9. Ask how the person usually handles these feelings and suggest he try that approach.

10. Discuss the person's behavior with him. Describe what you see but never scold, punish, threaten, or shame the person. Deal with the obvious, and here and now.

11. Assist in problem solving. The person may never have acquired good problem solving skills, which may be the reason he resorts to aggressive behavior. Help the person to identify the problem, look at options, set priorities, and make decisions.

12. Comply with reasonable requests. This builds trust and assures the person that you are willing to work with him.

13. Use the word "please" when making requests. This demonstrates respect and gives the person control through providing an option.

14. Avoid arguments or discussions that stimulate hostility and aggression. Use a matter-of-fact approach.

15. Give constructive feedback. If the person is gaining some insight into the behavior and change is apparent, he needs constructive feedback from caregivers. Use all positive reinforcers available to maintain the behavior changes.

16. Allow adequate personal space. The further the person moves up the escalation slope, the greater will be the need for more personal space. It is not wise to move toward or touch a person who is escalating. The gesture may be misinterpreted and responded to with aggression.

Communication Techniques for Use During Escalation (*Continued*)

17. Outline expectations in advance. Before a problem arises, set out the behavioral expectations in a calm manner.

18. Set limits. Do so politely, but firmly. Set limits in response to specific situations. Consistency is the key. Be sure all involved caregivers know the established limits.

19. Face verbal abuse, vulgarity, and profanity as a symptom of pathology (like coughing or muscle weakness), not as a personal affront. Help families to understand the behavior as a symptom of disease. If you are caught off guard or cannot think of how to respond therapeutically to a threat, accusation, or other angry, hostile remark it is better to ignore it than to allow yourself to become angry also. This will only add fuel to the fire.

20. Express your own feelings of discomfort with the behaviors (e.g., "I get scared when you double your fist and raise your hand") but at the same time outline the behavioral limits that the person is expected to maintain.

take it any more") and the earlier interventions have been ineffective, the following interventions are added:

Pay attention to your own impression that the person is growing hostile. One's own intuition at the scene is the best indicator of an impending aggressive act. Share your intuitions with family and other caregivers. Instruct family members and primary caregivers to share their intuitions when tense behavior occurs in a home setting.

Where the situation is volatile, arrange to have someone with you or nearby. This helps to moderate both the patient's and the caregiver's anxiety.

Whatever the setting, always arrange your position closer to the exit than the patient's.

Bear in mind that attention is reinforcing. At whatever point you begin to attend to the person, you are giving reinforcement to that behavior.

Talking with the person does little good at this point. As the situation escalates the individual becomes unable to cope with making choices so the caregiver must make the choices for him (e.g., "John, come, I will walk with you to the garden" or "Mary, come with me please"). Verbal interaction should be matter of fact and directed in short sentences.

Contract with him: I'll do something for you and you do something for me (e.g., "I'll get you some coffee and you come to your room to sit with me").

Help him save face by offering problem solving options that are more attractive than the option of assault.

CRISIS

When escalation continues to overt aggression such as kicking, pushing, hitting, biting, hair pulling, etc., there are additional intervention strategies the caregiver should add to the interaction:

Look for other people and let them know you are in trouble. Back up help does not have to be visible.

Scan the room for potential weapons that the person may pick up. It is best that the caregiver not have a weapon as the patient may grab it.

Do not point at the person as it may be perceived as intrusive and controlling.

Use short directive sentences without anger. At this point the person often is unable to make choices or follow lengthy explanations of why you are asking him to do something. Always include "please" with any request.

Clear the area of other people.

Avoid physically touching the person if possible. Physical contact will increase the probability of injury to both patient and caregiver.

Try a "show of force" (also known as a "show of support") if other persons are available at a time when the patient refuses your verbal request. This may instill a sense of relief in the person that there is help to care for him if he loses control and may in and of itself help him regain self-control. Seek a position of defense, do not attack. Approach in a semi-circle formation as a team. Try to avoid the area directly in front of the abusive person. Maintain visual contact of other team members so you can work together. One person will try to "talk him down." Approach slowly. Fast movements may increase the patient's perception of threat and increase the likelihood that he will strike out in defense.

Communicate with other team members by talking "to and through" the aggressive person. While maintaining eye contact and conversation with the person deliver messages and instructions to other staff or persons who have come to assist, e.g., "John, Bill, and I will walk with you to the blue chair in the TV room." In this manner everyone knows what to expect and the line of communication with the patient never has to be broken to consult with others.

Avoid arguing about strategy disagreements until after the patient is taken care of. Philosophies and approach of nurses may differ but to take issue with the person leading the team at the time of a crisis is poor judgment and will only add stress to the situation.

DEESCALATION

Deescalation is the emotional and behavioral movement back to the baseline. The behaviors exhibited in this phase of the crisis cycle are often similar to those demonstrated during escalation. The focus for the family or caregiver will be to facilitate the person's return to the baseline without retriggering another crisis. The following interventions are suggested:

Move the person to a quiet, private place.

Reassure the individual that the worst is over now. Convey in a nonthreatening manner that maintenance of self-control is expected.

Debrief the incident with the person. Ask which interventions and actions by caregivers were helpful during the incident and which were not. Note his responses for future use.

Again, do not pressure for answers that are not forthcoming. Use the deescalation phase for teaching prevention of future incidents.

Touch can be supportive and display caring.

Assess for any injuries that may have occurred during the incident.

POSTCRISIS DEPRESSION

Most persons experience some degree of regret, remorse, or guilt following an assault. Even persons with chronic confusion who are severely memory impaired often display behavior describing emotional discomfort following aggressive behavior. Depending on the degree of remorse, the person's perception of the severity of the incident, and the range of coping skills there may be withdrawal from others and from performing ADL tasks. In some cases the person may feel badly enough to attempt to hurt himself. The caregiver should:

Observe closely.

Provide verbal support (e.g., "Can I do anything to help you feel better?") and reassuring physical touch if this is acceptable to the individual.

Allow rest. Failure to allow the body this rest time may serve as another stressor.

Attempt to elicit information regarding the nature of the trigger. Be sensitive to the capacity to discuss it at this time.

EVALUATION

Evaluation of the nursing treatment can be measured by recording the frequency of combative, hostile episodes, the comfort of the staff, family, and friends with the person, the comfort of the person with himself, and the use of nonaggressive problem solving strategies.

CAREGIVER NEEDS

A debriefing for the caregivers is part and parcel of the process and should never be overlooked. This is the time to identify one's own feelings about the incident or behavior and to reflect on how these may interfere with the ability therapeutically to intervene. It is important to recognize that as one becomes more involved in an assault, the ability to make sound judgments may fluctuate, and as the stress increases that judgment may decrease. It is necessary for nurses to evaluate their own reactions and facilitate the debriefing of others to note their impressions and evaluate the effectiveness of their own behavior and interventions. Ask "What did we do right? What could we have done differently? What might we do if this occurs again?" The single caregiver needs to participate in this evaluative process as well, perhaps more than those who work in teams.

Family members may need to be helped to seek out feelings and to plan with each other.

Possibly one of the hardest parts of coping with aggressive behavior is taking care of oneself. There are patient evaluations, paper work, and the needs of other persons that may usurp all the time and energy the caregiver feels she has. Without debriefing as well as some routine measures of stress management (e.g., physical exercise, hobbies, music, etc.) the caregivers may carry the turmoil of the event or behaviors and thus set themselves up for ongoing difficulties in daily living.

Daily Living with Frequent Requests for Help or Attention

Extremely frequent requests for help can be due to the person's loneliness, anxiety, or need to feel more control over the environment. It may also be part of an irritability that can be associated with depression.

RISK FACTORS

Misdiagnosis (e.g., the person who has a clinical depression may be overlooked and not provided the assistance to treat the problem).
As with the person who continually yells, the one who is demanding of the caregiver's time and attention risks losing that person's interest and desire to respond, which becomes particularly critical when there is a genuine emergency or need.
Social isolation.

PROGNOSTIC VARIABLES

The person who has the capacity for insight and desire for behavioral change may be considered a good candidate for therapy and behavioral interventions. The success of such programs hinges on the commitment and consistency of the caregivers.

INTERVENTIONS

Some helpful concepts and approaches include the following:

1. Schedule one to one time on a daily basis with a person the patient trusts, in order to address loneliness.

2. Assist the older person to "repeople" his world. Older persons have been found to be most often lonely for someone who is deceased. Companions of the same age seem to be as important to older persons as to younger people. Women tend to find relief with their families; men more with friends. However, for either sex, living alone has been found to increase the likelihood of loneliness. Some options for repeopling may be found in retirement communities, day care centers, senior centers, senior citizen groups in churches, and classes open to older persons on college campuses. Nurses in long-term care settings may find that offering the older person special time with someone he enjoys to be a help. Whether a staff member, a volunteer, or a family member, the schedule should be designed so that it can be adhered to (i.e., the person must be able to visit with the frequency and duration that is scheduled). A calendar on the person's wall can have scheduled visits noted and serve as a reminder of upcoming times for special attention.

3. Use pets as surrogates for human intimacy. They can be a source of comfort during the high-risk evening and night hours or the Sunday afternoons when others are busy. Where human contacts are limited and the person's lifestyle and finances can accommodate a pet, this may be an effective way to offer a dependable living presence and help the person occupy time. The pet owner can feel needed, and there is a source of dependable affection.

4. Offering the person real choices about what to wear, what to eat, what to do for leisure activity, and when and where to do these things can help increase feelings of control.

5. Try setting up a check-in schedule with the person to indicate when someone will be available. Supplying paper and pen for jotting down concerns or needs to give to the caregiver at the designated check-in times can be quite effective. It is critical that the scheduled check-in times be strictly adhered to. Another variation of this approach may be found in the use of cards that may be used to "pay" for each check-in by the caregiver when summoned by the patient. The patient is given a certain number of cards at the beginning of each day to be used at his or her own discretion, but once the cards are "spent" the person may not call any more unless it is a true emergency.

Daily Living with Refusal to Do Personal Grooming and Hygiene

The refusal to perform personal grooming and hygiene care or cooperate with a caregiver to do these tasks may be a symptom of acute or chronic confusion. The person may not understand what is being asked of him. It may be a symptom of depression in which the person feels fatigued, uninterested, or overwhelmed by the request being made. It may be a reflection of personal preference and lifestyle. Or it may be demonstrative of the disorganization experienced by some persons with chronic schizophrenia or bipolar illness.

RISK FACTORS

Social isolation
Dental caries

PROGNOSTIC VARIABLES

The person who can see and value the consequence or reward of the behavioral change will be more likely to be interested in becoming involved in a program. Once again, the caregiver's patience and flexibility play key roles in the success of changing this type of behavior.

INTERVENTIONS

The person may be described as having the ability but "just won't do it." The first principle to keep in mind is that the label "lack of motivation" does not solve the problem. It can, in fact, make the situation worse by placing fault or blame and creating an adversarial relationship between the person and the caregiver. The following interventions may be of help:

1. A bargaining approach may be effective for some tasks such as grooming or dressing (e.g., "Would you please put your shirt on and I'll be there in a few minutes to help you with your pants").
2. A system of immediate rewards can be instituted for cooperation with care or completion of specific tasks with minimal prompts. It is important to identify what is rewarding to the person by asking him or someone who knows the person well. Generally an immediate payoff is appropriate, or if a points system is used (in which the person earns cred-

its toward some larger reward) the reward should be given at least every 24 hours.
3. Depending on the specifics of the behavior problem, it can be helpful for a staff person who has a special relationship with the person to work with him. The usefulness of this should be weighed against potential burnout for the staff member, if the patient is particularly difficult.
4. Use a reapproach technique if the person becomes angered by the caregiver's request to perform. Allow time to regroup and indicate in a calm matter-of-fact tone when you will be back. If behavior has transgressed appropriate or acceptable levels tell the person so in a straightforward manner.
5. Give the person some choice about the undesirable activity you are asking to be performed. For example, offer choices between a bath or shower and preferred time of day for bathing.
6. Attempt to give the person increased control and dignity in the situation. Assign a task and leave the room long enough to allow the person to perform independently.

Daily Living with the Person Who Stays in His Bed or Room and Refuses to Get Up or Participate in Activities

There are few things as frustrating to a caregiver as facing the person who refuses to get out of bed, leave his room, or do any activity despite having the capacity to do so.

RISK FACTORS

Refusing to participate in activities is often concomitant with depression but can also signal physical illness. It can also be a personal preference of the individual. It becomes difficult to sort out the possible causes and even more challenging to make determinations as to appropriate intervention. It is important to respect preference but equally important to realize the cascading detrimental physical and mental sequelae related to isolation and immobility.

PROGNOSTIC VARIABLES

Those persons with strong support systems and patient, tolerant caregivers will fare better and progress faster and further than those persons without this support. Accurate diagnosis and treatment of depression, if this is the etiology, is obviously critical to affecting change.

INTERVENTION

The caregiver may be left feeling helpless in such a situation, but it is generally not of any benefit to label the person as uncooperative or unmotivated. Reframing the caregiver's perception of the situation to allow the person the choice not to get up will help to remove negative feelings that the caregiver may have developed. The fact that the person "chooses" rather than "refuses" may be a step-off point for thinking about the behavior. These behaviors may be deliberate and related to personality and lifestyle preferences, but may be associated with paranoid disorders or depression and are often compounded by the fact that it may be easier for the family or caregiver to allow the person to stay in bed or isolate himself than it is to work toward getting the person up. Treatment of the underlying etiology will likely restore energy and purpose. However, in the meantime, for the physical health of the older person, it is very important to get him out of bed to prevent complications arising from the behavior that were not inherent in the underlying illness. The following strategies can be used:

1. Discuss with the person in a direct but caring manner the importance of getting up and staying active. This will be most effective if done by a person the patient likes and trusts. Avoid overconcern or false cheerfulness.
2. Be aware of the person's fears and sense of discomfort with physical and interpersonal closeness; maintain appropriate physical distance to avoid breaking in on his privacy.
3. Use brief statements (e.g., "I came to see you. I will stay with you for 5 minutes").
4. Provide time frames (i.e., tell the person when you are leaving and when you will return).
5. Do not expect or push the person to respond initially, but make general comments, pausing or asking questions occasionally to "open the door" for participation.
6. As the person's comfort level permits, gradually expand the amount of time you spend with him and as he improves introduce one-to-one activity with another resident if in a long-term care facility. In shar-

ing activities, even parallel activities (such as watching television) as opposed to interactive activities (such as card games), one gains the self-image of sameness with another.

7. Attempt gradually to increase the numbers of persons with whom the person can interact.
8. Verbal praise and recognition is always helpful. In providing this type of reenforcement, it is most meaningful to make "I" rather than "we" statements, e.g., "I am glad you joined us today," or "I feel proud of you," rather than "We are so glad you joined us."
9. A system of rewards may be useful in this situation also. The person can be rewarded with something meaningful when he gets up. In cases where the patient is particularly resistive and rewards are hard to come up with, the caregiver may resort to allowing the person to return to bed as a reward if he will get up and walk down the hall.
10. The person's movement in bed should be monitored, with positioning and active or passive exercising done when the person does not do it himself to prevent skin breakdown and minimize the effects of immobility.

Daily Living with the Person Who Refuses to Eat

The gravity of the situation for a person who refuses to eat is related to the age and health of the elderly person and the amount of food and fluids being consumed. The risks are greater if the person refuses all fluid or food and the refusal continues for a long time, increasing the risk of dehydration and malnourishment.

RISK FACTORS

Refusal to eat can signal a physical illness. It can be a symptom of depression or a result of a paranoid delusion when the person is suspicious of food and fears it is poisoned or hears a command hallucination not to eat. It may also be a manipulative gesture to gain attention.

INTERVENTION

The following interventions may be used to address the problem:

1. Do not nag at the person. Offer gentle, matter-of-fact encouragement. Observe intake for 1 to 2 days. Lack of food for this time will not likely be detrimental. However, lack of fluid is a critical situation. Dehydration can occur in an alarmingly short time in elderly persons.
2. Emphasize that food is nutritious and has not been tampered with.
3. Include the person in meal planning as much as is feasible.
4. Provide as much control for the person as is possible by allowing him to select meal time, dining site, portions of foods, etc.
5. Offer snacks and fluids between meals.
6. Tasting food or drinks to "prove" they are safe is not often helpful in that the person may design some reason why you are protected from harm but he is still threatened.
7. Persistent low intake will require a tray or plate monitor as well as specific recording of fluid intake.
8. Weigh the person daily.

Daily Living with Chronic Suspicion and Mistrust

Suspiciousness and paranoid thoughts are common in chronic schizophrenia as well as late onset of emotional disturbances, e.g., paraphrenia and dementia. The intensity or severity and duration of the symptoms fall along a continuum from mild to severe. Paranoid states may include delusions that are narrow and situational, e.g., others are taking the person's things or interfering with property. The individual can manage daily living and communications well outside of these areas. These older persons tend to live in the community; their neighbors tolerate them and their bizarre behavior as obviously abnormal but nonthreatening.

Another group of persons experience paranoid thoughts that are more widespread, e.g., their home is bugged with microphones or people are talking about them. For this group of persons, suspicion and chronic mistrust is more diffuse, general, and pervasive. It results in greater disorganization throughout their everyday lives. They tend to be loners and may continue in their disarray until someone discovers the effects their fears are having on their environment and health status.

A third group includes those persons with clear schizophrenic symptoms. The consequent impact of the symptoms on daily living falls along a continuum, though not necessarily congruent to the symptom intensity. For example, an involved fixed paranoid delusion can create dramatic distress for one individual while another person experiencing similar beliefs may not be particularly troubled by them.

RISK FACTORS

Those persons with hearing impairment are at high risk.

Those with frank psychotic pathology having elements of paranoid ideation.

Those who in earlier times have experienced (or perceived) personal (physical and/or mental) abuse or threats.

Those who have recently been threatened, robbed, or assaulted.

SIGNS AND SYMPTOMS

Signs and symptoms of mistrust and chronic suspicion can range from mild to severe. They also can become progressive. Early signs may include the following:

Unwillingness to open the door
Locking of all doors, windows, and drawers
Undue caution about answering questions
Behaving in secretive ways when relating to others
Limiting personal contacts to one or two people
Leaving blinds drawn or drapes closed at all times
Reporting that they feel others are talking about them
Phoning crisis clinics or emergency services to talk about perceived threats
Responding disproportionately to threatening noises, gossip, and misplaced objects
Tending to misinterpret input to support their sense of threat

All of these behaviors obviously alter the person's daily living and the ways in which the requirements of daily living are met.

Severe disability related to chronic mistrust and suspicion manifests itself in behaviors that include the following:

Accentuation of all early behaviors
Failing to shop for food or refills of medications

because of fear of harm if the person leaves his home

Hiding of possessions, e.g., jewelry, dentures, and glasses

Hoarding of supplies, garbage, papers, or other materials in the living space

Increasing avoidance of physical contact with others

Delusions of threat from people who "come through their walls or appliances," poisoning or gassing from heat outlets, and so on

Growing confusion or psychotic phenomena such as hallucinations

Increasing risk of abusive behavior if others ignore or deprecate their delusions

The increasing disruption to daily living and threats to health with this type of deterioration are easily seen.

PROGNOSTIC VARIABLES

Unless the threat to safety is actual and genuine security can be established, the prognosis for a good quality of life for elderly persons with chronic suspicion is poor. Their ideas tend to be firmly entrenched and rarely can be dislodged. These people tend to be able to continue to live in the community as others around them accommodate to their behavior. They can alienate and frighten others when they talk only about their fixed ideation.

TREATMENT

Since these older people will tend to continue to live in the community, nursing management concerns not only the suspicious persons but also those who must live near them.

For mistrustful older persons, the following guidelines may prove helpful to caregivers.

Understand that the behavior of these older persons is not rational; therefore, attempting to alter the thinking or behavior by using logic is not likely to be effective. The behavior is a symptom or sign just like an ulcer on the leg that does not heal.

Set limits on what they talk about. Suggest that they may need to talk about their concerns to the nurse or another designated person who will understand their situation, but that they may wish to limit discussions of their fears and suspicions with others who might not understand.

Behave nonjudgmentally. Do not put the person down.

Develop "scripts" in advance, ones they will then be available for use when particular situations arise.

Be alert to cues that the individual may be becoming combative (see signs and symptoms in the section on aggressiveness earlier in the chapter) and take seriously the prodromal signs. Teach caregivers the behaviors and safety guidelines for hostile combative behavior (see treatment of aggressiveness discussed earlier in the chapter).

In all stages of this behavioral style it is important for the nurse or family to determine the critical areas of daily living that are at risk because of the person's fears, e.g., shopping for food, cooking, eating, getting medication refills, taking medications, personal hygiene, and so on. When these areas have been identified, interventions and monitoring need to be scheduled to ensure that these activities and tasks are being maintained in a safe, effective way.

EVALUATION

Since this condition is chronic and tends to preclude help from others, by its very nature, evaluation is based on indicators of continued safety and well-being to the extent that trust can be established and protection and care can be given. Responses of family, neighbors, and caregivers to nursing management can be evaluated in terms of their comfort and success in relating to the individual and their confidence in the strategies and scripts they have developed.

Daily Living with a Chronic Negative Perspective

There is one group of older persons who create difficulties in daily living, not only for themselves but also for all those around them. They tend to be a souring, corrosive force. These are the older people who seem to find their pleasure in seeing the bleakest, the blackest, the most negative elements in any situation—even in the good things that happen to them. Their behaviors almost guarantee that their predictions become self-fulfilling prophesies as it relates to their own well-being. For them, the cup is always half empty, never half full. Their negativism is rarely related to their disabilities—it is a way of life. They are the ones who gossip, test limits, deprecate their own and others' efforts, seek special attention, and offer resistance to programs.

The following are some guidelines that caregivers and family members can use in dealing with these negative individuals:

Get them involved in doing an activity, even though they may complain the whole time. The first step is to ask the person if there is anything available that he does enjoy. If the person is able to identify something, try to increase the frequency or availability of it. If the person cannot identify anything enjoyable or pleasant, ask what he would like to have changed that would make the situation more tolerable. Attempt to address the person's wishes.

Accept the deprecating, complaining behavior, but continue to recognize positive contributions and outcomes, even as they negate them.

Agree on an approach in which all staff members and family members will behave consistently in responding to specified behavior. Routines are helpful.

Give honest feedback to the person regarding your feelings when he constantly complains or finds fault.

Be reliable and dependable. Do what you say you will do, when you said you would do it.

Set limits. For example, gossiping is not accepted behavior in this setting.

Try giving the person a scheduled time to voice complaints. Indicate that complaints will be discussed only at the scheduled time and that reminders will be given at designated times if he should forget. Try to discuss concerns at nondesignated times. Genuine attention should be given at the complaint time.

Use a firm but kind and caring approach.

EVALUATION

It is not reasonable to expect that long-standing negativism will be replaced by a positive style in daily living, even with skilled nursing intervention. Responses may occur in areas of continued functioning and participation in activities and events of daily living, despite the negative attitude. Nursing management may also lessen the effect of the negative behavior on others.

Responses to nursing management by family members and primary caregivers may occur in areas such as greater understanding of the older person's behavior and increased confidence and comfort in the strategies developed for dealing with the negative elements of the older person's lifestyle.

Daily living with wandering, pilfering, hoarding, and yelling are all behavior problems generally associated with dementia and are discussed in Chapter 18.

References and Other Readings

Abrahams J, Crooks V. Geriatric mental health. Orlando, FL: Grune & Stratton, 1984.

Aronson M, Gaston P, Merriam A. Depression associated with dementia. Generations 1984; 9:49.

Bennett R, Gurland B. The acting-out elderly. New York: The Haworth Press, 1983.

Berni R, Fordyce W. Behavior modification and the nursing process. St Louis: CV Mosby, 1973.

Bettis S. Depression: the "common cold" of the elderly. Generations 1979; 3:15.

Brower H. The alternatives to restraints. J Gerontol Nurs 1991; 17:18.

Campion M, Maletta G. Behavior: a symptom of cognitive and functional disorders. In: Gorden G, Stryker R, eds. Creative long-term care administration. Springfield, IL: Charles C Thomas, 1983:228.

Cassel CW, Walsh JR. Geriatric medicine (2nd ed.). New York: Springer-Verlag, 1990.

Cohen JD, Eisdorfer C. Major psychiatric and behavioral disorders in the aged. In: Andres R, Bierman E, Hazzard W, eds. Principles in geriatric medicine. New York: McGraw-Hill, 1985:867.

Cohen L: Coping with anxiety: a step-by-step guide. Nursing '79, 1979; 34.

Conney M, Nolan P. Management of the disturbed patient. Nurs Times 1979; 75:1896.

Evans L, Strumpf N. Tying down the elderly. Am Geriatr Soc 1989; 35:65.

Friedman J: Cry for help: suicide in the aged. J Gerontol Nurs 1976; 2:28.

Goldenberg B, Chiverton P. Assessing behavior: the nurses' mental status exam. Geriatr Nurs 1984; 5:94.

Gwyther L, Matteson M. Care for the caregivers. J Gerontol Nurs 1983; 9:92.

Katz S. Assessing self-maintenance: activities of daily living, mobility and instrumental activities of daily living. J Am Geriatr Soc 1983; 31:721.

Larson M. Violent behaviors: clinical practice in nursing assessment and intervention. In: Long D, Williams R, (eds): New York: Appleton-Century-Crofts, 1978:175.

Levine A. Visual hallucinations and cataracts. Ophthalmic Surg 1980; 11:95.

Mace N, Robins P. The 36-hour day (2nd ed.). Baltimore: Johns Hopkins University Press, 1991.

Mitchell-Pederson, et al: Reducing reliance on physical restraints. Today's Nurs Home 1986; 7:40.

Paykel E, Fleminger R, Watson J. Psychiatric side effects of antihypertensive drugs other than reserpine. J Clin Psychopharmacol 1982; 2:14.

Pisarcik G: The violent patient. Nursing '81 1981; 63.

Radar J, Harvath T. How to document difficult behaviors. Geriatr Nurs 1991; 12:231.

Reifler B, et al. Coexistence of cognitive impairment and depression in geriatric outpatients. Am J Psychiatry 1982; 139:623.

Reifler B, Eisdorfer C. A clinic for impaired elderly and their families. Am J Psychiatry 1980; 137:1300.

Requarth C. Medication usage and interaction in the long-term care of the elderly. J Gerontol Nurs 1979; 5:33.

Rosenthal R. Now hear this: that difficult patient may be hard of hearing. In: Inservice Training and Education, 1983.

Schafer A. Restraints and the elderly: when safety and autonomy conflict. Can Med Assoc J 1985; 132:1257.

Wurtman RJ. Alzheimer's disease. Sci Am 1985; 252:62.

Zimmer JG, Watson N, Treat A. Behavioral problems among patients in skilled nursing facilities. Am J Public Health 1984; 74:1118.

20
Parkinson's Disease

MARIA LINDE

Pathophysiology and Medical Management

Parkinson's disease (PD) is a progressive neurologic disorder primarily affecting people over 50 years of age (Hoehn and Yahr, 1967). However, an estimated 10% to 15% of the parkinsonian population have symptom onset before age 40. PD has been estimated to have a prevalence rate of 100 to 150 per 100,000, with an incidence rate of 20 cases per 100,000 annually (Yahr, 1982). With the world population showing an aging trend, PD can be expected to increase.

PD has existed in our society for a long time. It was not until 1817, however, that Dr. James Parkinson reported and described the signs and symptoms of parkinsonism (Parkinson, 1817).

The term *parkinsonism* is used to label a symptom complex that may develop secondary to known causes or appear as a feature among several diseases of the nervous system referred to as parkinsonism-*plus* (Jancovic, 1989). Parkinsonism may also develop as a manifestation of an idiopathic disorder referred to as PD.

The most common form of the symptom complex is idiopathic PD, the subject of most of this chapter. However, in the early stages and through the course of the illness, the neurologic conditions of the various forms of parkinsonism share many of the signs and symptoms and create some of the same difficulties in managing daily living. Atypical signs, accelerated rate of progression, and diminished efficacy of levodopa should always be cues to consider a diagnosis other than PD (Kedas et al, 1989).

On an initial evaluation a patient had all the typical symptoms of PD and was given a prescription for levodopa. In her visit to the clinic 6 months later, she had developed opthalmoplegia of vertical gaze and her family observed that levodopa was of little benefit. Her family reported that she now had problems in climbing stairs, had frequent falls, and spilled a lot when eating. The neurologist changed the diagnosis to progressive supranuclear palsy (Garland and Warner, 1988).

CAUSES OF PARKINSONISM

The causes of parkinsonism include drugs, neurotoxins, metabolic diseases, and structural changes.

Drugs	Neuroleptics: phenothiazines, thioxanthenes
	Antiemetics: metoclopramide, prochlorperazine
	Antihypertensive: reserpine
Neurotoxins	MPTP: methyl-14-phenyl 1-1,2,3,6 tetrahydopyridine
	Chronic manganese poisoning
	Chronic disulfide inhalation
	Acute cyanide poisoning
	Chronic carbon monoxide exposure
Metabolic	Hallervorden-Spatz disease
	Wilson's disease
	Hepatocerebral degeneration

...basal gan-

...phalus

...repeated head trauma (dementia pugilistica)

...EDITY

A positive family history is found in 15% to
20% of cases. PD occurs worldwide, but geographic and racial differences may exist. A similar incidence has been found in both sexes.

RISK FACTORS

The strongest known risk factor for PD is age,
indicating that the underlying process of the
pathology is time dependent. Other risk factors
include smoking (Rajput et al, 1987) and special
premorbid personalities who are introverted
and have a need for high achievement (Todes
and Lee, 1985), and familial history.

PARKINSONISM-PLUS

Parkinsonism-plus involves several syndromes
with parkinsonian features plus added symptoms and features. The differential diagnosis is
important in order to provide appropriate treatment.

PROGRESSIVE SUPRANUCLEAR PALSY

Parkinsonism plus supranuclear opthalmoplegia chiefly affects the vertical gaze. This condition is resistant to levodopa except in the early
stages. Findings indicating the presence of this
syndrome include reports of difficulty in climbing stairs and increasing messiness in eating.
This disorder is progressive and becomes terminal in a decade.

OLIVOPONTOCEREBELLAR ATROPHY

This condition presents with parkinsonian
symptoms plus ataxia. It includes upper and
lower motor neuron signs that may be sporadic.

SHY-DRAGER SYNDROME

The Shy-Drager syndrome involves parkinsonism plus dysautonomia. The signs and symptoms include orthostatic hypotension, impotence, incontinence, and intolerance to
levodopa (Polinsky, 1988).

PATHOLOGY

The pathology of parkinsonism is quite uniform. The substantia nigra and nigrostriatal fibers to the corpus striatum are destroyed.
There is depigmentation and loss and gliosis of
nerve cells in the basal ganglia, particularly in
the midbrain. The affected cells decrease their
normal production of the neurotransmitter
dopamine. Other neurotransmitters involved
include norepinephrine, serotonin, gamma-
aminobutyric acid, and glutamate decarboxy-
lase. Since all neurotransmitters interact in a
complex fashion, it can be understood how the
symptoms of PD appear to involve the entire
nervous system (Bennet, 1988). Mortality for
the disease is 1:1 (Martilla and Rinne, 1985).

DIAGNOSIS OF IDIOPATHIC
PARKINSON'S DISEASE

Until a specific biochemical, physiologic, genetic, or histologic marker is identified, it may
not be possible to clinically identify different
forms of parkinsonism at the onset of symptoms. Parkinsonian symptoms do not become
evident until the concentration of dopamine is
only about 20% of normal, suggesting a long
preclinical course. The diagnosis is dependent
on careful history taking and examination by an
experienced movement disorder practitioner.

Other conditions mimic PD, particularly in
later stages, so the differential diagnosis is difficult. The response to levodopa may serve as a
diagnostic tool.

MANIFESTATIONS

Disease manifestations vary considerably, with
symptoms occurring in any combination. Contrary to common belief, tremors may or may
not be present in PD. Primary symptoms are
bradykinesia (slowed movement), rigidity,
postural instability, and tremors.

MOTOR SIGNS OF BRADYKINESIA

The clinical manifestations of bradykinesia include the following:

Slowness in initiating movements, seen by patients as weakness (muscle weakness actually
   is absent in PD except from disuse in advanced PD)
Reduced spontaneous movement

"Freezing" during voluntary motor activity; short, slow steps when walking

Difficulty in arising from a chair or turning in bed; lack of arm swing when walking

Writing in very small letters (micrographia)

Loss of facial expression (hypomimia)

Staring expression, decreased blinking, and retracted eyelids

Impaired convergence in vision

Voice changes: abnormally weak voice due to incoordination in muscles of vocalization (hypophonia); absence of normal pitch, rhythm, and variation in stress (aprosody of speech); difficulty in articulation (dysarthritic speech)

Rapid eye movement (hypometric saccades)

FALLS

Because of the motor difficulties, falls are not unusual. It is important to get an accurate history of when falls are occurring: in the evening, suggesting medication complications such as dyskinesia? When the person changes from recumbent or a sitting to a standing position, suggesting postural hypotension? If falling cannot be attributed to the mentioned factors, the diagnosis must be reconsidered.

TREMORS

Tremors, present at rest, disappear during sleep. They are regular and rhythmic, with a frequency of 5 to 6 Hz beats per minute. It is not unusual to see intention tremors in addition to tremors at rest.

RIGIDITY

Patients experience rigidity as stiffness. The pain that many individuals with parkinsonism experience (e.g., headaches, back pain) may be directly related to rigid muscles. Rigidity of muscles of the chest and shoulders is sometimes felt as chest pain and that in the legs as leg cramps. These pains do not respond well to analgesia, but are helped by stretching, changing position, and to an increase or decrease in the amount of levodopa. Deep muscle aching may also be a side effect of Sinemet (carbidopa/levodopa), so evaluation of patient response to this drug would also be appropriate.

BRADYPHRENIA AND DEMENTIA

Differing types of PD may exist, with or without intellectual deterioration. Studies reporting a 15% to 40% incidence of dementia may be open to question (Mayeux et al, 1988).

Parkinson stated that the senses and intellect were unaffected, but 25 years later another physician disagreed (Ball, 1882). The controversy continues today. Some researchers attribute any detectable mental decline to psychomotor slowing or aging. Ballard (1987), in studies of young onset patients with parkinsonism and age-matched cohorts found no mental deterioration.

DEPRESSION

Depression is rather prevalent in PD. At times patients or their families recall that depression may have been the first noticeable symptom (Mayeux, 1982). Symptoms often respond to tricyclic antidepressant drugs, and these medications may also help the parkinsonian symptoms (Bunting, 1991).

SECONDARY MANIFESTATIONS IN THE AUTONOMIC NERVOUS SYSTEM

The following manifestations result from autonomic system effects of PD:

Low blood pressure, particularly postural hypotension

Neurogenic bladder (cystometrograms are needed when this symptom appears)

Difficulty in attaining and maintaining penile erection. Less is known about female dysfunctions in PD since there have been no studies (Lipe et al, 1990; Brown et al, 1990)

Constipation

Seborrhea, especially affecting face and scalp

Excessive sweating (infrequent, but not unusual)

SLEEP DISORDERS

Sleep disorders are common in PD. The etiology includes PD pathology, complications of treatments, and symptoms. The majority of patients with PD experience no rapid eye movement sleep as demonstrated on sleep electroencephalography. Sleep disorders may respond to either taking levodopa no later than 7 PM or taking small amounts of tricyclic antidepressant medications (starting with the smallest available dose).

ASSESSMENT OF THE PATIENT WITH PARKINSON'S DISEASE

A variety of assessment tools and rating scales exist to standardize observations of responses in PD. They assist in following patients over time, permitting perspective on progression of symptoms.

The best known scale for assessing five stages in PD is the Hoehn and Yahr scale (1967). These stages are

Stage 1: unilateral disease
Stage 2: bilateral disease
Stage 3: bilateral disease plus postural instability
Stage 4: severe disability, inability to walk or stand unassisted
Stage 5: wheelchair bound or bedridden, possibly with tracheostomy or gastrostomy

Two other scales are commonly used. The unified Parkinson's rating scale is found in Table 20-1. It was developed by an international committee of neurologists with experience in PD. Patients are rated by assignment of a score between 0 and 4 for each symptom. The scale measures mentation and mood, activities of daily living and subjective complaints, objective findings, and complications of treatment. Patients are rated for both "on" and "off" states. The unified rating scale is the most comprehensive scale for assessing response to the disease and treatment. The Schwab and England Activities of Daily Living Scale (Table 20-2) is useful in determining degree of general independence and areas for needed assistance. In addition to these instruments, nursing assessment will address eating difficulties and nutritional status, problems with fluid intake and hydration, and genitourinary and gastrointestinal problems that require nursing management.

MEDICAL TREATMENT

PD is unique among chronic neurologic diseases in that medication administration and monitoring are crucial, particularly as the disease progresses. *Treatment with antiparkinson medications is always symptomatic.* The role of the nurse in the medication treatment of PD is

crucial. Th...
be employee...
ions vary an...
practitioners a...
when therapy sh...

Health team de...
imparting knowle...
drugs are essential. It...
son being treated know...
treatment and why a par...
selected. Table 20-3 (p. 34...
tions presently used in treati...
dications, and the most comm...

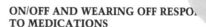

ON/OFF AND WEARING OFF RESPO... TO MEDICATIONS

These terms describe specific fluctuation in symptoms in response to medication. They generally are not apparent until a patient has been on levodopa treatment for several years. Definitions for these terms are

On — The patient is functioning at optimal level although it may be in the presence of dyskinesias
Off — The patient displays parkinsonian symptoms
Wearing off — The patient displays parkinsonian symptoms, typically 30 to 60 minutes before next dose is due (Nutter et al, 1984)

GUIDELINES FOR THE PATIENT OR PERSON RESPONSIBLE FOR MANAGEMENT OF MEDICATIONS

- Give on a *timed* rather than a *demand* schedule
- Remember, a delay of even 15 minutes can interfere with optimal response (alert hospitalized parkinsonian patients may be permitted self-medication)
- Give levodopa at least 30 minutes before meals (food volume and large neutral amino acids compete for absorption into the bloodstream. Neutral amino acids also use the same capillary carrier as levodopa entering the brain and can reduce the clinical response if taken together)
- Give levodopa with at least 8 oz of water (to ensure transport to small intestine where absorption takes place)

(*continued on p. 344*)

TABLE 20–1 *Unified Rating Scale for Parkinsonism: Definitions of 0 to 4 Scale*

Instructions: This scale is designed for recording information regarding a patient's functioning and symptoms. With the exception of the motor examination (items 18 to 31), the items in the scale area are to be quantified by using all the information available to the raters, including both clinical observations and information reported by the patient.

In rating the patient's current status, an arbitrary period of 1 week before the evaluation (for all items except 18 to 31) is adopted to standardize the data. In order to reinforce this, the interviewer should occasionally precede questions with, "During the past week, have you . . .?" The motor examination (18 to 31) should record the patient's status at the time of the examination only.

I. **Mentation, behavior, and mood**

Rate each item once on the basis of patient interview.

1. **Intellectual impairment**

    0—None

    1—Mild. Consistent forgetfulness with partial recollection

    2—Moderate memory loss, with disorientation and moderate difficulty handling complex problems. Mild but definite impairment of function at home, with need of occasional prompting

    3—Severe memory loss, with disorientation for time and often to place. Severe impairment in handling problems

    4—Severe memory loss, with orientation preserved to person only. Unable to make judgments or solve problems. Requires much help with personal care. Cannot be left alone at all

2. **Thought disorder (due to dementia or drug intoxication)**

    0—None

    1—Vivid dreaming

    2—"Benign" hallucinations with insight retained

    3—Occasional to frequent hallucinations or delusions; without insight; could interfere with daily activities

    4—Persistent hallucinations, delusions, or florid psychosis. Not able to care for self

3. **Depression**

    0—Not present

    1—Periods of sadness or guilt greater than normal, never sustained for day or weeks

    2—Sustained depression (1 week or more)

    3—Sustained depression with vegetative symptoms (insomnia, anorexia, weight loss, loss of interest)

    4—Sustained depression with vegetative symptoms and suicidal thoughts or intent

4. **Motivation/initiative**

    0—Normal

    1—Less assertive than usual; more passive

    2—Loss of initiative or disinterest in elective (nonroutine) activities

    3—Loss of initiative or disinterest in day-to-day (routine) activities

    4—Withdrawn, complete loss of motivation

II. **Activities of daily living (determine for "on/off")**

For items 5 to 17, rate each item twice: once for "on" periods and once for "off" periods, and the person should answer your questions about daily functional capabilities separately for "on" and "off" periods.

5. **Speech**

    0—Normal

TABLE 20–1 *(Continued)*

    1—Mildly affected. No difficulty being understood

    2—Moderately affected. Sometimes asked to repeat statements

    3—Severely affected. Frequently asked to repeat statements

    4—Unintelligible most of the time

6. **Salivation**

    0—Normal

    1—Slight but definite excess of saliva in mouth, may have nighttime drooling

    2—Moderately excessive saliva; may have minimal drooling

    3—Marked excess of saliva with some drooling

    4—Marked drooling, requires constant tissue or handkerchief

7. **Swallowing**

    0—Normal

    1—Rare choking

    2—Occasional choking

    3—Requires soft food

    4—Requires nasogastric tube or gastrotomy feeding

8. **Handwriting**

    0—Normal

    1—Slightly slow or small

    2—Moderately slow or small; all words are legible

    3—Severely affected, not all words are legible

    4—The majority of words are not legible

9. **Cutting food and handling utensils**

    0—Normal

    1—Somewhat slow and clumsy, but no help needed

    2—Can cut most foods, although clumsy and slow; some help needed

    3—Food must be cut by someone, but can still feed slowly

    4—Needs to be fed

10. **Dressing**

    0—Normal

    1—Somewhat slow, but no help needed

    2—Occasional assistance with buttoning, getting arms in sleeves

11. **Hygiene**

    0—Normal

    1—Somewhat slow, but no help needed

    2—Needs help to shower or bathe; or very slow in hygienic care

    3—Requires assistance for washing, brushing teeth, combing hair, going to bathroom

    4—Foley catheter or other mechanical aids

12. **Turning in bed and adjusting bed clothes**

    0—Normal

(Continued)

TABLE 20–1   *(Continued)*

    1—Somewhat slow and clumsy, but no help needed

    2—Can turn alone or adjust sheets, but with great difficulty

    3—Can initiate, but not turn or adjust sheets alone

    4—Helpless

13. **Falling (unrelated to freezing)**

    0—None

    1—Rare falling

    2—Occasionally falls, less than once per day

    3—Falls an average of once daily

    4—Falls more than once daily

14. **Freezing when walking**

    0—None

    1—Rare freezing when walking; may hesitate at start

    2—Occasional freezing when walking

    3—Frequent freezing. Occasionally falls from freezing

    4—Frequent falls from freezing

15. **Walking**

    0—Normal

    1—Mild difficulty. May not swing arms or may tend to drag leg

    2—Moderate difficulty, but requires little or no assistance

    3—Severe disturbance of walking, requiring assistance

    4—Cannot walk at all, even with assistance

16. **Tremor**

    0—Absent

    1—Slight and infrequently present

    2—Moderate, bothersome to patient

    3—Severe, interferes with many activities

    4—Marked, interferes with most activities

17. **Sensory complaints related to parkinsonism**

    0—None

    1—Occasionally has numbness, tingling, or mild aching

    2—Frequently has numbness, tingling, or aching, not distressing

    3—Frequent painful sensations

    4—Excruciating pain

III. **Motor examination**

    For items 18 to 31 rate each item once on the basis of the patient's status during examination. To the extent possible, sequential patient examinations should be carried out at the same time of day and/or equivalent intervals relative to dosing.

18. **Speech**

    0—Normal

    1—Slight loss of expression, diction, or volume

TABLE 20–1 (*Continued*)

  2—Monotone, slurred but understandable, moderately impaired

  3—Marked impairment, difficult to understand

  4—Unintelligible

19. **Facial expression**

  0—Normal

  1—Minimal hypomimia, could be normal "poker face"

  2—Slight but definitely abnormal diminution

  3—Moderate hypomimia, lips parted some of the time

  4—Masked or fixed facies with severe or complete loss of facial expression; lips parted $\frac{1}{4}$ inch or more

20. **Tremor at rest**

  0—Absent

  1—Slight and infrequently present

  2—Mild in amplitude and persistent. Or moderate in amplitude, but only intermittently present

  3—Moderate in amplitude and present most of the time

  4—Marked in amplitude and present most of the time

21. **Action or postural tremor of hands**

  0—Absent

  1—Slight; present with action

  2—Moderate in amplitude, present with action

  3—Moderate in amplitude with posture and action

  4—Marked in amplitude; interferes with feeding

22. **Rigidity (judged on passive movements of major joints. Cogwheeling to be ignored)**

  0—Absent

  1—Slight or detectable only when activated by mirror or other movements

  2—Mild to moderate

  3—Marked, but full range of motion easily achieved

  4—Severe, range of motion achieved with difficulty

23. **Finger taps (patient taps thumb with index finger in rapid succession with widest amplitude possible, compare sides)**

  0—Normal

  1—Mild slowing and/or reduction in amplitude

  2—Moderately impaired. Definite and early fatiguing. May have occasional arrests in movement

  3—Severely impaired. Frequent hesitation in initiating movements or arrests in ongoing movement

  4—Can barely perform the task

24. **Hand movements (patient opens and closes hand in rapid succession with widest amplitude possible, measure each)**

  0—Normal

  1—Mild slowing/reduction in amplitude

  2—Moderately impaired. Definite, early fatiguing. Occasional arrest in ongoing movement

  3—Severely impaired. Frequent hesitation or arrests

  4—Can barely perform the task

(*Continued*)

TABLE 20-1 *(Continued)*

25. **Rapid alternating movements of hands: (pronation-supination of hands, with as large an amplitude as possible, both hands simultaneously)**

    0—Normal

    1—Mild slowing and/or reduction in amplitude

    2—Moderately impaired. Definite and early fatiguing

    3—Severely impaired. Frequent hesitation in initiating movements or arrest in ongoing movements

    4—Can barely perform the task

26. **Foot agility (patient taps heel on ground in rapid succession picking up entire foot. Amplitude should be about 3 in)**

    1—Normal

    2—Mild slowing and/or reduction in amplitude

    3—Severely impaired. Frequent hesitation in initiating movements or arrest in movement

    4—Can barely perform the task

27. **Arising from chair (patient attempts to arise from a straightback wood or metal chair with arms folded across chest)**

    0—Normal

    1—Slow or may need more than one attempt

    2—Pushes self up from arms of seat

    3—Tends to fall back and may have to try more than one time; can get up without help

    4—Unable to arise without help

28. **Posture**

    0—Normal, erect

    1—Not quite erect, slightly stooped posture; could be normal for older person.

    2—Moderately stooped posture, definitely abnormal, can be slightly leaning to one side

    3—Severely stooped posture with kyphosis, moderately leaning to one side

    4—Marked flexion with extreme abnormality of posture

29. **Gait**

    0—Normal

    1—Walks slowly, may shuffle with short steps, but no festination or propulsion

    2—Walks with difficulty, but requires little or no assistance, may have festination or propulsion

    3—Severe disturbance of gait, requires assistance

    4—Cannot walk at all, even with assistance

30. **Postural stability (response to sudden posterior displacement produced by pull on shoulders while patient erect with eyes open and feet slightly apart. Patient is prepared)**

    0—Normal

    1—Retropulsion, but recovers unaided

    2—Absence of postural response; would fall if not protected

    3—Very unstable, tends to lose balance spontaneously

    4—Unable to stand without assistance

31. **Body bradykinesia and hypokinesia (combining slowness, hesitancy, decreased armswing, small amplitude, and poverty in general)**

    0—None

TABLE 20–1   *(Continued)*

    1—Minimal slowness, giving movements a deliberate character; could be normal for some. Possibly reduced amplitude

    2—Mild degree of slowness and poverty of abnormal

    3—Moderate slowness, poverty, or small amplitude of movement

    4—Marked slowness, poverty, or small amplitude of movement

IV. Complications of therapy (in the past week)

  A. *Dyskinesias*

  32. Duration: what proportion of the waking day are dyskinesias present? (historical information)

    0—None

    1—25% of day

    2—26%–50% of day

    3—51%–75% of day

    4—76%–100% of day

  33. Disability: how disabling are the dyskinesias? (historical information)

    0—Not disabling

    1—Mildly disabling

    2—Moderately disabling

    3—Severely disabling

    4—Completely disabling

  34. Painful dyskinesias: how painful are the dyskinesias?

    0—No painful dyskinesias

    1—Slight

    2—Moderate

    3—Severe

    4—Marked

  35. Presence of early morning dystonia (historical information)

    0—No

    1—Yes

  B. *Clinical Fluctuations*

  36. How are "off" periods related to time after a dose of medication?

    0—Always predictable

    1—Sometimes predictable

    2—Never predictable

  37. Do any of the "off" periods come on suddenly, e.g., over a few seconds?

    0—No

    1—Yes

  38. What proportion of the waking day is the patient "off" on average?

    0—None

    1—1%–25% of day

    2—26%–50% of day

    3—51%–75% of day

    4—76%–100% of day

(Continued)

TABLE 20–1 *(Continued)*

C. *Other Complications*

39. Does the patient have anorexia, nausea, or vomiting?

0—No

1—Yes

40. Does the patient have symptomatic orthostasis?

0—No

1—Yes

Record the patient's blood pressure, pulse, and weight on the scoring form.

- Be alert for any signs of increase in side effects from medications or decline in functioning and report them to the physician (antiparkinson medications, especially levodopa require periodic adjustment, preferably by a neurologist skilled in movement disorders)

Nursing Diagnosis and Management of High-risk Areas of Daily Living

Nurses and others who are helping individuals and families manage daily living with the diagnosis, treatment, and altered functioning associated with PD need to consider aspects of management beyond the medical treatment.

DAILY STRETCHING ACTIVITIES

Hospitalized patients should have written orders scheduling passive and active stretching exercises beginning on the first day of hospitalization. The patient and family need to become aware that daily stretching is often as important as medication in managing some of the PD symptoms. Individuals who accept and adhere to a regimen of stretching exercises tend to fare better.

TABLE 20–2 *Schwab and England Activities of Daily Living Scale*

100%	Completely independent. Able to do all chores without slowness, difficulty, or impairment. Essentially normal. Unaware of any difficulty
90%	Completely independent. Able to do all chores with some degree of slowness, difficulty, and impairment. Might take twice as long. Beginning to be aware of difficulty
80%	Completely independent in most chores. Takes twice as long. Conscious of difficulty and slowness
70%	Not completely independent. More difficulty with some chores. Three to four times as long in some. Must spend a large part of the day with chores
60%	Some dependency. Can do most chores, but exceedingly slowly and with much effort. Errors; some chores impossible
50%	More dependent. Help with half of chores, slower, etc. Difficulty with everything
40%	Very dependent. Can assist with all chores, but few alone
30%	With effort, now and then does a few chores alone or begins alone. Much help needed
20%	Nothing alone. Can be a slight help with some chores. Severe invalid
10%	Totally dependent, helpless. Complete invalid
0%	Swallowing, bladder, and bowel are not functioning. Bedridden

---

From Schwab RS, England AC. Projection technique for evaluating surgery in Parkinson's disease. In: Gillingham FJ, Donaldson IML, eds. Third symposium on Parkinson's disease. Edinburgh: Livingstone, 1968, pp. 152–157; with permission.

TABLE 20–3 *Medications Presently Available for Treatment in Parkinsonism*

Drug	Indications	Common Side Effects
ANTICHOLINERGICS		
Trihexyphenidyl (Artane)	Tremors	Dry mouth
Benztropine (Cogentin)	Drooling	Constipation
Procyclidine (Kemadrin)		Blurred vision
Ethopropazine (Parsidol)		Confusion, hallucinations
Carbidopa/levodopa (Sinemet)	Tremors/rigidity	Nausea, hallucinations, orthorstatic hypotension, restlessness, vivid dreams
Sustained release (Sinemet)	Bradykinesia	Dyskinesias
Amantadine (Symmetrel)	Tremors Bradykinesia Rigidity	Leg edema Livedo reticularis
DOPAMINE AGONISTS		
Bromocriptine (Parlodel)	Fluctuations "Wearing off" "On/off"	Same as carbidopa/levodopa
Pergolide (Permax)	Fluctuations	Same as carbidopa/levodopa
Seligiline* (Eldepryl)	"Wearing off"	Insomnia

*The hypothesis that seligiline slows the progression of PD has not been proven (Swanson, in press).

KNOWLEDGE OF THE DISEASE

Patients, with the current improved therapies, tend to live for a long time with PD. Therefore, having an accurate, current working knowledge about antiparkinson drugs is important. Patients and those who share in the caregiving need to know the names of the drugs, the dosage, the schedule, what to do if they miss a dose, what the side effects are, which side effects should be reported, note when PD symptoms begin to appear before the next drug dose, how to contact the prescribing clinician, etc.

Members of the health care team can increase and reinforce the knowledge and the importance of the therapy by asking patients questions and by helping them to use the precise language to describe their medications and what they are experiencing. Caregivers and family members can be helped in similar fashion.

DIETARY CONSIDERATIONS

Maintaining plasma levels of levodopa requires certain dietary considerations. Variations in gastric emptying time and in protein content of a meal can influence the plasma level. Taking the levodopa at least 30 minutes before the meal bypasses the problem. Only a very few patients in the advanced stages of PD need to limit their protein during the day and consume the bulk of it toward the end of the day (Pincus and Barry, 1987). Patients taking levodopa, except in the form of Sinemet, probably should avoid taking supplemental forms of vitamin B_6 because of problems with drug interaction.

Some patients with PD, especially those with autonomic nervous system involvement, may need to adjust their eating patterns. They may need to schedule more frequent smaller meals.

EATING

A recent study of videotaped eating among patients with PD identified a variety of specific difficulties. They included the following:

Problems in starting to eat, slow arm movements, changes in tempo, interruptions in eating, difficulties in preparing food, difficulties in concentrating on eating, strong focusing on the task

Handling food on the plate: disturbed hand position, holding utensils inappropriately, too much food on the utensil, raising an empty utensil to the mouth, using only one hand most of the time, seeking food outside the limits of the plate or tray

Transporting food into the mouth: spills, over- or undershooting the mouth, mouth not meeting the utensil, opening mouth too early, opening mouth when touched, difficulties in emptying glass

Manipulating food in the mouth and swallowing: difficulty in biting off pieces, chewing predominantly vertically, chewing without food in the mouth, pressing food instead of chewing, interrupting chewing, failing to lick lips when necessary, food pushing out of mouth, forcing swallowing, shivering when swallowing, coughing, swallowing late, swallowing ineffectively (Athlin et al, 1989)

When patients with PD become sufficiently impaired and have these kinds of eating difficulties, nursing assessment and a treatment plan are needed to provide for the environment and assistance to make eating as comfortable and effective as possible.

CONSTIPATION

Constipation occurs frequently in PD. Its causes include the disease process, drugs, or a combination of the two. Reduced physical activity may also contribute to the problem.

Strategies to combat the problem include the following:

Drinking six to eight glasses of water daily (an hourly schedule is easier than larger amounts at less frequent intervals)

Avoiding bulk formers in patients who have reduced gastric motility (they do not seem to help)

Using the following Craig Formula (provided by a caregiver) to increase gastrointestinal motility. It takes about a month to reestablish regular bowel movements on this regimen

    1 lb each: prunes, raisins, figs
    1 cup lemon juice
    1 cup brown sugar
    1 package senna tea (steep 5 minutes).

Makes 2.5 cups

Combine the above ingredients and cook for 5 minutes. Blend in a blender. Store in freezer. Take 1 to 2 teaspoons daily. *Modify amount depending on need.*

GUIDELINES FOR CAREGIVERS OF PARKINSONIAN PATIENTS AND THEIR FAMILIES

The following guidelines apply to nurses who care for these patients. Because this is a chronic disease, much of the care and management of problems in daily living occur in the home rather than the institutional setting. Therefore, in order to obtain accurate data and provide adequate treatment, caregivers and others who share the patient's daily living in the home setting frequently must be able to use these guidelines as well.

- Help the patient and others to understand the reality that the symptoms of PD are unpredictable. This **symptom uncertainty** creates anxiety and stress for each of the participants. Each person involved may handle the stress in a different way, but each will have an impact on the others.
- Periodically inquire about the presence of vivid dreams or hallucinations (some patients may not report these unless specifically asked; family members will not be able to report unless they realize that these symptoms may have significance in the drug therapy).
- Regularly take blood pressure in the prone, sitting, and standing positions (see Chapter 28).
- Monitor sleep patterns and the basis for sleep disruptions (e.g., nocturia due to neurogenic bladder, or taking levodopa after 7 PM).
- Teach the patient and others that any movement disorder will be magnified when the person feels stressed. Plan for adequate time to accomplish activities so that the patient does not experience the stress of feeling hurried.
- Teach the importance of time management and scheduling. Develop strategies for maintaining a regular and comfortable schedule involving medications, exercises, and usual and unusual activities. Such schedules are important to the ongoing well-being of the patient and others who share the daily living.

- Explain to those who share life with the patient that the symptom of loss of facial expression does not reflect diminution of intellectual powers or lack of responsiveness to others. Reading facial messages is such an ongoing unconscious part of everyday communication that the loss of it can cause misunderstandings and disrupted relationships. For example, a PD patient's wife, whose husband's first symptom was loss of facial expression, confessed to considering divorce because she thought her husband had "lost interest in me." It may be necessary for the nurse to check on difficulties in this area on more than one occasion since facial signals are so taken for granted.

References and Other Readings

Athlin E, Norberg A, Axelsson K, et al. Aberrant eating behavior in elderly Parkinsonian patients with and without dementia: analysis of videorecorded meals. Research in Nursing and Health 1989; 12:41.

Ball J. Agintante. Encephale 1882; 2:22.

Ballard PA. Young onset Parkinson's disease A: a neurological and neuropsychological study. Ann Neurol 1987; 22:173.

Bennet JP. Biochemical pathology and pharmacology of Parkinson's disease. Costa Mesa, CA: PMA Publishing Corp, 1988:63.

Brown RG, Jahanshahi M, Quinn N, Marsden CD. Sexual function in patients with Parkinson's disease and their partners. J Neurol Neurosurg Psychiatry 1990; 53:480.

Bunting L, Fitzimmons B. Depression in Parkinson's disease. J Neurosci 1991; 23:158.

Garland L, Warner J. Management of care of patient with progressive supranuclear palsy. Atlanta: Wesley Homes, Inc., 1989.

Hoehn MM, Yahr MD. Parkinsonism: onset, progression and mortality. Neurology 1967; 17:427.

Kedas A, Reed M, Lux W. Parkinson's mime. Geriatr Nurs 1989; 10:182.

Lipe H, Lonstreth W, Bird T, Linde M. Sexuality in PD. Neurology 1990; 10:1347.

Martilla RJ, Rinne U. Clues from epidemiology of PD. In: Advances in neurology, vol 45. New York: Raven Press, 1985.

Mayeux R. Depression and dementia in Parkinson's disease. In: Movement disorders. London: Butterworth, 1982:75.

Mayeux R, Rosenstein R, Stern Y, et al. The prevalence and risk of dementia in idiopathic Parkinson's disease. Arch Neurol 1988; 45:260.

Nutt JG, Woodward WR, Hammerstad JP, et al. The "on-off" phenomenon in Parkinson's disease. N Engl J Med 1984; 310:483.

Parkinson J. An essay on the shaking palsy. UK: Sherwood, Neely and Jones, 1817.

Pincus JH, Barry K. Influence of dietary protein on motor fluctions in Parkinson's disease. Arch Neurol 1987; 44:270.

Polinsky RJ. Shy-Drager syndrome. In: Jancovic J. Tolosa E. (eds.). Parkinson's disease and movement disorders. Baltimore: Urban and Schwarzenberg, 1988, pp. 153–166.

Rajput AH, et al. A control study of smoking habits in idiopathic PD. Neurology 1987; 37:226.

Swanson R: Drug treatment of Parkinson's disease. J Drug Ther, in press.

Todes CJ, Lees AJ. The premorbid personality of patients with Parkinson's disease. J Neurol Neurosurg Psychiatry 1985; 48:97.

Vernon G. Parkinson's disease. J Neurosci 1989; 21:273.

Yahr M. Parkinson's disease. Seminars in Neurology 1982; 2:343.

21
Strokes

MARIA LINDE

Pathophysiology and Medical Management

The risk of strokes increases with advancing age. In the over-75 age group the estimated prevalence is 95 per 1000. The most notable increase in incidence of strokes was among women 85 years and older (Broderick et al, 1989). No means has been found to alter these risks since strokes presumably result from the age-related, progressive changes in blood vessels. Because strokes in the elderly frequently result in prolonged adjustment in daily living, nursing management is a significant component of post-stroke health care.

There are two phenomena related to cerebrovascular incidents in the over-70 age group that the nurse must be prepared to recognize and manage: transient ischemic attack and stroke.

TRANSIENT ISCHEMIC ATTACKS

DESCRIPTION

Transient ischemic attack (TIA) is a central neurologic deficit lasting no more than 24 hours, caused by ischemia secondary to interruption of blood flow to a portion of the brain.

ETIOLOGIC FACTORS

The temporary ischemia occurs as a result of atherosclerotic plaques or spasm of blood vessels. Total or partial occlusion may be caused by emboli and interrupted or diminished circulation to a segment of the brain.

HIGH-RISK POPULATIONS

Persons at high risk of TIAs include those over age 65 with hypertension (140/95), diabetes, or clinical evidence of coronary artery disease. Both sexes are equally at risk among the elderly. This is in contrast to the younger age group where men have higher risk.

Times of higher risk of TIA occur when the individual changes position in such a way as to suddenly change the blood pressure, e.g., from supine to standing. Even sudden changes in positions may constitute a danger time for some individuals. Monitoring of blood pressure levels in different positions may give the nurse important clues as to risk.

DYNAMICS

As a result of a temporary failure to receive an adequate blood supply and, therefore, insufficient perfusion, the affected neurons fail to function or function at a lower level for a period of time.

SIGNS AND SYMPTOMS

Signs and symptoms give here (Table 21–1) for TIAs are localized to the carotid or vertebrobasilar system, or a combination of the two. As the label suggests, these signs and

TABLE 21–1 *Signs and Symptoms of Transient Ischemic Attacks*

Disturbance	Result
Communication disturbance	Unable to express or comprehend written or spoken language
Visual disturbance	Has double vision or temporary blindness in one eye
Loss of muscle control	Unable to use the leg and arm on one side of the body
Amnesia	Cannot recall brief periods of time
Sensory disturbance	Has lost sensation of pain or temperature on one side of the body
Numbness	Lacks feeling in face, arms, legs, and side, especially if only one side is involved
Loss of balance	Falls for no apparent reason, either with a blackout that goes away promptly or without any loss of consciousness
Lack of comprehension	Fails to recognize familiar objects or persons, even those that are quite familiar

symptoms are transient, tending to disappear within a day.

PROGNOSIS

TIAs involving the carotid territory carry a worse prognosis for occurrence of a major vascular accident than those in the vertebrobasilar area (Fig. 21–1). The appearance of TIAs in the carotid territory in a serious matter. One study showed that 76% of the persons who suffered TIAs of the carotid territory had only one or two of these transient prodromal warning attacks before their major episode. This is in contrast to 52% of patients with TIAs in the vertebrobasilar territory. Therefore, the decision as to what diagnostic tests to make and the

treatment to be initiated is a matter of some urgency.

MANAGEMENT

Medical management consists of surgical intervention as well as pharmaceutical therapy to prevent progression from temporary ischemic episodes to a stroke. The aggressiveness of diagnostic testing and management varies with the number of TIAs that have occurred, the blood vessels involved, and the individual physician's philosophy—and also whether or not the patient reports the incidents. Aggressive diagnosis and immediate surgical intervention are associated with lesions in the carotid system. Bypass of obstructed blood vessels is the most common surgical therapy.

Aspirin is being used increasingly as prophylaxis against strokes. Ticlopidine, an anticlotting agent, is under review by the Food and Drug Administration and may be found to be better than aspirin in preventing strokes (Grotta, 1987; Gent et al, 1989).

The use of anticoagulants is common, particularly if there are associated cardiac irregularities. The patient needs to know how to observe for bleeding, i.e., easy bleeding, bleeding gums, hematuria, and black or blood-streaked stools. If hypertension is present, anticoagulant therapy is contraindicated.

Drug interactions need to be taught because they are critical. Common drugs such as aspirin, salicylates, quinidine, and thyroid preparations will *potentiate* the drug's effects. Barbiturates, on the other hand, will inhibit the anticoagulant effect. The nurse needs to be aware of this and must make the patient and family aware of these drug interactions.

Hospitalization for TIAs may or may not be used, again depending on the location of the lesion, the physician's preference, and the support systems available to the patient in the home.

STROKES

DESCRIPTION

Strokes, or cerebrovascular accidents (CVAs), are dysfunctions in sensory, perceptual, communication, or motor function that result from impaired blood flow to a particular area of the brain. They may have a sudden and massive onset or may be slowly developing phenomena

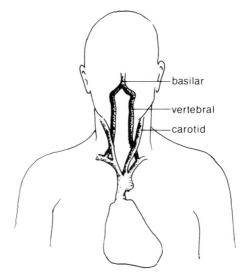

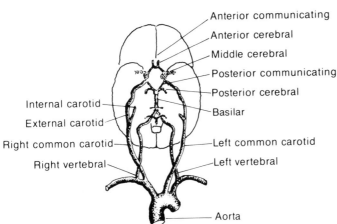

FIGURE 21–1   Carotid and vertebrobasilar vascular systems.

over a period of time. The individual may or may not recognize that changes are occurring; this is especially true if the right hemisphere is affected.

ETIOLOGIC FACTORS

Certain other conditions predispose to strokes. These include hypertension, atherosclerosis, mitral stenosis, and any type of cardiac disorder, including ischemic heart disease and atrial fibrillation (Wolf et al, 1987). Clinical experience indicates an increased risk of cerebral infarction with even modest impairments of glucose tolerance. In the older age group it is well to remember anemia as a cause for cerebral ischemia.

HIGH-RISK POPULATIONS

Populations at high risk for strokes include the elderly, African Americans, Japanese, smokers, cardiac patients, diabetics, persons with polycythemia vera and individuals with a family history of strokes. There is no difference in risk based on sex in the older age group.

DYNAMICS

Blood flow to the brain is interrupted or decreased as a result of gradual narrowing of the lumen, caused by obstruction from local thrombi or atherosclerotic plaques or from emboli from distant parts. Intracerebral extravasations and ruptured aneurysms are less likely to occur in the elderly. However, subdural hematomas resulting from falls do occur.

SIGNS AND SYMPTOMS

The signs and symptoms of stroke may occur as a very obvious, critical and massive event or may appear as subtle cues that occur in almost any area of function. When the onset is gradual or when the individual lives alone and is unaware of the growing deficits, or has a stroke and is found later, it is difficult to assess the time of the stroke.

SUBTLE SIGNS AND SYMPTOMS

For the older person in the home, the retirement center, the senior citizen center, or the clinic the following signs and symptoms may be indicative of the onset of a stroke:

- The homemaker burns herself when cooking but does not recognize that it has happened. Or the person gets a cigarette burn on the fingers and does not notice it (sensory stroke).
- The individual picks up the phone and cannot remember a phone number he has been using for many years.
- The person, in getting out of bed, finds himself on the floor but is able to get up.
- The woman takes out a comb and then forgets how to comb her hair (loss of recall in using a familiar object).
- The individual dials a number and, when the person being called answers, finds himself unable to speak.
- The person suddenly has difficulty in swallowing.
- The person has a sudden numbness in one of the extremities.
- The individual feels that a curtain has abruptly come across a portion of the visual field. (It usually involves one eye but many do not think to put a hand over each eye to test this.)
- The person riding the bus suddenly becomes aware that he does not know where he is.

The older individual who experiences these small manifestations of a stroke may be unaware of them and, therefore, unable to report them. Another common occurrence is the elderly person who would prefer to ignore the signs and symptoms and, therefore, does not report them. The history is important, and an effort needs to be made to obtain an accurate one. Sometimes this means obtaining data from others who have been in contact with the person—family, neighbors, friends, the mailman, the grocery clerk, and so forth.

MAJOR SIGNS AND SYMPTOMS

The signs and symptoms will be drastic and sudden when a large blood vessel is involved. This abrupt onset is one of the most devastating features of a major stroke—the individual is so totally unprepared.

The signs and symptoms in major lesions can be manifestations of unilateral or bilateral involvement, cerebellar involvement, or, when the anterior spinal artery is occluded, a quadriplegic pattern of involvement. The classic signs and symptoms of a stroke include hemiplegia, quadriplegia, hemianopsia, incontinence, sensory losses or alterations, dysarthria, dysphasia, and dysphagia.

Sensory Symptoms It is important to obtain specific data on the nature of the losses in the sensory area. Such data are necessary in considering prognosis and planning the management of the immediate environment in such a way as to protect the patient from elements that may cause additional injury. These data may be obtained from the medical data base, or the nurse who has competence may do a sensory examination. The interpretation of sensory data is difficult and takes practice. The sensory examination is subjective and therefore the least reliable: two examiners may obtain quite different "data."

There are times when an older person who has had a minor stroke may not wish to be hospitalized. It is important that an accurate sensory check be made in order to be certain that the individual will not be harmed in areas where he is unable to perceive injurious stimuli. The appreciation of sensory losses by the patient is often nonexistent due to the site of the neurologic lesion. It is extremely important that specific examination strategies for this type of dysfunction be established.

Language Dysfunction Language dysfunctions or deficits need to be plotted accurately. The deficits can include both comprehension and expression of language, reading, writing, and arithmetic. Because these capabilities and functions affect so many dimensions of daily living, it becomes crucial to collect accurate data on the areas and nature of the specific deficits in each of the five areas.

COMPREHENSION   The nurse is interested in discovering how much or how little the person can understand, since overestimation or underestimation of a problem leads to poor management. Data on the following areas of comprehension need to be collected.

Does the person respond to a *simple request?* "Close your eyes."

Can the person respond to a *two-step request?* "Close your eyes and touch your nose."

If the person does not respond to *verbal commands,* will he follow body language? Demonstrate an activity involving body parts. Touch your finger to your own nose.

Can the person *read* a newspaper heading? (Be sure he has on his reading glasses.)

Or the nurse could print a written request for him to carry out if he is unable to speak, e.g., "Touch your nose."

Can he carry out simple *arithmetic calculations?*

Can he make change? Give him a 50-cent piece and ask him to make change for a 15- or 25-cent purchase. (This is important because some individuals recover all functions except the ability to handle money.)

Can he *write* a sentence from the nurse's dictation? For example, "He shouted the warning."

EXPRESSION   Another facet in communication deficit is that of expression, or speech. Comprehension and expression need to be assessed separately. The person who understands but cannot speak must be both insulted and angered by the behavior of others who assume that the individual who cannot speak understandably cannot possibly understand what is being said to him. The two—comprehension and expression—do not necessarily go hand in hand. One or the other, or both, may be affected, depending on the location of the lesion.

When the *anterior portion of the frontal lobe* (Broca's area) is involved, comprehension is intact to varying degrees. However, speech is altered in several ways. In the most severe form the individual may be totally without expressive speech, or he may retain automatic speech, so that he can name the days of the week, his own name, and so forth. He may have restricted speech—he tends to leave out verbs, sentences are short, and he points to objects he cannot name (anomia). Such lesions also can cause profanity to become a predominant feature of speech; in fact, sometimes those are the only words an individual can say. This can occur in the vocabulary of someone who has never used profanity before. It may be a manifestation of frustration. It is something the individual cannot control, because of the lesion. Families, friends, and health care personnel need to be counseled to allow the behavior and not to censure someone who does it. The family and friends' frustration and embarrassment need to be dealt with so that they do not alienate themselves from the individual and cause him even more loneliness.

When the *posterior portion of the frontal lobe* (Wernicke's area) is involved, comprehension is more likely to be lost. This individual's speech is dysfunctional in several ways. He tends to talk a great deal, is difficult to understand because she makes up new words (e.g., pluber or pluver for plumber), says the opposite of what he means, and transposes words in sentences. Sentences do not make sense. Again, the dysfunction occurs in varying degrees.

COGNITIVE   FUNCTIONING   Cognitive dysfunction is closely associated with the brain hemisphere involved. Cognitive function among those who survive the acute stage is a crucial determiner of effectiveness in living after stroke. Because some of these deficits are subtle, it is important to be aware of the risks of cognitive deficits and the location of the associated lesion (Table 21–2).

Some people think that a person with right-sided hemiplegia, who has lost language function and who is so aware of his own deficit, is more disabled than the individual with left-sided hemiplegia. The latter can speak and usually talks a good game, denying disability. The reality is that the person with left-sided hemiplegia rarely is able to regain self-sufficiency. His symptoms of a stroke may be less visible, but if a major stroke has occurred, he could be devastated in terms of coping ability.

It becomes important for families and health care providers to differentiate the cognitive deficits associated with the location of the lesion. The patient's post-stroke behavior needs to be understood and indeed can be predicted

TABLE 21–2 *Relationship of Lesion Location to Type of Cognitive Dysfunction*

Left Hemiplegia (lesion in right hemisphere)	*Right Hemiplegia (lesion in left hemisphere)*

Spatial–perceptual deficits
    Loss of depth perception; loss of appreciation of distance, form, and rate of movement of objects
	Impaired language function
	    Reading, writing, speaking, understanding

Judgment problems
    Decrease in concern for personal safety; decreased ability to handle finances
	Perseveration
	    Repetitious speech and motor activities (e.g., washing face repeatedly)

Easy distractibility	
Short attention span	
Lack of awareness of deficit Talks a good game but performance does not match words	Extreme awareness of the deficits
Neglect of involved extremities Forgets the extremities that have been affected with sensory or motor loss	
Unable to transfer learning from one situation to another	
Behavioral style—quick, impulsive	Behavioral style—slow and cautious

based on the lesion's location. Because the behavior of the patient is beyond his control, knowing what to expect perhaps makes this behavior more acceptable even if it does not make it any easier to live with him.

Motor Function and Mobility Another obvious area for assessment is that of motor function. Strength, endurance, balance, and capability are affected by strokes. Therefore, assessments need to be made in all of these areas in order to develop valid plans for management of daily living.

HAND FUNCTIONING The individual whose lesion affects the dominant hand is much more devastated in daily living than other stroke victims and must learn to cope with usual daily activities in a variety of difficult and awkward ways. The adaptation of previous patterns in the use of one hand or both in activities is important in the post-stroke period. The devastation of being essentially right-handed and losing the function of that hand is a real barrier to independence in myriad daily functions. When both sensory and motor loss occur, the prediction can be made that the functional capacity

will be much less, making adjustments more difficult. Therefore, it becomes important to incorporate data on both sensory and motor functioning into the management plan. Hand function should be assessed in terms of finger-thumb opposition. If the patient has this, he can pick up and grip objects to some degree; without it the individual will not have functional use of that hand.

Another consideration in assessment is the care that is taken of the affected hand. Is it ignored? Is it exercised? Is it groomed? Is it allowed to be damaged? Is it owned or disowned? One may begin by asking, "Does this arm and hand feel like it belongs to you?" From this questioning a wealth of data may flow.

The individual's method of adaptation is an expression of his imagination and resourcefulness. One person may use his mouth to grasp or hold articles and to open packages. Another may use his functioning hand and increase its usefulness. Others will be devastated by their stroke and increase their dependence on their environment. It becomes important to assess not only the dysfunction but also the predicted or actual patterns of adaptation to the dysfunction. For example, ask the patient to open a package of salt or a carton of milk. Assessment of dressing and managing buttons could be made in the office situation by asking the patient to remove his coat or jacket (or observe coping with buttons and zippers). Stockings and shoes are a major problem—again, either ask him how he manages or observe the type of shoes he is wearing and how he removes them and puts them on.

BALANCE/COORDINATION   Muscle strength without balance does little for mobility in daily activities. Cerebellar lesions place balance and muscle coordination at high risk. If the patient has adequate speech, he may tell you about problems involving balance. Activities at high risk include any that require the individual to bend over (e.g., putting on shoes and stockings, picking up objects, getting in and out of the tub or shower, walking up and down stairs, opening drawers that are low, and getting out of bed). The most obvious objective datum is the *gait* of the person. *Whenever* the individual uses a wide stance in standing or walking there is a problem with balance. Coordination and balance may be tested with the finger-to-nose and heel-to-shin tests. Also ask the individual to stand and close his eyes; those with balance problems tend to fall to one side.

Where balance and coordination are at risk the individual must work much harder in many seemingly incidental or routine maneuvers. Therefore, *fatigue* becomes a factor to be considered in nursing management.

STRENGTH   Strength involves the capacity to engage in a particular physical demand. For example, can the individual come to a sitting or standing position by himself or does he require assistance? How much can he lift? Can he raise his legs enough to climb stairs or get on a bus? Objective data involves observation of the individual in these activities.

FATIGUE   Strokes tend to cause fatigue. The individual tires rapidly; this is particularly evident later in the day. One must learn how much the individual can accomplish before becoming fatigued. How long a rest period is required before he can engage in activities again? What kinds of activities can he engage in and for how long? How does he react to constraints on his endurance?

Vision   The most common dysfunctions in vision associated with strokes include loss of visual fields, seeing double, and, occasionally, nystagmus.

LOSS OF VISUAL FIELD   Visual field loss may be of several kinds: loss of half of the visual field in each eye, complete loss of vision in one eye, or loss of a quadrant in each eye. A visual field deficit causes many functional risks for the patient. An indication of the types of visual loss and the loss of function is given in Table 21–3.

Data on the patient's visual field are important to patient safety and effective living. These data may be obtained from the medical record. Where the data are not available it becomes important for the nurse to be able to do this testing. The following steps aid in testing visual fields:

1. Stand or sit about 2 feet away from the patient.
2. Have the patient cover one eye with his hand or a piece of paper.
3. Direct the patient to look at the nurse's nose.
4. Move an object (pencil or finger) from outside the visual field toward a point opposite the patient's nose, keeping the object equidistant from patient and nurse.
5. Direct the patient to indicate (verbally or by signal) when he first sees the object and when he loses sight of it.

Figure 21–2 indicates the directions of visual fields that need to be tested.

Frequently the patient is unaware of the loss of visual fields after a stroke. Without a diagnosis of this deficit, the patient may not observe it until he wonders why a paragraph he is reading does not make sense (he sees only half of it) or why he runs his wheelchair into a wall when he thinks he is going straight. Even then, the patient may connect these symptoms to some other aspect of his stroke and, therefore, not report it.

Part of the assessment involves direct observation of patient activity. Does he ignore objects on the right or left side? Does he bump into doorjambs or objects on a particular side? Another test situation is to ask the person to identify objects on a tray placed before him. He will ignore objects outside his field of vision. It is crucial to record not only the area of loss but also the patient's awareness or lack of it.

Part of patient management is to (1) create a conscious awareness of the deficits that exist in visual fields and (2) help the patient make the accommodations that must be built into his activities.

TABLE 21–3 *Loss of Visual Fields and Resultant Functional Losses*

Type of Deficit	Loss	Examples of Functional Risk
Homonymous hemianopsia*	*Right:* When person is looking straight ahead, vision loss is in right half of visual field in each eye	If unaware of visual field loss, the person fails to compensate by moving the head to see into the blind area
		Ignores objects or persons in the lost visual field—walks into walls, ignores food outside of available visual field, fails to notice people in lost field
	Left: Vision loss is in left half of visual field in each eye	Restricted from driving
		May have visual interpretive defects
Bitemporal hemianopsia	Peripheral half of visual field is lost in each eye	Failure to see objects (stationery or moving) until they reach the central area of vision
		Startle reaction as people or objects "pop" into view
Blindness in one eye		Loss of depth perception and as above

*If unresolved in 2 to 3 weeks, it becomes a permanent disability.

DIPLOPIA   Double vision usually is reported by the patient. Where there is a brain stem lesion it is a predictable symptom. An associated symptom of the diplopia is nausea.

NYSTAGMUS   Nystagmus (irregular jerking movement of the eyeball) can be observed. It can also be elicited by moving an object across the visual field and asking the patient to follow it with his eyes. Some patients are aware of the phenomenon and find it unpleasant. (There are also familial tendencies to nystagmus. In this case there is no stroke-associated pathology.)

Emotional Lability   Emotional lability is an organic problem associated with lesions in the pseudobulbar region, with bilateral hemisphere problem, or with interruption of both corticospinal tracts. However, because both emotional lability and depression frequently are manifested after a stroke, nurses and other health care providers often have failed to differentiate between them and because of this, management has not been effective.

Emotional lability is a phenomenon characterized by inappropriate ease of laughter and crying, mostly crying. Because crying is also a manifestation of depression, it becomes impor-

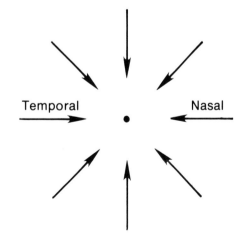

FIGURE 21–2   Testing visual fields.

tant to assess the presenting situation. The following pieces of data will help to make an accurate diagnosis of emotional lability:

1. Is the person aware of the behavior?
2. Can the behavior (crying) be interrupted by engaging in another activity such as getting a drink of water or grabbing the back of a chair?
3. Is the person embarrassed by the behavior?
4. Does the person wish to stop it?

Affirmative answers to these four questions would indicate the presence of emotional lability rather than, or in addition to, depression. (For signs and symptoms of depression, see Chapters 17 and 19.) Depression frequently occurs with strokes. Current medical thought is that it should be recognized and treated (Fuhrman, 1989).

Another aspect of assessment regarding emotional lability is the response of the family. Are family members aware that the behavior is an organic phenomenon? Do they have any knowledge about how to control it?

When family and patient understand that the behavior is not an unexpected response but is due to the stroke, the situation may become more tolerable for all concerned.

GRIEVING The individual who has had a stroke and suffers residual loss of function goes through the grieving process in coping with this loss. It is a normal and necessary response. Because the loss is ongoing, the grieving tends to be recurrent. The stages of denial, anger, bargaining, depression, and acceptance can all be seen. However, denial deserves particular consideration with some stroke patients. *Those who suffer from left hemiplegia will experience denial as an organic response.* It is more properly identified as *neglect,* because denial is a defense mechanism and has accrued negative social connotations.

As with the assessment of grieving in any loss situation, data are needed on the stages the individual is currently in and the patterns of coping with the grieving. It is important also to gather data on the response of individuals in the support system with regard to the stroke patient's grieving. Do they understand what is going on and its necessity? Do they understand the nature of movement from one stage to another? Do they realize it should not and cannot be short-circuited or avoided? Can they toler-

ate the discomfort of the individual's grieving? Do they have respite from it? What help do they wish?

STATUS OF SUPPORT SYSTEMS

Strokes tend to leave the individual with physical, cognitive, emotional, and communication dysfunctions at some level that remain fairly static for long periods. Many individuals can be quite dependent, but their status does not change. They do not deteriorate and die nor do they get a great deal better after they have achieved the initial major return of function. They present real challenges to those who care for them. Maintenance, and satisfaction with it, is crucial.

Information on the kinds of support systems available and the patient's attitude toward the use of support resources become very important. One difficulty is that the person who has had a stroke sees himself as deviant from others, a minority. For some persons this results in an isolation from others, including available support systems. Data on these areas are needed if a usable plan of management of daily living is to be developed.

The family who sees its loved one disabled tends to equate helping with caring. Therefore, it becomes very difficult not to "do for" the person what is difficult for him to do for himself. Family members may need help to work through the realization that the individual may have to struggle, be frustrated, be angry, and be slow as he does things for himself.

The highest form of loving may be that of keeping hands off.

COMPLICATIONS

High-risk Physical Complications After surviving the acute stage, there are still complications that are a high risk for the person who has had a stroke. These complications are both physical and psychosocial (Table 21–4) and are a result of the residual functional deficit.

PROGNOSIS

According to the American Heart Association, the incidence of strokes in 1989 was 500,000, with a death rate of 29.4%. There are now almost 3 million Americans alive who are victims of stroke.

In terms of pathology and pathophysiology, those individuals who have only motor losses as

TABLE 21–4 *High-risk Physical and Psychosocial Complications*

Physical Complications	Psychosocial Complications
Joint contractures on the affected side	Body image greatly affected when major portions of the body lack sensation or cease to function normally
Shoulder separation on the affected side	
Constipation—related to less activity, decreased appetite and fiber/fluid ingestion, drugs, and depression	Social isolation at high risk, particularly when the individual has an expressive or comprehension communication deficit; sees himself as deviant or a tremendous burden to others; or when others communicate to him that he is an unwanted burden
Atonic bladder	
Trauma to areas with decreased sensation	
Edema in flaccid extremities that are allowed to dangle for long periods of time in a dependent position	Depression—hopelessness of any improvement in one's status. Sadness at one's state in life
	Anxiety over the risk of using up one's social and economic resources as the disability drags on
Sensory deprivation—in terms of the sensations available in the environment, if the person becomes more socially isolated (e.g., people don't talk to you if you can't talk with them or don't understand). Whole areas of the body fail to sense stimuli from the environment or proprioceptive impulses	Living with fear of another stroke
	Shifting from independence to dependence—can be catastrophic for individuals who value highly their independence
Fatigue and major increased amounts of time required to accomplish routine activities of daily living	Frustration and anger over dysfunction and its limitations—"why me?"

a residual tend to do very well. They have almost complete recovery within a year or so. Those with both sensory and motor losses have a less favorable prognosis. Right-sided hemiplegic patients, despite their communication difficulties, tend to be able to care for themselves and live independently. They are aware and alert, and a communication system can be developed. Those with left-sided hemiplegia are less likely to be able to maintain an independent lifestyle because of spatial-perceptual deficits in particular.

Factors affecting long-term prognosis negatively include increased age, cardiac disease, hypertension, leg weakness, male sex, cardiovascular disease, arthritis, or neurologic disorder. Poor outcome is also associated with altered consciousness, dysphasia, and visual field defects in the first 12 hours (Chambers et al, 1987).

MEDICAL MANAGEMENT

Acute The initial medical management is concerned with assessing the damage and preventing complications. This includes careful work-up to determine the etiology and nature of the pathology. It will include computed tomography (CT) scan or magnetic resonance imaging (MRI) study, cerebral arteriography, electrocardiography, Doppler flowmeter studies, and laboratory studies such as electrolytes, arterial blood gases, complete blood count, and erythrocyte sedimentation rates.

There is no medical treatment that will predictably improve long-term recovery. General guidelines include starting treatment as soon as possible (within 24 hours of stroke), avoiding hypotension and hypoxia, careful expansion of volume to best use cardiac output, care in feeding, and respiratory treatments to avoid aspiration.

Treatment includes the use of heparin if the pathology is embolic in origin. Blood pressure is controlled for adequate brain perfusion (avoiding hypotension). Bed rest is used for up to 72 hours. Fluids are controlled in terms of overall need versus minimizing the risk of increased intracranial pressure. Increased intracranial pressure is controlled with drugs such as mannitol. Vital signs and serial neurologic assessments are done every 30 to 60 minutes until findings are stable. Airways are maintained and catheters are usually in place.

Hemodilution by reducing hematocrit to 30% to 33% is being studied. Calcium channel blockers are also being researched. The rationale is that increased intracellular levels of calcium after ischemia are caused by ion flux into neurons and release of intracellular stores (Grotta, 1987).

Long-term Management Ongoing medical care tends to address the problems associated with hypertension, further clotting risks, and symptom management. The services of other disciplines such as speech, occupational, and physical therapy may be prescribed.

Hearing loss is a concomitant deficit in some patients that may compound deficits in comprehension and should receive attention.

Nursing Diagnosis and Management of High-risk Areas in Daily Living

DAILY LIVING WITH FAILURE TO RECOGNIZE TRANSIENT ISCHEMIC ATTACKS

TIAs may be forerunners of strokes. Individuals who ignore or fail to recognize and seek medical treatment place themselves in greater jeopardy of disabling strokes than if they did not use the medical technology that is currently available. Helping the high-risk elderly person to be aware of both manifestations and treatment options is a nursing responsibility.

RISK FACTORS

Certain older persons are at greater risk of managing daily living by not dealing with the signs and symptoms of TIAs. These include persons who

Attribute the signs and symptoms of TIAs to aging

Avoid taking "minor complaints" to the doctor for financial reasons or personal preference

Have an unclear mental state

Are loners with few close associates to recognize changes in their physical and mental state

SIGNS AND SYMPTOMS

Direct questioning regarding the occurrence of specific symptoms of TIAs may yield data that episodes of TIA have occurred and were unrecognized or ignored. Persons in contact with the older person may report observing the associated changes or statements the person has made to them indicating TIAs.

PROGNOSTIC VARIABLES

Negative prognosis for managing daily living with TIA symptoms is associated with minimizing or denying signs and symptoms, lack of belief in medical treatment, unclear mental status, and being socially isolated.

COMPLICATIONS

Without treatment, TIAs normally progress to strokes.

TREATMENT

Nursing intervention is primary educative. It includes:

Alerting high-risk persons or their families and close associates to the signs and symptoms of TIAs and the significance of these manifestations that appear and then rather rapidly disappear

Educating potential candidates for TIAs about the recent advances in medical treatment that prevent or delay the progression from TIAs to strokes

Helping the elderly person or primary caregiver to have a plan for accurately reporting episodes in such a way as to obtain effective health care

EVALUATION

Evaluation of response to nursing intervention is based on the incidence of prompt accurate reports of TIAs.

DAILY LIVING WITH ACKNOWLEDGED TRANSIENT ISCHEMIC ATTACKS

Living with recognition of the unpredictable occurrence and recurrence of TIAs and with the symptoms in the attacks represents an uncertainty and loss of control in daily living. Knowing that the condition represents a chronic atherosclerotic condition and is a precursor to strokes adds an ever-present threat of major disability or death. Living each day with both the unpredictability of the episodes and the predictability of the outcome (when treatment is not effective) adds a new serious dimension to daily living.

RISK FACTORS

Older persons who face the greatest difficulty in managing daily living with both the symptoms and threat of TIAs include those who:

Have had repeated episodes of TIAs

Have had previous CVAs and now have renewed signs and symptoms of further pathology and risk

Live alone and have limited predictable and consistent human contacts

Are fearful because they know the implications and threat of stroke associated with TIAs

Are very old and feel they have little credibility when they report the signs and symptoms of TIAs

SIGNS AND SYMPTOMS

Those who are not managing daily living effectively with TIAs may present with:

Failure-to-thrive syndrome—growing apathy, self-neglect, and depression

Increasing levels of anxiety

Bruises, abrasions, burns, and fractures secondary to accidents occurring in an unsafe environment during TIAs

Lack of any plan or resources for daily contacts to check on their well-being

Lack of knowledge of strategies to minimize the hazards of daily living with TIAs

Retreat to a very circumscribed form of daily living due to fears of TIAs

PROGNOSTIC VARIABLES

Poor prognosis for the effective management of daily living attaches to:

Being totally preoccupied with the threat and risks of TIAs

Having no backup support system or plan for checkups on health status

Having poor skills or an inadequate plan for reporting the symptoms they are experiencing

COMPLICATIONS

Failure to manage daily living effectively with the stress and manifestations of TIAs can lead to alcoholism or suicide. The dysfunction during attacks may result in trauma. The untreated pathology will lead to a stroke. Fear of attack may reduce daily living to a homebound, narrow existence.

TREATMENT

Nursing intervention addresses several areas of daily living: mobilizing acceptable, predictable external resources, modifying the environment, and teaching some coping skills. These interventions may include the following activities:

Mobilizing a personal support system of individuals who will make a daily contact or of technology such as Life-line, Medic Alert, or other electronic devices to alert assistance and reduce the risk of being left unattended for prolonged periods

Encouraging or assisting the older person to find a physician or clinician in whom they have confidence and with whom they are comfortable

Planning with the elderly person regarding engaging in more activities, diversions, and distractions to limit time for preoccupation with TIAs and their risks

Posting the telephone numbers of the doctor, nurse, or hospital on the telephone

Obtaining a long telephone cord or locating the phone at the bedside

Obtaining and using antiembolic stockings if the individual has postural hypotension

Encouraging the person to change positions slowly from lying or sitting to standing and to avoid sudden rapid changes of position and movement

Improving the safety of the environment in the home. Remove small rugs, on which the person could easily slip; remove furniture in way of passage; add support bars in bathroom and safety strips in the tub. Some medical supply houses have consultants on the staff who, without a fee, will make a home assessment. An occupational therapist also is an excellent resource

Nursing management of the person with TIAs also includes contacts with the family and friends. Obtain the confidence of the patient to share data on these attacks with the nurse. Work with the family on explaining the importance of reporting them or what to do when they occur. Their knowledge of the dynamics of the situation and their understanding and support for the person provide immeasurable sustenance.

EVALUATION

Response to nursing intervention may be seen in the elderly person's reports of regular contacts with support persons, accurate and prompt reporting of attacks, absence of signs and reports of trauma, and a level of activity and diversion appropriate to his or her capabilities.

DAILY LIVING WITH THE SYNDROME OF IMPAIRED JUDGMENT, IMPAIRED SPATIAL-PERCEPTUAL DEFICITS, AND INABILITY TO TRANSFER LEARNING (RIGHT HEMISPHERE LESIONS)

Common residual dysfunctions of right hemisphere CVAs (left hemiplegia) profoundly affect the capacity of individuals to manage daily living independently. Their self-perception is one of competence—to drive, to manage money, to cook a meal for guests—but their performance does not match this self-image. Spatial-perceptual deficits involve distance, depth perception, balance, form, and movement—all capacities intimately involved with managing routine tasks of daily living such as walking, reaching for objects, and so forth. Tasks that are learned in one setting cannot be repeated in a different setting. There is easy distraction. *Comprehension is not affected,* but performance is. Another deficit is associated with the inability to own the affected side of the body; thus neglect of this side is common.

Deficits of this nature present uncommon difficulties not only to the person who has them but also to those who have responsibility for providing care and companionship.

RISK FACTORS

Elderly people with right hemisphere CVAs who have the greatest difficulty in managing daily living are those who

Have the additional deficit of a visual field cut
Are unable to understand or accept the deficits
Are unable to learn accommodative strategies

Are unable to learn the skills and behaviors in each of the settings where they must take place
Do not have primary caregivers who can understand and adapt to the deficits in the elderly person
Do not have a structured, consistent environment

Individuals with significant infarctions in the right parietal lobe are at greatest risk of suffering prolonged alterations in judgment involving overestimation of personal capabilities. They then encounter major problems in managing daily living safely.

SIGNS AND SYMPTOMS

Manifestations that the elderly person is not managing daily living effectively or safely come in many forms. They are observed to place themselves in unsafe situations such as attempting to drive a car, reaching for hot objects on a stove with their impaired depth perception, and not protecting the ignored affected side from cold or heat. They are observed to walk into objects. They show evidence of falls, burns, or other trauma. They neglect personal hygiene on the affected side such as combing their hair only on the unaffected side. They talk confidently about their capabilities and make plans or take action based on their self-perception, but their performance does not match their expectations. They learn a behavior in one setting or context and then are unable to repeat it in any other setting. They become angry with constraints.

Since the primary caregivers are so critical to the well-being of these elderly persons, their physical and emotional status is of importance. Signs and symptoms of burnout or the inability to manage daily living with these constant burdens are important (see the section in Chapter 13 on monitoring the status of primary caregivers).

PROGNOSTIC VARIABLES

The ability to manage daily living effectively with ongoing impaired judgment varies with the insight the person is able to achieve and the acceptance of the disability together with its restrictions and the availability of consistent, skilled companions and caregivers in a safe structured environment. ·

COMPLICATIONS

The complications for individuals include trauma to themselves and occasionally endangering others by their behavior and activities. For companions and primary caregivers the complication tends to be burnout.

TREATMENT

Management of daily living for the left-sided hemiplegic individual must overcome perceptual-spatial deficits, insufficient judgment in decision making, and the inability to follow through and must meet the need to learn each behavior in every required context since often he is unable to transfer learning. Additionally, the failure to "own" the affected parts of the body creates difficulties. The person tends to overestimate his abilities.

In general it helps to have a structured routine and environment that is consistent and predictable. It is also important to find the strategies that work best in dissuading the person from unsafe behavior. Observe the extent to which performance matches what the person indicates he can do, but be sensitive about the timing of making the person aware of the discrepancies. There are times when this insight would be too devastating.

There are several other areas where the person's self-concept may be threatened by the need for supervision and constraints. One is in the control of finances. Another is in the use of a car. The elderly person may take the car out for a drive because he honestly does not recognize the extent of his deficiencies. (Some states require retesting for relicensure following a stroke.) The losses in competence need to be compensated for by genuine appreciation of them as persons and by regular, realistic, and positive acknowledgment of their accomplishments.

Treatment for the Inability to Transfer Learning
The inability to replicate learned behavior in a new setting dictates particular treatment. Comprehension is not affected; therefore, oversimplification may be seen as a put-down. There may be a tendency to be easily distracted, so those involved in the teaching should minimize the number of stimuli operating at one time (e.g., no television or background noise, no extra people); teach the person alone in a quiet setting. Break the teaching into small steps. Teach and get return performance in each of the settings where it is most likely to be used rather than expect the individual to be able to transfer learning from one situation to another. Overteaching, overpracticing, and overlearning become important in the performance area. Repetition makes for a safer, more predictable performance.

One general device that uses comprehension is the placement of written reminders or instructions in strategic places in the environment, e.g., on the shower door, post transfer instructions broken into steps:

Lock the brake of the wheelchair.
Look at your left foot as you stand up.
Grasp the safety bar with your right hand.
Pull yourself to a standing position.

Treatment for Deficits in Spatial Perception
Managing daily living with changes in the ability to judge distance, depth, form, and movement and with balance deficits creates persistent difficulties. Use the teaching strategies discussed in the previous section.

Treatment for Neglect of the Affected Side
Left-sided hemiplegic persons need to reintegrate the affected side as a very conscious experience. They need to look at it regularly, touch it, and name the parts. It is important to use the functioning arm to do range of motion and passive exercises on the affected side. In order to minimize trauma it is necessary to get into a pattern of visually checking the position of affected limbs, particularly in high-risk areas such as the kitchen. In colder climates attention needs to be paid to preventing exposure—mittens may be easier than gloves. Or, where coat pockets are available, pulling the affected hand into the pocket not only affords protection but also may contribute to maintaining balance.

Neglect may be compounded also by loss of visual fields. It is helpful here to place objects, furniture, clothing in the closet, food, and so forth on the side where it is most likely to be seen and noticed. This can reduce neglect to some degree. On the other hand, contractures of the neck toward the unimpaired side are at greater risk in left hemiplegic persons, particularly those with neglect, where they tend to keep the head turned away from the affected side. Teaching them to deliberately turn their heads to the point where they can see areas on the impaired side will do two things: reduce the risk of contracture and maintain awareness of their body and environment.

Prompt cueing of a positive nature is important (Kalbach, 1991). Where visual neglect is noticed, avoid an approach such as, "Why don't you turn your head so you can see?" Instead, say, "Mary, turn your head (right/left) and you'll see the grandchildren coming." Give positive feedback as the steps are proceeding during an activity. Do not wait till the end. If something is not going well, ask a question that calls attention to the problem, e.g., "Carl, are you matching the buttonhole to the right button?" Praise is important: "You do well."

Treatment for Primary Caregivers   Living closely with or having responsibility for a person with left hemiplegia is a demanding situation. Since the hemiplegic's well-being depends to a great extent on structure and consistency, care for the mental and physical health of those involved in the person's care becomes critical. It is important to

Monitor the well-being of the persons most closely involved with the patient. Legitimize their emotional responses. Learn their goals and values. Work with them to find satisfying activities with the patient and with others.

Provide and arrange for or help them to arrange for scheduled predictable periods of respite from caregiving responsibilities and even the presence of the patient. Determine the length of time needed for the person to be able to return to the tasks somewhat refreshed.

For other options and problems, see Chapter 13 on families of the elderly.

DAILY LIVING WITH ALTERED COMPREHENSION AND DYSPHASIA (LEFT HEMISPHERE LESIONS)

Individuals with significant infarction in the left hemisphere (right hemiplegia) do not have the degree of spatial–perceptual or judgment deficits of the left hemiplegic. However, they are at risk of prolonged deficits in language function. Given the difference in deficits, the person with right hemiplegia is much more likely to resume more independent functioning, despite the discouraging awareness of the difficulties. Again, there is no loss of mental acuity.

Trying to manage daily living with limited or altered speech creates major difficulties and adjustments in getting one's needs met at even the most basic levels—to say nothing of the higher levels of needs for acceptance, affection, and esteem. Further, the often invisible slowed response time to the speech of others plus the need for added time to find the words to make responses tends to limit the ability to keep pace with the speech of others in business transactions (e.g., shopping and traveling) and to enter into conversations.

RISK FACTORS

Individuals who are at higher risk for not being able to manage daily living with altered speech and comprehension are those who

Live with people or in a community where there is little understanding of the dynamics of the pathology (e.g., that aphasia does not signify impaired mental status)

Go out into the community where the condition is not recognized or understood

Lack a consistent companion who has come to understand the alternative communication patterns used by the dysphasic person ·

Were highly verbal before their stroke

SIGNS AND SYMPTOMS

Manifestations of failure to manage daily living with dysphasia emerge from both patients and those around them. The dysphasic person may present a neglected appearance, lose weight, cease to try to communicate in any way and at any level, or withdraw from human contact. Former activities and diversions, even those not involving speech, may be avoided. There is a sense of giving up.

Family members, friends, or neighbors may be observed to diminish or avoid visiting, talk to them as if they were children, cease talking to them, or talk about them as if they were not there. They may fail to touch them and show signs of affection. The risks of depersonalization are high.

PROGNOSTIC VARIABLES

A poor prognosis is associated with

Lacking a caring, skilled personal support system of individuals with knowledge, skill, creativity, affection, and staying power

Living in an environment where there is lack of knowledge regarding dysphasia and strategies for living with it

Having less obvious comprehension deficits that further interfere with keeping up with verbal input

Living in an environment that overestimates or underestimates the deficit

Having a premorbid personality that lacked humor, ego strength, and independence

COMPLICATIONS

Major complications tend to be linked. They include inability to get basic needs met, sensory underload, and depersonalization. Such deprivation can lead to serious depression and suicide, either sudden or slow.

TREATMENT

In the immediate post-stroke phase it becomes important to foster return of speech and comprehension as soon as the person is responsive. In the early stages this includes the following:

Encouraging the use of the individual's available speech or comprehension. For example, if the person can read words or sing, but not speak, use that capability to maintain the capacity to produce these sounds and respond to symbols of printed or spoken sounds.

If a visual field deficit has been diagnosed or recognized, position yourself where sight is possible before communicating with the patient.

Take time to listen. *Do not rush the person* or communicate a sense of impatience.

Help relatives to understand what is happening and the important role they can play. Assist them to engage in effective strategies.

Several hazards exist for individuals who experience a residual deficit in communication. Their self-concept can change. They may see themselves as stupid or feel they are losing their minds because they cannot understand or speak. The nurse needs to reassure the patient that there is no decrease in intellectual powers, nor is the individual out of touch with reality, but that the nurse understands why the person may feel that way. Families and other health care providers also need to be included in this preparation (see boxes on pp. 364 and 365).

In speaking to the patient it is important to realize that he does not have a hearing deficit; speaking loudly is inappropriate.

Alternatives to Speech for Long-term Dysphasics Some patients never recover the ability to speak. Realization of this brings a strong reactive depression and grieving. A high-risk time is the point when the high-intensity speech therapy or rehabilitative efforts are terminated and the realization comes that others have given up on him. It becomes crucial that the transition to nonspeech-oriented communication systems be in full use to minimize the shock of loss. Alternatives include (1) pointing, gestures, and pantomime; (2) cards with common requests or words; and (3) encouraging nonverbal activities with others so that they can feel self-worth and companionship without words.

It is important to continue expectations for functioning. A person cannot retain integrity and feelings of self-worth if there is no obligation, responsibility, or demands placed on him.

The use of speech pathologists and speech therapists can be very helpful. However, it still may fall to the nurse to determine how the speech exercises and activities can be incorporated into daily living and can involve other people in the environment. It also will be incumbent on the nurse to help to create situations and environments in which the individual can learn from others with the same problems and continue to practice speaking over long periods of time—groups in senior citizen centers, visitors into the home or nursing home, and so forth.

Treatment of Perseveration For the few individuals with motor and sensory perseveration (persistent repetition of the same verbal or motor response to varied stimuli), management involves calling it to their attention when it occurs and interrupting the activity, e.g., "Mrs. Johnson, you already washed your face." While the motor perseveration tends to have disappeared by the time the individual reaches convalescent or home care settings, it can recur. The sensory component (repetitive speech) continues longer. It is well for health care provider and family to be aware of this behavior. An example of this might be

Nurse: Good morning, Mrs. Johnson.
Mrs. J.: Good morning.
Nurse: What did you have for breakfast today?

Guidelines for Communicating to the Individual with Poststroke Communication Deficits

Talk to the person.

Use normal volume—do not shout

Get the patient's attention before speaking

Face the patient and be sure the light is on your face

Have only one person talk at a time

Use short sentences

Speak more slowly—it may take more time to process thought

Use concrete language

Ask questions that require a yes-or-no response

Avoid double questions (Is it this or that?)

Do not change the subject matter quickly

Allow plenty of time for answers (schedule enough time for each encounter and do not give cues of impatience)

Engage only in conversations you have time to finish

Do not correct mistakes

Ignore profanity

Express your pleasure when the person communicates, but do not praise in a patronizing way

Do not send mixed messages in which your words say one thing and your body says another—nonverbal language is well understood by the patient

Be honest. Do not pretend you understand if you do not. Share the person's frustration. "It's very frustrating to try to talk and not be understood"

Mrs. J.: Good morning.
Nurse: It's good to see you all dressed today.
Mrs. J.: Good morning.

It may or may not be possible to interrupt this pattern immediately. Sometimes changing the motor behavior will serve to change it. These episodes of sensory perseveration tend to be isolated blocks of behavior rather than ongoing.

Treatment for the Primary Caregiver Role relationships may be altered and, at a minimum, need to be assessed in terms of the impact of changed communication patterns between husband and wife, family members, and companions. Despite loss or alterations of speech and comprehension, many couples and families have found ways to compensate and

maintain their relationships in premorbid roles. Since intellectual acuity is not usually affected, capacity for participation in decision making and other family activities is quite possible.

The partner in a relationship that has been close and characterized by verbal sharing may feel a tremendous loss and ongoing loneliness associated with the patient's dysphasia. The grief and sometimes anger over the loss may be more bearable if it can be seen as normal and legitimate. The nurse may be helpful in predicting this potential response and legitimizing the emotional reactions that are associated with it. Suggesting that the person seek someone with whom to share the experiences, someone who can be a nonjudgmental sounding board, can prove helpful. It is important to teach the partner that the trajectory for im-

Guidelines for Helping the Patient Communicate

Do not persist if the person becomes frustrated in attempts to communicate

Use nonverbal communication such as pointing and gestures

Use a series of flash cards or list of words or pictures to reduce frustration

Communication is easier when the person is not tired, morning is easier than night

Touching is helpful for a frustrated person

"No" does not always mean no; it may also mean yes

Facilitate the use of gestures, pantomime, or other signals if there is a major language deficit. Do not mix speech with a nonverbal communication system

Keep trying; improvements in speech can occur months and even years after the stroke

Explore the ability to sing or read aloud (part of automatic speech). Some persons who can not speak can regain communication skills through singing and records. Use familiar songs, ones the person knows well and enjoys. First languages are more easily used than those acquired later

Express for the patient your understanding of the difficulty of being unable to speak for himself. Indicate that being angry and frustrated is normal

Include the dysphasic person in decision making in the home as much as possible. (One wife indicated that in 10 years she never made a decision without discussing it with her dysphasic husband)

Letters from distant relatives or friends may take the form of tape recordings

---

provement of speech is a long one (even years) so that the course can be put into perspective.

EVALUATION

Responses indicating that the person with dysphasia is managing daily living can be seen in continued involvement with others. Alternative ways for communicating are found or accommodations are being made by others. Basic needs are being met and failure-to-thrive does not occur. Frustration decreases. Family members and companions spend time with the person and continue to enjoy his company and show affection and esteem.

DAILY LIVING WITH SENSORY–MOTOR DYSFUNCTION (RIGHT OR LEFT HEMIPLEGIA)

Transient or long-term sensory–motor dysfunction is an element of most strokes. The impact on daily living is related to the location and degree of residual deficit. See Figure 21–3 for a diagram used to communicate loss of sensation and motor function.

RISK FACTORS

Sensory Persons who are not aware of the nature and extent of sensory deficits are at risk for trauma and greater than usual problems in managing daily living. When visual field deficits are also present there is double jeopardy because they are unable to use vision as a compensatory mechanism for sensory losses.

Motor Persons who not only have motor losses but also sensory losses will encounter greater difficulty. The spatial–perceptual deficits and impaired judgment of the person with left hemiplegia also add greatly to the risks.

Sensory and Motor Architectural barriers and a living environment that does not lend itself to alterations to accommodate to the post-stroke deficits make daily living more difficult. Lack of money to make changes or purchase helpful equipment is an added risk factor. Lack

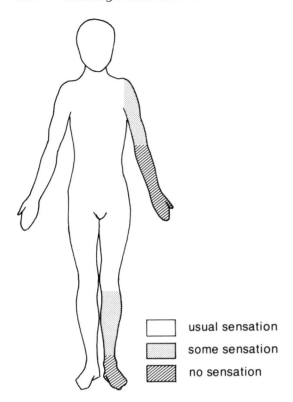

usual sensation

some sensation

no sensation

FIGURE 21–3   Body diagram for communicating areas of loss of sensation (see text).

of an acceptable, consistent primary caregiver is a major factor in producing both ineffectiveness and unhappiness in daily living with poststroke disabilities.

SIGNS AND SYMPTOMS

Lack of effectiveness in managing daily living with sensory and motor deficits can be manifested in the patient by the following:

Reports of dissatisfaction
Bruises, abrasions, burns, joint dislocations, and decubiti—signs of trauma, accidents, or failure to change position or receive appropriate skin care
Underuse of an extremity in the activities of daily living, when capability exists
Less active participation in daily living than would be expected from apparent potential
Reluctance to be seen by others

The primary caregiver is also a source of signs and symptoms of daily living that is not going

well. Data from this source include the following:

Reports of areas of dissatisfaction with daily living given patient status and the kinds of responsibility
Reports of sleep deprivation
Strength and endurance insufficient to carry out the physical tasks to be done
Signs of burnout
Absence of others to provide respite on a regular basis
Absence of activities outside of the caregiving role

PROGNOSTIC VARIABLES

The likelihood that an older person will manage daily living following a stroke depends on a supportive physical environment and acceptable skilled, capable support figures or caregivers. A premorbid personality of drive, persistence, ego strength, and humor contribute to managing daily living with residual disability. Adequate finances for equipment, services, and transportation are always a factor.

COMPLICATIONS

The complications associated with trying to manage daily living with sensory and motor deficits following a stroke include the downward spiral of failure-to-thrive, a high risk of contractures with increasing immobility, and further difficulties with daily living. Social isolation, either self-imposed or the result of changes in others, is a third complication (Table 21–4).

TREATMENT

The development of a plan for effective management of daily living for the older individual following a stroke is contingent on accommodating to, substituting for, or supplementing the areas of identified functional deficit.

Awareness of Sensory Losses   In order to compensate for loss of sensation, an individual has to become aware of what the specific losses are. A diagram of the body showing the areas of loss of sensation (Fig. 21–3) may be useful in making the ideas more concrete. If the patient and family or caretakers have the information in written form, it allows them to refer to it whenever they wish.

Daily exercises in which the part of the body (e.g., the hand) that has lost sensation may be touched, rubbed, and handled as well as named are important. This may assist the person in remembering to own it.

Compensating for the Loss of Sensation

Because the body is not sending messages regarding the position of a part of the body and the forces that are impacting on it, *the eyes must be used as a compensatory mechanism.* Patients need to be taught to *watch the affected extremity*—noting the position it is in and anything in the environment that is acting on it, such as heat, sharp surfaces, or impact. The patient who has been in a rehabilitation setting before discharge will have been taught to do this. If the individual has not been exposed to this teaching, it is important for the home health nurse or the nurse in the clinic or senior center to check on whether the individual and caregivers know about this and are remembering to do it.

Where a hand has lost sensation, a bath thermometer, or checking water temperature with the unaffected hand, is important in setting water temperatures for bathing, showering, and hand washing. The use of gloves or protection from the cold would be important in very cold climates.

Motor Function

Nursing management of motor function is concerned with maintaining joint motion, preventing stretching of supporting joint structures, preventing contractures, and maintaining or improving muscle strength and endurance.

To maintain joint mobility, it is thought to be sufficient for most people to engage in range of motion activities twice each day, with each joint being put through full range of motion to the point of pain three times per exercise period.

It is important that patients and families understand that the range of motion activities are done in order to prevent loss rather than to restore voluntary muscle function. If they believe that the purpose of the range of motion exercises is to return muscle function, they have been known to quit doing them when voluntary movement fails to return. The result is that the patient develops major contractures that further complicate his or her life.

Positioning of affected limbs is important in both daytime and nighttime activities. If a flaccid upper extremity exists, an arm sling should be worn whenever the person ambulates to prevent stretching of the shoulder ligaments with greater risk of shoulder dislocation. A hand splint for maintaining a functional position is important at night. If there is a sensory loss, it is recommended that the individual not sleep more than 20 minutes on the affected side. To prevent turning over to that side during sleep, a pillow may be set behind the patient's back (for those who sleep on the unaffected side). This will avoid injury to the affected side where sensory loss exists. For the individual with a flaccid foot, a stack of books wrapped in a towel makes a good foot support in bed.

Where some function remains, the management plan may be directed toward maintaining and increasing the *strength and endurance* by activities and exercise. Persons over age 70 need some strength for what they *want* to do. They need to learn to judge when they are tired and stop before then. This is very hard to do. The nurse may be helpful in working this through. Many communities have programs of group exercises for stroke patients at the local YMCA or YWCA, senior citizen centers, and day-care centers. Nurses in the community should learn about these available resources. For those who enjoy swimming there are sessions for the handicapped in some local community pools. Engaging in activities with others having the same problems may decrease the sense of deviance and social isolation. It may also add incentive to continue to participate in exercises or activities in the home in the interim between sessions.

Booklets and audiovisual material indicating exercise and activity programs are listed at the end of this chapter.

One of the problems that stroke patients face as they return to engaging in the activities of daily living is that *they are slower in all of their physical activities. Everything takes longer and requires more effort.* Caregivers should plan a sufficient block of time in any encounter to permit patients to accomplish the needed activities at the pace they must set. Impatience, hurrying them, or stepping in and doing what they should do for themselves is not therapeutic. It is important also for the nurse to help the individual verbalize problems and to communicate an understanding of what he is experiencing as well as to work with him to develop acceptable plans of a balance of activity and rest that is satisfying to him.

It may be helpful for the nurse to tell the patient and support persons that they will experience frustration in doing things because it takes longer, so that they need to allow more time for activities and, at least initially, a rest period after an activity.

Older persons who have had strokes have told nurses that venturing out into large gatherings is particularly taxing. Often those who try to reenter into social activities prematurely have a very trying and unsuccessful experience. They then become much more reluctant to try it again and may become more isolated socially. A wiser course may be a deliberately gradual increase in the size of social groups, building up to the larger size ones as tolerance increases. They should arrange with a family member to take them out of the social situation early, before they get tired. If the person knows of this option in advance, he is more likely to be willing to go out.

Where motor strength is missing, there are some *assistive devices* that can make it possible for individuals to engage more successfully in daily activities. Short leg braces, tripod canes, hemiwalkers, and walkers can add to the individual's capacity for mobility.

A wheelchair is contraindicated if an individual has the potential for walking. It has been found to be a real barrier for regaining the ability to walk. The patient becomes dependent on it and it inhibits learning to walk. However, for going out to places where substantial walking is required, a wheelchair can be used, e.g., to airports or for shopping. Then the wheelchair increases endurance and provides social outlets.

Persons who have had strokes can expect *falls to occur more often.* It becomes a practical issue to give them some control over falls in knowing the best way to fall and how to get up. The individual should be taught to fall toward the unaffected side whenever possible. This allows him to edge himself across the floor using his elbow, hip, and knee (resting as needed) until he comes to a heavy piece of furniture—a sofa or bed. Usually he can use this to brace himself and work up to a standing position.

Patients and their families can be alerted to the increased need to *balance activities with rest.* With each activity being more demanding because of the dysfunction, it becomes more work and endurance is reduced. Most elderly people find that they have greater energy earlier in the day, so those activities that require greater concentration of energy should be scheduled during late morning and early afternoon hours, e.g., visits to the doctor's office.

Family Members and Caregivers For the care and treatment of family members and caregivers, see Chapter 13.

EVALUATION

Evidence that nursing interventions in the area of sensory–motor deficits are having a positive effect are seen in the home environment, the patient status, and the status of the caregivers and family. The patient has minimal signs of trauma and engages in activities to the extent of his capacity. Levels of frustration and emotional responses are appropriate to the achievements being made or problems being encountered. Patterns of socialization are commensurate with energy and desires. The living environment is made as accommodating to deficits as the structure and finances permit.

For caregivers, effective management includes having the physical strength and endurance to supplement or substitute for the sensory–muscular deficits of the patient. It also includes the wisdom and restraint to assist only with those activities that the patient cannot or should not do. Where the caregiver's strength and endurance are not adequate, there is some form of supplementary help. A respite schedule is in place and is used. If there is a spouse or ongoing companion, that person has an external support person who is a satisfying listener.

Family members engage with the patient and caregiver in ways that are mutually helpful and healthy.

DAILY LIVING WITH VISUAL FIELD DEFICITS

Changes in visual fields drastically affect what persons will attend to and therefore how they will behave in daily living. The visual field cut will *totally block out* any objects outside of that range. Thus, if objects, food, furniture, or people are in the area of the visual field cut they will not be noticed. Unless the person can be taught to be aware of this deficit and adopt a changing head position and scanning movements, the implications for daily living are formidable.

RISK FACTORS

The person with a left visual field cut will be at greater risk because it is associated with decreased capacity for recognizing the deficit.

The time period of greatest risk occurs before the elderly person has learned that a problem exists and has integrated the compensatory scanning behavior into daily living. On an ongoing basis, going into a strange environment will always present greater risks.

Certain situations regularly carry higher risks for trauma. These include crossing streets, handling hot pots on a stove, and being around toddlers as examples.

SIGNS AND SYMPTOMS

Indications that daily living is not being managed well with visual field cuts include observing falls, near falls, or walking into objects. These persons may be observed not to eat or take fluids independently. They may have bruises, burns, and abrasions. They may complain about the loss of ability to read or play solitaire because portions of each page or the card display are "missing."

PROGNOSTIC VARIABLES

Managing daily living with visual field cuts is dependent on learning efficient and consistent scanning behaviors.

COMPLICATIONS

Complications include visual underload from taking in only fractions of presenting situations, inadequate eating or drinking, and trauma.

TREATMENT

Since the individual usually is not aware of the visual field deficits, the first step is to make him aware of the blind area and the implications this has for daily living. Once he knows where the losses are, he can be taught to turn his head to compensate for loss of vision. In addition, it is important to teach the family and friends about the limitations of visual field. Then they can anticipate that they and objects in the environment will not be seen in certain positions, and they will place themselves within the patient's visual field when they wish to be noticed. A diagram of the blind areas will help both the patient and family see what the problem is and be more active in accommodating to it.

To teach a person with field deficits how to accommodate, the nurse may show him how to deliberately set up an obstacle course using furniture. As he learns to navigate it in the privacy and safety of his own home he learns what he must do to scan the situation to move about more freely.

Reading presents particular problems to the individual with field deficits. He tends to lose his place. A ruler placed immediately beneath the line he is reading, or the use of the finger moving along the line, assists in keeping his place.

The balancing of figures as in checking accounts also is a problem, again because of the inability to keep one's place in the book. The individual may need the assistance of another person to balance his accounts.

Driving privileges are revoked in many states for individuals with visual field deficits. The individual may have to be helped to readjust to life without the usual form of transportation.

Diplopia is managed by covering one eye. The patch is changed from one eye to the other every 2 to 4 hours to keep eye muscles active.

DAILY LIVING AS A PRIMARY CAREGIVER TO A STROKE PATIENT

One of the most difficult tasks in long-term management is helping the person who lives with the stroke victim. Living with profound, or even moderate, cognitive sensorimotor deficit 24 hours a day, 7 days a week for months and years taxes the emotional and physical stamina of any human being.

Nurses need to play a role in trying to recruit others to provide regularly scheduled "time off" from each other for these two people. Both persons need it; however, it may be difficult for each to accept. The patient may be embarrassed to have other persons see his disability and he may feel comfortable only with his accustomed companion. On the other hand, the spouse or other care person may experience guilt at leaving the patient and may worry that a "stranger" won't know how to manage.

One approach that has worked to the benefit of both individuals is encountering different people. Where mobility permits, day care centers offer a useful service and therapeutic environment. Home health care aides, volunteer visitors from church groups or clubs, retired persons, and neighbors—all could be tapped to visit a few hours occasionally. Often the nurse is the catalyst who sets this in motion.

Try leaving the patient with others. When the visiting nurse comes to give care, the spouse leaves. When visitors come, the spouse leaves. If the spouse can manage a vacation or trip of several days, checks can be made regularly to reassure that things at home are going well.

There is no question that the spouse needs to get out to regroup and revitalize. Respite is critical to maintaining the strength to manage long-term chronic disability on a round-the-clock basis. Nursing plans of management need to address as much attention to the support persons as to the one who has had the stroke. For the best outcome, neither can be neglected, even though their needs are quite different.

THE NURSING CHALLENGE

The nursing management of the older person who experiences a stroke presents a real challenge to nursing. Obviously, skilled nursing is important in the acute phase and early convalescence—ultimate progress is affected by the quality of nursing care given in this stage. But probably more demanding nursing occurs as the long road of living with the residual deficits of stroke and aging is encountered (Hodgins, 1964). To be effective the nurse must remain alert to small and slow changes, must consider creative options for dealing with continuing or new problems, and must maintain a professional, positive attitude that, in turn, helps the patient and those who surround him. All these require a special kind of nursing.

The areas to be addressed in nursing diagnosis and management are broad. They touch on almost every aspect of daily living and on coping resources that may be diminished in so many dimensions—physical, communication, sensory, and emotional. The long, unabated stress on support systems demands that they, too, receive critical nursing attention. The nursing expertise requires a working knowledge not only of the pathophysiology, complications, and rehabilitation phenomena but also of the resources in the community that may be used by the patient and family to share the experience and to gain support.

Satisfaction for the patient, family, and nurse often must be found in slow, tiny gains or, perhaps, in holding one's own. It becomes critical for the nurse to notice and interpret data indicating even small changes so that each participant (including the nurse) has realistic data to document the results of their efforts. It is a major achievement if the nurse is genuinely satisfied with these rewards and helps patients and families find a comparable sense of accomplishment.

All in all, it takes a broad, skilled, perceptive, creative, persistent, and positive nursing approach, one that realistically buoys up and maintains those involved as long as necessary. Such a demanding task over a long period of time logically suggests that even the best and strongest of nurses will need to have their wellsprings renewed and their perspective freshened. It suggests that the nurses should as carefully document their own ongoing professional and personal resources and arrange for the personal and professional support systems that will enable them to maintain the kind of an approach with the stroke patient and family that will be most effective. Currently there are nurses who are delivering this high-quality nursing care to stroke patients; there are more who can.

ONGOING EVALUATION

The person who recovers from a major stroke faces a long rehabilitation period. He may become discouraged frequently by the very gradual recovery he experiences. Recovery does take place and this is important to keep in mind. It is helpful to document the changes that occur. The nurse may suggest and implement a flow sheet whereby the stroke victim and his family can follow the progress. The record keeping may be designed according to the person's functional limitations on day 1 following the stroke. The Evaluation Flow Sheet (see box on p. 371) is an example of what can be used. These are sample items. The increments could be smaller or greater, depending on the need to see progress with limited or major recovery. The deficits also will determine the

Evaluation Flow Sheet

ACTIVITY	DATE	COMMENTS
Turn self in bed		
Control bowel and bladder function		
Swallow without choking		
Handle oral secretions		
Feed self		
Transfer onto chair, commode, or wheelchair		
Bathe self		
Take shower or tub bath		
Dress in street clothes		
Apply short leg brace		
Do range of motion exercises for upper extremity		
Walk aided		
Walk unaided		
Write letters		
Read a newspaper		
Handle checking account		
Take own medications		
Operate a motor vehicle		
Attend a concert or public event		
Go out to visit		
Use a bus (if done premorbidly)		
Use a satisfactory communication system		
Develop lifestyle and support systems that allow for satisfactory time apart and together with caregiver		

variables. The nurse, the patient, and the family should identify the variables that are important to them at a point in time. The items can be updated and new examples added according to the status of the situation.

Rationale for use of the Evaluation Flow Sheet is the following:

1. To assess the improvements of functions
2. To give evidence that changes occur
3. To allow the patient and family responsibilities and an active role in management
4. To enhance self-esteem and body image
5. To recall how much progress has been made since the onset of disability
6. To have a data base for short-term goal setting

Literature for Patients and Families

American Heart Association National Center
7320 Greenville Ave
Dallas, TX 75231
    Caring for the Person with Stroke
    Facts about Stroke (English and Spanish)
    Strokes, a Guide for the Family
    How Strokes Affect Behavior

National Stroke Association
1420 Ogden
Denver, CO 80218
(303) 839–1992

BE STROKE SMART ARTICLES

Activities of Daily Living
Aphasia—Prison Without Walls
Bladder Problems Following Stroke
Communication Difficulties (3 articles)
Depression—A Natural Reaction to Stroke
Emotional Aspects (5 articles)
Home and Work Adaptations (5 articles)
Home Exercises for Stroke Patients
Household Barriers Confronting the Stroke
  Survivor
Let's Give Stroke the Kind of Treatment
  It Deserves
One-Handed Activities
Open Channels
Positioning the Stroke Survivors with Paralysis
Rehabilitation—Guidelines & Resources
  (9 articles)
Returning to Work After a Stroke
Self-Help Devices for the Kitchen
Stroke: A Main Cause of Death Surrounded
  by Myths
Stroke Prevention: Reducing Your Risk
Stroke: Questions and Answers
Suggestions for Communication with the
  Right Hemisphere Damaged Patient (left
  hemi)
Suggestions for Effective Communication
  with the Aphasic Patient
The Importance of Proper Diet After Stroke
Therapeutic Recreation
Therapy & Long Term Care in Stroke
  Recovery
There Is Sex After Stroke
Understanding Speech & Language Problems
  After Stroke
Use of Braces to Help Regain Control of the
  Foot/Ankle
What Every Family Should Know about
  Stroke
What Is a Stroke?

PAMPHLETS

Living at Home After a Stroke
Stroke: What Is It, What Causes It
  The Road Back—A Stroke Recovery Guide

BOOKS

The Road Ahead: A Stroke Recovery Guide
Stroke—From Crisis to Victory
  (by John H. Lavin)

PERSONAL EXPERIENCE
WITH STROKES

McBride C: Silent Victory. Nelson Hall Co,
  1969.
Dahlberg C: Stroke—A Doctor's Personal
  Story and His Recovery. New York: WW
  Norton, 1977.
Hodgins E: Episode: Report on the Accident in
  My Skull. New York: Atheneum Publishers,
  1964.

OTHER LITERATURE

Bahr R, Hess L: What every family should
  know about strokes. New York: Appleton-
  Century-Crofts, 1981.
Freese A: Stroke: The new hope and the new
  help. New York: Random House, 1981.
Sarno J, Taylor M: Stroke: A guide for patients
  and their families, 2nd ed. New York:
  McGraw-Hill, 1979.
Sessler G: Stroke: How to prevent it/how to
  survive it. Englewood Cliffs, NJ: Prentice
  Hall, 1981.

MEDIA RECOMMENDATIONS

Stroke (flip chart and slides)
  Robert J. Brady Co., Bowie, MD 20715
"I Had a Stroke" (film and videotapes)
  Film Makers Library
  133 East 58th St. Suite 703 A
  New York, NY 10022
Stroke (video, film, slides)
  Medfact Inc.
  1112 Andrew N.E.
  Massillon, OH 44646

References and Other Readings

Adams R, Victor M. Principles of neurology, 3rd ed.
  New York: McGraw-Hill, 1985.
American Heart Association. 1992 heart and stroke
  facts. Dallas: AHA, 1992.
Barnett H, Mohr J, Stein B, et al. Stroke: pathophys-
  iology, diagnosis and management, vols 1 and 2.
  New York: Churchill Livingstone, 1986.
Broderick J, Phillips S, Whishnant J, et al. Incidence

rates of stroke in the eighties: the end of the decline in stroke? Stroke 1989; 20:577.

Chambers B, Norris J, Shurvell B, et al. Prognosis of acute stroke. Neurology 1987; 37:221.

Core Curriculum for Neuroscience Nursing, 3rd ed. Chicago: American Association of Neurological Nursing, 1990.

Fuhrman M. Mood changes after cerebrovascular accidents: depression. Stroke Connection, 1989.

Gent M, Blakely J, Easton J, et al. The Canadian American ticlopidine study (CATS in thromboembolic stroke). Lancet 1989; 1:1215.

Grotta J. Medical progress. Current medical and surgical therapy for cerebrovascular disease. N Engl J Med 1987; 317:1505.

Kalbach L. Unilateral neglect: mechanisms and nursing care. Am J Neurol Nurs 1991; 23:125.

Springer S, Deutsch G. Left brain—right brain. Salt Lake City: Freeman and Co, 1981.

Wolf P, Abbott R, Kannel W. Atrial fibrillation: a major contributor to stroke in the elderly. The Framingham Study. Arch Intern Med 1987; 147:1561.

PART FIVE

High-Risk Pathophysiology in the Elderly: Medical and Nursing Management

The 13 chapters in Part Five apply the daily living model to selected *high-risk* pathologic conditions in the elderly. The chapters, arranged alphabetically, each include both medical and nursing information. The nursing sections systematically address the problems in daily living associated with the pathophysiology and its treatment. For individualized nursing diagnoses the reader can use the information from the book and the data about the person's specific requirements of daily living, specific functional strengths and deficits, and external resources.

Chapter 22 (Cancer) presents content on biases and values affecting cancer diagnosis and treatment, biology of cancer in the elderly, updated material on cancer by sites, screening schedules for older individuals, factors that influence treatment decisions as well as specific therapy including biotherapy, and a new section on clinical trials. Daily living with dysfunctions associated with the pathology of cancer and its treatment are included. Chapter 23 (Cardiovascular Problems) has added valvular heart disease and arrhythmias to information on other cardiac problems and management of daily living with them.

Chapter 24 (Diabetes Mellitus) provides current insights on the nature of diabetes in the elderly and presents medical and nursing management approaches. The contributors' ongoing nursing care of older diabetics and their families gives this chapter both solid substance and practical ideas. Chapter 25 (Gastrointestinal Problems) has been updated to provide the most recent research and treatment of gastrointestinal problems in the older individual. Chapter 26 (Genital Problems) deals with selected common genital problems of older men and women, including prostatic cancer, benign prostatic hypertrophy in males, and vaginal atrophy and infections in women.

Chapter 27 (Hearing Loss) has been revised to strengthen the section on daily living with hearing loss, including expansion of hearing examination and rehabilitation with hearing loss. Chapter 28 (Hypertension) is written by an experienced nurse practitioner with a large caseload of patients in an ambulatory care setting. This chapter has been revised to incorporate the latest research and norms of treatment for hypertension in the older person. Chapter 29 (Incontinence and Urinary Problems) deals with nursing management to prevent and rehabilitate patients with incontinence and to help older individuals live with incontinence that cannot be reversed. It also presents the current knowledge and treatment options for the common and debilitating problem of urinary tract infections.

Chapter 30 (Musculoskeletal Problems) has been extensively revised to address common problems of gait, falls, and fractures, as well as osteoporosis and osteoarthritis. Chapter 31 (Renal Failure: Acute and Chronic) discusses both the nature of acute and chronic renal failure and its medical treatment, but also the problems associated with decisions about moving to dialysis as a treatment, living with the demands of dialysis, and decisions about discontinuing the treatment. Chapter 32 (Respiratory Problems) focuses on pneumonia and chronic obstructive pulmonary disease. Current medical therapy and nursing management of daily living with the symptoms and the demands of the treatment are discussed.

Chapter 33 (Common Skin Problems) deals with common skin conditions that can occur in older persons. This chapter covers infectious conditions and problems such as dryness and itching and trauma. It examines strategies for managing the discomforts associated with skin problems. Chapter 34 (Vision Problems) is written by a gerontological nurse practitioner actively involved in clinical practice. This chapter provides current knowledge on eye conditions and their treatment including cataracts, macular degeneration, glaucoma, and inflammations, as well as nursing management of problems of living with impaired vision.

22
Cancer

VERA S. WHEELER

Cancer is a complex disease with an increasing incidence in the elderly. Age is one of several major risk factors for developing cancer (Oleske and Groenwald, 1990). Cancer can potentially arise from every tissue and organ system in the body and can affect all aspects of an individual's physiologic, emotional, and social functioning. This chapter highlights aspects of cancer care pertinent to the elderly patient. The reader is referred to the references for a more comprehensive review of specific aspects of cancer care. The specific purposes of this chapter are as follows:

1. To identify the magnitude of the cancer problem in the aged population as it may be encountered in both the inpatient and ambulatory care settings.
2. To provide pertinent insights and application of cancer knowledge to understanding the elderly person with cancer.
3. To confront the "give up" attitude toward cancer management in the elderly and to identify a more rational basis for decision making that can be used by nurses and their elderly patients.

Part of this chapter is based on the Second Edition with credit to Doris Molbo.

Age-related Biases

When cancer literature is reviewed, reference is often given to the fact that the incidence of cancer increases with age. Fifty percent of all cancers occur after age 65 (Oleske and Groenwald, 1990; Dellefield, 1986). In spite of this statistic, although many texts may include information on childhood cancers, little attention is specifically given to the problems of the elderly patient with cancer. The elderly can be as vulnerable as the infant with organ system impairments, changes in mentation, and communication.

As cancer and the elderly patient are considered in this chapter, it is necessary to realize that health care professionals as well as the public may have different attitudes about cancer in the young and economically productive than they do about cancer in the elderly. When a malignancy occurs in the child, young adult, or parent, the health care professional may express anger and a feeling of tragedy at the loss to a family and community of a productive life. When an elderly person is diagnosed with a malignancy, the health care professional may express dismay or frustration, but not the same directed anger. There tends to be a fatalistic submissiveness to the presence of the cancer and a sense of the inevitable death.

377

Effect of Professional Bias

Health professionals who lack knowledge and training in geriatric medicine may influence and restrict the elderly patient's opportunities for diagnosis and cure. Their ignorance of the significant risks for development of cancer in the older person and an age-related bias may influence whether they promote and initiate screening tests or postpone them, "not wanting to burden" the older person. They may ignore or delay acting on signs and symptoms or avoid treatment measures, adopting a "wait and see" approach until the source of the symptoms is clearly apparent. Although these actions may be well-intentioned initially, their overall effect is to prevent the elderly person from having a cancer diagnosed early and therefore receiving potentially more effective, less toxic treatment.

Effects of Societal Biases

Health care professionals are not alone in this pervasive feeling about cancer in the elderly person. The general public and the family—even the elderly person himself—may feel and display a "give-up syndrome" when cancer is suspected. As Dellefield (1986) points out, attitudes and health beliefs of the older patient may be based on outdated beliefs about cancer and its treatment, fears of pain, mutilation, and death. When cancer is suspected, one may see nothing, expect nothing, and do nothing.

Values Affecting Diagnostic and Treatment Decisions

It is true that persons over age 70 have made delicate compensatory adaptations within the physical, psychological, and social spheres of their being. They have an accumulation of life's stressors before the time they encountered cancer. Therefore, their management is more complex, requiring concomitant management of their other health problems such as diabetes, mobility limitations, and anxiety.

The oft-heard phase "He's old, let him be. He's lived his life; he shouldn't have to have more pain or suffer anymore" must be counterbalanced, however, with the knowledge necessary to answer honestly the following questions:

Will the person suffer more or less in the future if treatment or rehabilitation are denied now?

What are his goals? What tasks of life are left to be completed?

What do his perceived loved ones understand of the answers to the previous questions? What can they give? What do they want? What does he want?

Cancer Biology

To the public, cancer is one disease. However, cancer is many diseases that vary in etiology, symptoms, growth rate, response to treatment, and prognosis. Any organ and tissue in the body can give rise to a malignancy, even within one site. In the lung, for example, there can arise several cancers having different growth patterns, etiologies, and treatment strategies.

Although a malignancy may be first detected as a single lump, cancer is frequently not a localized disease. It is a systemic disease. Cancer is defined as an uncontrolled growth of cells. What characterizes it as cancer is the malignant ability for cancer cells to break off from the primary tumor and establish secondary sites of growth (Kupcella, 1990). Metastatic cells use natural routes of communication within the body such as the circulatory system or lymphatics. The immune system, located in lymph nodes and the bloodstream, functions to recognize and destroy altered or metastatic cells. It is still unclear why this immune surveillance function fails and cancers are able to successfully metastasize and establish new sites of disease.

How does age affect the growth rate of the malignancy and patient survival? Do patients live longer? Holmes (1989) has suggested that some evidence points to many cancers being relatively indolent when compared with the cancers of younger adults. For example, 20% to 36% of undiagnosed cancers were found at autopsy in an elderly group ranging from ages 66 to 86. Other studies suggest the site of cancer origin within an organ may change with increasing age. For example, there is an increased incidence of medially located breast cancers in the elderly population versus lateral breast cancers in younger adults (Holmes, 1989). It has also been reported (Holmes, 1989) that increasing age is positively related to an increasing stage of disease except in lung cancer. In other words, the older patient with cancer of the breast, cervix, endometrium, ovary, or bladder is more likely to be diagnosed at an advanced stage of disease. Although there is considerable variability between cancers, breast cancer demonstrates one pattern of change in tumor aggressiveness with age. Older women survive longer with lower stage disease compared with younger women. However, younger women survive longer with high stage or advanced disease (Holmes, 1989).

Certain cancers appear to have an affinity for specific sites of new growth. Prostate cancer, for example, often metastasizes to the pelvis and spine; breast cancer to sites in bone, lung, or brain; colon cancer to liver; and lung cancer to brain. These patterns can be explained partly by available routes of metastasis and a downstream capillary bed. This may act as a filter, enabling a malignant cell to escape the circulation and establish a new growth (Kupcella, 1990). There is also a "seed and soil" theory. Those organs that are common sites of metastasis have special characteristics that favor the establishment of new growth. Studies also have demonstrated that cancer cells do not necessarily stop at the first capillary system (Kupcella, 1990). Health care practitioners can use this information when sorting out a patient's signs and symptoms. For example, there may be an increased chance of malignancy in an elderly man who presents with an expected enlarged prostate, but also complains of back pain.

Many cancers have the ability to produce systemic bodily symptoms that mimic nonmalignant diseases. For example, hypercalcemia in a patient with normal parathyroid function and without metastasis to the bone; skin changes such as hyperpigmentation, flushing, or pruritis; or a cushingoid syndrome secondary to increased ACTH. These are called paraneoplastic syndromes and are frequently caused by specific mediators such as hormones, inappropriately made by the malignant tumor itself. These syndromes can precede, follow, or present at the same time as the malignancy (DeWys and Killen, 1983). Paraneoplastic syndromes are associated with a variety of cancers such as lung, breast, ovarian, lymphoma, and kidney cancer. Effective control of the particular syndrome often requires primary control of the cancer itself. Recognition of the more common syndromes such as unexplained hyperpigmentation prompt the health care professional to recommend an evaluation for an occult malignancy. Symptoms in a nonmalignant disease such as parkinsonism that appear resistant to common therapy may have their origins in an occult malignant process (Huang, 1990).

Incidence

Before reviewing specific high-risk sites of disease in the elderly population, there are some overall facts about the incidence of cancer that should be kept in mind (Cancer Statistics Review—1973 to 1987):

1. Heart disease is the leading cause of death except in women 35 to 75 years and older (American Cancer Society, 1991).
2. A contributing factor to the increased incidence of cancer is the likewise increase in the number of older persons in the total US population.
3. Mortality for children and persons under 45 years of age have declined while overall cancer deaths have increased.
4. Each sex and race show significant increases in the incidence of cancer between 1973 and 1987.

Etiology

The age of a person is a well-known, major risk factor for the development of a malignancy. The incidence of all cancers, in general, increases with age. At age 25, the risk of cancer is 1 in 700; at age 65, it is 1 in 14 (Vannicola, 1988). Why do the elderly have such an increased risk for cancer?

One of the most prevalent theories is that the elderly person has lifelong exposure to environmental carcinogens. By living longer, the total dose he receives is greater than the younger adult. Epithelial tissue cancer from glandular and mucous membrane tissues have a greater incidence in the elderly population (Anisimov, 1989). These tissues are also the body surfaces having increased contact with carcinogens such as cigarette smoke, alcohol, radiation, and various food substances. Evidence for this theory might be illustrated by a cancer age and incidence curve that has the peak incidence at the oldest age groups such as in colon cancer (Newell et al, 1989) (Figure 22–1).

There are other factors that may also be interrelated with environmental exposure to carcinogens. Somatic cells undergo an aging process with an altered enzyme process. This results in a lessened ability to repair DNA mutations and an accumulation of damaging free radicals from oxygen metabolism (Lipschitz et al, 1985; Crawford and Cohen, 1984). Another theory suggests that the elderly person has an increased susceptibility to carcinogens compared with a younger adult (Schwab et al, 1989). These possible factors may combine with genetic susceptibility in some malignancies to increase the potential for the occurrence of a cancer (Lipschitz et al, 1985).

Finally, another theory proposed to explain the increased incidence of cancer in the elderly is immune senescence. The thymus, responsible for T-lymphocyte maturation, begins involution at sexual maturity, about age 15. At age 50, thymic hormones are no longer detectable in the bloodstream (Lipschitz et al, 1985). Although the total number of T-lymphocytes remains constant, the ratio of helper T cells increase compared with the number of cytotoxic T cells. The responsiveness of T cytotoxic cells also decreases as there is an increase in the number of immature cells in the bloodstream. This may affect the person's immune surveillance or the ability to recognize mutant or virally altered cells and destroy them (Schwab et al, 1989).

There are also humoral immunity changes with aging, including a decrease in the antibody response, decrease in the serum antibodies to foreign antigens, and an increase in autoantibodies. The overall effect of these immune system changes is a moderate immunodeficient state (Schwab et al, 1989). This may explain an increased susceptibility to viral and mycobacterium, resulting in an increased incidence of tuberculosis and herpes zoster and a decreased response to mutant cells with an increase in malignant growth.

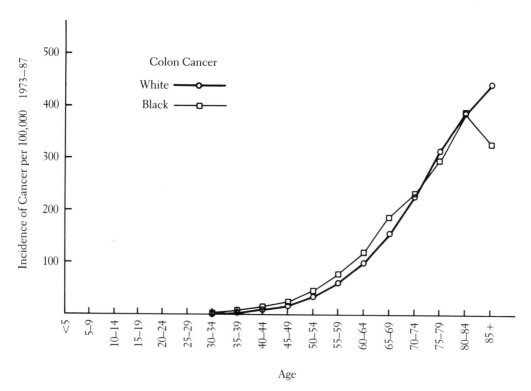

FIGURE 22–1   Incidence of colon cancer per 100,000 population for both sexes, blacks and whites, 1973–1987. (Cancer Statistics Review, 1973–1987; National Cancer Institute, NIH.)

Signs and Symptoms

PROBLEMS ASSOCIATED WITH THE ELDERLY

Patients, their families, and health professionals alike are regularly exposed to the American Cancer Society's message, "Know Cancer's Seven Warning Signals." These warning signs are:

A change in bowel or bladder habits
A sore that does not heal
Unusual bleeding or discharge
A thickening or lump in the breast or elsewhere
Indigestion or difficulty swallowing
Obvious change in wart or mole
Nagging cough or hoarseness

The elderly as a group, however, may receive different responses from health professionals when they present themselves with the signs or symptoms suggestive of malignancy. One individual indicated that she had been trying to find a gynecologist who did not regard the seven danger signals as a sign of her old age. At the point when she was writing about her experiences, she had contacted four physicians who assured her that her condition was nothing more than the result of her advancing age (Cullen et al, 1976).

It is true that some of the warning signs cannot be used as exclusive signals of malignancy for the elderly. An increasing number of debilitating diseases present in the older person tend to confound or mask the presence of the usual symptoms of malignancy. For example, a person already may have degenerative bone disease, pulmonary disease, and impaired bowel and urinary functions. The person may have lived many years with unhealed leg ulcers or with loose, uncomfortable dentures, with resulting traumatic ulcers. Thus, it is more difficult to recognize the pattern of new signs against the background of preexisting illness and debility.

It becomes important then for the patient and the family to identify to the health care providers all of the signs and symptoms present, both old and new, at the time of a physical examination. The professional can then logically study the significance of the newly presenting symptoms in light of previous ones. The task for the professional will be to sort out

progressive chronic disease from the possibility of a malignancy.

The use of an ongoing, well-documented problem-oriented health record can be of tremendous value for this purpose. In the present health care environment, patients frequently do not see the same practitioner twice. They may not have enough time with the health care practitioner to state symptoms in their own way. The health record can partially speak for the patient. It allows the health professional to assess the patient's totality of symptoms with an economy of effort and then focus on what is most important at the moment.

The health care provider must be prepared to view the patient with an open mind in order to consider new possible diagnoses or correct past errors. For example, does the fatigue, anemia, and gastric discomfort signal another small hemorrhage from the hiatal hernia or do they suggest new disease, such as a malignancy? Or, does the enlarged prostate of the elderly man suggest a benign aging process or an occult malignancy?

There are some signs and symptoms definitive of malignancy that are more easily located and defined in the elderly. For example, the atrophy of the mammary or glandular tissue of the breast in the woman over age 65 minimizes the amount of palpable normal tissue in the breast. The woman who has had earlier premenopausal benign cystic disease will, if she has not had exogenous estrogen replacement, be completely free of any palpable remnants of the cystic disease by age 65. Therefore, when the breast is examined in older women, **any** palpable lesion that is not normal fat tissue is likely to be a malignant lesion. Further, when hormonal stimulation decreases and vaginal secretions cease, any vaginal discharge must be suspect even if the patient has had prior vaginal infections.

Thus, it becomes important, particularly in the elderly, with their coexisting diseases, to record all signs and symptoms observed in the patient. The health practitioner should review them at appropriate intervals (biweekly or monthly) and observe for their continued presence, exacerbation, or the appearance of new symptoms. These changes, when considered over time, can indicate the increasing probability of malignant lesions (see Scheduling Screening Programs later in this chapter).

SPECIFIC SIGNS AND SYMPTOMS IN HIGH-RISK ORGANS

The elderly are a high-risk group for malignancy. Therefore, the common signs and symptoms of malignancy must be kept in mind at all times. In the following section, pertinent risk factors for particular target organs that are at highest risk for malignancies in the elderly are presented.

BRAIN

The incidence of brain tumors of all types show an early peak in childhood, with medulloblastoma as the predominant cancer, and a latter peak in the 50- to 70-year age group, with predominately glial cancers (Grieg et al, 1990). Brain tumors show the second biggest increase in mortality of older persons after lung cancer (Fig. 22–2). The significant rise in incidence of brain tumors may be partly explained by improved technology and ease of use in the computerized tomography scan (Grieg et al, 1990).

Brain tumors are malignant in that they can reoccur and cause the person's death if not controlled. However, unlike other cancers, primary CNS tumors rarely metastasize outside the brain (Robinson et al, 1991).

The etiology of adult brain tumors is unclear at present. Exposures to environmental carcinogens, viruses, chemicals, and radiation have been proposed, but no causative associations have been proven (Robinson et al, 1991).

Clinical signs and symptoms suggestive of brain cancer are nonspecific and often can be misdiagnosed as stroke (hemiparesis, sensory change, and hemianopia). Other symptoms may include lethargy, intellectual decline, immobility, and incontinence. Headache, vomiting, and seizure occur in only 10% of patients (Stewart and Caird, 1991). In the setting of the elder patient who is at great risk of a variety of neurologic and physical changes, brain tumors may not be diagnosed until after death.

The treatment of the majority of brain tumors is palliative. Steroid therapy may provide temporary symptomatic relief in the elder pa-

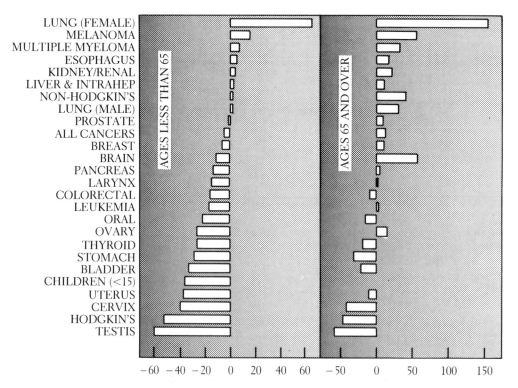

FIGURE 22–2 Cancer mortality rates. Changes by percent from 1973 to 1987 for ages less than 65 and ages 65 and older. (Cancer Statistics Review, 1973–1987; National Cancer Institute, NIH.)

tient (Stewart and Caird, 1991). The prognosis continues to be poor for patients diagnosed with primary brain tumors.

LUNG

Lung cancer continues to be the most common cancer in men. Since 1986, it has exceeded breast cancer as the most common cancer in women. The incidence of cancer rises rapidly starting at age 45, with the peak incidence at ages 70–74 for females and 75–79 for males (Fig. 22–3).

The risk factors for developing lung cancer are exposure to cigarette smoke and industrial and environmental pollutants. The risk of cancer is also increased when the person has been a smoker and has had exposure to a carcinogen such as asbestos. Other lung carcinogens include ionizing radiation, metals such as chromium and nickel, and alcohol consumption (Lindsay, 1991).

Although there are four histologic types of lung cancer, all follow a relatively silent developmental course until the disease is well advanced. Symptoms that might be suggestive of lung cancer include hemoptysis, persistent cough, vague chest pain, and increasing breathlessness (Canning and Caird, 1991). Weight loss and fatigue, at the time of diagnosis, are poor prognostic signs and may indicate a large tumor burden. Clubbing of the fingers occurs in about 30% of patients. Finally, many lung cancer patients first present with an ectopic paraneoplastic hormone production, leading to hypercalcemia, Cushing's disease, and inappropriate antidiuretic hormone production (Lindsay, 1991). There are no recommended screening tests for early detection of lung cancer.

BREAST

Female breast cancer is a heterogeneous disease combining premenopausal and postmenopausal women who may have different etiologic origins to their disease. Age is a significant

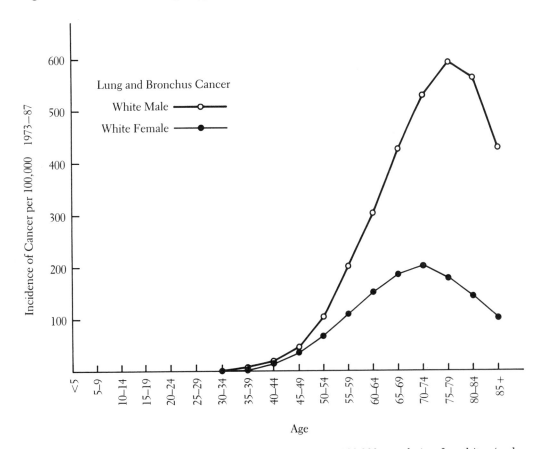

FIGURE 22–3 Incidence of lung and bronchus cancer per 100,000 population for whites (males and females), 1973–1987. (Cancer Statistics Review, 1973–1987; National Cancer Institute, NIH.)

risk factor for the development of breast cancer (Fig. 22–4). The older the woman, the greater risk for developing breast cancer. The risk for developing breast cancer from birth to age 50 is 2%, from birth to age 70 it is 7%, and from birth to age 85 it increases to 11%. In 1991, approximately 175,900 new cases of breast cancer will have been diagnosed (Morra and Blumberg, 1991). From another perspective, Stewart and Foster (1989) note that 70% of breast cancers are diagnosed in women 50 years or older compared with fewer than 2% before age 30. This has significant implications for focusing breast screening and education about breast self-examination.

Other risk factors for developing breast cancer include the following:

1. History of breast cancer: Persons with a prior history are more likely to have a second cancer in the breast.
2. Age at menarche and menopause: Women with an earlier menarche and later menopause have a greater lifetime hormonal ex-

posure and are more likely to develop breast cancer.
3. Familial history: There may be a predisposition to breast cancer at menopause and increased incidence of bilateral disease. The influence of family heredity is expressed before age 65 (Stewart, 1989).
4. Body mass and obesity: High-fat diet has been suggested as related to an increased risk for postmenopausal women. Further studies to fully explain this relationship are needed (Stewart, 1989; Morra and Blumberg, 1991).
5. Hormonal usage: Use of oral contraceptives and postmenopausal estrogen use have unclear relationships to the risk of breast cancer in the elder patient and further studies are needed (Stewart, 1989).

Additional risk factors may include exposure to ionizing radiation, reproductive history, and alcohol consumption.

As the breast ages, glandular tissue is replaced by fatty tissue. There is less incidence of

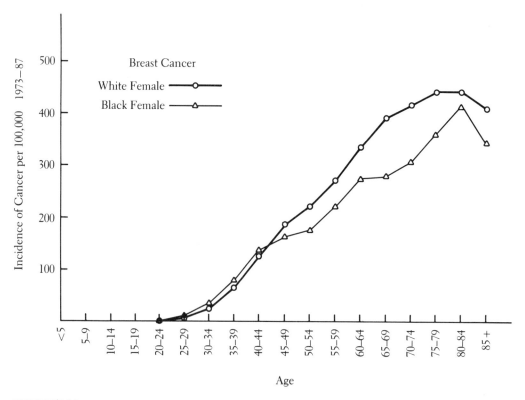

FIGURE 22–4   Incidence of breast cancer per 100,000 population for females, blacks and whites, 1973–1987. (Cancer Statistics Review, 1973–1987; National Cancer Institute, NIH.)

fibrocystic and fibroadenoma benign breast disease. The replacement of glandular and connective tissue with fat makes mammography even more effective in detecting breast lesions. However, there is an increased chance that breast masses in the elderly person are malignant (Stewart, 1989).

The elderly person also has a higher incidence of estrogen receptor–positive cancer. This may increase the chance of effective use of hormonal therapy such as tamoxifen.

It is recommended that women over the age of 50 have monthly breast self-examinations and annual mammography and clinical examination. However, studies show that up to 70% of women over 60 years of age and Hispanic women of all ages have not had a mammogram (Morra and Blumberg, 1991). What are the barriers to the use of breast screening? Cost and availability have been cited as the most frequent barriers. Second, physicians treating the elderly patient group "forget" or simply do not initiate mammography screening. Elderly patients when asked indicated that they would have a mammogram if their physician ordered it and explained its importance (Weinberger, 1991).

Finally, the public and patients falsely believe that older women, aged 75 or older, are at decreased risk for breast cancer. However, the peak incidence is in the 80 to 85 age group and only decreases after age 85 (Fig. 22–4). In spite of this, screening by mammography appears to be relatively nonexistent for this group.

Prognosis of women diagnosed with breast cancer varies according to age and stage at diagnosis. In a Swedish study comparing survival from breast cancer in different age groups, Adami (1986) found that the cohort of women aged 45 to 49 were more likely to survive compared to women aged 50 to 59. Those women aged 75 or older had the worst prognosis.

OVARIAN CANCER

It is estimated that there were 20,500 new cases of ovarian cancer diagnosed in 1990. White women have a 46% greater incidence than African-American women of ovarian cancer with the peak incidence at ages 70 to 74 years (Cancer Statistics Review, 1973–1987).

Survival is correlated with age. Ovarian cancer is the fourth leading cause of death in the age group 55 to 74 (Boring et al, 1991). While deaths from this cancer have declined in women under age 65 years, it has increased nearly 25% in women greater than 65 years as shown in Figure 22–2. This may be explained by stage of presentation or diagnosis, the type of treatment offered and the ability of older women to tolerate curative therapy.

Ovarian cancer is one of many abdominal cancers that presents itself at an advanced stage of malignancy. Often the cancer has spread beyond the ovary itself involving pelvic and abdominal organs particularly the bowel. Early signs and symptoms of this cancer are nonspecific. They include intermittent indigestion or flatulence, urinary frequency, abdominal pressure, and increasing abdominal girth with ascites (Diekmann, 1988; Otte, 1990). There is at present no recommended screening tests for early detection.

The etiology of ovarian cancer is unknown. Women with a familial history of ovarian cancer are at increased risk as well as are women with a history of breast or colon cancer. Some researchers suggest a link with the high-fat diet common in highly industrialized countries where the incidence is the greatest (Otte, 1990).

In postmenopausal women, an ovarian mass detected on routine pelvic exam is less likely to be a benign process and should be evaluated further with ultrasound, CT scan, or MRI (Otte, 1990). The usual route of metastatic spread is by local extension into the pelvic and abdominal areas causing major problems with maintaining bowel function and patency of ureters.

The mainstay of treatment in ovarian cancer is systemic or intraperitoneal chemotherapy. For women with good functional status, many of these regimens may provide good palliation and quality of life.

PROSTATE

Cancer of the prostate is one of the most common malignancies in elderly men. The incidence actually increases with age and is the second leading cause of cancer mortality in men aged 75 years or greater (Moon, 1992). Mortality from prostate cancer varies widely throughout the world. Japan, Hong Kong, and Singapore report some of the lowest rates compared with the four to five times greater incidence in the United States, England, France, and Sweden. African-American men have a 40-fold increased incidence compared with Japanese men, who have the lowest incidence (Perez et al, 1989).

Many elderly men have occult prostate cancer without clinical symptoms. One study reported by Harbitz and Haugen (1972) showed that in autopsies from all causes, 10% of men aged 50 to 59 and 50% of men older than 70 years had evidence of adenocarcinoma of the prostate.

Signs and symptoms of prostate malignancy are similar to those of benign prostatic hyperplasia: frequency, nocturia, and difficulty starting and stopping urinary flow. Chronic urinary retention with overflow may also be present with urinary infection.

Although 75% to 80% of patients are diagnosed with localized disease, occasionally patients may present with signs of advanced metastatic disease (List et al, 1989). The clinical symptoms that might indicate significant metastatic disease include back pain or other bony pain, particularly in the pelvis or lower extremities, hypercalcemia, weight loss, anemia, or lower extremity weakness (Lind, 1990).

With the introduction of the transrectal ultrasound for screening, more tumors are being diagnosed earlier. Also, a blood test for prostate-specific antigen has been recently investigated for its role in early detection of prostatic cancer. Levels of prostate-specific antigen increase when a prostatic malignancy is present. However, the test still has a significant error rate (Catalona et al, 1991; Mettlin and Dodd, 1991).

It has been said that many elderly men die *with* prostate cancer rather than *from* it (Kaplan and Bagshaw, 1990). It is a therapeutic dilemma to decide whether the patient's prostate cancer will cause local or systemic complications if left untreated. In spite of recent diagnostic advances, it is unclear what the best treatment option might be in the older patient.

COLON AND RECTUM

Cancer of the colon and rectum are found most often in the elderly. It is the second leading cause of cancer-related mortality in patients 55 to 74 years of age. Cancer of the colon is more common in women, whereas cancer of the rectum is more common in men (Schofield, 1990).

The clinical symptoms associated with colon malignancy vary with the location. Right-sided colon cancer is usually a silent disease, manifesting itself only as a dull pain, unexplained weight loss, or anemia secondary to gastrointestinal bleeding. A disturbance in bowel habits with increasing constipation alternating with diarrhea, lower abdominal pain, or blood in the stool are typical symptoms of left-sided colon cancer. Patients with rectal cancer may report a sensation of incompletely evacuated stool and rectal bleeding and mucous discharge.

Changes in bowel habits and character of stool require the older person to be a good observer and historian. One also must remember other coexisting factors such as the following:

1. The amount of water and other fluids taken during the time period.
2. Type and amount of foods eaten, e.g., increased fatty foods, low-fiber foods, or only carbohydrates.
3. Changes in activity and exercise patterns.
4. New medications such as iron, tranquilizers, large doses of aspirin, or antacids.
5. Periods of depression or emotional crises.

In addition to periodic health checkups through visits to the physician, many cancer control associations such as the American Cancer Society sponsor screening programs as demonstration projects with high-risk populations. These may involve colon cancer screening by examining stool specimens for occult blood, using an inexpensive Hemoccult test.

In order to achieve an accurate finding, the participating person should follow a restricted diet for 3 days before the test to prevent false-positive results. This diet typically restricts the eating of red meat. When such screening programs are instituted in nursing homes it becomes important that all residents be reminded at each meal the reason for the temporary change in the menu.

Occult stool blood testing is reported to yield approximately 2% of persons with a positive test result. At least one fourth of these have an adenoma or cancer on further work-up (Winawer et al, 1991). However, 30% of cancers may be missed by a single screening using standard guiaic slide tests. Cancer control organizations also recommend a flexible sigmoidoscopy every 3 to 5 years beginning at age 50. Patients whose colon cancers are detected at an earlier stage have an 85% 5-year survival versus a 38% 5-year survival for more advanced disease (Winawer et al, 1991).

PANCREAS

The incidence of pancreatic cancer has increased 300% in the last 40 years. Persons aged 80 years are four times more likely to develop pancreatic cancer than an adult half their age (Diekmann, 1988).

Like many abdominal tumors, cancer of the pancreas can be a silent disease, having few specific signs and symptoms to alert the host until the malignancy is well advanced. When the tail of the pancreas is involved, patients may experience worsening epigastric pain radiating to the back along with an acute onset of unstable diabetes and weight loss. If the cancer is located in the head of the pancreas, jaundice, pale stools, dark urine, pruritis, and weight loss may occur (Frogge, 1990).

Risk factors associated with the development of pancreatic cancer include cigarette, cigar, and pipe smoking, exposure to industrial pollutants such as benzidine, chronic pancreatitis and alcohol use, and high fat diets (Spross et al, 1988). Jewish men and African-Americans also have an increased incidence of pancreatic cancer.

The prognosis for pancreatic cancer is poor. Treatment is often palliative and the majority of patients die within 1 year of diagnosis.

LYMPHOMA

Lymphomas are cancers arising from immune cells and organs such as lymph nodes, bone marrow, spleen, or liver. The majority of lymphomas derive from B-cell lymphocytes in various stages of development (Carson and Callaghan, 1991).

It is unclear what etiologic factors contribute to the incidence of lymphomas. Age-related immune dysfunction may predispose a person to the development of non-Hodgkin's lymphoma. The role of viruses as a causative agent still remains unclear (Diekmann, 1988).

Non-Hodgkin's lymphoma occurs more often in men than women. The incidence rises steadily with age, with the peak incidence in the eighth decade (Fig. 22–5). The incidence in the elderly population has shown nearly a 50% increase from 1973 to 1987 (Fig. 22–2).

There are various classifications of lymphoma, both Hodgkin's and non-Hodgkin's. They range from low-grade indolent types in non-Hodgkin's lymphoma that are relatively symptom-free to aggressive moderate- or high-grade variants with rapid doubling times.

Clinical symptoms include palpable, painless node enlargements usually in the cervical region. Other lymph node areas may also be in-

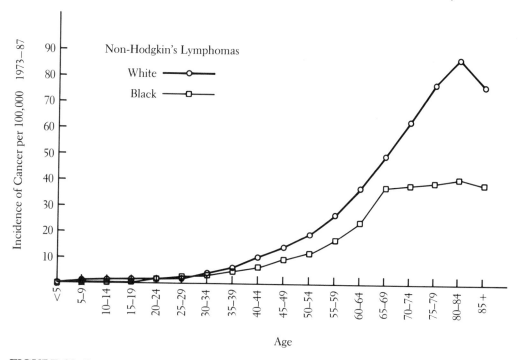

FIGURE 22–5 Incidence of non-Hodgkin's lymphoma per 100,000 population for both sexes, blacks and whites, 1973–1987. (Cancer Statistics Review, 1973–1987; National Cancer Institute, NIH.)

volved such as the groin and axilla. Fever, night sweats, and weight loss, known as B symptoms, occur in many patients. There is also an increased incidence of herpes zoster in the elderly patient with non-Hodgkin's lymphoma due to immune deficiencies. Often elderly patients present with an advanced stage of intermediate or high-grade lymphomas (Diekmann, 1988). Prognosis depends on a number of factors, such as the grade of lymphoma, the ability of the patient to receive chemotherapy, and the response to this therapy.

MELANOMA

Malignant cutaneous melanoma arises from the melanin-producing skin cell, the melanocyte. It is one of the most serious primary skin cancers that occur in the elderly. Approximately 32,000 persons will be diagnosed in 1991 with this skin cancer, with a greater proportion of men than women. There is an increased incidence in all age groups, especially in men over 40 years of age (Fig. 22–6). As shown in Figure

22–2, there is a 50% increased incidence of mortality in persons 65 and over.

Risk factors for the development of melanoma include a fair complexion and red hair; exposure to ultraviolet radiation, chronic sunburn and a previous history of a malignant melanoma. There is also a familial association of incidence with dysplastic nevi. These are precursor skin lesions that may, under unknown influences, develop into melanoma (Fraser et al, 1991).

Malignant melanoma lesion can be identified as having any of the following characteristics:

Ink-black, raised mole with irregular borders
Scaly, ulcerated, bleeding surface
Areas of multiple colors in the mole with blue, red, or amelanotic areas
Flat, brown irregular spreading lesion with raised areas

The elderly person should be taught to do self-examination of all skin areas and have a person assist in looking at areas such as the

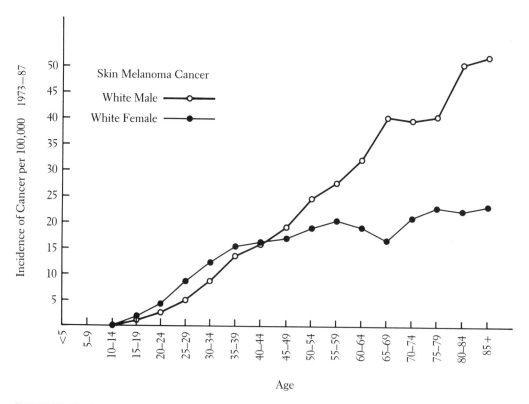

FIGURE 22–6   Incidence of melanoma of the skin per 100,000 population for whites, males and females, 1973–1987. (Cancer Statistics Review, 1973–1987; National Cancer Institute, NIH.)

back that are hard to see. They also should be provided informational pamphlets describing the type of changes they are looking for. Any recent change in mole color or characteristics should be referred to a specialist for further evaluation. Patient education materials are available from the National Cancer Institute Office of Cancer Communications and from many drug companies manufacturing skin protectant products. Early detection and surgical resection of malignant lesions is essential to prevent metastasis and widespread disease. Good prognosis is directly related to diagnosis of an early stage of disease.

Prognosis

Cancer is a chronic disease. It does have remissions, and some types of malignancies have been successfully treated and cured with primary therapy. Often, malignancies in the older person progress more slowly (Holmes, 1989), and management of complications of treatment is an essential feature of care. An elderly person may die as a result of infection, bleeding, or blood clot as a direct result of the cancer itself. However, when primary therapy has not been given, obstruction, ulcerating tumor masses, overwhelming odor, isolation, and pain will impair the quality of life for the elderly person.

SCHEDULING SCREENING PROGRAMS

Screening programs for the early detection of malignancies such as breast, colon, oral cavity, and skin are useful and economically justified when carried out in a high-risk population. Table 22–1 identifies some common warning signs and typical screening tests that might be performed. Figure 22–7 shows a sample schedule that might be used by retirement homes, ambulatory care clinics, and nursing homes.

In the absence of monthly examinations, at least the patient's record should be reviewed for reported signs and symptoms. This record review may pick up symptoms suggestive of malignancies of other conditions that have not improved with the current treatment plan and need reevaluation. The record analysis is purposely staggered throughout the year for increased vigilance of all areas.

DIAGNOSTIC TESTS

Sometimes diagnostic tests are avoided by both professionals and family. The feeling that "she can't take any more suffering" can be valid; however, it must be appraised carefully. Most important, the patient should be included in any decision making. It could be that the present suffering might be relieved once the problem is more fully understood.

The decision to withhold information regarding diagnosis, diagnostic tests, and treatment options is a formidable responsibility for any individual or professional to assume. The right of any individual to make these decisions for another is increasingly being held in question. With the concept of informed consent comes the right to know and to receive information without prejudice.

Some diagnostic tests are simple and cause no physical problems other than anxiety regarding the outcome or the uneasiness of strange interpersonal contacts, the absence of familiar supportive persons, and the strange foreboding environments. Such problems can be mediated by health care professionals.

Other tests may be more difficult for the elderly, either because they entail detailed instructions, energy draining preparation, difficult maneuvers, or pain. These procedures should be explained *without personal bias* toward the elderly person on his level of comprehension. The patient costs of fatigue, stressors, pain, anesthesia, and difficult or long positioning (e.g., proctoscopy, tomography, magnetic resonance imaging [MRI], angiography) must be balanced against the next set of questions: If it is cancer, what then? What physical and emotional strength does the person have to live with the treatment protocols and effects? Which will cause the least harm: the treatment or allowing the disease to take its course? Do we know enough about the malignancy to predict which course of action will give the greatest quality of life to the remaining time? If the primary disease is so overwhelming to contemplate, certainly the prospect of living with metastatic complications is even more difficult. Untreated tumors can cause ulceration, overwhelming odor, unremitting pain, and obstruction.

The following is a cogent example of what can happen to an elderly person with a paternalistic, avoidance approach to decision making:

TABLE 22–1   *Cancer Detection*

Site	Common Warning Signals	Screening Tests	Differential Diagnostic Tests
Breast	Lump or thickening in breast, dimpling of breast	Breast self-examination monthly, annual clinical examination, mammogram	Aspiration of fluid from breast masses, breast biopsy, chest radiography, skeletal survey
Colon and rectum	Change in bowel habits and character of stool, rectal bleeding	Annual checkup with digital examination, annual occult blood stool examination, proctosigmoidoscopy in persons over 50 years	Colonoscopy with biopsy, barium enema
Kidney and bladder	Change in bladder habits, urinary difficulty, hematuria	Annual checkup with urinalysis, occasionally exfoliative studies	Intravenous pyelogram, abdominal CT scan, renal arteriography, venacavogram, MRI
Lung	Persistent cough or hoarseness, hemoptysis	No recommended screening	Roentgenography, chest tomograms; CT scan, MRI, bronchoscopy including bronchial washings, sputum cytology, mediastinoscopy scalene node biopsy
Prostate	Difficulty in voiding	Annual checkup including digital examination, transrectal ultrasound	Prostate-specific antigen, serum acid phosphatase, bone scan, needle biopsy
Uterus	Unusual vaginal discharge or bleeding, pelvic pain	Annual checkup including pelvic examination and Pap smear, exfoliative studies	Chest radiography, tissue biopsy, fractional D & C, CT scan, intravenous pyelogram, colposcopy, barium enema
Skin	Sore that does not heal, color change or bleeding of mole	Skin self-assessment	Excisional biopsy
Stomach	Indigestion, meal intolerance, anorexia	Annual checkup, occult blood stool test	Upper gastrointestinal series, gastric analysis, exfoliative studies, endoscopy, chest radiography

Adapted from Otte D. Gynecologic cancers; and Frank-Stromberg M, Cohen R. Assessment and interventions for cancer prevention and detection. In: Groenwald SL, et al, eds. Cancer nursing, principles and practice, 2nd ed. Boston: Jones & Bartlett, 1990; with permission.

Mrs. A, aged 82, is alert, communicative, and had been a very active person. Now she lay on the examination table in the emergency room gasping for breath. She was anxious and fearful as she grasped for supportive hands nearby. Mrs. A had cancer of the thyroid, a constantly growing mass at the base of her neck. At first her family thought she was developing a goiter. But then they considered the question, "What if it's cancer?" Their response to this question was to ignore the condition. Some months later Mrs. A found breathing increasingly difficult. Because her earlier fears about the obviously enlarging neck mass had received no recognition or help, she began to withdraw from communication about herself with the daughter and son-in-law with whom she lived. She felt neglected, helpless, and isolated from her only perceived loved ones.

	Jan	Feb	Mar	Apr	May	Jun	Jul	Aug	Sep	Oct	Nov	Dec
Breast	Y X R	X	X	X	X	X	X R	X	X	X R	X	X
Cervix	Y R						R					
Colon-Rectum	Y		R					R				
Lung		R					Y					R
Oral	X		X	Y R	X		X	R	X		X	R
Prostate	Y	R						R				
Uterus	Y R						R					

FIGURE 22–7 An examination and record assessment schedule for systematic surveillance for malignant disease. Y, yearly screening or examination; X, examination by patient or staff; R, record.

This malignancy could have been diagnosed by the use of a radioactive isotope and the procedure would have been a very simple one. Her particular cancer could have been successfully treated with a *therapeutic* dosage of the same isotope, with possible adjuvant radiation therapy. Here the balancing of the stress of diagnosis and treatment versus the stress of watch and wait obviously falls on the side of treating the disease.

All patients and their families have the right to make informed decisions. Therefore, nurses should see and assess for themselves what the impact will be of the various diagnostic and treatment protocols recommended by the physician. Nurses are often in a position to give accurate neutral information about the options and clarify information that the physician has given. The relative payoff, the discomforts, and the ways in which these discomforts can be modified are all issues that should be discussed.

Professionals who work regularly in diagnostic treatment areas also need to be conversant with the particular needs and problems of the elderly. How can one manage the need for toileting, the coughing, and the dry mouth during tomography, with its long periods of immobility? The unknown, isolation, preparation for the tests, sensory assault of the environment, procedure, awkward, embarrassing, or painful positioning, and lengthy time involved take their energy toll on the elderly patient.

The technicians in diagnostic areas need to plan additional time and interventions to decrease the impact of these tests on the elderly patient. Careful positioning should be performed before the examination that is consistent with the patient's peculiar anatomy and respiratory or skeletal comfort. Insensitive preexamination positioning leading to pain, chilling, and a full bladder will eventually disrupt the test and lead to costly rescheduling.

Elderly patients require food and water (if permitted) during lengthy testing; they also should be offered an opportunity and assistance to use the toilet. Elderly patients often may require pain medication *before* coming to the radiology department or other diagnostic area. Personnel in these areas are not prepared to administer any medications other than those required for the testing procedure. Elderly patients also require relief of anxiety with explanation and reassurance before being transported to a strange area for a strange examination. The patient should know why the test is necessary and be promised continuing communications about the condition. The patient should know the time dimensions of the examination, including the estimated or real waiting times involved. For instance, a bone scan might take 1 hour and 30 minutes, *but* there is a 3 hour wait between injection and scan.

In many large medical centers, a full-time professional nurse is employed in diagnostic radiology and radiation therapy. The nurse can anticipate the needs of such patients and support them when they are in the department. Nursing care is frequently needed by patients in diagnostic radiology departments. The patients' needs are not and cannot be met by radiology technicians or physicians intent on their priority task of getting a good film. Regular nursing staff cannot be dispatched for long periods of time from patient units to stay with patients in the radiology area. Yet patients' needs continue and even increase during these studies.

FACTORS THAT INFLUENCE TREATMENT DECISIONS

Once the diagnosis of cancer has been made, the patient receives further evaluation to determine the appropriate treatment plan. This also includes the possibility of a recommendation of no treatment. All patients should be assessed for the specific type of cancer and the extent of its spread. This is called staging. The patient is also assessed for performance status. This is defined as the patient's level of daily activities of living, ranging from no impairment to total bedrest. Another area of assessment is the functional status of the patient's major organ systems. How well do the kidneys function as evidenced by a creatinine clearance test? How well will the patient be able to metabolize and excrete chemotherapy drugs? Finally, the patient should be assessed for nutritional status. Nearly all cancer therapies affect the patient's ability to eat and place a demand on current nutritional stores.

STAGING

An evaluation of the patient should be done at diagnosis to classify and stage the cancer. It may seem pointless or cruel to pursue tiresome studies to determine the source of the cancer or whether there are any sites of distant metastasis. This information is essential to selecting the most effective treatment plan. Some cancers, although presenting with metastatic disease, may be very treatable, whereas others have limited options for therapy.

Staging a malignancy is a way to describe the individual patient's disease state by classification of the anatomic spread of the tumor (O'Mary, 1990). The internationally recognized TNM system evaluates a cancer according to three categories: the primary tumor (T) or $_pT$, the adjacent lymph nodes (N), and the presence of any metastasis (M). This is a shorthand method to allow more objective description of a patient's cancer and better selection of a treatment found to be effective in patients with a similar stage of disease. The T_0, T_1, T_2, T_3, and T_4 indicate the increasing size of the primary tumor from absent to extending beyond the primary organ of occurrence. N_0, N_1, N_2, and N_3 indicate the quantity or location of nodes involved, depending on the specific cancer. Finally, M_0 or M_1 indicate the absence or presence of distant metastasis. Occasionally, the M will be further designated with an abbreviation for common sites such as pulmonary (PUL), brain (BRA), or skin (SKI).

Each malignancy has its own characteristic growth pattern. Some cancers metastasize to distant sites early; others often spread first to regional lymph nodes before extending to bone or brain. An example of the TMN system of classification of melanoma is shown in Display 22-1 (pp. 419-420) in a format appropriate for a physical evaluation. Staging systems are individualized to specific cancers and include combinations of TMN. There are also other systems such as the Dukes' classification of stages of colon cancer.

If the nurse is to be an accurate interpreter of information to the patient or the patient's advocate, it is important for her to be knowledgeable about staging systems and their significance for treatment considerations. Several comprehensive oncology textbooks such as De-Vita, Hellman, and Rosenberg (1989) or Beahrs' *Manual for Staging of Cancer* (1988) can provide further information on staging specific cancers.

PERFORMANCE STATUS

There are several performance classification scales commonly in use in cancer care. Table 22-2 shows two of these scales, the Karnofsky Performance Scale and the Zubrod or Eastern Cooperative Oncology Group scale. Both scales are used to indicate the patient's ability to perform activities of daily living and burden of symptoms. They range from total independence with symptoms to completely bedridden and moribund. Clinical trials often use these scales to select patients most likely to tolerate the proposed therapy. Patients with low performance status, who are bedridden greater than 50% of their day tolerate rigorous treatment poorly and have a high rate of complications. A performance scale may be used as a measure of the impact of a therapy on the patient's quality of life.

TABLE 22–2 *Assessment of Performance Status by the Karnofsky and Zubrod (ECOG*) Scales*

Patient's Performance Status	Rating	
	Karnofsky	Zubrod (ECOG)
Normal, with no complaints; no evidence of disease	100	
Able to carry on normal activity; minor signs or symptoms of disease	90	0
Normal activity with effort; some signs or symptoms of disease	80	
Cares for self; unable to carry on normal activity or to do active work	70	1
Requires occasional assistance but is able to care for most of needs	60	
Requires considerable assistance and frequent medical care	50	2
Disabled; requires special care and assistance	40	
Severely disabled; hospitalization is indicated, though death is not imminent	30	3
Very sick; hospitalization is necessary; active supportive treatment is required	20	
Moribund; fatal processes are progressing rapidly	10	4
Dead	0	

*Eastern Cooperative Oncology Group.
From Balducci L, et al. Cancer chemotherapy in the elderly. Am Fam Phys 1987; 35:139; with permission.

MAJOR ORGAN FUNCTION

The older patient often has preexisting chronic illness with deficits in kidney, lung, liver, or heart function before the diagnosis of cancer. For example, the patient may have recently recovered from a myocardial infarction, have emphysema, or adult onset diabetes with renal insufficiency. It is important to fully clarify these impairments when one considers which is the best cancer treatment for this patient. For example, a patient with a history of myocardial infarction may have serious problems when given a cisplatin-based chemotherapy regimen requiring saline diuresis and adequate kidney function. However, they may receive an alternate regimen of chemotherapy and achieve a disease remission.

NUTRITION

There is an increasing recognition that patients who are malnourished before the start of cancer therapy respond less well and have an increased number and duration of complications. Some of these problems can be poor wound healing and fistula formation, infection, and slowed bone marrow recovery from chemotherapy. A pretreatment nutritional assessment may be useful in identifying persons with a marginal nutritional status who when stressed with a major therapy may develop problems. Supplemental diet changes and needed dental work can be done before the therapy. Anorexia, nausea, fatigue, and pain are common therapy-related symptoms that will affect the patient's nutritional status. The elderly person may have low caloric intake and unbalanced dietary choices, which combine with the previously mentioned problems to create serious nutritionally based complications. There are two excellent resources for patients and their families. *Eating Hints* from the National Cancer Institute and Aker and Lenssen's *Guide to Good Nutrition During and After Chemotherapy and Radiation* (1988) both provide simple recipes and suggestions for maximizing caloric intake during therapy.

CANCER THERAPY

The treatment of cancer today is a complex, multimodality approach that may combine surgery, chemotherapy, and radiation therapy. Each of these therapies offer effective methods to control primary tumors and their systemic metastases. The choice of a specific treatment plan should be based on the patient's performance status, type and stage of disease, and prior experience with this regimen in patients of similar age.

With the older patient, age itself appears to preclude a comprehensive plan of therapy. The attitudes of the physician, family, and even the patient himself may reflect ageism ("old people will only die of another disease, why not cancer?") or preempting concern combined with ignorance ("The treatment is worse than the disease"). Treatment goals need not always be curative ones, but they need to be humane. The patient should be evaluated for his "biological age," preexisting status, and life goals, i.e., how the patient wants to spend the remainder of his life. An appropriate treatment plan is then selected based on these findings. The following sections examine major cancer therapies as they can be used in the elderly population.

SURGERY

Surgery is the oldest form of cancer therapy. It can be used for both curative intent or palliation. For example, a bowel resection and anastomosis can be a palliative removal of an obstruction or it can be curative if the cancer is localized.

Surgery with a curative intent is best used when the malignancy is small and no distant metastases have been identified. Occasionally, the surgeon may resect wide margins of normal tissue to prevent local recurrence. This may involve the loss of a limb, lung, stomach, or multiple organs as in an abdominoperineal resec-

tion (uterus, bladder, and rectum). The chances for cure must be weighed against the quality of life, coping with functional loss, preexisting disease, and the patient's goals. The loss of a limb may be a difficult decision at any age. For an elderly person, it may also mean the loss of independence and the risk of poor wound healing due to diabetes and vascular disease.

Chronologic age is not in itself a contraindication to major surgery (Bowles, 1983; Santo and Gelperin, 1975). It does, however, require a more extensive preoperative evaluation and preparation, with attention to patient symptoms that may have an effect postoperatively. At age 70, heart and pulmonary function are diminished, with renal function being approximately one half the renal function of a middle-aged adult (Bowles, 1983).

All elderly patients should be carefully evaluated for the successful resectability of their cancer. Patients who are found to be unresectable in surgery often have a rapid deteriorating postoperative course (Bowles, 1983).

Postoperatively, all elderly patients are at increased risk of respiratory compromise, hypoxia, and emboli secondary to deep vein thrombosis. These patients have less compensatory capacity in kidney, lung, and heart function and are intolerant of overhydration. Their preexisting immune function senescence provides increased opportunity for sepsis when physical barriers are broached with Foley catheters, intravenous lines, drains, and incisions. Finally, the stressful environment of an intensive care unit setting can disorient the elderly, leading to confusion and feelings of hopelessness and depression.

Some authorities have questioned the appropriateness of intensive care unit admissions for elderly cancer patients. One study conducted at a major cancer medical center surprisingly found that elderly patients with solid tumors, 65 to 75 years of age, had a lower inpatient mortality than patients under 65 years. There was also no increased use of intensive care unit resources with prolonged stays by the elderly group compared with the younger group (Chalfin and Carlon, 1990). Age was not associated with a negative outcome.

CHEMOTHERAPY

Chemotherapy is one of the few systemic treatments available for the control of cancer. Its effectiveness is based on cell kinetics, targeting malignant cells as they undergo the reproductive cell cycle. Many toxicities associated with chemotherapy are caused by normal cells in a reproductive cycle being damaged by the effects of these drugs. Normal cells such as myeloid, mucous membrane, and hair follicle cells can regenerate from unaffected stem cells; malignant cells often have fatal genetic damage.

Chemotherapeutic regimens vary considerably in schedule, dosage and drug combinations, depending on the malignancy being treated. Drugs are frequently given in combinations to achieve multiple, synergistic effects on malignant cells as they reproduce. Drugs are also selected to decrease excessive toxicity on any one body system, particularly the bone marrow. The reader is referred to various cancer textbooks listed in the references for more information on specific chemotherapeutic drug regimens.

How well do elderly patients tolerate chemotherapy? Walsh et al (1989) noted that the elderly are less likely to receive effective chemotherapy. Doses are frequently reduced or eliminated in treatment regimens of elderly patients.

Many physicians are reluctant to prescribe chemotherapeutic drugs because of a belief that the elderly person cannot tolerate them. Myelotoxicity is a major concern in the elderly patient. With aging, there is a loss of proliferative capacity of the bone marrow stem cells and a replacement with fibrotic tissue (Vannicola, 1988; Walsh et al, 1989). This may affect the elder person's ability to regenerate adequate numbers of neutrophils and platelets due to fewer functional stem cells. This could result in a greater incidence of infection and bleeding, two leading causes of death in cancer patients of all ages. Balducci et al (1987) also point out that malnutrition, common in the elderly, may also be a factor contributing to myelotoxicity.

Retrospective studies have confirmed an increased incidence of hematologic toxicity in patients older than 70 years in a wide variety of studies, particularly chemotherapy regimens using methotrexate and methyl-CCNU (Begg and Carbone, 1983). Walsh et al (1989), however, note that many studies do not clearly evaluate the toxicity according to age group and are difficult to evaluate for care recommendations.

Other age-related changes, as described in Table 22–3, need to be considered when planning chemotherapy in the elderly. Decreased lean body mass, hypoalbuminemia, and a reduction in total body water will significantly

TABLE 22–3 *Physiologic and Metabolic Changes of Aging*

Body composition
  Increased adipose tissue

  Decreased protein and water

Liver
  Decreased hepatic blood flow

  Decreased ability to activate carcinogens and drugs

  Decreased ability to conjugate drugs (Phase II reactions)

  Increased ability to deactivate carcinogens

Kidney
  Decreased glomerular filtration rate

  Decreased renal blood flow

Hematopoietic system
  Decreased hematopoietic stem cell reserve

From Balducci L, et al. Cancer chemotherapy in the elderly. Am Fam Phys 1987; 35:135; with permission.

change how water-soluble drugs affect the elderly patient (Balducci et al, 1989). Decreased renal function will slow the excretion of some cytotoxic drugs, contributing to increased toxicity. However, when these age-related alterations are recognized in the elderly patient and treatment regimens are planned accordingly, excessive toxicity can be avoided. When doses of cyclophosphamide and methotrexate were adjusted to each patient's rate of creatinine clearance, no excessive toxicity to the bone marrow in the elderly patients was found (Balducci et al, 1987).

Table 22–4 outlines some of the major chemotherapeutic drugs and major toxicities. There are selected drugs that have shown significant toxicity in the elderly patient. For example, bleomycin can cause excessive pulmonary toxicity, and doxorubicin is associated with cardiomyopathy with increasing doses. However, there are other drugs and regimens that may not use these drugs and may still be effective in controlling cancer in the elderly person.

Another factor important in the planning of treatment is the great variability in elderly persons. Treatment decisions need to be based on a patient's physiologic functioning, performance status, and personal life goals instead of

TABLE 22–4   *Common Toxicities of Major Chemotherapeutic Drugs*

Drug	Common Side Effects and Potential Toxicities
Bleomycin	Fever and chills, skin hyperpigmentation, stomatitis, pulmonary fibrosis
Cisplatin	Renal failure if not hydrated, hearing loss and peripheral neuropathy, nausea and vomiting, electrolyte imbalance
Cyclophosphamide	Myelosuppression, nausea and vomiting, alopecia, immunosuppression, potential hemorrhagic cystitis
Doxorubicin	Nausea and vomiting, myelosuppression, cardiomyopathy in higher doses, alopecia, radiation recall skin reaction
Fluorouracil	Nausea and vomiting, myelosuppression, diarrhea and gastrointestinal ulceration, photosensitivity and increased pigmentation of skin, stomatitis
Methotrexate	Myelosuppression, nausea and vomiting
Vincristine	Alopecia, constipation and possible ileus, peripheral neurotoxicity
Tamoxifen	Nausea and vomiting, mild myelosuppression, vaginal bleeding, bone pain
Megace	Vaginal bleeding, weight gain, potential thrombophlebitis, nausea and vomiting
Prednisone	Cushing's syndrome, weight gain, electrolyte disturbance, mental changes and mood changes, osteoporosis
Leuprolide	Vasomotor hot flashes, increased bone pain, peripheral edema

Adapted from Knobf TMK, et al. Cancer chemotherapy, treatment and care, 2nd ed. Boston: G.K. Hall Medical Publishers, 1984; with permission.

chronologic age (Walsh et al, 1989). Few clinical studies review toxicities according to age stratification and these other contributing factors. Walsh et al (1989) state that more work needs to be done to both identify those drugs that contribute to increased toxicity in the aged person as well as what factors in the aging process are causally related to toxicity. Finally, additional work is needed to educate physicians as well as the public on the experience of the elderly person receiving chemotherapy, the limitations as well as the benefits to quality of life.

RADIATION THERAPY

Radiation therapy is a versatile therapy for both primary and palliative cancer treatment. It uses ionizing radiation to produce intracellular damage, leading to tumor cell destruction. It can be delivered to the patient by a variety of methods. External beam radiation uses high-energy beams targeted at the tumor site and delivered in fractionated doses over a prescribed period of time. Internal implants can be used to deliver a dose of radiation to a specific area with the temporary placement of an applicator. Finally, radiation can be delivered to metastatic thyroid cancer by administering radioactive isotopes such as I_{131} orally. The tumor picks up and concentrates the radioactive isotope at the tumor sites and is damaged by the radiation. None of these methods are contraindicated in the elderly patient.

Radiotherapy can be useful for palliative care of the cancer patient for controlling troublesome, cancer-related symptoms. Some of these situations include imminent bone fracture and pain from bone metastasis, spinal cord compression and imminent paralysis in a patient who is not a candidate for surgery, and controlling tumor growth, hemorrhage, and odor. Treatment courses are short, directed at the problem and can be invaluable in improving the quality of life.

Radiotherapy used with curative intent differs from palliative treatment with longer treatment courses and overall higher doses. Curative therapy can be used in localized cancers such as laryngeal, skin, early stage breast cancer, or prostate cancer (Hilderley and Dow, 1991).

Side effects of therapy depend on the selected treatment area. Normal cells in this area are not spared the effects of the radiation. However, unlike malignant cells, normal cells are capable of intracellular repair and regeneration, depending on the total radiation dose delivered.

Typical side effects of radiotherapy include nausea, vomiting, fatigue, diarrhea if the abdominal area is treated, esophagitis, and various skin reactions, ranging from mild erythema to moist desquamation (Hilderley and Dow, 1991). Elderly persons need considerable support to manage these symptoms and still come in for treatment 5 days a week.

Age-related changes in the bone marrow reserve can contribute to increased toxicity in radiotherapy. Many radiation fields will involve large bony areas that can affect hematopoiesis. Anemia will contribute to low oxygenation of cells, altering the therapeutic effects of therapy. Patients sometimes require transfusion support if there is a significant effect on the bone marrow.

The elderly person's skin and mucous membranes may also be particularly vulnerable to radiation therapy. Aging produces a loss of subcutaneous fat and dermal tone with increased atrophy. Although high-energy external beam radiotherapy has significantly decreased skin toxicity, it can still be a problem for the elderly person (Blesch, 1988).

Finally, does the age of the patient affect the treatment course of radiotherapy? Steinfeld et al (1989) investigated the role of ageism in the treatment plan of patients receiving palliative therapy or curative therapy for breast cancer. They did not find, in a retrospective study, any evidence of dose reduction according to the patient's age in either group. For the elderly patient, even the oldest age groups, radiotherapy can be useful as primary or adjunctive cancer therapy.

BIOTHERAPY

Biotherapy is a rapidly expanding field in cancer therapy. It uses new technologic advances in molecular biology such as recombinant DNA techniques to create immunologically active agents or approaches that can stimulate or augment a host's responsiveness to cancer (Mayer, 1991). At present, many of these biologic agents are still being investigated. However, alpha interferon and several colony stimulating factors that act on bone marrow to increase neutrophil and macrophage cell lines have found useful roles in cancer therapy.

There are several classifications of biologic agents. These are

1. **Monoclonal antibodies:** Antibodies directed against specific tumors, possibly combined with a radioactive substance
2. **Tumor vaccines**
3. **Activated cytotoxic lymphocytes (TIL or LAK cells)**
4. **Growth factors:** Cytokines such as interleukin-2, interferons, and colony-stimulating factors.

Common side effects to many of these agents include a flu-like syndrome with fever, chills, rigors, headache, and overall malaise. Other symptoms that may occur with some agents include nausea, vomiting, anorexia, diarrhea, fatigue, hypotension, skin rash, mental status changes, and oliguria. These biologic agents affect nearly all bodily systems, but all of these effects are reversible when the agent is discontinued. Elderly persons already have pre-existing impairments of many major organs. Therefore, biologic agents must be used with caution in patients with cardiovascular, renal, or pulmonary compromise.

Alpha interferon is a biologic agent shown to have therapeutic effect in hairy cell leukemia. This is an uncommon cancer, with an increased incidence in the elderly. A treatment plan using alpha interferon may require daily subcutaneous injections for 3 months or longer. Initially, patients experience fever and chills. However, after a few days of daily treatment, other symptoms predominate including fatigue, anorexia, weight loss, and changes in mental status, hematopoietic, and cardiovascular changes. Although few patients have a complete remission, many patients can have a partial response or stable disease for months or years (Schiffer, 1991).

Currently, biotherapy has many limitations as a cancer therapy in the elderly population. However, as clinical trials of these new agents define the usefulness and applicability in cancer therapy, there may be benefits for the elderly patient to control cancer with lowered or reversible toxicities.

CLINICAL TRIALS

Until recently, elderly persons have been excluded from research trials by chronologic age. This made it difficult to generalize the findings of these trials to the management of the elderly population, ironically the population with the highest incidence of cancer.

Efforts have now been made in the United States and Great Britian to remove chronologic age barriers to clinical trials. A change in attitude now requires special studies of new drugs to be used by the elderly to evaluate their vulnerability to toxicity. More studies are also needed of overall response of the elderly population to existing drug regimens and other therapies.

PHYSICIAN DATA QUERY

The most up-to-date and comprehensive resource on cancer treatment is PDQ or Physician Data Query. It is available to both health care professionals and the public, anyone who needs timely information about cancer.

PDQ contains three categories of information. First is the Cancer Information File with the latest information on prognosis, staging, and treatment for the health professional. It also contains Patient Information statements in easy-to-read language. A second category of information is the Protocol File. These are brief statements on active clinical trials in the United States and other countries. Finally, the Directory File is a listing of physicians and organizations active in cancer treatment and research. The PDQ can be accessed through a medical librarian or through the National Cancer Institute's Cancer Information Service (1–800–4–CANCER).

Nursing Diagnosis and Management of High-risk Areas in Daily Living

From the perspective of the patient's daily living, there are some high-risk areas that are commonly shared by older persons having cancer despite the variations in diagnoses and treatment regimens. These are areas where nurses need information as a basis for:

Diagnosing each presenting daily living situation accurately and precisely
Developing a predictably effective treatment plan in collaboration with the older person and the primary caregivers
Evaluating the responses to the nursing interventions made by the older person, the caregiver, and/or family and the satisfaction of these three groups with daily living activities and outcomes in health status
Adjusting the plan as situations change or new daily living situations are superimposed

DAILY LIVING WITH LOSS OF DESIRE AND/OR ABILITY TO EAT

Many persons diagnosed with cancer often lose the desire to eat at various points in the course of the disease or its treatment. This anorexia may be related to the cancer pathology itself, to effects of treatment, to related pain or fatigue, or to associated emotional responses.

Malignant lesions or various treatment modalities to the mouth and throat can create major problems in appetite and nutrition (Schulmeister, 1991). Tumors in the mouth, gums, or pharynx can make chewing and swallowing difficult and painful. Esophageal lesions can obstruct the passage of food and result in regurgitation of all but liquid nourishment. Major surgical resections of the mouth, tongue, and neck region to remove oral malignancies can result in problems with chewing and swallowing food effectively (Parzuchowski, 1991). Radiation therapy to the oropharynx and salivary glands as well as some chemotherapeutic drugs can cause stomatitis or oral ulcerations, xerostomia or inadequate and ropey saliva, and/or infections. "Taste blindness" may also occur in which taste is peculiarly altered or lost (Billings, 1985; Schulmeister, 1991; Parzuchowski, 1991).

Treatment regimens to other parts of the gastrointestinal tract may also cause difficulty in eating. Surgical resection of the stomach and portions of the small intestines and pancreas can lead to "dumping syndromes" or malabsorption (Schulmeister, 1991). Intense nausea and vomiting is frequently a temporary side effect associated with chemotherapy. Sometimes the remembrance of it will cause patients to develop anticipatory nausea and vomiting just before the next treatment. Radiation to the abdomen may also lead to temporary nausea and vomiting depending on the treatment port and dosage (Iwamoto, 1991; Schulmeister, 1991). High-dose radiation to sites that include the intestines may lead to chronic malabsorption of nutrients and problems with nutrition (Szeluga et al, 1990).

Many patients with advanced cancer report a change in the taste of favorite foods. Meats often taste bitter and sweets are less sweet. Also, some chemotherapeutic drugs such as cyclophosphamide and cisplatin may cause a temporary metallic taste (Szeluga et al, 1990; Billings, 1985).

Fatigue (see later section on low energy) is an ever-present companion of cancer and its treatment. Older people, with their normally diminished energy, may find it even more difficult to continue their former routines of shopping and food preparation as well as simply eating the meal.

Fear and anxiety, which directly affect appetite, will occur at various periods in the course of living with cancer (Szeluga et al, 1990). High-risk times occur first when the patient is undergoing tests for suspicious symptoms and awaiting a diagnosis. Anxiety and depression may also affect nutritional status at the time of cancer recurrence, the very real prospect of more treatment and the loss of hope for a cure.

These then are the range of cancer-related situations that directly impact on the patient's desire to eat. Rarely do they occur all at one time. This nursing diagnosis concerns itself with managing daily activities in the presence of intermittent or long-term eating and nutritional difficulties. Optimal nutritional intake is often especially important to the cancer patient's recovery from treatment such as postoperative wound healing or bone marrow recovery from chemotherapy (Szeluga et al, 1990; Otto, 1991). It is also important for maintenance of the patient's energy level and a physical and emotional sense of well-being. However, maintaining a satisfactory nutritional intake in the older person with cancer whose premorbid baseline was barely adequate can be a special challenge to caregivers.

RISK FACTORS

Older persons who have no desire to eat or experience difficulty with ingesting adequate amounts of food are at the greatest risk of not managing their nutrition well in daily living if they:

Have a solitary life with few personal support systems
Are previously malnourished as a consequence of alcoholism or similar disease
Maintained poor oral hygiene before, during, or after chemotherapy or radiation therapy to the oropharynx

Are reluctant to ask for or accept help with shopping or food preparation
Are avoided during mealtimes because they make unacceptable eating sounds, swallow with obvious difficulty, or emit offensive odors
Are discouraged by their disease and its treatment and no longer care about living

SIGNS AND SYMPTOMS

Older persons who do not feel like eating or physically cannot eat, as a rule, do not volunteer complaints about it. When questioned, their responses tend to be positive or neutral. For example they might respond: "I eat all right," "I eat when I feel like it," "I nibble all day, but never much at a time." Sometimes, however, they reply with more candor: "Food doesn't appeal to me much," "I used to like meat, but now it tastes like it is rotten," and "It really hurts to chew or swallow."

Care providers report concern about the small amount that is eaten by the older person. They also report frustration about being unable to cook certain foods with strong odors for the rest of the family because the food aroma may cause anorexia or nausea. Also, the patient's diet may become monotonous, with only certain foods he can "get down" that do not cause nausea or diarrhea. The person may refuse to try other foods altogether. Caregivers can feel frustrated when they work hard to prepare something special, perhaps something the patient requested, and then he refuses to eat more than a bite or two. For the caregiver and the older person, the daily living elements of food preparation and eating can become tiresome and discouraging.

Signs of unsuccessful management of daily living with eating problems include weight loss and progressive weakness, muscle wasting, confusion, dehydration (dry mouth and skin), constipation and lowered urine output, poor wound healing, increased infections, and possible oral lesions secondary to vitamin deficiency (Aker and Lenssen, 1988; Szeluga et al, 1990).

PROGNOSTIC VARIABLES

Daily living with anorexia and difficulty in eating tends to be managed better if the person:

Has a strong desire to survive
Has definite goals to accomplish

Has received rehabilitation for surgical resections of the oropharynx

Expects to conquer the disease and accepts the treatment and the need to eat despite the difficulties

Has a reliable support system

Has effective strategies for managing difficulties in eating, swallowing, and gastrointestinal symptoms

COMPLICATIONS

Failure to eat in the presence of malignancy and the demands of therapy rapidly lead to malnutrition, decreased immune status, infection, progressive weakness, electrolyte imbalance, and death.

Depression may occur due to increasing isolation and the absence of previously remembered pleasures associated with eating. The pain and feelings of helplessness may result in the patient's giving up. (For complications associated with enteral feedings, see chapters on nutrition and gastrointestinal problems.)

TREATMENT

When the older person is seeking possible cure or palliation from treatment, the formal nutritional assessment is useful in establishing a baseline and comprehensive plan for nutritional support (Schulmeister, 1991; Szeluga et al, 1990). Less extensive nutritional planning can be helpful and less costly when the patient is not in active treatment and is experiencing fewer impacts on appetite or food intake.

Some older persons do not understand the relationship of nutrition to their treatment outcome and sense of well-being. Individual plans should be negotiated with patients and their caregivers that include written materials explaining the role of food in their treatment as well as personal food preferences. The plan should also consider the balance and texture of food as well as the person's income. It must also take into account the specific status of the patient such as

Difficulties wearing dentures due to oral ulcerations

Need for fineness of texture of the food to facilitate swallowing when the oropharynx or

esophagus is affected by the disease or its treatment

Loss of saliva and inability to masticate dry foods

Taste alterations

Analgesia before eating. This can be given topically (dyclone or viscous xylocaine applied to painful areas) or systemically

Premeal oral hygiene to remove debris, tenacious secretions, or bad odors

When cancer patients' distortions in eating tend to cause others to want to avoid them during mealtime, they can be taught the most effective way to eat, chew, and swallow. They can learn ways of managing to eat in front of others, given their own disabilities. One creative approach to this problem might be going to eat lunch with a nurse in the hospital cafeteria. Cancer patients may also need help in learning how to eat out in a restaurant or in social situations if this has been part of their lifestyle.

Every attempt should be made to assist the patient to eat to support his nutritional needs. However, alternative methods of feeding should be explored when the patient is unable to swallow, or when the gastrointestinal tract cannot accept food due to chronic obstructions or fistulas. When the patient experiences a weight loss greater than 10% of normal body weight even when eating the patient is in need of nutritional support by enteral or parenteral nutrition (Chernoff and Ropka, 1988). These methods might include nasogastric or gastrojejunostomy feedings or total parenteral feeding (Schulmeister, 1991). Alternative methods of feeding should be integrated into the patient's lifestyle with support from home care agencies to provide supplies and assist the caregivers and the cancer patient to administer the feedings.

Finally, spouses, families, and other primary caregivers also need attention. For the one who prepares the food and gets discouraged and frustrated when the older cancer patient refuses to eat, the nurse can serve as a safe sounding board. She can also assist the care provider to consider other options as well as remind the care provider not to badger the cancer patient to eat. Mealtimes should not become battlefields between the patient who may have little appetite and be depressed about his situation, and his family who fear he may die if he does not eat.

EVALUATION

To evaluate the older person's effectiveness in managing living every day with a lack of desire to eat, consider:

Nutritional status of the person

Adjustments being made in eating patterns to accommodate the lack of interest in eating

Satisfactions by patient and caregiver with adjustments being made

Effectiveness of support in obtaining and preparing food

Areas of frustration or satisfaction by the caregiver in interacting with the patient about food

Evaluating the patient's response to an inability to eat involves collecting information on the following:

Status of the oropharynx including mucosa, gingiva, and the ability to wear dentures

Assessment of the patient's nutritional status

Status of oral hygiene pattern

Status of analgesia in relationship to eating times and effectiveness of analgesia to permit eating

Degree of satisfaction with the nursing treatment plan and the current quality of life in eating

Ability of patient and caregivers to administer enteral or parenteral feedings in the home setting

DAILY LIVING WITH CHRONIC LOW ENERGY AND FATIGUE

In people over 70, even uncomplicated and successful surgery for cancer results in prolonged low energy levels (Nail and King, 1987). It is theorized that wound healing is given priority by the body and thus energy expenditure for anything else is lessened. For those in whom the tumor mass remains, it "steals" food from the body to continue its own growth and leaves the body deprived. In chemotherapy and radiation treatment, one has both tumor and normal cell kill, resulting in an increased need for nutrients for healing. When wound infection is a complication, the body's nutritional needs are in even greater jeopardy. These demands for nutrition coupled with a lack of desire or ability to eat create conditions for intense, continuous, physiologically based fatigue. In addition to the ongoing sense of tiredness, fatigue in the elderly cancer patient is characterized by sudden unexpected bouts of total exhaustion.

Other factors that may also contribute to the problem of fatigue are uncontrolled pain, anxiety, and depression and hopelessness.

RISK FACTORS FOR FATIGUE

Certain factors can be predicted to produce periods of low energy. These are the following (Nail and King, 1987; Aistairs, 1987; Piper et al, 1987):

The presence of other chronic diseases

The loss (or functional loss) of a limb, requiring the use of assistive devices for mobility

Malignancies in which fatigue is an initial and ongoing feature, e.g., leukemia

Advanced cancer with large tumor burden and cachexia

Anorexia and/or poor diet choices

Chronic pain

Insomnia or sleep interruptions

Cancer treatment regimens (chemotherapy, biotherapy, surgery, or radiation therapy)

Unrelieved symptoms such as nausea, vomiting, or pruritis

Anemia

Demands of diagnostic tests

Emotional components that contribute to low energy include the following (Aistairs, 1987):

Feeling abandoned by the family or health care providers

Time of first diagnosis

Time of recurrence of malignancy

Depression

Anxiety

Grieving

Unpleasant interpersonal relationships

RISK FACTORS FOR DAILY LIVING WITH LOW ENERGY AND FATIGUE

The levels of energy that may range from tiredness to intense exhaustion create obvious threats for managing daily living. Indicators that daily living is likely to become ineffective are the following:

Unavailability or unpredictability of physical and emotional support, living alone without family support

Lack of convenient transportation for health care or other necessary services

Lack of money for support services

Unmanageable distances to medical services and facilities

Stair climbing required to access essential rooms

Lack of pleasant events to anticipate

SIGNS AND SYMPTOMS

Manifestations that daily living is not being managed well with the level of energy the older person has include the following:

Changes in personal appearance and that of the environment, e.g., the person is less well "put together" or no longer gets dressed; housekeeping declines

A negative spiral in eating, e.g., failing to prepare nutritious meals, snacking on convenience foods

Decreased participation in health care, e.g., missed appointments

Decreased energy for going to the bathroom, leading to less fluid intake, constipation, and dehydration

Decreased participation in social interactions

Changes in speech patterns. The person is quieter, speaks with an energy-sparing style of no extra words or utterances, omits social amenities in speech, adopts a style of speech using half sentences and shifts rapidly from one subject to another, e.g., "I need oranges . . . and I forgot to feed the cat when I was up . . . have to get Kleenex"

Decrease in planning ahead for combining activities to save energy—thinks only of the present tasks

Occurrences of sudden, severe incapacitating exhaustion that can progress to feeling of faintness, tears, muscle weakness—"the bottom just drops out"

PROGNOSTIC VARIABLES

Managing daily living with chronic fatigue is basically contingent on having appropriate assistance, both physical and emotional, particularly in the "valley times."

COMPLICATIONS

Complications of daily living with chronic fatigue involve complete breakdown in basic activities of daily living, including hygiene, nutrition, and elimination. Depression is a frequent component of fatigue as well as hopelessness.

TREATMENT

Nursing interventions include educating the patient to be energy efficient and legitimize aspects of this behavior. It may deal with mobilizing and maintaining support systems that will supplement the person's own energy resources. The treatment may also deal with the needs of primary caregivers, who also run the risks of running out of physical and emotional energy.

Teach patients to recognize the body cues that signal the beginning of the sudden exhaustion phenomenon and to plan for strategies for removing themselves from the social or physical activities in which they are involved

Plan with the patients how to arrange their rooms for the least expenditure of energy, minimizing reaching, bending, walking, and carrying

Help them to devise specific reminders for activities they can combine in order to save energy: putting up reminders on the refrigerator door, the bathroom mirror, and so forth

Give patients a *script* for how to respond in common social situations so that there is a good fit with their energy level and the maintenance of positive relations with others. Teach them how to talk to visitors, doctors, or spouse. For example, a script for setting up visitors and their expectations in a positive way:

"Please don't be disturbed when I . . .
  have to go to the bathroom
  take my pill
  get up and move about, etc."

"I'll be back shortly, so please don't go away. I do so enjoy your company."

"My doctor is keeping me on a rather tight schedule these days and I'll have to take a nap in 45 minutes. I'm glad you came early enough so we can have this time together."

These scripts are used to help the individual to save energy by planning actions ahead and rehearsing speeches. This, in turn, reduces the amount of stressors produced in interacting with the visitor, getting off schedule, and being too fatigued.

EVALUATION

Evaluation of response to the nursing treatment plan and the ongoing situation is concerned with the following areas:

Status of basic and emotional needs and the current capacity and strategies for meeting these needs

The pattern of energy (up, down, rate of change) and the need to alter activities in a compensatory manner

The nature and number of satisfying experiences the person is having each day, despite low energy levels

Status of eating

Status of sleeping (e.g., daytime naps of sheer exhaustion vs. normal sleep cycles)

An evaluation of the person's support system is also needed. The following questions can be asked:

Is the support person working effectively?

Is there a change in the support person's effect?

Does the caregiver have a pattern of normal sleep each night?

Is there a downward trend in the caregiver's weight pattern?

What are the arrangements for respite? Is the respite predictable? Is it dependable? Is it being genuinely used?

Are any additional resources needed?

LIVING WITH CANCER PAIN EVERY DAY

Cancer pain is one of the most urgent and important health care problems of modern society. It is responsible for one of the greatest fears connected with living with cancer. It involves high costs in physiologic, psychologic, economic, and social expenditures. It is inadequately managed in many patients. And the inadequacy of health professionals in managing cancer pain continues to perpetuate fear in the general public as they view the suffering in their loved ones (Bonica, 1984).

Pain in cancer can be an element of both early and late disease as well as of treatment and its sequelae. Daut and Cleeland (1982) reported that 6% of patients with nonmetastatic disease and 33% of patients with metastatic disease were found to have pain associated with cancer. These were 667 patients with breast, prostate, colorectal, and three gynecologic cancers, in both inpatients and outpatients (Daut and Cleeland, 1982). Patients with metastatic disease have higher reports of pain problems, particularly if the sites of metastatic disease include bone involvement or nerve

compression (Coyle and Foley, 1987). Further, pain control has been found to be inadequate in hospitalized patients and home care despite the availability of active narcotic and nonnarcotic drugs and increased technology of delivery systems (Howard-Ruben, 1987). Responsibility for inadequate pain control rests with both doctors and nurses. Physicians were found to be prescribing 50% to 65% of an effective dosage for analgesia, and nurses were giving as little as 20% to 30% of the already inadequately prescribed medication (Marks and Sachar, 1973; Spross, 1992).

For the elderly, managing daily living with pain can be even more difficult when influenced by misconceptions about how the elderly experience pain. Some of these misconceptions are that pain is a natural outcome of growing old, that pain perception decreases with age, or that the potential side effects of narcotics make these drugs too dangerous for use in the elderly (McCaffery and Beebe, 1989). Other problems common to the elderly may make the usual methods of assessment and evaluation ineffective. Patients may have coexisting sensory deficits, memory impairment, or frank confusion and dementia. As a result, the elderly patient may not verbalize pain clearly or may be misunderstood regarding whether the intervention has been effective in relieving the pain (McCaffery and Beebe, 1989). Also, patients who have chronic pain may not exhibit some of the pain behaviors and bodily changes that nurses usually associate with pain. Figure 22–8 outlines the differences in presentation between acute and chronic pain. Thus, elderly persons in the United States today have a high risk of having to live with severe pain if they have cancer.

The dynamics of pain in cancer arise from multiple sources. They include:

The malignancy itself: Primary and metastatic tumors cause pressure on organs or structures near the tumor mass with
  Necrosis within an organ system or structure
  Obstruction of an organ system (e.g., the colon)
The treatment itself: Surgical incisions, amputations, sequelae to treatment
  Phantom limb pain
  Postthoracotomy pain syndrome
  Radiation therapy and/or chemotherapy related skin desquamation
  Stomatitis of the mouth; mucositis of the gastrointestinal tract, vagina, and genitourinary tract

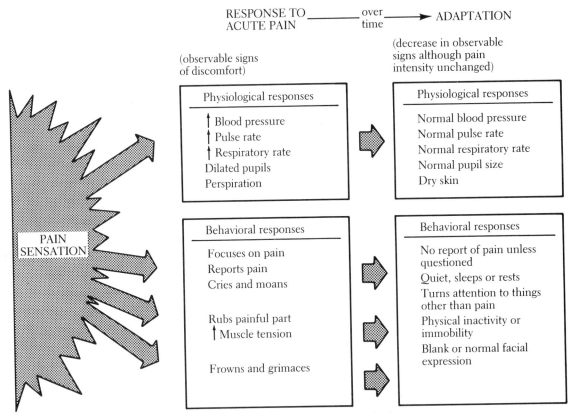

FIGURE 22–8 Adaptation to acute pain. (Modified from Smeltzer S, Bare B. Brunner and Suddarth's textbook of medical–surgical nursing, 7th ed. Philadelphia: J. B. Lippincott, 1992; with permission.)

Radiation-induced myelopathy
Concomitant disease unrelated to malignancy:
  Arthritis, bursitis, neuropathies, diaphragmatic (hiatal) hernia, fractures

RISK FACTORS

Three categories of variables are associated with the patient's difficulty in managing daily living with pain. These are:

Intensity and constancy of the pain
Factors that decrease the tolerance for pain
Inhibitors for adequately managing pain

  Factors that increase the intensity of pain include the tumor sites, e.g., bone and pancreas, or a multiplicity of sites as in metastatic, end-stage, or terminal illness. Intensity of pain can also be increased by multiple treatment modalities. Coexistent pain from concomitant problems form additional risks.
  Conditions or situations that decrease the

ability to tolerate the pain include the following:

Presence of gastrointestinal symptoms, e.g., nausea, vomiting, diarrhea, constipation, impactions
Emotional stressors such as anxiety, depression, fear, and anger
Inadequate pain management in the past
Inability to sleep
Confusional states, dementia
Giving up

  Risk factors associated with inhibiting adequate management of the pain include the following:

Inadequate support system
Cultural deterrents to verbalizing pain
Refusal to control pain or want it eliminated because of the pain's meaning to the patient
Inadequate knowledge or expertise by primary caregivers in pain control measures

Caregiver values that inhibit giving adequate medication for pain control including a potential fear of creating drug addiction

SIGNS AND SYMPTOMS

The pain of cancer and its treatment interfere with daily living in all its aspects. Manifestations may be either reported by the patient or observed by caregivers.

Crucial to the management of pain in daily living for the older cancer patient are the attitudes and well-being of their primary caregivers. Thus, in seeking data on the management of daily living with pain, it is important also to gather evidence on attitudes toward pain, analgesics, and pain alleviation. Are the attitudes of the cancer patient and caregivers regarding pain alleviation congruent? Does the caregiver acknowledge the presence and intensity of pain reported by the patient? How are the family and primary caregivers managing their own daily living in the face of the patient's pain and altered daily living? What respite and opportunities for genuine rest do the primary caregivers have?

PROGNOSTIC VARIABLES

Daily living with acute or chronic pain is likely to be managed better if there is:

Good knowledge of the nature of acute and chronic pain, what can be done about it, and who will do it

Good family and professional supports regarding pain alleviation and pain communication

Objective observation, assessment, and reporting of pain using a common basis of expression (see Treatment of Cancer Pain)

Understanding by physicians and nurses of the use of various combinations of medications, e.g., nonnarcotic analgesics, nonnarcotic analgesics with a psychotropic medication, or other combinations

Adequate support and respite for primary caregivers and family in dealing with their own feelings and physical well-being

COMPLICATIONS

Chronic and persistent cancer pain results in progressive physical deterioration due to sleep deprivation, fatigue, debilitation, poor nutri-tion, and diminished social contact. This impact is greater and more severe in cancer patients than chronic pain in any other disease.

Psychologic changes of helplessness, loss of capacity for self-care, giving up, and a desire to die are complications of unmanaged pain in daily living.

Analgesia causes its own complications. It can result in constipation, drowsiness or dizziness that may lead to falls, mental status changes including confusion and forgetfulness in medication taking and recording, dry mouth, nausea and vomiting, decreased rate and depth of respirations, and nightmares.

TREATMENT

Managing daily living with the pain of cancer involves the establishment of an accurate data base for ongoing assessment of pain and the effectiveness of treatment as well as sound knowledge of the options in medication management. The treatment plan considers both the patient and the family, particularly those who are primary caregivers.

It is important to have a consistent and reliable pain reporting system used by the patient, caregiver, and health professional. This system should first include an initial assessment of the pain problem using a method acceptable to the patient for communicating about the pain experience. Second, a diary or journal should be used by the patient or primary caregivers to regularly record progress, or lack of it, toward achieving pain-free living.

Knowledge of analgesic equivalents, combination analgesics, and the principles of pain management, including dose titration, is a prerequisite for professionals caring for elderly cancer patients. Such understanding is important as well for those patients and families able to participate and manage daily living with pain in the home. It is not possible to provide complete information on all aspects of pain management in this section. The reader is referred to cited pain references for further details on the methods introduced in the following sections.

Observing and Documenting Pain There are many pain assessment tools available to the health professional by experts in the field of pain control. One tool created by McCaffery and Beebe (1989) combines both descriptions for assessing one or more pains that the patient is experiencing as well as describing its effects on daily living (see Display 22–2, pp. 421–422).

The intensity of pain in this tool is measured with the use of a vertical analog scale (shown in Fig. 22–9). Many patients learn to succinctly report their pain by the numbers. However, if the patient is unable to describe his pain using the numerical system, words can be substituted such as "No pain, a little pain, a lot of pain, too much pain" (McCaffery and Beebe, 1989). This scale is also used in ongoing evaluation of the effectiveness of the pain treatment plan.

Finally, the pain diary or journal is a written account that correlates the analgesic with time and the pain intensity rating. An example of this tool is given in Figure 22–10. Additional columns may include whatever information will be useful in evaluating the pain control plan. In an acute care setting, hourly recording of respirations and the level of sedation may be important along with pain relief. In the home care setting, the level of patient activities of daily living will provide essential information to determine whether mutual goals for pain control have been achieved.

The changing patterns of pain over time should emerge from this written journal and support the patient's subjective appraisal. Although it may seem burdensome to maintain this written record, the investment can pay off in proving or disproving the effectiveness of a medication and helping to devise a better pain control plan. It is especially valuable to the nurse who may visit the home only biweekly to try to determine what changes to make to achieve better pain control for the patient.

Pharmacologic Management of Pain   Effective management of pain in daily living usually centers on the use of one or more medications along with nonpharmacologic methods. Combinations of medications may include the following:

Nonnarcotic analgesics (aspirin, acetaminophen, indomethacin)
Narcotic analgesics (morphine sulfate, codeine, hydromorphone)
Adjuvant medications (amitriptyline, dexamethasone, phenytoin)

An adjuvant analgesic medication is a varied group of agents with the capability to enhance the actions of the narcotic or nonnarcotic medications or provide added analgesic effect via a different mechanism (McCaffery and Beebe, 1989). These may include a tricyclic antidepressant such as amitriptyline (Elavil) to decrease anxiety and increase sleep, a corticosteriod that may decrease inflammation, or an anticonvulsant useful in neuropathic pain. Other agents such as caffeine, ritalin, or alcohol may have surprisingly beneficial effects on pain (McCaffery and Beebe, 1989).

Oral administration is the preferred route if possible. If the pain is out of control and severe, a continuous intravenous administration of a narcotic such as morphine may be used in a closely monitored setting. Once the dose of medication that will provide pain relief is achieved, the medication can be converted to an oral route if the patient is able to take food or fluid by mouth. The equianalgesic chart shown in Table 22–5 (McGuire and Scheidler, 1990) provides information on how these transitions can be made with little loss in pain control. After each transition, individualization of the dose is needed, with small increases or de-

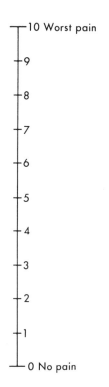

FIGURE 22–9   Vertical visual analog scale. (Modified from McCaffery M, Beebe A. Pain: Clinical manual for nursing practice. St. Louis: C. V. Mosby, 1989; with permission.)

Name _____ Date _____

Time	Pain rating scale	Medication type & amount taken	Other pain relief measures tried or anything that influences your pain	Major activity being done: lying sitting standing/walking
12 MIDNIGHT				
1 AM				
2				
3				
4				
5				
6				
7				
8				
9				
10				
11				
noon 12				
1				
2				
3				
4				
5				
6				
7				
8				
9				
10				
11				

Comments: _____

_____

_____

FIGURE 22–10   Daily diary. (Modified from McCaffery M, Beebe A. Pain: Clinical manual for nursing practice. St. Louis: C. V. Mosby, 1989; with permission.)

creases. Note that the oral doses of morphine are six times greater than the equianalgesic dose given intramuscularly (10 mg intramuscularly to 60 mg orally). One common error is to undermedicate the patient with oral medication because the milligram amounts seem very high. Oral morphine solutions such as Roxanol and sustained release morphine tablets (MS Contin) are now available to facilitate oral administration and increase the interval between medication times.

Oral medication may also be useful in providing a more balanced level of analgesia than when it is given parenterally. As shown in Figure 22–11, intermittent parenteral medication is characterized by peaks and valleys; however,

TABLE 22–5   *Equianalgesic Chart: Relative Potencies of Commonly Used Analgesics*

Mild to Moderate Pain			Oral Dose (mg)*	
	Codeine		30	
	Meperidine		50	
	Propoxyphene		65	
	Acetaminophen		650	
	Sodium salicylate		1000	

Severe Pain	IM (mg)†	PO (mg)†	Plasma Half-life (hr)	Average Duration of Action (hr)
Codeine	130	200	2.5–3	3–5
Meperidine	75	300	3–5	2–4
Oxycodone	15	30	2–3	3–5
Hydromorphone	1.5	7.5	2–3	3–6
Morphine	10	60*	2–3.5	4–5
Levorphanol	2	4	11–16	4–5
Methadone	10	20	15–30	4–6
Oxymorphone	1	—	2–3	4–5

*Approximately equal to aspirin 650 mg.
†Approximately equivalent to morphine 10 mg IM.
These values were determined from and based on clinical experience and single-dose studies of patients in acute pain.
For chronic dosing, some pain experts believe that the oral morphine dose is approximately 20 to 30 mg, but this has not been demonstrated in any controlled trial.
From McGuire DB, Scheidler VR. Pain. In: Groenwald SL, et al, eds. Cancer nursing, principles and practice, 2nd ed. Boston: Jones & Bartlett, 1990; with permission.

oral absorption more closely resembles a continuous plasma level.

Medications should be given on a regularly scheduled basis, *not as needed*. The patient should not have to ask for pain medication. However, medication times should be arranged to allow uninterrupted periods of sleep (e.g., administering morphine, sustained release, one 30 mg tablet every 8 hours, at 10 PM and at 6 AM, or every 12 hours at 9 AM and 9 PM as appropriate).

Sleeping patients are often considered to be pain free. This is not true. Often they awaken in severe pain as the plasma levels of the analgesic is cleared by the liver and falls to low levels. It will now require substantially more analgesic to achieve pain relief than if the patient regularly received the medication around the clock even if the patient had to be awakened to take the medication.

Titration of Narcotic Dosage   For effective pain management, the initial dose is purposely set a little high to achieve an immediate control of pain. The dosage is then administered on a regularly scheduled basis (every 4 or 8 hours), not as needed. Titration is achieved by lowering the dosage (not altering the time interval), until the optimal effective dosage is achieved, the last effective dosage before insufficient control (Fig. 22–12) with manageable side effects. When the optimal pain management has been effective on this level for a period of time and then pain once again appears, this may indicate physical tolerance or a change in condition, and an adjustment must be made.

Combinations of nonnarcotic and narcotic analgesics may be useful in providing increased pain relief using different avenues of action. For example, acetaminophen has a different mechanism of action than codeine and does

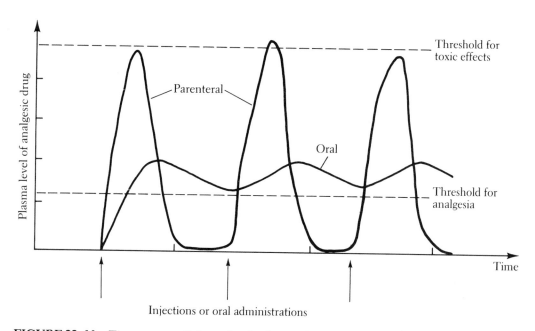

FIGURE 22–11   Time courses of plasma levels of an analgesic drug given parenterally or orally. The threshold for toxic effects could mean the onset of respiratory depression, for example. Because of slow resorption from the gastrointestinal tract, variations in serum concentration are much lower with oral than with parenteral administration. Analgesic levels are easier to maintain. (From Zimmermann M, Drings P. Guidelines for therapy of pain in cancer patients. Recent Results Cancer Res 1984; 89:10; with permission.)

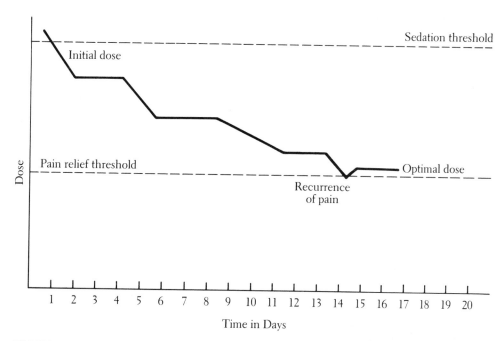

FIGURE 22–12   Method of titrating narcotic dosage for a patient with chronic cancer pain. (From Lipman AG. Drug therapy in cancer pain. Cancer Nurs 1980; 3:44; with permission.)

not add to sedation or constipation. Adjuvant medications such as amitriptyline may also be added to the plan and are useful in managing specific problems such as anxiety and insomnia.

The use of aspirin, acetaminophen, or liquid morphine solution may also be helpful in controlling a sudden episode of pain, possibly associated with increased activity, without changing the primary analgesic. If the patient, however, requires more than the occasional supplement, the dose of the primary analgesic should be increased, but not the interval.

Oral morphine carefully titrated to the elderly person's need is a safe narcotic for severe pain, providing relief in the majority of cases. Chronic ventilatory failure seems not to be a problem with oral morphine used in the aged with chronic cancer pain, even when there is existing respiratory tract pathology (Walsh and Saunders, 1984).

Tolerance versus Addiction   Many professionals equate drug tolerance (need for a larger dose of medication to achieve optimal pain relief) with addiction (compulsive use of habit-forming drugs to satisfy psychological and physical needs). In one study most physicians were found to underestimate the effective dose range of narcotics, to overestimate the effective duration of action, and to exaggerate the dangers of addiction (Marks and Sachar, 1973; Spross, 1992). Professional education continues to be needed if effective pain management in daily living with cancer is to be achieved.

Understanding of Pain Principles by Patient and Family   The following guidelines should prove helpful to the patient and primary caregivers:

Admit when you have pain. Keep a pain journal. Describe how it feels, how severe, where, when, and how long
Do not allow the pain to get severe before taking action
Take pain medications on a regular, round-the-clock schedule and try to prevent pain before it starts
Be aware of what precedes pain attacks and what makes pain worse, especially fatigue, sleep loss, anxiety, and depression. Ask for help in managing these problems before your pain becomes severe
Know what relieves the pain

Know how to adjust your pain plan for periods of increased activity. Also plan for how to make adjustments for times of bad news, acute pain from new diagnostic tests, etc. Have additional medications or relaxation tapes available for these stressors
Know the potential side effects of all the medications you are taking and how to get help (who to contact and how to reach them at any hour)

Regular Scheduling of Evaluation of the Pain Management Regimen   Regular review of the medications being used and the pain journal are needed to avoid incompatibility in drugs, duplications, and evaluation of effectiveness and side effects. If these are scheduled at present intervals, better control is more likely.

Other Dimensions of Pain Management in Daily Living   Analgesia is a critical element in managing pain in daily living, but it is not the only focus in the nursing treatment plan. Some other areas useful in pain control the nurse can teach the patient and caregiver include the following:

Relaxation techniques: Scripts can be recorded specifically for the patient or prerecorded tapes are available
Helping the patient and family to discover and use distractors, e.g., music, surprises, friends, slides and movies of family activities, and telephone calls
Use of warmth or ice to reduce pain in a local area
Talking with the patient and family in order to discover what they fear the most. Provide information and support to put their fears into perspective
Use of imagery to control fear and anxiety: Prerecorded audiotapes can be used as needed by the patient
Helping the patient and family to arrange for a pleasant environment (e.g., sounds, light, warmth, pictures, plants, fish, birds, other pets)
Discovering the way in which spiritual beliefs or support will prove useful to the patient and caregivers
Mobilizing acceptable additional resources as needs change (e.g., Meals on Wheels, hospice, home nurses, chore persons)
Helping the person to participate in at least one satisfying activity each day

Negotiating with the patient and family for responsibilities in daily living that the patient can assume, e.g., in a nursing home walk a blind friend to dinner, feed a pet, care for plants, or cut flowers

Negotiating for the patient to contribute to daily living and maintain as much of the usual role in activities of daily living of the household as possible. The patient can make the shopping list, sort the mail, or fold the laundry

Determining important goals in the person's remaining days and trying to help him or her find ways to achieve them

Supporting the primary caregivers and family in their goals and needs with particular attention to genuine respite

Alternative Medical Options for Pain Management Patients and their families need to be aware of the other medical options for pain management. These include sympathetic nerve blocks, hormone therapy or chemotherapy, palliative surgery or radiation therapy, and local anesthetics. When patients cannot use oral medication, analgesics can also be administered either subcutaneously or via an implanted catheter in the home care setting with small continuous infusion pumps. Intrathecal analgesic administration is also possible in some medical centers.

In order to make informed decisions, the patient and family need to know what each of the appropriate proposed treatments can and cannot do and what their side effects will be. They also need health care professionals to advocate on their behalf when usual pain control methods do not work and innovative methods need to be attempted.

EVALUATION

The pain plan should be evaluated at regular intervals such as every week. If changes are made in the plan, more frequent evaluation is necessary. No patient should have to resign himself to living with unrelenting pain or consider suicide to gain relief from suffering.

DAILY LIVING WITH VULNERABILITY TO INFECTION

Infection is a major cause of death in the cancer patient. It is also an area of high vulnerability for the elderly cancer patient. First, the tumor appears to impair host defense mechanisms and second, cancer therapies directly affect infection fighting potential as well as normal physiologic barriers such as intact skin.

The elderly patient is particularly susceptible to infection due to normal aging effects on body systems such as fragility of skin, decreased sensation, decreased lung function, potential diabetes, potential visual impairment, impaired urinary bladder function, and decreased bone marrow reserve. The immune system is also less responsive to foreign invaders with aging. Often the infection is discovered late. The elderly patient may live alone, be less attentive to infection prevention, and have no assistance to obtain help. The diminished body defenses may lead to few early signs of infection before septicemia occurs. Since the activities of daily living may be influential in preventing infections in the ambulatory patient, they become an area for nursing management.

RISK FACTORS

The factors in cancer and its treatment that may increase an elderly person's vulnerability to infection include the following:

Breakdown of skin and mucosal barriers due to:
   tumor mass eroding skin, bowel, or creating fistulas
   chemotherapy and radiation therapy effects on skin, oral, or rectal mucous membranes
   nonhealing surgical wounds or fistula development
Treatment-related neutropenia
Impaired antibody production
Iatrogenic factors including poor handwashing, equipment such as humidifiers and catheters (Foley catheters, intravenous catheters)
Personal hygiene and oral and perineal care, handwashing, food handling habits

SIGNS AND SYMPTOMS

Managing daily living to prevent or manage infections requires the ability to recognize manifestations of infection in themselves. The signs can be ambiguous: fever, redness, swelling, and pain may or may not be present. For example, a urinary infection may be present without symptoms of pain on urination due to an impaired immune response. Occasionally, subjective symptoms of increasing restlessness, irritability, malaise, anorexia, and a sudden onset of confusion may give the best clues to early sepsis.

Patients who are suspected of having early signs of sepsis should be evaluated by their physician immediately. With decreased immune defenses, the patient can rapidly progress to septic shock, which can be fatal if the person does not receive prompt supportive care with antibiotics, fluids, and close monitoring (Klemm and Hubbard, 1990).

Evidence that the person and family can manage or are managing daily living in such a way as to minimize risks would include data that they

Understand the risks of infection and sites at high risk for infection

Use good handwashing techniques

Wash vegetables and fruits thoroughly, and store foods at the proper temperature

Maintain adequate protein and calorie intake during periods of increased susceptibility to infection

Know how to minimize contact with infected persons without alienating them

Report potential signs and symptoms of infection to the physician promptly in order to get immediate treatment

PROGNOSTIC VARIABLES

Poor prognosis for preventing and managing infections in everyday living is associated with ignorance about strategies for prevention, unwillingness to take precautions, dehydration, malnutrition, delay in reporting symptoms of infection to the physician, depression, poor self-care routines, and hopelessness.

COMPLICATIONS

The complications of infection are increased morbidity, hospitalization, and mortality.

TREATMENT

The best treatment for infection in older persons with cancer is prevention. The nursing regimen for this includes involving the patient and family in:

Understanding the risks of infection and the potential outcomes

Learning effective handwashing and oral hygiene techniques

Learning how to clean humidifiers and respirators, oxygen tubing, or other treatment instruments used in daily home care

Developing scripts for dealing with visitors who might expose the patient to infections

Developing alternatives of care if the primary caregiver develops an infection

When there are indications of a possible infection, both the patient and family need to know that early reporting is important. They also need to know who to contact and how to report the symptoms in a manner that will lead to an appropriate response

EVALUATION

The effectiveness of the nursing treatment plan in helping the patient and family to manage daily living with an increased potential for infection will be shown in decreased hospitalizations for infections, their understanding of the importance of the problem, and their skill in detecting and reporting infections at an early stage.

DAILY LIVING WITH LONELINESS AND SEPARATIONS

The older person with cancer experiences multiple separations in daily living with the disease and its treatment. Some of these separations occur because of physical barriers or geographic distances associated with treatment. There is a form of societal separation. There are separations of a close personal nature. There is also a separation from one's physical self.

The nature of cancer tends to frighten others, even the family. That fear sets the person on the periphery of the family group, sometimes in subtle unspoken ways, at other times overtly. Being subjected to another's pity separates an individual. So does reduced communication. There is a continuing belief (usually unspoken) that cancer is contagious, and the result is physically distancing.

The rigorous diagnosis and treatment activities, if carried on throughout the course of the disease, separate the patient in the following ways:

Socially because of the ensuing fatigue, pain, nausea, alopecia, and stomatitis

Socially from friends who may identify too closely with the illness or are afraid of "catching" the cancer

Geographically if the treatment is inpatient and the location is any distance from family and friends, or if they are unable to use transportation systems to come to visit. Hospitalization also means separation from favorite things and pets

Physically, even from health care professionals. External beam radiation requires remaining isolated in the treatment room 5 days a week often for 4 to 6 weeks. Brachytherapy involves not only inpatient status for 4 to 5 days, but also means that people may come only as close as the doorway while the patient feels totally radioactive—not just the cancer site—but all of him. Chemotherapy also involves separation, when nurses administering the therapy wear gloves and gown and possibly goggles and a mask

Enclosures and doors have a finality, giving a message that isolation and control is in the hands of someone else. Certain therapies have consequences that separate:

Head and neck dissection surgery may change forever the familiar sound of one's voice, or may remove the voice, or the ability to whistle or sing like others. It also changes one's familiar facial appearance

Chemotherapy or radiation therapy also limits the ability to talk because of temporary, but painful mucositis, a swollen tongue or lips, and "unspittable" saliva

Chemotherapy and radiation therapy may change the person's head of hair to no hair or strange-colored hair, or even straight hair from once curly hair. This separation, even though anticipated, is a shock when one morning hair falls out in bunches and one must face a bald head.

Fatigue and pain make cowards of us all. When these are present in the elderly, their world shrinks to a small sphere of self with very limited forays out of it to visit, shop, or even just walk around. Such limitations may separate them from experiences that others take for granted or do not even notice, the ability to go for a walk or browse through a shopping mall.

RISK FACTORS

The persons at greatest risk of not handling the separations associated with cancer are those who:

Feel helpless or hopeless

Live alone or have diminishing contact with family and friends, particularly age-mates or favorite people

Suffer severe pain or intractable nausea and vomiting

Are in the advanced stages of terminal cancer

SIGNS AND SYMPTOMS

Manifestations that older persons are not managing the separations inherent in having the diagnosis, disease, and treatment of cancer include the following:

Comments about missing certain people or things in their lives

Avoidance of strangers who require special effort with interactions and who appear uncomfortable with the diagnosis of cancer

Withdrawal and apathy

Growing inability to handle the pain and other physical symptoms

Depression

Suicide language or attempt (usually successful even when the person would seem to have little energy either to plan or implement the act)

PROGNOSTIC VARIABLES

Managing separations is more likely if the person has a desire to survive and a strong ego. It is also helped by the presence of at least one dependable committed person and the availability of expert health care professionals to lend perspective and options of action to both the patient and the companion.

COMPLICATIONS

Failure to manage the separations as they occur and allowing them to accumulate tends to result in a downward spiral toward lonely dying.

The complication of suicide cannot be overlooked. There is a higher incidence of male suicides with cancer than in the general population (Blazer et al, 1986).

TREATMENT

An important feature in a nursing treatment regimen is a high level of awareness of the alienating features in the older person's cancer and cancer experience. This includes understanding the separating features of the disease, its treatment, and the response of family and friends. It involves knowing this older person's strengths and resources (internal and external) as well as the deficits as a basis for planning with that person how to handle daily living with the high-risk separations and crises these may precipitate. Because the person's closest companion, caregiver, or family members are going to be key figures in helping to prevent separations, they too are a target for diagnosis and treatment. The family members may also be having their own difficulties dealing with the physical and emotional changes accompanying the disease and its treatment. At times they will be the primary targets for diagnoses and nursing management (McCabe, 1991).

Elements of the nursing treatment plan include helping the older patient and primary caregiver or family to:

Be aware of the high-risk times for feeling isolated and lonely

Be aware of the areas in which separations can occur

Be aware that some of these areas will be so sensitive that the older person will have great difficulty in initiating discussion of them, even as intense suffering over them is being experienced

Learn strategies for sharing the sense of separation and the feelings that are generated

Learn strategies for preventing, circumventing, or overcoming the separating features (e.g., loss of touch in a treatment room, loss of ability to communicate with one's voice)

Both the older patient and the one who assumes responsibility for maintaining him need external support in daily living throughout the course of the illness experience. Just as the patient needs consistency in the person giving that support, so also does the caregiver require a consistent and dependable professional consultant.

EVALUATION

Response to the nursing treatment plan for managing separations in daily living can be evaluated in terms of:

The person's and caregiver's ability to verbalize high-risk areas of separation and identify when they are occurring

The consistency and dependability of a primary caregiver, one who is willing to deal with the separation issues in the daily living of the older cancer patient

The evolving of successful strategies for preventing or managing the separations

Evidence of both individuals maintaining some equilibrium in the face of separation crises

The consistency and dependability of a nurse or other professional to relate to the patient and caregiver over the duration of the experience

The willingness of the patient and caregiver to consult with "their" nurse

Expressions of the patient and caregiver over the successful way they have managed the separations or have managed to avoid them

DAILY LIVING WITH CANCER TREATMENT AND HEALTH PROFESSIONALS

Cancer in older persons is a disease that can place them in a difficult relationship with health care professionals. Cardiovascular or renal diseases are viewed in terms of worn-out parts that can be patched up, resected, or replaced. Cancer, on the other hand, is spoken of as body betrayal, bad cells spreading out and destroying good cells. It is a war in progress. The strategists in this war are the physicians, often oncologic specialists interested in using and refining treatments to win the war, if not this particular patient's battle.

The decisions regarding diagnostic and treatment activities for cancer in the older patient, 70 years or greater, require some individual attention. Diagnostic work-ups can be strenuous on all patients, especially the elderly patient. Age may be used as a basis for flatly refusing to treat even when the patient is willing to undergo the therapy. The elderly patient who has always approached problems directly and is prepared to conquer cancer, may be frustrated by the approach of "let's wait and see what happens," which is often no treatment. The patient's family may also favor a no treatment approach.

Likewise, although an elderly patient with good performance status may qualify for an aggressive research treatment protocol, he may be unprepared for the morbidity associated with the therapy. A protocol treatment plan is usually modified only by physiologic changes in body weight, and laboratory results such as the complete blood count. Once treatment is begun, older persons may have to drop out of the study if they are unable to cope with the side effects of the drugs or other treatments. Older persons have been devastated at being dismissed and told "You failed treatment," without further explanation (i.e., the treatment has failed to help your disease and it is inappropriate to continue it). Persons who withdraw from treatment protocols risk censure and potential for lack of supportive care.

The older person, like their younger counterparts, have goals and a sense of how they want to live their life. In order to make informed decisions, they need to know what it is like to live with the treatment and what changes in their life may occur as a result of treatment. On the other hand, they also need to know what living without treatment is like. For example, breast tumors tend to break down, ulcerate, and produce uncontrollable offensive odors; a simple lumpectomy or mastectomy will avoid this problem. Thus, they need at least one person who is a *neutral* sounding board who has expertise in neoplastic disease in the elderly and the treatment options and outcomes in order to talk about their goals and ask questions.

When there is the threat to one's well-being as it is represented by a progressive disease such as cancer, physicians are seen as the holders of the keys to life and comfort. The relationship of the older person to the physician is one of significant dependence on that person's medical wisdom, interest, responsiveness, and compassion. If the patient drops out of a research protocol or chooses not to go through the proposed treatment regimen, there may exist some legitimate concern about some level of abandonment by the physician or health care professions. If the specialist physician is primarily focused on treatment, it may be most helpful to request a referral to another physician who can provide supportive palliative care rather than curative treatment.

The patient may also need assistance in working through with the family his decisions for nontreatment and the right to make this decision. The family may desire to "do everything possible for Dad" and may have urgent issues in loss and grief that do not allow them to honor their parent's decision against treatment. In all family discussions, patients should be watched closely for cues that they are "giving in" to the desires of the family over their own wishes. Separate discussions with the patient and family may be another way to evaluate the situation.

Cancer support groups can be a helpful adjunct for both the elderly person and family members. The companionship of others facing the same decisions and problems in daily living can relieve some of the sense of aloneness and helplessness. It must be recognized that some people are not "groupy" and will not choose to join with strangers. A group of friends or age mates may be of more assistance. Also, some older persons and their families may be drawn to spiritual resources and be able to find considerable support through their minister or other spiritual leader.

The nurse who is perceptive to the issues discussed and knowledgeable about the health system can prove to be a valuable ally to the older patient and family. Some of the steps older persons can be advised to follow are:

Work through his own physician (internist or family physician) and ask that the doctor continue to serve as overall coordinator of care

Continue to see the family physician for ongoing care. Ask that physician to serve as spokesperson to the specialty team if the patient feels he is unable to speak for himself

Suggest the patient or family take a tape recorder to sessions with the physician or oncology nurse. Tape the discussion in order to take it home and remember what was said

Summary

Progress in the management of the elderly oncology patient first begins with the health care professional. Both physicians and nurses should become knowledgeable about the effectiveness and toxicities of major cancer therapies. They also need to know how these treatments specifically affect the elderly person and their physiologic, emotional, and social circumstances.

Increasing chronologic age is not a sufficient reason to not give the elderly person information on which he can make an informed decision and participate in how his illness will be treated. Although the "no treatment option" should be included in the plan, the elderly person and the family should be presented with realistic options and possible outcomes of treatment, including potential side effects.

Patients who are old and have cancer are not always afraid of dying. They do fear pain and being separated. Both of these fears can be prevented and may be the cornerstone to effective daily living for the cancer patient.

References and Other Readings

Adami HO, et al. The relation between survival and age at diagnosis in breast cancer. N Engl J Med 1986; 315:559.

Aistairs J. Fatigue in the cancer patient. Oncol Nurs Forum 1987; 14:25.

Aker S, Lenssen P. A guide to good nutrition during and after chemotherapy and radiation, 3rd ed. Seattle: Fred Hutchinson Cancer Research Center, 1988.

American Cancer Society, Inc. Cancer facts and figures—1991. Atlanta, 1991.

Anisimov VN. Age-related mechanisms of susceptibility to carcinogenesis. Semin Oncol 1989; 16:10.

Balducci L, et al. Cancer chemotherapy in the elderly. Am Fam Phys 1987; 35:133.

Balducci L, et al. Pharmacology of antineoplastic agents in the elderly patient. Semin Oncol 1989; 16:66.

Beahrs O, et al. Manual for staging of cancer, 3rd ed. Philadelphia: JB Lippincott, 1988.

Begg CB, Carbone PP. Clinical trials and drug toxicity in the elderly. Cancer 1983; 52:1986.

Billings JA. Outpatient management of advanced cancer. Philadelphia: JB Lippincott, 1985.

Blazer DG, Bachar JR, Manton KG. Suicide in late life. J Am Geriatr Soc 1986; 34:519.

Blesch KS. The normal physiological changes of aging and their impact on the response to cancer treatment. Semin Oncol Nurs 1988; 4:178.

Bonica JJ. Management of cancer pain. Recent Results Cancer Res 1984; 89:13.

Boring CC, et al. Cancer statistics, 1991. CA 1991; 41:19.

Bowles LT. Surgical essentials in the care of the elderly cancer patient. In: Yancik R, et al, eds. Perspectives on prevention and treatment of cancer in the elderly, aging series, vol. 24. New York: Raven Press, 1983.

Burklow J. Cancer rates higher in older people: But, why? JNCI 1990; 82:17.

Cancer Statistics Review, 1973–1987. National Cancer Institute, National Institutes of Health, Bethesda, MD., Publication No. 90-2789.

Canning GP, Caird FI. Lung tumours. In: Caird FI, et al, eds. Cancer in the elderly. London: Wright, 1991.

Carson C, Callaghan ME. Hematopoietic and immunologic cancers. In: Baird S, et al, eds. Cancer nursing, a comprehensive textbook. Philadelphia: WB Saunders, 1991.

Catalona WJ, et al. Measurement of prostate-specific antigen in serum as a screening test for prostate cancer. N Engl J Med 1991; 324:1156.

Chalfin DB, Carlon GC. Age and utilization of intensive care unit resources of critically-ill cancer patients. Crit Care Med 1990; 18:694.

Chernoff R, Ropka M. The unique nutritional needs of the elderly patient with cancer. Semin Oncol Nurs 1988; 4:189.

Cohen R, Frank-Stromberg M. Assessment and interventions for cancer prevention and detection. In: Groenwald SL, et al, eds. Cancer nursing, principles and practice, 2nd ed. Boston: Jones & Bartlett, 1990.

Coyle N, Foley K. Prevalence and profile of pain syndromes in cancer patients. In: McGuire DB, Yarbro CH, eds. Cancer pain management. Orlando, FL: Grune & Stratton, 1987.

Cullen JW, Fox BH, Isom RH. Cancer: the behavioral dimensions. New York: Raven Press, 1976.

Crawford J, Cohen HJ. Aging and neoplasia. In: Eisdorder C, ed. Annual review of gerontology and geriatrics. New York: Springer Publishing, 1984.

Daut RL, Cleeland CS. The prevalence and severity of pain in cancer. Cancer 1982; 50:1913.

Dellefield ME. Caring for the elderly patient with cancer. Oncol Nurs Forum 1986; 13:19.

Derby SA. Cancer in the older patient. In: Ashwanden P, et al, eds. Oncology nursing—advances, treatments and trends into the 21st century. Rockville, MD: Aspen Publishers, 1991.

DeWys WD, Killen JY. The paraneoplastic syndromes. In: Rubin P, ed. Clinical oncology, a multidisciplinary approach, 6th ed. New York: American Cancer Society, 1983.

DeVita V, Hellman S, Rosenberg S. Cancer, principles and practice of oncology, 3rd ed. Philadelphia: JB Lippincott, 1989.

Diekmann J. Cancer in the elderly: systems overview. Semin Oncol Nurs 1988; 4:169.

Fraser MC, Hartge P, Tucker MA. Melanoma and nonmelanoma skin cancer: epidemiology and risk factors. Semin Oncol Nurs 1991; 7:2.

Frogge MH. Gastrointestinal cancer: esophagus, stomach, liver and pancreas. In: Groenwald SL, et al, eds. Cancer nursing, principles and practice, 2nd ed. Boston: Jones & Bartlett, 1990.

Grieg NH, et al. Increasing annual incidence of primary brain tumors in the elderly. JNCI 1990; 82:1621.

Guy JL. Medical oncology—the agents. In: Baird S, et al, eds. Cancer nursing, a comprehensive textbook. Philadelphia: WB Saunders, 1991.

Hahn MB, Jassak PF. Nursing management of patients receiving interferon. Semin Oncol Nurs 1988; 4:95.

Harbitz TB, Haugen OA. Histology of the prostate in elderly men. Acta Path Microbiol Scand, Section A 1972; 80:756.

Harmer MH, ed. TNM, classification of malignant tumors. UICC- International Union Against Cancer, 3rd ed. Geneva, 1982.

Hilderley LJ, Dow KH. Radiation oncology. In: Baird S, et al, eds. Cancer nursing, a comprehensive textbook. Philadelphia: WB Saunders, 1991.

Holmes FF. Clinical evidence for a change in tumor aggressiveness with age. Semin Oncol Nurs 1989; 16:34.

Howard-Ruben J. Issues in cancer pain. In: McGuire DB, Yarbro CH, eds. Cancer pain management. Orlando, FL: Grune & Stratton, 1987.

Huang C. Paraneoplastic CNS syndromes. In: Caird FI, et al, eds. Cancer in the elderly. London: Wright, 1990.

Isom RN. Inferences and synthesis of significant results. In: Cullen JW, et al, eds. Cancer: the behavioral dimensions. New York: Raven Press, 1976.

Iwamoto R. Principles of radiation therapy. In: Otto S, ed. Oncology nursing. St. Louis: Mosby Year Book, 1991.

Jassak PF. Biotherapy. In: Groenwald SL, et al, eds. Cancer nursing, principles and practice, 2nd ed. Boston: Jones & Bartlett, 1990.

Jewkes AJ, Rowley S, Priestman TJ. Gastric cancers. In: Caird FI, et al, eds. Cancer in the elderly. London: Wright, 1990.

Kaplan ID, Bagshaw MA. Cancer of the prostate. In: Caird FI, et al, eds. Cancer in the elderly. London: Wright, 1990.

Klemm PR, Hubbard SM. Infection. In: Groenwald SL, et al, eds. Cancer nursing, principles and practice, 2nd ed. Boston: Jones & Bartlett, 1990.

Knobf TMK, Fisher DS, Welch-McCaffrey D. Cancer chemotherapy, treatment and care, 2nd ed. Boston: G.K. Hall Medical, 1984.

Kupcella CE. The spread of cancer: invasion and metastasis. In: Groenwald SL, et al, eds. Cancer nursing, principles and practice, 2nd ed. Boston: Jones & Bartlett, 1990.

Lind BS. Surgical management of the elderly cancer patient. In: Zenser TV, et al, eds. Cancer and aging, progress in research and treatment. New York: Springer, 1989.

Lind JM, Nakao SL. Urologic and male genital cancers. In: Groenwald SL, et al, eds. Cancer nursing, principles and practice, 2nd ed. Boston: Jones & Bartlett, 1990.

Lindsey AM. Lung cancer. In: Baird S, et al, eds. Cancer nursing, a comprehensive textbook. Philadelphia: WB Saunders, 1991.

Lipschitz DA, et al. Cancer in the elderly: basic science and clinical aspects. Ann Intern Med 1985; 102:218.

List ND, et al. Age factors in management of prostate cancer. In: Yancik R, et al, eds. Cancer in the elderly. New York: Springer, 1989.

Marks RM, Sachar EJ. Undertreatment of medical inpatients with narcotic analgesics. Ann Intern Med 1973; 78:173.

Mayer DK. Biotherapy: recent advances and nursing implications. Nurs Clin North Am 1991; 25:291.

McCabe MS. Psychological support for the patient on chemotherapy. Oncology 1991; 5:91.

McCaffery M, Beebe A. Pain, clinical manual for nursing practice. St. Louis: C.V. Mosby, 1989.

McGuire DB, Scheidler VR. Pain. In: Groenwald SL, et al, eds. Cancer nursing, principles and practice, 2nd ed. Boston: Jones & Bartlett, 1990.

Mettlin C, Dodd GD. The American Cancer Society guidelines for the cancer-related checkup: an update. CA 1991; 41:279.

Moon TD. Prostate cancer. J Am Geriatr Soc 1992; 40:622.

Morra ME, Blumberg BD. Women's perceptions of early detection in breast cancer: how are we doing? Semin Oncol Nurs 1991; 7:151.

Nail LM, King KB. Fatigue. Semin Oncol Nurs 1987; 3:257.

Newell GR, Spitz MR, Sider JG. Cancer and age. Semin Oncol 1989; 16:3.

Oleske D, Groenwald SL. Epidemiology of cancer. In: Groenwald SL, et al, eds. Cancer nursing, principles and practice, 2nd ed. Boston: Jones & Bartlett, 1990.

O'Mary SS. Diagnostic evaluation, classification, and staging. In: Groenwald SL, et al, eds. Cancer nursing, principles and practice, 2nd ed. Boston: Jones & Bartlett, 1990.

Otte DM. Gynecologic cancers. In: Groenwald SL, et al, eds. Cancer nursing, principles and practice, 2nd ed. Boston: Jones & Bartlett, 1990.

Otto S. Chemotherapy. In: Otto S, ed. Oncology nursing. St. Louis: Mosby Year Book, 1991.

Parzuchowski J. Head and neck cancer. In: Otto S, ed. Oncology nursing. St. Louis: Mosby Year Book, 1991.

Perez CA, Fair WR, Ihde DC. Carcinoma of the prostate. In: DeVita, et al, eds. Cancer, principles and practice of oncology, 3rd ed. Philadelphia: JB Lippincott, 1989.

Piper BF, et al. Fatigue mechanisms in cancer patients: developing nursing theory. Oncol Nurs Forum 1987; 14:25.

Robinson CR, Roy SC, Seager ML. Central nervous system tumours. In: Baird S, et al, eds. Cancer nursing, a comprehensive textbook. Philadelphia: WB Saunders, 1991.

Santo AL, Gelperin A. Surgical mortality in the elderly. J Am Geriatr Soc 1975; 23:42.

Schiffer CA. Interferon studies in the treatment of patients with leukemia. Semin Oncol 1991; 18:1.

Schofield P. Colon, rectum, anus. In: Caird FI, et al, eds. Cancer in the elderly. London: Wright, 1990.

Schulmeister L. Nutrition. In: Otto S, ed. Oncology nursing. St. Louis: Mosby Year Book, 1991.

Schwab R, Wallers CA, Weksler ME. Host defense mechanisms and aging. Semin Oncol 1989; 16:10.

Spross JA. Cancer pain relief: An international perspective. Oncol Nurs Forum 1992; 19[suppl 7]:5.

Spross JA, Manolatos A, Thorpe M. Pancreatic cancer: nursing challenges. Semin Oncol Nurs 1988; 4:274.

Steinfeld AD, et al. Patient age as a factor in radiotherapy. J Am Geriatr Soc 1989; 37:335.

Stewart DA, Caird FI. Brain and spinal cord. In: Caird FI, et al, eds. Cancer in the elderly. London: Wright, 1991.

Stewart JA, Foster RS. Breast cancer and aging. Semin Oncol 1989; 16:41.

Szeluga DJ, Groenwald SL, Sullivan DK. Nutritional disturbances. In: Groenwald SL, et al, eds. Cancer nursing, principles and practice, 2nd ed. Boston: Jones & Bartlett, 1990.

Vannicola P. An overview of the physiologic changes of aging and their effects on cancer. American Cancer Society reprint, 1988.

Walsh SJ, Begg CB, Carbone PP. Cancer chemotherapy in the elderly. Semin Oncol 1989; 16:66.

Walsh TD, Saunders SM. Hospice care. The treatment of pain in advanced cancer. Recent Results Cancer Res 1984; 89:201.

Weinberger M, et al. Breast cancer screening in older women: practices and barriers reported by primary care physicians. J Am Geriatr Soc 1991; 39:22.

Winawer SJ, Schottenfeld D, Flehinger BJ: Colorectal cancer screening. JNCI 1991; 83:243.

Display 22–1 Melanoma of the skin (excluding eyelid). (From Beahrs et al. TNM system for staging of cutaneous melanoma. In: Manual for staging of cancer, 3rd ed. Philadelphia: J. B. Lippincott/American Joint Committee on Cancer, 1988, pp. 143–144.)

MELANOMA OF THE SKIN (EXCLUDING EYELID)

Data Form for Cancer Staging

Patient identification
Name _____
Address _____
Hospital or clinic number _____
Age _____ Sex _____ Race _____

Institution identification
Hospital or clinic _____
Address _____

Oncology Record

Anatomic site of cancer _____
Histologic type _____
Grade (G) _____
Date of classification _____

Chronology of classification
(use separate form for each time staged)
[ ] Clinical (use all data prior to first treatment)
[ ] Pathologic (if definitively resected specimen available)

Definitions

Primary Tumor (pT)

[ ] pTX   Primary tumor cannot be assessed
[ ] pT0   No evidence of primary tumor
[ ] pTis   Melanoma *in situ* (atypical melanotic hyperplasia, severe melanotic dysplasia), not an invasive lesion (Clark's Level I)
[ ] pT1   Tumor 0.75 mm or less in thickness and invades the papillary dermis (Clark's Level II)
[ ] pT2   Tumor more than 0.75 mm but not more than 1.5 mm in thickness and/or invades to papillary-reticular dermal interface (Clark's Level III)
[ ] pT3   Tumor more than 1.5 mm but not more than 4 mm in thickness and/or invades the reticular dermis (Clark's Level IV)
  [ ] pT3a   Tumor more than 1.5 mm but not more than 3 mm in thickness
  [ ] pT3b   Tumor more than 3 mm but not more than 4 mm in thickness
[ ] pT4   Tumor more than 4 mm in thickness and/or invades the subcutaneous tissue (Clark's Level V) and/or satellite(s) within 2 cm of the primary tumor
  [ ] pT4a   Tumor more than 4 mm in thickness and/or invades the subcutaneous tissue
  [ ] pT4b   Satellite(s) with 2 cm of primary tumor

Lymph Node (N)

[ ] NX   Regional lymph nodes cannot be assessed
[ ] N0   No regional lymph node metastasis
[ ] N1   Metastasis 3 cm or less in greatest dimension in any regional lymph node(s)
[ ] N2   Metastasis more than 3 cm in greatest dimension in any regional lymph node(s) and/or in-transit metastasis
  [ ] N2a   Metastasis more than 3 cm in greatest dimension in any regional lymph node(s)
  [ ] N2b   In-transit metastasis
  [ ] N2c   Both (N2a and N2b)

Distant Metastasis (M)

[ ] MX   Presence of distant metastasis cannot be assessed
[ ] M0   No distant metastasis
[ ] M1   Distant metastasis
  [ ] M1a   Metastasis in skin or subcutaneous tissue or lymph node(s) beyond the regional lymph nodes
  [ ] M1b   Visceral metastasis

Stage Grouping

[ ] I	pT1	N0	M0
[ ] II	pT2	N0	M0
[ ] III	pT3	N0	M0
	Any pT	N1	M0
	Any pT	N2	M0
[ ] IV	Any pT	Any N	M1

Histopathologic Grade (G)

[ ] GX   Grade cannot be assessed
[ ] G1   Well differentiated
[ ] G2   Moderately well differentiated
[ ] G3   Poorly differentiated
[ ] G4   Undifferentiated

Histopathologic Type

The types of malignant melanoma are as follows:

Lentigo maligna (Hutchinson's freckle)
Radial spreading (superficial spreading)
Nodular
Acral lentiginous
Unclassified

  A rare desmoplastic variant also exists.
  Melanomas are identified according to site (mucosal, ocular, vaginal, anal, urethral, and so forth). The staging classification described in this chapter applies only to those arising in the skin.

Sites of Distant Metastasis

Pulmonary   PUL
Osseous   OSS
Hepatic   HEP
Brain   BRA
Lymph nodes   LYM
Bone marrow   MAR
Pleura   PLE
Peritoneum   PER
Skin   SKI
Other   OTH

Staged by _____ M.D.
_____ Referral
Date _____

(Continued)

Display 22-1 *(Continued)*

Illustrations

Indicate on diagrams primary tumor and regional nodes involved.

Depth of Invasion
[ ] Level I (not a melanoma and further characterization is not necessary)
[ ] Level II   [ ] Level IV
[ ] Level III   [ ] Level V
Other description _____
Maximal thickness (mm) _____
Site of primary lesion (check diagram)
_____
Extent of primary lesion (include all pigmentation)
_____
Size in greatest diameter _____ cm

Display 22-2 Initial pain assessment tool. (Modified from McCaffery M, Beebe A. Pain: Clinical manual for nursing practice. St. Louis: C. V. Mosby, 1989; with permission.)

INITIAL PAIN ASSESSMENT TOOL   Date_____

Patient's Name_____ Age_____ Room_____

Diagnosis_____ Physician_____

                                        Nurse_____

I. LOCATION: Patient or nurse mark drawing.

II. INTENSITY: Patient rates the pain. Scale used _____

    Present:_____

    Worst pain gets:_____

    Best pain gets:_____

    Acceptable level of pain:_____

III. QUALITY: (Use patient's own words, e.g. prick, ache, burn, throb, pull, sharp) _____
_____

IV. ONSET, DURATION VARIATIONS, RHYTHMS:_____
_____

V. MANNER OF EXPRESSING PAIN:_____
_____
_____

VI. WHAT RELIEVES THE PAIN?_____
_____
_____

VII. WHAT CAUSES OR INCREASES THE PAIN?_____
_____
_____

VIII. EFFECTS OF PAIN: (Note decreased function, decreased quality of life.)

    Accompanying symptoms (e.g. nausea)_____

    Sleep_____

    Appetite_____

    Physical activity_____

    Relationship with others (e.g. irritability)_____

    Emotions (e.g. anger, suicidal, crying)_____

    Concentration_____

    Other_____

IX. OTHER COMMENTS:_____
_____

X. PLAN:_____
_____

(Continued)

Display 22–2 *(Continued)*

INITIAL PAIN ASSESSMENT TOOL FOR MRS. P.   Date 5/2/87

Patient's Name Mrs. P.   Age 62   Room Home care

Diagnosis Breast cancer with bone metastases   Physician _____
to ® rib and lumbar spine. Arthritis in both   Nurse _____
knees and shoulders

I. LOCATION: Patient or nurse mark drawing.   A = Rib pain B = Back pain C = Knee pain D = Shoulder pain

II. INTENSITY: Patient rates the pain. Scale used   Unable to use numbers, prefers to use: no pain
a little pain, a lot of pain, too much pain.
    Present: a little pain.
    Worst pain gets: a lot of pain.
    Best pain gets: a little pain.
    Acceptable level of pain: a little pain.

III. QUALITY: (Use patient's own words, e.g. prick, ache, burn, throb, pull, sharp) A and B are constant aching
pain. C and D are inconsistent throbbing pain.

IV. ONSET, DURATION VARIATIONS, RHYTHMS: A and B started about 1 week ago. "X-ray shows I
have more cancer in the bones there." C and D—had for about 15 years. Worst when first wakes up—
stiffness.

V. MANNER OF EXPRESSING PAIN: Reluctant to "bother" nurses.

VI. WHAT RELIEVES THE PAIN? A and B—medication. Movement of R arm makes rib pain worse.
Lying still helps. Heating pad to shoulder pain helps some.

VII. WHAT CAUSES OR INCREASES THE PAIN? Movement makes rib and back pain worse—sitting
upright in chair ↑ back pain. Damp weather makes shoulders and knees ache more.

VIII. EFFECTS OF PAIN: (Note decreased function, decreased quality of life.)
    Accompanying symptoms (e.g. nausea) None.
    Sleep Falls asleep easily. Awakens every 1–2 hr. because can't get comfortable.
    Appetite Not much interest in food since chemotherapy treatments 4 months ago.
    Physical activity Tries to sit in recliner in living room as much as possible.
    Relationship with others (e.g. irritability) Feels "a bother" to daughter who she lives with.
    Emotions (e.g. anger, suicidal, crying) Tries to "keep going".
    Concentration Alert, pain interferes with interest in her grandchildren.
    Other_____

IX. OTHER COMMENTS:_____

X. PLAN: Evaluate pain medication. Possibly add nonsteroidal anti inflammatory
medication. Improve sleep by improving pain control.

23
Cardiovascular Problems

DEANNA RITCHIE

Cardiovascular disease (CVD) in western cultures increases in prevalence and incidence in the elderly population. However, aging and CVD are not synonomous. Recent studies of aging populations have shown, through exclusion of individuals with CVD, that there are certain changes in the cardiovascular system that occur normally as one ages chronologically (Fleg et al, 1988). These changes affect how the presence of CVD is accepted by the body. The signs and symptoms, prognosis, complications, and clinical treatment of CVD are significantly altered by the normal changes of aging (see box on p. 424).

The CVD diagnoses most common in elderly people include

Ischemic heart disease
Angina pectoris
Myocardial infarction (MI)
Congestive heart failure (CHF)
Valvular heart disease
Arrhythmias
Hypertension (see Chapter 28)

Both the medical and nursing management of elderly patients with aforementioned cardiovascular problems offer a unique challenge to the practitioner.

Pathophysiology and Medical Management

CORONARY HEART DISEASE

Coronary heart disease (CHD) occurs when the coronary arteries are not able to meet the demand of the myocardium for blood supply. The atherosclerotic process in the coronary arteries and vessel spasm are contributing factors in the development of CHD. Myocardial ischemia is reversible if the blood supply is only reduced temporarily. This may be an acute or chronic situation. A myocardial infarction (MI) occurs when, in addition to the atherosclerotic process and spasm, there is the organic problem of a thrombus formation at the site of the atheromatous lesion. The myocardium relying on this obstructed blood flow suffers cell death, and an MI occurs.

CHD increases in frequency and severity in the elderly population (Wenger et al, 1987). This increased occurrence is due to pathologic changes in the coronary arteries, an accumulation of coronary risk factors over time, and the influence of other systemic diseases.

CHD can present in the elderly in several different forms: angina pectoris, MI, congestive heart failure, or arrhythmias. There is also the additional asymptomatic coronary disease, later proven by diagnostic tests. For example,

---

Normal Changes in the Cardiovascular System in Elderly Persons

Increased left ventricular wall thickness

Increased aortic stiffness

Early diastolic filling is slowed

Incidence of arrhythmias is increased

Thickening of the endocardium

Increased collagen and fat in heart

Decreased ejection fraction with exercise

Reduced responsiveness to catecholamines

---

an elderly person may have had an MI without the typical overt signs and symptoms and a later electrocardiogram confirms the diagnosis. Silent MIs and asymptomatic CHD are common in the elderly population due to decreased sympathetic response.

RISK FACTORS

The risk factors for CHD in the elderly population are essentially the same as for the younger population. Patients and/or practitioners often tend to overlook coronary risk factors in the elderly as too late to change or insignificant. Reducing alterable risk factors in elderly persons impacts coronary artery disease (CAD) as strongly as it does in younger age groups (Kannel et al, 1987). Changes in risk factors for the elderly may include age-specific guidelines that make alteration easier, but are still beneficial (Table 23–1).

SIGNS AND SYMPTOMS

In evaluating an elderly patient for suspected or worsening CHD it is extremely important to consider two things: (1) other disease entities may mask or confuse signs and symptoms of heart disease and (2) mental status may be altered due to illness, medications, or dementia (Gerber, 1990). A complete, verified, and accurate history is extremely important. Signs and symptoms of CHD are often masked by signs and symptoms of alcohol abuse and/or medication toxicity. Diet history may also be helpful if

digestive complaints are included in the history.

CHD may be symptomatic or asymptomatic in the elderly. In 80% of symptomatic patients angina pectoris is the primary presentation (Wenger et al, 1987). Complaints of dyspnea and/or fatigue in inactive patients is a signal that ischemia may be the primary cause. Other common complaints due to altered pain pathways are syncope with exertion, palpitations with effort, abdominal complaints, flu-like symptoms, jaw pain, activity limits, and unexplained behavior. Signs of decreased oxygenation, i.e., skin and mucous membrane pallor, edema, decreased, increased, or irregular pulse, and an initial extremely low blood pressure can indicate an ischemic event (Frishman et al, 1987; Hurst, 1990).

Elderly patients with multiple risk factors of CAD should alert the practitioner to CHD even in the absence of symptoms. Patients with diabetes often are asymptomatic with their heart disease. Extreme fatigue may be the only presenting symptom in that group (Frishman et al, 1987; Hurst, 1990).

DIAGNOSIS

The electrocardiogram (ECG) is still the primary indicator of changes in the cardiovascular system. Acute ischemic events, arrhythmias, medication effects, the establishment of old ECG changes, or a normal ECG give the practitioner valuable information. However, the specificity of the ECG of elderly patients is limited. Often they show ST-T wave abnormalities not specific to myocardial ischemia and may represent normal aging changes of left ventricular hypertrophy, interventricular conduction defects, or bundle branch block (Fleg et al, 1988).

An exercise thallium test may help demonstrate ischemia, particularly in patients who increase their heart rate to at least 60% of predicted maximum for their age. In elderly persons inappropriate blood pressure and/or heart rate responses to exercise may occur even without CAD (Fleg et al, 1988).

Use of coronary angiography for further diagnosis of CHD, particularly in healthier elderly people who have performed an exercise tolerance test where positive data were obtained, is increasing. Patients over 70 years of age have an increased incidence of complica-

TABLE 23–1 *Risk Factor Reduction in the Elderly*

Risk Factors	Guidelines for Reduction	Methods for Reduction
Nonmodifiable		
Age	N/A	
Sex	N/A (postmenopausal women have an increased risk for developing CVD)	
Family history	Probably not a factor if CAD occurs after age 65. Family history is a risk factor for those who have immediate family members who have had CAD, hypertension, CVA before age 65	
Modifiable		
Smoking	Less a risk factor after 65 than in young. Research shows risk disappears after age 65 (Kannel et al, 1987). Modification more important for oxygen use. There is an influence on other vascular problems, claudication, CVA	Counseling, classes, nicotine gum or patches
Hypertension	If inherited or present with aging. Control to < 160/95 and systolic < 160. Hypertension and hyperlipidemia: risk of MI increased 15 times	Diet, exercise, medication (see Chapter 28)
Hyperlipidemia	Check fractionations: LDL increase has been predictive of CAD in men > 50 years old. In women > 50 years old, triglycerides are a better predictor. HDL < 50 mg/dL in men to age 79 and women to age 69 is an increased risk. Men with triglycerides > 150 mg/dL and HDL < 40 mg/dL are of special concern	Diet is first choice for elevated LDL. If other fractions abnormal, consult endocrinologist for the appropriate medications. Most medications have not been researched in the elderly or in women. Many influence liver metabolism or are prone to gastrointestinal side effects
Diabetes	Independent risk factor, particularly in older women; they have two times the risk for MI and with hyperlipidemia, 15 times the risk for MI	Control of blood sugar and weight. Check blood sugar before and after exercise and offer snacks as needed (see Chapter 24)
Physical inactivity	Impacts other risk factors (hypertension, weight, stress, diabetes, hyperlipidemia. Improves functional aerobic capacity	Some exercise is better than none in the elderly. An exercise tolerance test is useful for writing an exercise prescription (adaptation may be needed from the usual Full Bruce treadmill symptom limited test) (Balady and Weiner, 1989). Heart rate does not increase as much, but end-diastolic volume increases more (stroke volume) to maintain cardiac out-

(Continued)

TABLE 23–1   *(Continued)*

Risk Factors	Guidelines for Reduction	Methods for Reduction
		put. Writing an exercise prescription for a patient includes even those who are limited to low levels of activity and the table is useful with these people even in the later stages of cardiac rehabilitation (Table 23–8). Also the rate of perceived exertion is useful for those who cannot take their own pulse or pulse limitations are not adequate, for instance those with shortness of breath due to chronic CHF or chronic obstructive pulmonary disease
Obesity	Obesity and increased body mass distribution particular risk in women	Give careful guidelines. Rapid weight loss problems can outweigh benefits.
	Weight loss favorably affects other risk factors. Definitions of ideal weight and regional fat distribution are unclear in elderly	Encourage by assisting with monitoring. Calorie requirements are less as we age. Frequent smaller meals help. Discourage abnormal obsession with food likes and dislikes. Increase activity.
Psychological stress	Related risk factor, may be signal to other problems, i.e., asymptomatic disease. Impacts other health maintenance problems, i.e., medication compliance	Use geriatric counseling services where available. Sleeplessness is common and may require medication use. Seek psychiatric advice and follow guidelines. Some antidepressants have cardiac effects, i.e., Nortriptyline can prolong the QT interval. Monitor ECGs. Be aware of medication interactions, when first starting medications

tions with coronary angiography (O'Rourke et al, 1987).

COMPLICATIONS

Complications of CHD in the elderly include MI, CHF, and arrhythmias. The resultant MI compounds the situation by adding the potential for cardiac rupture, pulmonary embolism, and death.

PROGNOSIS

Elderly patients who are treated medically and have one- or two-vessel disease have a 6-year survival rate (76% and 69%, respectively). The 6-year survival for three-vessel disease is considerably less, 40%. This is significant in that these statistics show a greater survival with one-, two-, or three-vessel disease in the older than 65 age group than in younger patients. The elderly pa-

tients in this study had normal ejection fractions and coronary arteries similar to the younger participants (Fleg et al, 1988; Gerber, 1990; O'Rourke et al, 1987; Wenger et al, 1987).

TREATMENT

The treatment of both young and older patients with symptomatic CHD is similar. Special considerations are advised with particular modes of therapy and decisions for further intervention are considered individually on the basis of the physiologic versus chronologic age.

Medical Therapy   The primary aim of treatment for the patient with ischemic heart disease is to decrease the myocardial oxygen demand and increase the coronary blood flow and oxygen supply. Selected therapies to accomplish this goal are presented in Table 23–2.

Commonly used antianginal drugs have spe-

TABLE 23–2 *Selected Therapies to Reduce Ischemia and Infarction*

Decrease Myocardial O_2 Consumption	Increase Coronary Blood and O_2 Supply
Rest with backrest elevation 20–30°	Oxygen
Selected diet (small, frequent, easily digested meals; no caffeine)	Nitroglycerin
Nitroglycerin and long-acting nitrates	Calcium channel blocking agents
Narcotic analgesics	Revascularization
Beta-blocking agents	Thrombolysis
Calcium channel blocking agents	Percutaneous transluminal coronary angioplasty
Vasodilators	Coronary artery bypass surgery
Sedatives and tranquilizers	Vasoactive drugs that improve systemic hemodynamics
Stool softeners and laxatives	Anticoagulants and antiplatelet agents
Diuretics	Antilipid agents (long-term)
Antihypertensive agents	Exercise program
Stress management	Risk factor modification
Exercise program	
Risk factor modification	

From Patrick, Woods, Craven, et al. Coronary heart disease. In: Medical–surgical nursing. Philadelphia: J. B. Lippincott, 1986, p. 525; with permission.

cial considerations for the elderly population, such as lower initial doses and careful observation for interactions with other medications and toxicity side effects (see box on p. 428) and (Table 23–3).

Coronary Arteriography Coronary arteriography is indicated in patients who continue to have angina that occurs at rest, interferes with their lifestyle, and occurs despite implementation of maximal medical therapy. The risks of this procedure should be carefully weighed against the benefits. Consideration must be given to what will occur if significant stenoses are found (i.e., is this an elderly patient who would be a safe candidate for further interventional therapy, coronary angioplasty, or coronary artery bypass graft surgery [CABGS]?).

Percutaneous Transluminal Coronary Angioplasty Percutaneous transluminal coronary angioplasty has been successfully performed in many elderly patients over the past few years. The success rate in patients older than 60 years is no different than in younger people. Success is defined as the reduction of the coronary artery stenosis by at least 20%, no occurrence of MI, and no need for emergent CABG. There is also no difference in the complication rate or death in elderly patients of whom 70% had single-vessel disease (O'Rourke et al, 1987).

Coronary Artery Bypass Graft Surgery Elderly patients have an increased operative risk with CABG surgery. Long-term survival, however, is excellent in specific subgroups of patients (Figs. 23–1 and 23–2). Five-year survival is 90% in those with good left ventricular function and no other complicating medical illnesses. Elderly women do not benefit from decreased angina as well as men do. Physiologic age is an important variable to consider in elderly candidates for CABG surgery (O'Rourke et al, 1987). In a study of elderly patients recovering from CABG surgery, Gortner et al (1988) found an increase in activity as well as perceived general strength 3 to 6 months following the surgery.

Characteristics of Elderly People Relative to Drug Disposition and Responses

1. Reduced renal function: Accumulation of renally cleared drugs
2. Reduced serum albumin and increased alpha$_1$-acid glycoprotein levels: Changes in percentage of free drug, volume of distribution, and measured levels of bound drugs
3. Relative increase in body fat: Increased distribution volume of fat-soluble drugs
4. Reduction in lean body mass and total body water: Decreased distribution volume of water-soluble drugs
5. Reduction in liver metabolizing capacity: Accumulation of metabolized drugs
6. Decreased cardiac reserve: Potential for heart failure
7. Decreased baroreceptor sensitivity: Tendency to orthostatic hypotension
8. Concurrent illnesses: Disease interactions
9. Multiple drugs: Drug interactions
10. Large interindividual variation: Wide dose range

From Rocci ML, Vlassis PH, Abrams WB. Geriatric clinical pharmacology. Geriatr Cardiol 1986; 4:54; with permission.

Myocardial Infarction Disease Form of CAD

The diagnosis of an acute MI may be an elderly person's initial CHD event. The patient may or may not have experienced angina or other symptoms of CAD. The MI may be silent, i.e., discovered weeks or months later when an ECG is performed. The presentation may be dramatic, accompanied by CHF and possibly pulmonary edema. As is the case for CHD, the presence of other diseases confusing historical presentation may mask an MI.

TREATMENT   Treatment of elderly patients with an MI is essentially the same as for younger patients, with special consideration given to age-related changes in the cardiovascular system that affect medication metabolism and risks from interventional procedures. More elderly patients are being treated initially with thrombolytic agents (streptokinase or tissue plasminogen activator) if they have none of the contraindications and it is thought that the benefits will outweigh the risks for the treatment. The primary risk from these agents is that of cerebral bleeding, which is often unknown. However, in a previously healthy elderly person with a large anterior MI the risk may be worth the intervention. More study in the use of thrombolytic agents in the elderly is needed. In the past they have been excluded from experimental trials of these drugs.

DIAGNOSIS   Diagnosis of an MI is often difficult due to age-related changes in the ECG and cardiac enzyme misrepresentation. The ECG in elderly individuals, as mentioned previously, is not as specific as with the young population. Also cardiac enzymes may not identify infarctions due to normal or lower total creatinine phosphokinase (CPK) levels with elevated cardiac isoenzyme fractions. Many institutions do not even run isoenzymes on total CPK samples if they are below the rather high range. The normal range for total CPK levels in the elderly have not been determined and levels often vary, due to changes to muscle mass with aging (Wenger et al, 1987). The three criteria usually relied on for diagnosis of MI—presentation of chest pain, ECG changes, and CPK enzyme elevations (Wenger et al, 1987; Gerber, 1990)—therefore, have lower specificity for the elderly patient. This should remind practitioners to be aware of those elderly patients at risk for MI and to suspect MI in some instances where factual information is not available. In cases where suspicion is strong, cautious prophylactic post-MI treatment, i.e., vasodilators, beta-blockers, and aspirin therapy may be advisable.

TABLE 23–3 *Representative Cardiovascular Drugs Exhibiting Age-related Alterations in Disposition or Response*

Drug	Principal Age-related Factor	Pharmacokinetic Changes			Comments
		V_D	Half-life	CL	
Digoxin	Renal clearance	↓	↑	↓	Reduce dosage
Diuretics	Renal site of action	—	—	—	Reduced effect; volume and/or metabolism disturbance
Lidocaine	Liver clearance	↑	↑	NSC	Reduce dosage
Procainamide	Renal clearance	—	—	↓	Reduce dosage with compromised renal function and CHF
Quinidine	Liver and renal clearance	NSC	↑	↓	Individualize dosage
Disopyramide	Renal clearance; anticholinergic side effects	—	↑	↓	Reduce dosage with compromised renal function; check bowel and bladder function
Tocainide	Renal clearance	—	↑	↓	Reduce dosage with compromised renal function
Cibenzoline	Renal clearance	↓	↑	↓	Reduce dosage
Beta-blockers, lipid-soluble	Liver clearance	NSC	↑	↓	Decreased response; individualize dosage
Beta-blockers, water-soluble	Renal clearance	—	↑	↓	Decreased response; individualize dosage
Prazosin	Liver clearance; reduced bioavailability	↑	↓	NSC	Individualize dosage
Warfarin	Protein binding; tissue sensitivity	NSC	NSC	NSC	Reduce dosage

CL, total clearance (hepatic and renal); NSC, no significant change; V_D, volume of distribution is a ratio of the amount of drug in the body to its plasma concentration at a time when the amount of drug in the tissues is directly proportional to the amount in the plasma; —, no information or not relevant; ↑, increased; ↓, decreased.
From Rocci ML, Vlassis PH, Abrams WB. Geriatric clinical pharmacology. Geriatr Cardiol 1986; 4:54; with permission.

CONGESTIVE HEART FAILURE

Heart failure is a syndrome where the heart cannot pump an adequate supply of blood, in relation to venous return, to meet the metabolic needs of the tissues. The condition may be brought on by increased activity or exercise or in later stages it may occur at rest. The prevalence of heart failure increased with age as much as eightfold in the seventh as compared with the fifth decade of the Framingham population (Wenger et al, 1987). At all ages men have a higher incidence of heart failure than women.

RISK FACTORS

The primary causes of CHF are CHD and hypertensive heart disease. Age-related factors influence the course of the illness and response to therapy (Wenger et al, 1987; Weisfeldt et al,

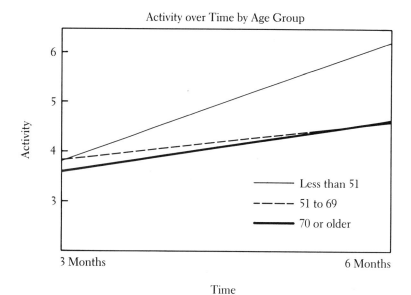

FIGURE 23–1   Increase in patient activity scores during a 3- to 6-month interval after surgery. (From Gortner SR, Rankin SH, Murphy M. Elders' recovery from cardiac surgery. Prog Cardiovasc Nurs 1988; 3:58; with permission.)

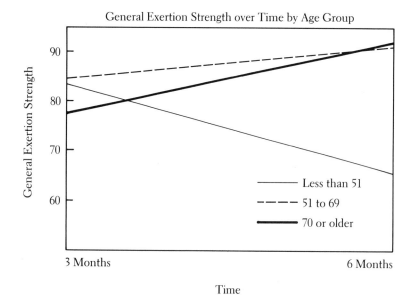

FIGURE 23–2   Self-reported percent confidence in general exertion strength at 3 to 6 months postsurgery. (From Gortner SR, Rankin SH, Murphy M. Elders' recovery from cardiac surgery. Prog Cardiovasc Nurs 1988; 3:54; with permission.)

1990). Other less common causes of CHF are valvular heart disease, cardiomyopathy, and particularly amyloid heart disease.

The age-related factor that influences CHF is impedence to left ventricular ejection occurring with exercise or stress. In more severe cases this can occur at rest as well. CHF is often brought on by bradyarrhythmias or tachyarrhythmias, particularly atrial fibrillation with loss of the atrial contribution to ventricular filling and in some cases complete atrioventricular (AV) block. CHF may also be precipitated by anemia, fever, hyperthyroidism or hypothyroidism, renal insufficiency, dietary sodium excess, alcohol abuse, fluid overload, drugs that depress myocardial function (beta or calcium channel blockers) or promote sodium retention (nonsteroidal and anti-inflammatories), or the patient's inability to follow prescribed therapy.

SIGNS AND SYMPTOMS

Physical signs of heart failure involve the cardiovascular and pulmonary systems. These signs and symptoms are best characterized by dividing them into four categories:

Right ventricular failure
Left ventricular failure
Pulmonary venous congestion
Systemic venous congestion

Right-sided heart failure includes an increase of the systemic venous pressure represented by jugular venous distention, hepatomegaly, dependent edema, and ascites. Left-sided failure is characterized by elevated pulmonary venous pressures and decreased cardiac output. Clinical manifestations include breathlessness, weakness, fatigue, dizziness, confusion, pulmonary congestion, hypotension, and possible death (Table 23–4) (Laurent-Bopp, 1991). Acute pulmonary edema usually develops suddenly and presents with marked dyspnea and orthopnea, pink frothy sputum, pallor and cyanosis, hypotension, obtundation, and confusion. Cardiogenic shock is brought on by decreased myocardial contractility, which markedly depresses cardiac output. Hypotension, tachycardia, decreased mentation, oliguria, and peripheral vascular collapse occur (Laurent-Bopp, 1991) (see Fig. 23–3).

The physical examination of the cardiovascular and pulmonary systems gives the practitioners important signs of CHF. Cardiac auscultation may reveal an S_3, S_4, or summation gallop, indicating excess volume and myocardial stretching. Cardiac palpation often reveals a displacement of the point of maximal impulse and a cardiac lift, suggesting cardiac enlargement and hypertrophy, respectively. Chest radiography may also show cardiac enlargement. Jugular venous distention may be present and should be quantified. Peripheral or central edema may be noted and if it occurs often pitting may result.

Pulmonary signs of CHF include presence of diffuse crackles heard on auscultation. Inspiratory and expiratory wheezes may also be present due to bronchiolar constriction. The lungs usually appear highly vascular on the chest radiographic study.

The liver edge may be palpable in the right upper quadrant as a result of right ventricular failure and hepatic engorgement. Measurement of abdominal girth may indicate abdominal distention and ascites.

DIAGNOSIS

Diagnosis of CHF is made by physical examination and is discussed under signs and symptoms. Diagnostic studies commonly used to supplement the signs and symptoms for accurate diagnosis and to direct treatment of heart failure syndrome include:

Chest radiography: positive findings include cardiomegaly, prominent pulmonary veins, and interstitial pulmonary edema
ECG: the practitioner examines for patterns of ventricular hypertrophy, arrhythmias, degree of myocardial ischemia, injury, or infarction
Right-sided heart catheterization: the indication for this procedure will depend on how aggressive the therapy will be for the elderly patient and the patient's physical, psychological, and mental condition. Hemodynamic variables to assess the severity of failure can be obtained and appropriate medical therapy prescribed for manipulation of these parameters
Laboratory tests: arterial blood gases are helpful in assessing the oxygenation status of the patient. Blood chemistries, hematologic screen, urinalysis, blood urea nitrogen, creatinine, and uric acid are all important tests to be done in the elderly patient in whom fluid and electrolyte imbalances and decreased renal function are common occurrences

TABLE 23–4   *Clinical Indicators of Left and Right Ventricular Failure*

Left Ventricular Failure	Right Ventricular Failure
OBJECTIVE FINDINGS	
Tachycardia	Neck vein pulsations and distention
Decreased S_1	
S_3 and S_4 gallops	Increased jugular venous pressure
Crackles (rales)	Edema
Pleural effusion	Hepatomegaly
Diaphoresis	Positive hepatojugular reflux
Pulsus alternans	Ascites
SUBJECTIVE FINDINGS	
Breathlessness	Weight gain
Cough	Transient ankle swelling
Fatigue and weakness	Abdominal distention
Memory loss and confusion	Gastric distress
Diaphoresis	Anorexia, nausea
Palpitations	
Anorexia	
Insomnia	

From Laurent-Bopp D. Heart failure. In: Patrick M, et al (eds.). Medical–surgical nursing: pathophysiological concepts, 2nd ed. Philadelphia: J.B. Lippincott, 1991; 752; with permission.

PROGNOSIS

The medical prognosis for elderly persons with CHF is limited. For most older individuals, CHF represents end-stage heart disease.

Overall, the ability of older persons to accept the limitations associated with the dysfunction and comply with the treatment regimen affects prognosis. The quality of life will vary depending on their expectations and previous lifestyle.

COMPLICATIONS

The most severe complication associated with CHF is the development of other end-stage organ diseases, as a result of chronic perfusion reduction. Hepatic or renal failure can result from end-stage CHF.

Other complications include fluid and electrolyte imbalances and the secondary effects of medications. An increased susceptibility to infections, especially pneumonias, complicated by the coexistence of CHF produces another vicious cycle. The older person is more prone to infections, and infections worsen the existing CHF.

TREATMENT

The goals of treatment are to (1) reduce cardiac workload, (2) improve contractility, and (3) reduce sodium and water retention. Treatment modalities include pharmacologic agents, activity prescriptions, and dietary manipulation.

Reduction in Cardiac Workload   In order to reduce the workload of the heart, activity restrictions may be necessary. Strenuous activities are limited in both duration and frequency,

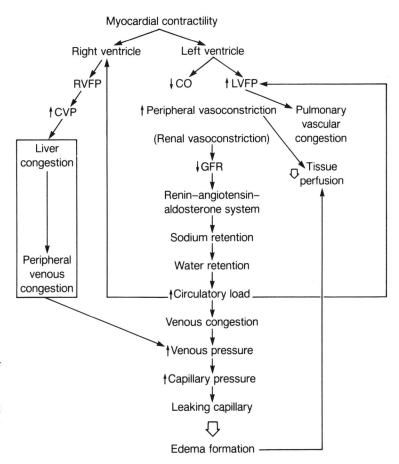

FIGURE 23-3 Dynamics of congestive heart failure. RVFP, right ventricular filling pressure; LVFP, left ventricular filling pressure; CVP, central venous pressure: CO, cardiac output; GFR, glomerular filtration rate.

or completely eliminated depending on the severity of CHF. A graded exercise program may be developed to maintain physical conditioning in the older person. It may incorporate many routine activities of daily living. In general, older persons with CHF should be encouraged to plan activities and exercise carefully, allowing for frequent rest periods as needed. Fatigue or exhaustion should be avoided. With severe CHF, the person may be restricted to sitting or even complete bed rest.

Weight reduction in obese elderly will also help to reduce the cardiac workload. Older persons with their established eating patterns may benefit from supportive nutritional counseling to maintain adequate nutrition during weight loss efforts.

Pharmacologic agents used to decrease cardiac workload include vasodilators that

Reduce peripheral vascular resistance (forces the heart must pump against)
Redistribute blood volume by changing the venous capacity (reduce the volume of blood the heart has to pump)

Table 23-5 shows common vasodilators with their recommended dosages, actions, side effects, and implications for daily living.

Improve Contractility Digitalis, a cardiac glycoside, is the standard treatment for increasing the force and velocity of each contraction. Factors influencing the individual's sensitivity to digitalis include the following (Braunwald, 1988):

Fluid and electrolyte balance, particularly sodium and potassium

TABLE 23–5   *Vasodilators*

Drug/Dosage/Route	Actions	Side Effects	Precautions
Hydralazine (Apresoline) 50–300 mg orally every day	Directly relaxes arterial smooth muscle. Increases cardiac output due to reduced peripheral resistance	Reflexive tachycardia, fluid retention	Monitor heart rate and weight
Minoxidil (min.) Initial dose, 5 mg every day Range: 10–40 mg every day	Similar to hydralazine. More potent long-acting vasodilator		
Prazosin (minipres) 1–20 mg orally every day 1 mg twice or three times a day to start; adjusted to increase dose over following few days	Blocks alpha-adrenergic receptors. Exerts direct vascular-smooth-muscle relaxation. Works equally on arteries and veins	First-dose effect may include postural hypotension, faintness, dizziness, and palpitations. Effects abate after several doses	Give first dose in safe environment with close observation. Take Rx when activity level is low. Warn about postural hypotension effects and position changes to prevent falls
Nitrates			
Nitroglycerin Topical: 0.5–4 inches (15 mg/inch) Transdermal: 5–20 cm^2	Venodilation; reduces preload	Headaches, dizziness	Application site may relate to symptoms. Apply to chest or abdomen. Abdominal application may reduce dizziness. Application before retiring may reduce paroxysmal nocturnal dyspnea
Isosorbide dinitrate (Isordil) Sublingual, 5–10 mg; Orally, 5–30 mg three times a day	Same as nitroglycerine	Frequent headache, postural hypotension	May require dose adjustment
Captopril (Capoten) 25–150 mg three times a day Begin with 25-mg dose or less Also, Lisinopril 5–10 mg every day Enalapril 5–10 mg twice a day	In CHF reduces peripheral resistance and preload. Increases cardiac output and stroke volume	Mouth sores, skin rash, nausea/vomiting, diarrhea, postural hypotension, taste disturbances, diaphoresis, hyperkalemia, false-positive urine test for acetone	Take 1 hour before meals—30% will not be absorbed if taken with meals. Serum potassium may rise if taken with K^+-sparing diuretics. Avoid sudden changes in posture. First-dose effect may occur within 3 hours of initial dose (see prazosin for explanation of first dose)

Concomitant drug therapies, e.g., antiarrhythmics, catecholamines
Altered thyroid or renal function
Acid–base imbalances

Elderly people are more sensitive to the toxic side effects of digitalis as they are with other medications. In addition, a reduced glomerular filtration rate, common among older adults, prolongs the drug's half-life. Periodic evaluation of digitalis blood levels is used to monitor therapy.

Sympathomimetic agents can also improve myocardial contractility. These include the following:

Dopamine and dobutamine (for intravenous use)
Amrinone (vasodilator and inotropic agent)

Reducing Sodium and Water Retention Dietary restriction of sodium is still the best way to reduce sodium and water retention. Older persons are asked to do the following:

Remove salt shakers from the table (added salt accounts for up to 2 g of sodium per day)
Use herbs, spices, and lemon juice as a substitute for salt in cooking

Many former salt users who have been weaned attest to the improved flavor of foods without a blanket of salt.

Older persons also need to know about the high sodium content of foods. Most ready-to-eat fast foods or processed foods are high in sodium. Typically, frozen foods contain little or no added sodium. Fresh fruits and vegetables contain no additional sodium. When older persons are unable to obtain and cook fresh foods, the frozen alternative is preferred over canned or other fast food processing.

Diuretic therapy is commonplace in elderly patients to prevent sodium and water retention. Although the benefits of diuretic therapy are many, medications are not the panacea of treatment modalities. It is essential that individuals using diuretics understand what their "water pill" is doing and what it has the potential to do. Diuretics decrease sodium reabsorption, increase urine output, and allow potassium loss in the urine. Urinary potassium loss enhances hydrogen ion loss, producing metabolic alkalosis. If the kidneys are unable to dilute urine adequately, hyponatremia can result. Fluid and electrolyte imbalances resulting from diuretic therapy can potentiate congestion, fatigue, and weakness.

Other Measures Palliative measures may be used to improve the quality of life. Oxygen therapy may be used during activity and also at rest. Antiembolic hose may reduce the risk of thrombus formation and possible embolization resulting from venous stasis.

VALVULAR HEART DISEASE

Although valvular heart disease may originate in early life, the cardiopulmonary problems often do not become apparent until late adulthood. The appearance of signs and symptoms may be compounded by the presence of other diseases common among elderly patients. Rheumatic heart disease (RHD) is the most common cause of valvular heart disease in the world, degenerative calcification is the most common cause in the United States and Great Britain (Levine and Underhill, 1991; Rahimtoola et al, 1987; Weisfeldt et al, 1988). Aortic stenosis and mitral valve prolapse, resulting in mitral stenosis, are the most common acquired valvular dysfunctions.

AORTIC STENOSIS

The most common valvular heart disease in the elderly is calcific aortic disease. In the sixth and seventh decades aortic stenosis is due to a congenitally bicuspid aortic valve but in older (70 years or older) individuals it is most likely due to primary aortic degenerative changes. This can occur rapidly due to abrupt calcification and scarring. In 6 to 8 months mild aortic stenosis (AS) can become severe obstruction.

AORTIC REGURGITATION

Aortic regurgitation may result from a congenital valve abnormality, myxomatous degeneration, systemic arterial hypertension, RHD, or infective endocarditis.

MITRAL STENOSIS

Mitral stenosis does not present until old age. The cause is predominantly RHD. Calcification is a less common cause.

MITRAL INSUFFICIENCY
OR MITRAL REGURGITATION

Mitral insufficiency, or chronic mitral regurgitation, is often caused by papillary muscle dysfunction in CHD in elderly patients just as in young patients. Heart failure and acute bacterial endocarditis can also be causes of mitral insufficiency. As the heart enlarges and the atrial annulus becomes dilated, leaflets are misaligned. In elderly patients three causes of mitral regurgitation are often seen: CHD and its complications, and two degenerative causes, myxomatous degeneration MVP, and mitral annulus calcification. Both cause rupture of chordae tendinae. Mitral annulus calcification occurs commonly in the elderly. It may obstruct left ventricular inflow, and conduction abnormalities are common.

Risk Factors   Risk factors for valvular heart disease in the elderly population include CHD, RHD, calcific disease, and congenital disease.

Signs and Symptoms   These are discussed under diagnoses in this section.

Complications   The primary complications of valvular heart disease are CHF, arrhythmias, pulmonary emboli, cerebral vascular accidents, and bacterial endocarditis. Bacterial endocarditis can cause any of the embolic events, as well as valvular failure. The prophylactic protocol from the American Heart Association should be followed in all patients at risk for development of bacterial endocarditis (Table 23–6).

Treatment   Treatment of valvular heart disease in elderly patients is similar to what is done for younger patients. This includes treating acute pulmonary edema or heart failure, controlling atrial fibrillation, and treating and preventing embolization, bronchopulmonary infections, and bacterial endocarditis. Atrial fibrillation should be restored to normal sinus rhythm if the patient is symptomatic. Anticoagulation may be indicated to prevent thromboembolic dispersion. Thromboemboli are more likely to develop with conversion to a normal sinus rhythm if atrial fibrillation has been present for 2 weeks or longer. Chronic atrial fibrillation is also an indication for anticoagulation for the same reason.

INDICATIONS FOR SURGERY   Indications for surgery are a severe valvular lesion and symptomatic presentation. Patients with extremely

reduced left ventricular function and those undergoing CABG for angina may also have severe valvular disease. The valvular repair with the CABG may benefit the patient more than the CABG alone. Operative mortality is increased when the patient has the following:

Severe ventricular dysfunction
Inoperable CAD
Moderately severe heart failure
Pulmonary hypertension
Other associated disorders, i.e., chronic obstructive pulmonary disease, renal failure, peripheral vascular disease, renovascular disease, and carotid artery disease
Poor overall psychological and functional status
Poor nutritional state

In some instances conduction abnormalities require a permanent pacer placement before surgery.

Coronary arteriography should be performed to identify the need for CABG. The evaluation of elderly patients for cardiac surgery should consider the physiologic and psychological age as well as the chronologic age.

VALVULAR SURGERY   Due to the normal aging changes and the presence of other disease processes, elderly patients are at increased risk for heart surgery. However, when surgery is feasible it often improves the patient's condition and more importantly the quality of life.

A bioprosthetic valve can be appropriate for elderly patients who have fewer years left to live and no need for anticoagulant therapy. The decision needs to be made carefully because many elderly patients live over 10 years after surgery. The prospect of a reoperation is not attractive in an 80 year old. Older patients may require smaller valves in which case a bioprosthesis may become stenotic. A prosthetic valve usually requires anticoagulant therapy. Many elderly patients need anticoagulant therapy for other conditions. Management of anticoagulant therapy is basically the same regardless of the precipitating event when monitored carefully by a knowledgeable practitioner. Each case requires individual judgment in the choice of prosthesis.

BALLOON VALVULOPLASTY   This is a newer technique that has been used quite effectively in elderly patients in whom surgery is deemed high risk. A balloon-tipped catheter is passed

TABLE 23–6 *Regimens for Dental, Oral, or Upper Respiratory Tract Procedures and Genitourinary/Gastrointestinal Procedures in Patients Who Are at Risk**

Drug	Dosing Regimen
RECOMMENDED STANDARD PROPHYLACTIC REGIMENS FOR ORAL, DENTAL, AND UPPER RESPIRATORY TRACT	
Standard regimen	
Amoxicillin	3.0 G orally 1 hour before procedure; then 1.5 g 6 hours after initial dose
Amoxicillin/penicillin-allergic patients	
Erythromycin	Erythromycin ethylsuccinate, 800 mg, or erythromycin stearate, 1.0 g,
or	orally 2 hours before procedure; then half the dose 6 hours after initial dose
Clindamycin	300 mg orally 1 hour before procedure and 150 mg 6 hours after initial dose
ALTERNATE PROPHYLACTIC REGIMENS FOR ORAL, DENTAL, AND UPPER RESPIRATORY TRACT	
Patients unable to take oral medications	
Ampicillin	Intravenous or intramuscular administration of ampicillin, 2.0 g, 30 min before procedure; then intravenous or intramuscular administration of ampicillin, 1.0 g, or oral administration of amoxicillin, 1.5 g, 6 hours after initial dose
Ampicillin/amoxicillin/penicillin-allergic patients unable to take oral medications	
Clindamycin	Intravenous administration of 300 mg 30 min before procedure and an intravenous or oral administration of 150 mg 6 hours after initial dose
Patients considered high risk and not candidates for standard regimen	
Ampicillin, gentamicin, and amoxicillin	Intravenous or intramuscular administration of ampicillin, 2.0 g, plus gentamicin, 1.5 mg/kg (not to exceed 80 mg), 30 min before procedure; followed by amoxicillin, 1.5 g, orally 6 hours after initial dose; alternatively, the parenteral regimen may be repeated 8 hours after initial dose
Ampicillin/amoxicillin/penicillin-allergic patients considered high risk	
Vancomycin	Intravenous administration of 1.0 g over 1 hour, starting 1 hour before procedure; no repeated dose necessary
REGIMENS FOR GENITOURINARY/GASTROINTESTINAL PROCEDURES	
Standard regimen	
Ampicillin, gentamicin, and amoxicillin	Intravenous or intramuscular administration of ampicillin, 2.0 g, plus gentamicin, 1.5 mg/kg (not to exceed 80 mg), 30 min before procedure; followed by amoxicillin, 1.5 g, orally 6 hours after initial dose; alternatively, the parenteral regimen may be repeated once 8 hours after initial dose
Ampicillin/amoxicillin/penicillin-allergic patient regimen	
Vancomycin and gentamicin	Intravenous administration of vancomycin, 1.0 g, over 1 hour plus intravenous or intramuscular administration of gentamicin, 1.5 mg/kg (not to exceed 80 mg), 1 hour before procedure; may be repeated once 8 hours after initial dose
Alternate low-risk patient regimen	
Amoxicillin	3.0 g orally 1 hour before procedure; then 1.5 g 6 hours after initial dose

*Includes those with prosthetic heart valves and other high-risk patients.
From Dajani S, et al. Prevention of bacterial endocarditis: Recommendations by the American Heart Association. JAMA 1990; 264:919; with permission. Copyright 1990, American Medical Association.

through the femoral vein (for the mitral valves) or artery (for the aortic valve) and across the valvular area. The balloon is inflated to decrease the stenotic area (Levine and Underhill, 1991). The procedure is performed in the catheterization laboratory and the patient is maintained on aspirin therapy following the procedure.

PROGNOSIS

The treatment of valvular disease not only involves the interventions mentioned previously, but more importantly treating each sequela, such as arrhythmias and CHF. Valvular disease in elderly patients can be managed by moderating lifestyle as necessary and complying with treatment.

DIAGNOSIS

Common tests used to diagnose valvular heart disease include cardiac catheterization, radionuclear imaging, echocardiography, ECG, exercise tolerance testing, and chest radiography.

Physical Assessment

AORTIC STENOSIS A fourth heart sound and left ventricular hypertrophy are common findings for conditions other than aortic stenosis in the elderly. This often presents a diagnostic dilemma and thus more definitive tests, i.e., echocardiography or cardiac catheterization, are necessary.

MITRAL STENOSIS Patients with mitral stenosis are often asymptomatic for years. Symptoms of CHF may be seen with exercise, fever, and emotional stress. Often the symptoms are precipitated by atrial fibrillation with a rapid ventricular response. The disease may further decrease blood pressure and cardiac output as the left atrial pressure increases and the stenotic mitral valve fails to allow passage of blood to the left ventricle and into arterial circulation. On auscultation there is an apical diastolic rumble, which, in later stages with decreased blood flow, may decrease altogether. With exercise the rumble may increase again. Some patients progress to right-sided heart failure, and increased jugular venous pressure, signs of liver enlargement, and peripheral edema ensue.

Cardiac catheterization is the definitive diagnostic test. The pressure gradient across the mitral valve is measured, as well as left atrial size and pulmonary artery wedge pressure.

MITRAL INSUFFICIENCY OR REGURGITATION An S_1 is often followed by a mitral click and a crescendo-decrescendo murmur is often auscultated throughout S_2. The late systolic murmur is indicative of regurgitant flow through the prolapsed mitral valve. M-mode and two-dimensional echocardiography are of value in defining clues about diagnosis, assessing size and function of the left ventricle, and diagnosing associated conditions. Doppler echo is of value in quantifying the regurgitation. Left ventricular function assessment is important in evaluating patients considered for surgery. Exercise capacity needs to be documented as well with an exercise tolerance test.

AORTIC REGURGITATION Diagnosis of aortic regurgitation is usually not difficult. With a recent onset, infective endocarditis is considered and may progress to AV block. Peripheral signs are often hidden by a rigid arterial system. Echocardiography, with or without Doppler ultrasound, defines the extent of the lesion, establishes a diagnosis and evaluates the etiology and other associated diseases of the heart. Again, left ventricular function assessment is important in evaluating potential surgical candidates (Levine and Underhill, 1991; Rahimtoola et al, 1987).

ARRHYTHMIAS

RISK FACTORS

As a person ages the risk of developing arrhythmias increases. The electrophysiologic changes that occur with aging are caused by several pathologic changes. There is an increase in elastin and collagen in all parts of the heart. Fat accumulates around the sinoatrial node, sometimes separating the node from the atrial musculature. In extreme cases this causes sick sinus syndrome (Fleg et al, 1988). In addition to the fibrosis of the sinoatrial node, there is a decrease in the number of pacemaker cells (Levine and Underhill, 1991). By the age of 60 the number has decreased and by age 75 less than 10% of the cell number found in young adults remains. Also a degree of calcification is found in the left side of the cardiac skeleton (aortic and mitral annuli, central fibrous body, and the summit of the intraventricular septum). This affects the atrioventricular (A-V) node, A-V bundle, bifurcation, and proximal and right bundle branch. If these areas are damaged or destroyed, an idiopathic block occurs (Fleg et al, 1988). In addition, the increasing prevalence of coronary atherosclerosis, ventricular hypertrophy, atrial dilatation, myocardial fibrosis, and lipofuscin and amyloid deposits increase the possibility of ECG changes and arrhythmias.

SIGNS AND SYMPTOMS

When elderly persons are screened for cardiac disease, normal healthy persons are not found to have arrhythmias (Table 23-7). As mentioned previously, however, the incidence in the overall elderly population is increased when compared with the younger group. One explanation for this increased incidence is that practitioners see more elderly with arrhythmias, such as atrial fibrillation, because they become symptomatic due to other changes, i.e., decreased cerebral blood flow and reliance on an atrial "kick" (Fleg et al, 1988).

ECG Changes In the normal aging process the resting heart rate is not changed, but RR and QT intervals in healthy men show small but significant increases with age (Markus et al, 1987). The PR interval also increases due to conduction delay proximal to the bundle of His. Conduction time through the bundle to the ventricles is not affected. With age there is a leftward shift of the QRS axis, a variable degree of fibrosis in the anterior fascicle of the left bundle branch, and mild left ventricular hypertrophy. Despite the increase in left ventricular mass in elderly clients QRS voltage decreases. This paradox has been explained several ways. Extracardiac factors such as changes in the heart's position in the thorax, senile emphysema and chest wall deformities, and partial replacement of cardiac muscle by fat or amyloid also occur. The most readily observed ECG changes occur with the repolarization process; ST flattens and the amplitude of the T wave diminishes. Therefore, when observing the ECG of an elderly person to determine the pathologic condition, the practitioner should keep normal aging changes in mind (Markus et al, 1987; Fleg et al, 1988).

Syncope In the elderly patient one of the most common symptoms associated with arrhythmias is syncope. In one study 21% of the etiology was cardiac in origin, 48% noncardiac, and 31% was unexplained. Susceptibility to

TABLE 23-7 *Ambulatory ECG Findings in Elderly Subjects with No Clinical Heart Disease*

Heart rate (beats/min)	34–180
Longest sinus pauses (seconds)	1.8–2
Supraventricular premature complexes (>20/h)(%)	66
Paroxysmal supraventricular tachycardia (%)	13–28
Ventricular premature complexes (>10/h)(%)	32
Ventricular couplets (%)	8–11
Ventricular tachycardia (%)	2–4

Reprinted with permission from the American College of Cardiology (Journal of the American College of Cardiology), 1987; 10:66a.

syncope in elderly people occurs primarily because of decreased cerebral blood flow. Syncope is the first symptom to be manifested for several serious illnesses including

Cerebrovascular atherosclerosis
Calcific aortic stenosis
Obstructive cardiomyopathy
Pulmonary embolism (13%, initial symptom)
Acute volume depletion (bleeding, diuresis, dehydration)
Hypotension (orthostasis, varicose veins, anemia, or hyponatremia)
Autonomic insufficiency (diabetes)
Sick sinus syndrome, tachycardia-bradycardia syndrome
Intraventricular conduction disturbances, supraventricular
Tachyarrhythmias and ventricular tachyarrhythmias

Medications may also precipitate syncope in elderly people. Drugs such as beta-blocking agents, vasodilators, calcium blockers, antihypertensive agents, and lithium all can cause syncope in elderly people when dosage is not carefully adjusted.

Sick Sinus Syndrome Sick sinus syndrome is a collection of abnormalities of the sinoatrial node and atrial function that is classified into three major groups:

1. Persistent, unexplained sinus bradycardia
2. Intermittent or sustained sinus arrest
3. The bradycardia-tachycardia syndrome, characterized by the presence of no. 1 or 2 in association with episodes of paroxysmal atrial tachyarrhythmias.

Many patients with sick sinus syndrome remain asymptomatic. When symptomatic these patients present with (1) conscious disturbances (dizziness, presyncope, or syncope) due to bradyarrhythmias and (2) less commonly palpitation, fatigue, exacerbation of angina or CHF, or sequelae of thromboembolism.

DIAGNOSIS

The ECG is only helpful with the initial evaluation of symptoms of arrhythmias in elderly patients. The ambulatory ECG is used most often in the diagnosis and management of cardiac arrhythmias and unexplained central nervous system symptoms. When ECG data of ambulatory monitoring are evaluated, it is important to keep in mind the findings attributable to the normal aging process. Practitioners should be cautious about always associating syncope with asymptomatic tachyarrhythmias in ambulatory recordings of elderly patients. In patients with heart disease, however, there is a higher diagnostic yield with ambulatory ECG recordings and unexplained syncope, especially with ECG abnormalities at rest such as bradycardia, first-degree AV block, bundle branch block, or an intraventricular conduction defect. Invasive electrophysiologic (EPS) testing is not highly sensitive or specific in sick sinus syndrome and the arrhythmia is rarely reproduced. If a cardiac cause of syncope is likely, then EPS may be useful in diagnosis. It has been found that structural heart disease and a previous MI are predictive of a positive response to EPS testing.

PROGNOSIS

The prognosis of syncope is related to the severity of heart disease. One study found that in patients with cardiovascular syncope, the 1-year mortality was 24%, in patients with noncardiovascular syncope it was 2% to 4%, and in those with syncope of unknown cause it was 3%. In the Framingham study, left bundle branch block was associated with a worse prognosis in subjects with a preexisting ECG abnor-

mality or a superior QRS axis (Markus et al, 1987).

TREATMENT

In severe aortic stenosis, aortic valve replacement frequently cures syncope and increases life expectancy. Drugs used merely to slow the rate of ventricular tachyarrhythmias are often successful in suppressing syncope.

Pacemaker therapy is indicated in patients with syncope or near syncope who have second-degree or complete AV block and those with sick sinus syndrome and documented symptomatic bradycardia. Patients with hypersensitive carotid sinus syndrome with repeated symptoms and whose syndrome is of the cardioinhibitory type are eligible for a pacemaker. In patients who have symptomatic bradycardia with atrial fibrillation, a ventricular demand pacemaker, or one that responds with increasing rate to activity, is indicated. In patients with bradyarrhythmias, there is an increasing trend toward the insertion of a dual-chamber pacemaker (DDD). This pacemaker permits normal AV sequence and a cardiac rate proportionate to activity needs. The normal AV sequence is important in patients with decreased left ventricular compliance and will improve left ventricular filling and thus enhance cardiac output. DDD pacemakers are used primarily for patients who are ambulatory and physically active, whereas ventricular-inhibited pacemakers are generally reserved for patients who have a shorter anticipated life span and who are sedentary or bedridden. The cost of DDD pacemakers is greater and the life of the generator is shorter. Premature ventricular complexes on a single ECG were not predictive of increased risk of death during a 5-year follow-up in a large elderly population (Markus et al, 1987).

There is no evidence that antiarrhythmic drug therapy is useful for treatment of ventricular ectopic activity in an asymptomatic elderly person; in fact, it may be harmful and worsen the arrhythmias. Aspects to consider in the pharmacologic treatment of ventricular arrhythmias include the following:

1. Pharmacokinetics of these drugs differ considerably in older subjects compared with younger subjects. There is a longer elimination half-life, due to decreased rate of renal excretion or hepatic metabolism or both.

2. The elderly person is usually taking other medications that may cause drug interactions. Some common interactions include:

Digoxin and quinidine: increased digoxin levels with concomitant quinidine

Increased digoxin levels occur with amiodarone or verapamil

Cimetidine has been shown to decrease the elimination half-life of both procainamide and quinidine

Phenytoin may increase the metabolism of quinidine

Nifedipine with quinidine may decrease the serum concentrations of quinidine and reduce its antiarrhythmic effect

Increased quinidine plasma concentrations with verapamil due to a decrease in quinidine clearance (Markus et al, 1987)

Increased plasma concentrations of phenytoin and carbamezepine with concomitant use of calcium channel blockers (Bahls et al, 1991)

3. There are dynamic interactions of antiarrhythmic drugs with morphologic or physiologic alterations in the elderly

Sick sinus syndrome may be worsened by most antiarrhythmic drugs

CHF may be precipitated by disopyramide, flecainide, or propafenone, or any sodium-retaining medication

Treatment of ventricular arrhythmias in the elderly is difficult due to lack of data. Anticoagulant therapy for elderly patients with atrial fibrillation in the absence of valvular disease must await results of ongoing trials.

Nursing Diagnosis and Management of High-risk Areas in Daily Living

DAILY LIVING WITH SHORTNESS OF BREATH AND REDUCED STRENGTH AND ENDURANCE

CHF and valvular disease commonly result in shortness of breath and reduced strength and endurance. Not only is the cardiac output changed, but enlargement of the heart and engorgement of the liver cause these organs to occupy more space and restrict breathing. Fluid retention and electrolyte imbalance further compromise tissue perfusion. The resultant symptoms have an impact on most aspects of daily living, such as moving about, carrying objects, maintaining the living environment, eating, sleeping, dressing, bathing, elimination, and social–activities, all can be disrupted—sometimes drastically.

RISK FACTORS

Obviously severity of the pathophysiology is a basic risk factor, breathing and oxygenation may be so compromised as to preclude the effect of other risk factors. The presence of other major pathology, e.g., diabetes, stroke and arthritis, compounds the loss of energy and endurance.

Most elderly persons with altered cardiac function are not in the terminal stages of the disease, so that factors other than, or in addition to, physical status play a role. Risk factors that predict increased difficulty in managing daily living effectively with shortness of breath and cardiac-related fatigue include the following:

- Obesity
- Lack of "body sense." There are those who do not pay attention to the body signals indicating that the end of endurance is close. The result is that they totally exhaust their energy resources and become immobilized for longer periods
- Having responsibilities for the care of others who are dependent
- Extremes of temperature
- Architectural barriers or energy-expensive environment, e.g., living in a second floor apartment or a house where getting to the bathroom, bedroom, or laundry requires stair climbing; storage shelves for commonly used objects are too high or too low; there is lack of a washer or dryer; low, "squashy" chairs make prolonged sitting impossible; hilly terrain in neighborhood; long distances to stores
- Lack of family, friends, and neighbors or primary caregivers able and willing to give predictable, consistent assistance with tasks that are "too much" for the older person
- Lack of ability in the older person either to request or accept help
- Lack of available or usable transportation

SIGNS AND SYMPTOMS

The most common symptoms of ineffective daily living with shortness of breath and lost endurance are complaints such as the following:

Everytime I do *anything* I get exhausted, but I've got no one else to depend on

I get so frustrated with all the things I see that need to be done—it's all going downhill

I can't even pick up the grandchildren any more

I can't bend over to get things out of the bottom cupboards or to tie my shoes, much less take care of my feet

I need help carrying the groceries

I'm going to have to move soon—I just can't manage the stairs anymore

The kids would help, but they're so busy

Nurses may observe signs of changes in the person and the environment. Speech may sound "choppy" as the person breathes in mid-sentence or consistently uses short sentences. Shoes may be loosely tied, untied, or may appear too tight. Clothing may appear tight in the waist and abdominal areas. These persons may be observed to scan a room for places to sit or "hang onto" in any new situation. They may be seen to sit near open areas, "for better air."

In the living situation, trash and papers may be piling up, dust and dirt accumulating, and the bed may go unmade. The individual may be occupying a smaller part of the house than formerly was used.

PROGNOSTIC VARIABLES

Negative prognosis for managing daily living with shortness of breath and associated fatigue is associated with the following:

Premorbid living patterns that did not accommodate to limitations without generating feelings of undue hardship

Inadequate personal assistance and support figures or inadequate finances to purchase services

Lack of understanding of pathology and its relationship to activity, stressors, diet, and medications, as producers of shortness of breath and fatigue

The presence of ongoing infectious processes

COMPLICATIONS

Complications in daily living that may occur if shortness of breath and fatigue are not managed effectively include the following:

Discouragement and depression leading to slow suicide by misuse of medications, sodium consumption, not eating, and self-neglect

Malnutrition secondary to anorexia and the inability to shop for or prepare food

Use of high sodium convenience foods

Sleep deprivation

Inactivity and the complications of immobility

TREATMENT

Nursing treatment involves addressing a variety of areas in daily living. It may include the following:

Promoting understanding of the relationship of cardiac function and its treatment to the status of shortness of breath and energy levels being experienced under various circumstances, e.g., activity greater than oxygen supply (Table 23–8), increases in sodium intake, altering medications, or emotional stresses

Negotiating an acceptable schedule for activities and rest periods as well as energy-saving options for participating in activities and events. For example:

Social activities or travel may be avoided because of the effects of diuretics. Learning when to take the diuretic so they can attend activities and events can keep the person more involved. Locate the bathroom in each setting. Take aisle seats on buses or planes

Helping the person to identify the early cues of fatigue and to understand the benefits of resting before exhaustion occurs. Gathering data on how long a period of rest is needed before activity can resume as a basis for planning schedules

Mobilizing acceptable resources to take up the activities the elderly person is unable to satisfactorily accomplish (see Chapter 13, Families of the Elderly)

EVALUATION

Evaluation of the effectiveness of daily living will be associated with patient reports of satisfaction with schedules and activities. The status of the environment will give cues. Respiratory status, status of edema, and electrolyte values will be indicators as to whether the daily living is contributing to a positive health status.

TABLE 23–8   *Metabolic Units Table*

1 to 2 Metabolic Tasks	*2 to 3 Metabolic Tasks*
Activities of Daily Life	**Activities of Daily Life**
1. Sleeping	1. Dressing and undressing
2. Bed rest	2. Sitting in a chair
3. Lying quietly	3. Standing quietly
4. Feeding oneself in bed	4. Walking to the bathroom
5. Brushing one's teeth	5. Bathing in the bath tub
6. Washing the upper body while supported	
7. Shaving	**Work around Home**
8. Combing one's hair	1. Walking around the house
9. Washing one's hair	2. Pushing or propulsion of a wheelchair
10. Sitting on the edge of the bed	3. Fixing breakfast or lunch
11. Washing the entire body at the bedside	4. Machine washing and drying
12. Bedside commode use after transfer	5. Folding clothes
	6. Machine sewing
	7. Riding in a car
Work around Home	8. Driving a car
1. Conversation	
2. Use of light hand tools	**Occupation**
3. Hand sewing	1. Light desk work
	2. Typing
Occupation	3. Light repair work
1. Paperwork	
	Recreation
Recreation	1. Wood carving
1. Reading in a chair	2. Metal work
2. Picture painting	3. Weaving
3. Leather punching	4. Leather carving
4. Belt making	5. Piano playing
5. Rug hooking	6. Using small power tools
6. Knitting	7. Horseshoes
7. Embroidery	8. Pool
8. Card games	9. Golfing—riding a power cart
9. Walking 1 mph	10. Bicycling 5 mph

(Continued)

TABLE 23–8 *(Continued)*

3 to 4 Metabolic Tasks	4 to 5 Metabolic Tasks
Activities of Daily Life	Activities of Daily Life
1. Showering, standing	1. Use of a bed pan
Work around Home	Work around Home
1. Bending and stooping	1. Carrying light objects
2. Making a bed	2. Changing a bed
3. Fixing dinner	3. Grocery shopping
4. Washing dishes	4. Vacuum cleaning
5. Cleaning around the kitchen	5. Mopping
6. Dusting	6. Hanging out the wash
7. Sweeping the floors	7. Lifting 0–25 pounds
8. Window cleaning	8. Weeding
9. Washing clothes by hand	9. Mowing, using a power, push mower
10. Ironing clothes	10. Using a wheelbarrow
11. Planting	
12. Mowing, using a power, riding mower	Occupation
	1. Light manual work
Occupation	2. Driving a vehicle
1. Office work	3. Auto repair
	4. House painting
Recreation	
1. Sexual activity	Recreation
2. Riding a motor bike or motorcycle	1. Ping pong
3. Hammering	2. Fishing
4. Shuffleboard	3. Bowling
5. Badminton	4. Archery
6. Golfing, walking with a pull cart	5. Golfing, walking and carrying the clubs
7. Walking 3 mph	6. Dancing
8. Bicycling 7.5 mph	7. Walking 4 mph

1 MET (metabolic unit) = 3.5 mL O^2/min/kg of body weight (3 to 4 METs is the energy requirement for most activities of daily living. 5 METs is the completion of the low-level Bruce Treadmill Protocol).
From Hall LK, et al. Cardiac rehabilitation: exercise testing and prescription. New York: Spectrum Publications, 1984; with permission.

DAILY LIVING WITH THE ANOREXIA OF CHRONIC HEART FAILURE AND ITS TREATMENT

Chronic CHF and its treatment affect appetite and digestion in several ways. Failure of the heart as an effective pump and the associated hemodynamics result in an enlarged heart size and engorgement of the liver; these in turn encroach on stomach space. The dyspnea and fatigue can make shopping, food preparation, and even eating difficult. Decreased blood flow to the gastrointestinal tract interferes with digestion and absorption.

Treatment also affects appetite and comfort with food. Obese cardiac patients are urged to restrict caloric intake. Sodium is restricted, so that those accustomed to salt use and high sodium foods find meals unpalatable. Some medications result in a queasy feeling. If they are taken before meals there is less incentive to eat; after meals they make patients wish they had not eaten.

RISK FACTORS

Certain factors will increase the problems experienced with food and eating. These include the following:

Hepatic engorgement and enlarged heart
Dyspnea and decreased energy for eating
Persistent electrolyte imbalances
Therapy with medications such as bronchodilators (Theo-dur); diuretics, which have resultant hyponatremia; and potassium supplements, which cause resultant gastric burning
Restricted income and an inability to buy appetizing foods
Restricted capacity and need for assistance for shopping or preparing appetizing meals
Lack of motivation to maintain a positive eating pattern due to loneliness, fear, or despair
Obesity and the mandate to lose weight

In many situations multiple risk factors are present.

SIGNS AND SYMPTOMS

Lack of enjoyment in eating and inadequate nutrition are evidenced by comments the person makes and by increasing abnormal electrolyte values, edema, and exacerbation of symptoms.

The nurse may hear comments such as the following:

Nothing tastes good. The food is so bland without salt.
I just don't feel like cooking anymore. My wife always did all the cooking.
If I cook the kitchen's a mess.
Coffee and toast fill me up.
Those pills always make me . . . (queasy, burpy, feel a burning sensation, constipated, loose in the bowels, and so forth). They make the food taste terrible.
I hate to eat alone.
I don't have the energy to go to the store. I can't carry the bag up the stairs into the house (apartment).

When patients make no comments, nurses can raise questions about shopping, meal preparation, how mealtimes are managed, and the amount of pleasure or satisfaction derived from meals. A diary of what foods are eaten and related problems recorded for several days may yield a data base for diagnosis and treatment.

PROGNOSIS

Managing eating with the side effects of CHF can be predicted on the basis of the person's

Capacity and external resources for purchasing and preparing meals
Understanding and acceptance of diet as an important factor in health status and relative well-being
Companionship at meals if this has been a previous pattern
Desire to live
Severity of disease

COMPLICATIONS

Failure to incorporate appropriate eating into daily living with CHF can produce a downward spiral in which not eating results in even lessened hunger, leading to malnutrition, growing weakness, infections, and growing cardiac and serum chemistry imbalances.

TREATMENT

Helping older persons and those who participate in their care to maintain some degree of good nutrition and pleasure in mealtime with the problem of anorexia is based on specific data from the situation.

Any deficits in the ability to purchase, obtain, and prepare food need to be matched with acceptable, consistently available alternatives (e.g., food stamps, Meals on Wheels, and relatives, friends, and neighbors who could prepare a number of meals to be frozen, stored, and reheated.

Loneliness at meals might be alleviated by planning for shared meals on several occasions per week, and use of diversion, e.g., TV, reading, and radio during meals.

Where eating patterns reflect lack of knowledge, appropriate teaching supported by pamphlets or tapes can be used together with follow-up using food diaries.

Where energy for eating is low and digestion is disrupted, sample menus of easily eaten and digested foods may help.

Where a spouse or housemate is preparing food that is consistently rejected, the nurse may need to deal with their discouragement, anger, or guilt. The caregiver's feelings need an outlet or the situation can have negative consequences for both caregiver and recipient.

EVALUATION

Areas for evaluating patient response to nursing intervention are reported satisfaction with meals, adequacy of assistance in obtaining and preparing food, patterns of shared meals or other strategies to reduce loneliness at mealtimes, serum chemistries that are not increasingly abnormal, and the responses of the person who has been preparing the meals.

DAILY LIVING WITH CHEST PAIN (ANGINA)

The presence of pain related to coronary insufficiency can produce not only discomfort but also a level of anxiety that is even greater than that seen in patients with shortness of breath. It is seen as an ominous sign, a threat to life. Since it is most frequently brought on by physical activity or emotional stressors, it influences what elderly persons can or will do and what they can allow themselves to experience. For some individuals it becomes an overriding controller of their daily living.

RISK FACTORS

Those who are at greater risk of not managing daily living well in the presence or threat of angina include older persons who:

Enjoy physical activity, recreation, and hobbies

Have responsibility for the care of others

Are exposed to emotionally stressful situations, have a high basic level of anxiety themselves, or have spouses or housemates who are frightened and anxious about the threat angina presents

Have limited access to competent emergency care

Live alone

Have had uncontrolled angina episodes or previous MIs with cardiac arrests

Have little understanding of the pathology of angina and its relationship to activity and stressors

Live with escalating numbers of episodes and amount of discomfort

Lack of understanding about the use of antianginal medications, i.e., nitroglycerin preparations

SIGNS AND SYMPTOMS

Ineffective management of daily living with angina is reflected in comments and complaints of the inability to engage in desired or needed activities:

I can't do . . . anymore. I don't dare to try to . . . anymore.

The reverse symptom may also present when the elderly person reports engaging in activities despite the angina produced. There are varying patterns of nitroglycerine use—either overuse or reluctance to use it appropriately (*e.g.*, before activity, early in the angina, or repeating a dose when needed).

Some elderly people are quite able to monitor and understand the implications of their chest pain, calling on their physicians, emergency support vehicles, or emergency rooms at appropriate times. Others may either overuse or underuse medical and emergency care. Some fail to seek medical assistance when infarction occurs, either because of not knowing the difference between symptoms of angina, temporary ischemia and the syndrome of symptoms indicating infarction, or because of fear of what that diagnosis represents.

Housemates, family members, and primary

caregivers also present signs and symptoms indicating ineffective living with an older person who has angina. They may express high levels of fear or carry an aura of high anxiety. They may avoid learning cardiopulmonary resuscitation or the appropriate actions to take in cardiac emergencies. They may be calling for medical support with every episode of angina. Some may discontinue having any life of their own, fearing to leave their partner alone. A few may try to deny the existence of angina and urge the person with cardiac disease to engage in inappropriate activities. Whether frightened or too casual, whether overprotective or too demanding, the emotional status and behavior of a person sharing living space or major blocks of time with the older person with coronary insufficiency can significantly affect that person's daily living.

PROGNOSTIC VARIABLES

Beyond the status of coronary insufficiency, variables indicating the likelihood of managing daily living with chest pain involve both the person with the angina and those closest to them. These variables include the following:

Understanding of the nature and causes of angina and the range of interventions available
Willingness to use the available actions, behavior, and medications and personal support systems for assistance with activities of daily living
Past patterns of accommodating to alterations in lifestyle
Attitude toward death

COMPLICATIONS

Overcautiousness in structuring life to minimize angina and preoccupation with cardiac status can create the "cardiac cripple." Patients who overuse medical and emergency services risk losing credibility in addition to generating health care costs for themselves and others. Failure to seek help appropriately can result in delayed treatment of an infarction, leading to greater morbidity and possibly a premature death.

TREATMENT

Treatment in helping the elderly person to manage daily living with chest pain is directed to the patient and spouse or those who share the person's life most closely. It involves the following:

Helping each person involved to understand what the cardiac changes represent and the available strategies for best managing the chest pain
Working through *acceptable* activities and behaviors that each party will agree to integrate into daily living related to the cardiac pathology, its symptoms, and crisis management
Helping those involved to learn how to discriminate between angina attacks and the onset of an infarction
Giving emotional support as needed to both patient and primary caregivers (legitimizing fears and anxieties, helping them to locate a personal sounding board and helpful support figure with whom to share ongoing experiences and their reactions)

EVALUATION

The effects of nursing intervention can be judged in terms of the following:

Patterns and appropriateness of use of medical and nursing care to manage cardiac symptoms and problems in daily living
The degree of control the person has over pain and the ability to live a preferred lifestyle
The degree of satisfaction that the patient and partner are having in daily living

DAILY LIVING WITH THE INCREASED RISK OF SYNCOPE OR THE RISK OF DIZZINESS AND WEAKNESS

Presyncope encompasses feelings of dizziness, impending doom, heart rate and rhythm irregularities, nausea, and near loss of consciousness. Often the description is one of a combination of vague physiologic changes as well as fear of something happening out of control.

RISK FACTORS

The severity of the syncopal episode depends on the person's environment, i.e., bedridden, active, or living independently. It also depends on frequency of occurrence and accompanying symptoms. If the syncope is incapacitating, frequent, or limits function, the living situation will have to be adapted. Risk factors that would indicate this change are

Continuation of syncopal attacks
Degree of change in consciousness
Interference with quality of life

SIGNS AND SYMPTOMS

The signs and symptoms of syncope are important to elicit in order for medical and nursing interventions to be effective in decreasing and hopefully eliminating the attacks. Elderly people frequently present with syncope as an initial symptom described as "dizziness, about to faint or blackout." Accompanying symptoms may include nausea ("sick to my stomach") or palpitations ("heart fluttering in chest or skipping beats or weak pulse"). These descriptions enable the practitioner to direct the diagnosis of the syncope.

PROGNOSIS

If the person is willing to comply with medical diagnostic techniques, i.e., electroencephalography, ECG, ambulatory ECG monitoring, exercise tolerance test, and EPS, treatment can usually be implemented to eliminate the syncope. However, there are those who cannot tolerate the appropriate medications, such as antiarrhythmics. Pacemaker implantation may be too high of a risk in some older patients. In such cases living with the syncope is the only option. Also there are those who cannot give an adequate history due to confusion so that the diagnosis cannot be determined for appropriate medical treatment.

COMPLICATIONS

Complications of syncope include the following:

Complete loss of consciousness and lethal arrhythmias
Falls, causing neuromusculoskeletal injuries
Severe reduction in activity, causing the consequences of inactivity and immobility

TREATMENT

Nurses play a key role in the identification of signs and symptoms to diagnose the problem, monitoring of the medical treatment, and doing the patient education. Nurses often help patients describe their symptoms in relation to their daily life, i.e., activity or inactivity and meals or medication use or omission.

Nurses assist in ensuring that the elderly patient comprehends as much as possible about the physical problem, diagnostic tests, and prescribed treatments, i.e., medications or pacemaker. Timing of medication dosages is extremely important with antiarrhythmics, and adjusting these to an individual's lifestyle is often necessary for compliance. If a pacemaker has been implanted, appointments by phone or in person must be kept to ensure proper function. In addition, the nurse may be instrumental in helping the person adjust to living with the syncopal episodes when no medical treatments are deemed appropriate or effective. This may involve identifying the syncope in a noncommunicating patient and adapting and setting mobility limits for safety, and providing for a safe environment by making necessary changes in the home or providing support systems.

EVALUATION

Continuing to evaluate function based on a history of syncopal attacks is a nursing function, particularly in a long-term care facility. Nurses may also assist elderly patients in evaluating themselves for future attacks. Whether they have to deal with treatment for syncope or accept that there is no treatment, syncope is frightening for patients and those close to them.

DAILY LIVING WITH ALTERED HEALTH MAINTENANCE RELATED TO THE NUMBER OF CORONARY RISK FACTORS NEEDING REDUCTION

RISK FACTORS

As elderly persons are told to reduce risk factors for heart disease they feel years of a stable lifestyle pattern are threatened. The disruption of life patterns in the elderly patient is directly correlated with the number of cardiac risk factors in need of reduction. The threat of several lifestyle changes places the elderly person in a state of disequilibrium that, depending on the medical and psychological history, can cause only further chaos.

SIGNS AND SYMPTOMS

The signs and symptoms of disruptive altered health maintenance include:

Giving up
Anger

Depression
Blaming others
Disorientation

Telling elderly persons with smoking, eating, inactivity, and stress reaction patterns built up over 40 to 50 years that they need to change the way they live can be both difficult and futile. Many younger people cannot handle the overwhelming mandate to change their lifestyle. The elderly are often more symptomatic and have pressure from others to reduce and change lifestyle patterns and perhaps pleasures. Substitutes for previous patterns may not be as available:

Decreasing fat in diet has few immediate rewards
Smoking addiction may have no substitute other than eating
Weight loss is more difficult as age increases
Exercise may be painful, if alternative modes are not recommended

PROGNOSIS

If the elderly patient cannot reduce cardiac risk factors, the risk for increased chronic disability from cardiac disease exists. Elderly patients, however, are not destined to develop cardiovascular disease due to the aging process alone; but cardiac risk factor reduction is still important in the elderly. Risk factors for CHD are usually highly prevalent in elderly people. Smoking normally tends to decline in the elderly (Kannel et al, 1987). Data from the Framingham study and other epidemiologic studies indicate that most risk factors continue to contribute to the incidence of CHD in older persons.

COMPLICATIONS

The complications of overwhelming the elderly patient with changes in lifestyle have devastating effects on both mental stability as well as overall quality of life.

TREATMENT

Several suggestions for dealing with elderly people needing risk factor modification are mentioned. When using behavior modification in the elderly, the nurse must keep in mind that the same rewards for achievement used in younger patients may not work with elderly patients. Ideas for working with the older adult when helping them to reduce cardiac risk factors are listed:

Go slow
Select one risk factor at a time to work on
Set goals with them that they can attain
Reward small steps of improvement
Educate and enlist help of spouse, children, and friends
Find out what is most important to them (i.e., to play some golf, lose 5 pounds, attend family and friend gatherings, feel better) and assess what that means

EVALUATION

Evaluation is difficult for the cardiac rehabilitation practitioner working with elderly because the rewards are small and the same references for success in cardiac rehabilitation do not always apply. Elderly people cannot use an increased training heart rate as an indication of success with exercise and they may not progress to higher levels of exercise. Weight loss is probably one of the biggest problems for elderly in cardiac rehabilitation. The older adult may have been successful in quitting smoking, setting a regular exercise program, lowering blood pressure, relaxing to decrease stress, but eating often remains "the one joy I have left." Some have had alcoholic problems in the past that they have conquered, but eating what they want is difficult to give up. Strategies for dealing with this are not readily available. Sometimes role models help, particularly people their own age who have lost weight. However, it is difficult for them and for practitioners. Concentrating on other successes must be encouraged. The elderly cardiac rehabilitation patient population will only increase over time and practitioners must continue to find new and innovative ways to help this group achieve cardiac risk factor reduction.

There is an increasing amount of empirical evidence on circadian rhythms and their influence on cardiac pathology and drug management. There are differences in circadian rhythms in the time of day as well as in seasons on factors such as blood pressure, pharmacodynamics of drugs, laboratory values, thrombolic stroke, myocardial infarction, and sudden cardiac death. Each factor has its own rhythm. The references under Circadian Rhythms discuss the details.

References and Other Readings

American College of Sports Medicine. Guidelines for exercise testing and prescription, 4th ed. Philadelphia: Lea & Febiger, 1991:183.

Bahls F, Ozuna J, Ritchie D. Interactions between calcium channel blockers, carbamazepine, phenytoin: a retrospective analysis of 43 patients. Neurology 1991; 41:740.

Balady GJ, Weiner DA. Exercise testing in healthy elderly subjects and elderly patients with cardiac disease. J Cardiopulmonary Rehabil 1989; 9:35.

Beckman B, et al. Predicting hospital readmission of elderly cardiac patients. National Association of Social Workers Inc., 1987:221.

Borg AV. Perceived exertion: a note on "history" and methods. Medicine and Science in Sports 1973; 5:90.

Braunwald E. Clinical manifestations of heart failure. In: Braunwald E, ed. Heart disease, 3rd ed. Philadelphia, JB Lippincott, 1988.

Bruce RA, Larson EB, Stratton J. Physical fitness, functional aerobic capacity, aging and responses to physical training or bypass surgery in coronary patients. J Cardiopulmonary Rehabil 1989;9:24.

Buckley MJ, et al. Cardiac surgery and noncardiac surgery in elderly patients with heart disease. JACC 1987; 10:35A.

Burrows B, Alpert JS, Ross JC. Pulmonary heart disease. JACC 1987; 10:63A.

Dajani AS, et al. Prevention of bacterial endocarditis: recommendations by the American Heart Association. JAMA 1990; 264:2919.

Emery CF, Pinder SL, Blumenthal JA. Psychological effects of exercise among elderly cardiac patients. J Cardiopulmonary Rehabil 1989; 9:46.

Fleg JL, Gerstenblith G, Lakatta, EG. Pathophysiology of the aging heart and circulation. In: Messerli FH, ed. Cardiovascular disease in the elderly, 2nd ed. Boston: Martinus Nijhoff, 1988: 17.

Frishman WH, DeMaria AN, Ewy GA. Clinical assessment. JACC 1987; 10:48A.

Gentry WD, Aronson MK, Blumenthal J, et al. Behavioral, cognitive and emotional considerations. JACC 1987; 10:38A.

Gerber RM. Coronary artery disease in the elderly. J Cardiovasc Nurs 1990; 4:23.

Gortner SR, Rankin SH, Murphy-Wolfe M. Elders' recovery from cardiac surgery. Progress in Cardiovascular Nursing 1988; 3:54.

Hall LK, et al. Cardiac rehabilitation exercise testing and prescription. New York: Spectrum Publications, 1984.

Harris R. Exercise and physical fitness for the elderly. In: Reichel W, ed. Clinical aspects of aging, 3rd ed. Baltimore: Williams & Wilkins, 1989:86.

Herd JA, et al. Medical therapy in the elderly. JACC 1987; 10:29A.

Hurst JW. The physician's approach to the patient: goals and cardiac appraisal. In: Hurst JW, ed. The heart, 7th ed. New York: McGraw-Hill, 1990:115.

Imperial ES, et al. Graded exercise testing protocol for the elderly. J Cardiopulmonary Rehabil 1990; 10:465.

Jessup M, Lakatta EG, Leier C, et al. CHF in the elderly: is it different? Patient Care 1990; March 15:39.

Kane RL, Ouslander JG, Abrass IB. Essentials of clinical geriatrics, 2nd ed. New York: McGraw-Hill Information Services, 1989.

Kannel WB, et al. Prevention of cardiovascular disease in the elderly. JACC 1987; 10:25A.

Lakatta EG, et al. Human aging: changes in structure and function. JACC 1987; 10:42A.

Larson EB, Bruce RA. Health benefits of exercise in an aging society. Arch Intern Med 1987; 147:3.

Laurent-Bopp D. Heart failure: In: Patrick M, et al, eds. Medical surgical nursing: pathophysiological concepts, 2nd ed. Philadelphia: JB Lippincott, 1991.

Levine BS, Underhill SL. Valvular heart dysfunction. In: Patrick M, et al, eds. Medical surgical nursing: pathophysiological concepts, 2nd ed. Philadelphia: JB Lippincott, 1991:776.

Levy WC, et al. Supine, stroke volume, and cardiac dilatation in elderly. J Nucl Med 1990; 5:838.

Markus FI, Ruskin JN, Surawicz B. Arrhythmias. JACC 1987; 10:66A.

Messerli FH, ed. Cardiovascular disease in the elderly, 2nd ed. Boston: Martinus Nijhoff, 1988.

Nickel JT, Chirikos TN. Functional disability of elderly patients with long-term coronary heart disease: a sex-stratified analysis. Journal of Gerontology 1990; 45:S60.

Opie LH. Drugs for the heart, 3rd ed. Philadelphia: WB Saunders, 1991.

O'Rourke RA, Catterjee K, Wei JY. Coronary heart disease. JACC 1987; 10:52A.

Pollock ML, Wilmore JH. Exercise in health and disease, 2nd ed. Philadelphia: WB Saunders, 1990:128.

Posner JD, Gorman KM, Klein HS, et al. Exercise capacity in the elderly. Am J Cardiol 1986; 57:52C.

Rahimtoola SH, Cheitlin MD, Hutter AM. Valvular and congenital heart disease. JACC 1987; 10:60A.

Rocci ML, Vlassis PH, Abrams WB. Geriatric clinical pharmacology. Geriatric Cardiology 1986; 4:54.

Schulman SP, Gerstenblith G. Cardiovascular changes with aging: the response to exercise. J Cardiopulmonary Rehabil 1989; 9:12.

Shephard RJ. Habitual physical activity levels and

perception of exercise in the elderly. J Cardiopulmonary Rehabil 1989; 9:17.

Tedesco C, et al. Functional assessment of elderly patients after percutaneous aortic balloon valvuloplasty: New York Heart Association classification versus functional status questionnaire. Heart Lung 1990; 19:118.

Vetter NJ, Ford D. Smoking prevention among people aged 60 and over: a randomized controlled trial. Age Aging 1990; 19:164.

Wei JY. Use of calcium entry blockers in elderly patients: special considerations. Circulation 1989; 80(suppl IV); IV–171.

Weisfeldt ML, Lakatta EG, Gerstenblith G. Aging and cardiac disease. In: Braunwald E, ed. Heart disease: a textbook of cardiovascular medicine, 3rd ed. Philadelphia: WB Saunders, 1988:1650.

Weisfeldt ML, Gerstenblith G. Cardiovascular aging and adaptation to disease. In: Hurst JW, ed. The heart, 7th ed. New York: McGraw-Hill, 1990: 1488.

Wenger NK, Marcus FI, O'Rourke RA. Cardiovascular disease in the elderly. JACC 1987; 9:80A.

Wenger NK. Exercise for the elderly: highlights of preventive and therapeutic aspects. J Cardiopulmonary Rehabil 1989; 9:9.

Wenger NK, Franciosa JA, Weber KT. Heart failure. JACC 1987; 10:73A.

Wild LR, Craven RF, Cunningham SL. Assessment of vascular function and nursing strategies for common vascular problems. In: Patrick M, et al, eds. Medical surgical nursing: pathophysiological concepts, 2nd ed. Philadelphia, JB Lippincott, 1991:802.

Williams MA, et al. Early exercise training in patients older than age 65 years compared with that in younger patients after acute myocardial infarction or coronary artery bypass grafting. Am J Cardiol 1985; 55:263.

Williams MA, Sketch MH. Guidelines for exercise training of elderly patients following myocardial infarction and coronary bypass graft surgery. Geriatric Cardiovascular Medicine 1988; 1:107.

Wolfel EE, Hossack KF. Guidelines for the exercise training of elderly healthy individuals and elderly patients with cardiac disease. J Cardiopulmonary Rehabil 1989; 9:40.

Woods SL, Underhill SL. Myocardial ischemia and infarction. In: Underhill SL, Woods SL, Sivarajan ES, et al, eds. Cardiac nursing, 2nd ed. Philadelphia: JB Lippincott, 1989; 488.

CIRCADIAN RHYTHMS

Arendt J, Minors DS, Waterhouse JM. Biological rhythms in clinical practice. Boston: Butterworth & Co. Ltd., 1989.

Floras JS. Antihypertensive treatment, myocardial infarction and nocturnal myocardial ischaemia. Lancet 1988; 2:994.

Hjalmarson A, Gilpin EA, Nicod P, et al. Differing circadian patterns of symptom onset in subgroups of patients with acute myocardial infarction. Circulation 1989; 80:267.

Lucente M, Rebuzzi AG, Lanza GA, et al. Circadian variation of ventricular tachycardia in acute myocardial infarction. Am J Cardiol 1988; 62:670.

Muller JE, Lunder PL, Willich SN, et al. Circadian variation in the frequency of sudden cardiac death. Circulation 1987; 1:131.

Muller JE, Stone PH, Turi ZG, et al. Circadian variation in the onset of acute myocardial infarction. N Engl J Med 1985; 313:1315.

Peters RW, Muller JE, Goldstein S, et al. Propranolol and the circadian variation in the frequency of sudden cardiac death: the BHAT experience. Circulation 1988; 76(suppl IV):364.

Peters RW, Muller JE, Goldstein S, et al. Propranolol and the morning increase in the frequency of sudden cardiac death (BHAT Study). Am J Cardiol 1989; 63:1518.

Pickering G. Diurnal variations in cardiovascular morbidity. Ambulatory monitoring and blood pressure variability. London: Science Press, 1991.

Rocco MB, Barry J, Campbell S, et al. Circadian variation of transient myocardial ischaemia in patients with coronary artery disease. Circulation 1987; 75:395.

Twidale N, Taylor S, Heddie WF, et al. Morning increase in the time of onset of sustained ventricular tachycardia. Am J Cardiol 1989; 64:1204.

Willich SN, Levy D, Rocco MB, et al. Circadian variation in the incidence of sudden cardiac death in the Framingham Heart Study population. Am J Cardiol 1987; 60:801.

Willich SN, Linderer T, Wegscheider K, et al. Increased risk of myocardial infarction in the morning (abstract). J Am Col Cardiol 1988; 11:28A.

Willich SN, Pohjola-Sintonen S, Bhatia SJS, et al. Suppression of silent ischaemia by metoprolol without alteration of morning increase of platelet aggregability in patients with stable coronary artery disease. Circulation 1989; 79:557.

24
Diabetes Mellitus

CAROL A. BLAINEY   SHARON FILIPCIC

Diabetes mellitus can be defined as a genetically and clinically heterogeneous group of disorders characterized by glucose intolerance, with hyperglycemia present at the time of diagnosis. It is known that patients with diabetes have a higher risk of chronic microvascular, macrovascular and neurologic disorders, and it is widely assumed that chronic hyperglycemia is contributory to the development of these complications (Guthrie, 1988).

In the fall of 1990, the nation's Disease Control Center in Atlanta, Georgia released new statistics indicating that 14 million Americans have diabetes, half of whom are not as yet diagnosed. Approximately 700,000 cases of diabetes are diagnosed each year and diabetes causes more than 12,000 cases of new blindness in adults each year (American Diabetes Association WA NEWS, 1991).

In the strict sense diabetes mellitus is a syndrome rather than a disease because there are no clear-cut definable pathogeneses, etiologic factors, consistent clinical findings, or laboratory tests. In 1979, the National Diabetes Data Group established the currently accepted classifications of diabetes (Table 24–1). Of the seven classifications of diabetes, insulin-dependent diabetes mellitus (IDDM) and non–insulin-dependent diabetes (NIDDM) represent the majority of cases. About 20% of the cases are IDDM and approximately 70% to 80% of the cases are NIDDM. The abnormalities

of insufficient insulin production and/or aberrant use of insulin result in alterations in the metabolism of carbohydrates, proteins, and fats.

Blood glucose levels are age-related, with a gradual increase occurring with increasing age. Fasting blood sugar levels increase by 1 to 2 mg/dL per decade after age 30. Blood glucose levels 1 hour after glucose loading have been reported to increase by 6 to 14 mg/100 dL per decade. The variation is due to differences in results, a reflection of investigators using a variety of test doses of glucose and conditions (Jackson, 1990).

Pathophysiology and Medical Management

ETIOLOGIC FACTORS

Causes of diabetes have not been completely established at this time. Components of etiology include (1) genetic transmission, (2) environmental factors such as virus and lifestyles, and (3) autoimmune responses.

ETIOLOGY OF IDDM

The etiology of IDDM is thought to be a triad of genetic susceptibility, viral attack, and autoimmune responses. Specific genes of the chromosomes have been associated with IDDM.

452

TABLE 24–1 *Classification of Diabetes Mellitus and Other Categories of Glucose Intolerance*

Current Names	Previous Names	Clinical Characteristics
Insulin-dependent diabetes mellitus (IDDM), type I	Juvenile diabetes (JD), juvenile-onset diabetes (JOD), ketosis-prone diabetes, brittle diabetes	Little or no endogenous insulin: requires exogenous insulin for survival. Onset at any age, usually at young age (<25). Causes believed to be genetic, environmental, or acquired, probably involving abnormal immune responses
Noninsulin-dependent diabetes mellitus (NIDDM), type II	Adult-onset diabetes (AOD), maturity-onset diabetes (MOD), ketosis-resistant diabetes, stable diabetes, maturity-onset diabetes of the young (MODY)	Rarely develop ketosis except during infections or severe stress. Produce varying amounts of endogenous insulin, occasionally require exogenous insulin. Most are obese and over 40 years of age at onset. Cause thought to be genetic coupled with environmental factors
Diabetes mellitus associated with other conditions or syndromes	Secondary diabetes	Accompanied by conditions known or thought to cause diabetes mellitus: pancreatic or hormonal disease, drugs or chemical toxicity, abnormal insulin receptors, or certain genetic syndromes
Impaired glucose tolerance (IGT) Nonobese Obese	Asymptomatic diabetes, chemical diabetes, subclinical diabetes, borderline diabetes, latent diabetes	Glucose levels are between normal and diabetic levels. Increased susceptibility to atherosclerotic disease
Gestational diabetes (GDM)	Gestational diabetes	Women whose diabetes begins or is noted during pregnancy
Previous abnormality of glucose intolerance (PrevAGT)	Latent diabetes, prediabetes	Past history of elevated blood glucose, now have normal levels
Potential abnormality of glucose intolerance (PotAGT)	Potential diabetes, prediabetes	Never had glucose intolerance but considered at high risk due to several reasons, including relatives with diabetes, mothers of babies who weigh more than 9 lb at birth, obesity

Adapted from Medical World News, pp 52–53, October 29, 1979.

These genes (HLA antigens) are part of the major histocompatibility complex and act to aid in the regulation of the body's immune responsiveness. Ninety percent of people with IDDM in western countries have been found to have one or both of the genes associated with IDDM, DR3 or DR4 (Madsbad, 1990).

Islet cell autoantibodies have been found at the time of diagnosis of IDDM in 90% of the cases (Madsbad, 1990). This finding indicates that an autoimmune response is present and may be responsible for the destruction of the beta cells, resulting in the inability to produce insulin. Few individuals over 65 years of age develop IDDM and individuals who have IDDM have a shortened life expectancy. Therefore, the majority of elderly individuals have NIDDM.

ETIOLOGY OF NIDDM

The etiology of NIDDM differs from that of IDDM. The elements of causation are thought to be a combination of insulin insensitivity and insufficient production of insulin. With time there seems to be a progressive decline in the production of insulin. The genetic transmission of NIDDM is unclear, certainly there is a strong evidence to support the recurring presence of NIDDM in families; however, whether that is related to obesity, eating habits, or a NIDDM gene is not known. If standards of carbohydrate tolerance that are usually achieved by young healthy adults are applied to the elderly, the prevalence of abnormal glucose tolerance is greater than 60% for adults greater than 60 years of age (Porte and Kahn, 1990). It is imperative that practitioners differentiate changes in metabolism that occur with normal aging and changes in metabolism that are related to NIDDM. Onset of NIDDM can be insidious and noted only serendipitously when blood glucose level is measured in a routine examination or the onset may seem abrupt when stress from some event, such as cerebrovascular accident, stroke, infection, or medication, causes a transient major elevation in blood glucose level.

HIGH-RISK POPULATION OR SITUATIONS

Advanced age is in itself a risk factor for the development of NIDDM. Over 40% of individuals aged 65 to 74 and 50% of individuals aged 80 to 89 have either impaired glucose tolerance or diabetes mellitus (Minaker, 1990). *Obesity*, (body mass index ≥ 27 kg/m^2 in men and ≥ 25 kg/m^2 in women) and *central obesity* (waist-hip ratio ≥ 0.98 in men and ≥ 0.89 in women) doubled the prevalence of impaired glucose tolerance or NIDDM (Mykkanen et al, 1990). Obesity, a sedentary lifestyle, and relatives who have diabetes all contribute to increasing the likelihood of an individual developing NIDDM.

DYNAMICS

Maintenance of adequate glucose levels in blood flow to the brain is a prerequisite of life. Throughout the life of a normal healthy individual the extracellular glucose concentration is confined within narrow limits. The fasting blood glucose level is normally between 70 and 100 mg/100 mL plasma and in normal young adults never exceeds 150 mg/100 mL plasma even after a large carbohydrate meal. Blood glucose levels measured after eating or after a glucose challenge must be adjusted for the elderly. Table 24–2 depicts the criteria for age-adjusted

TABLE 24–2   *Criteria for Age-adjusted Oral Glucose Tolerance*

Age	Fasting	1 hr	2 hr	Summary OGTT/2 hr
50–60	116	203	195	514*
60–70	118	209	205	532*
70–80	120	215	215	550*

*Values above these levels would be considered in the range of abnormal blood glucose.
Adapted from Andres R. Aging and diabetes. Med Clin North Am 1971; 55:835.

oral glucose tolerance tests as determined by Andres (1971).

NORMAL FUNCTION

The regulation of plasma glucose levels is controlled primarily by three organ systems. One is the liver as the producer of glucose in the fasting individual. A second is muscle tissue as the major insulin-sensitive user of glucose in the body. The third is the endocrine pancreas, which produces insulin and glucagon (Porte and Kahn, 1990).

Varying circumstances such as exercise, stress, or high carbohydrate meals work to change the level of glucose in the extracellular fluid. In the normal basal state, the action of glucagon serves to mobilize fuel from cell stores (glycogenolysis), from newly formed glucose from the liver, and from free fatty acids and glycerol from adipose tissue (gluconeogenesis). These processes function to elevate the blood glucose level. Insulin, in contrast to the catabolic function of glucagon, has an anabolic action and serves to store food substrates in muscle, liver, and adipose tissue. The amount of glucose entering the extracellular fluid from the liver is balanced by the amount going to the brain and to the liver, fat, and muscle in the basal state.

Exercise   During exercise the balance between glucagon and insulin changes. Increased secretion of glucagon results in a greater amount of glucose in the extracellular fluid, which in the presence of insulin, is taken up by muscle to meet the increased need.

Food A high carbohydrate meal resulting in increased exogenous glucose causes the extracellular glucose level to increase, glucagon secretion ceases, and insulin secretion increases to cause the storage of excess food substrates in liver, muscle, and fat tissue.

Stress Situations of either physical or psychological stress result in the system striving to maintain cerebral glucose levels in circumstances that threaten to decrease blood flow to the brain and muscles. Hence, the extracellular level of glucoses is elevated through the glucagon-insulin balance. The action of glucagon continues to cause the liver to deliver glucose to the extracellular fluid, while insulin secretion decreases, but never ceases, to keep the glucose in the extracellular fluid at an elevated level. Stress situations point out the direct influence that hormones from the anterior pituitary have on blood glucose, specifically, (1) growth hormone, (2) corticotropin, controlling the secretion of some of the adrenocortical hormones, which in turn affect the glucose, proteins, and fats, and (3) thyrotropin, which controls the rate of secretion of thyroxine by the thyroid gland, which determines the rate of most of the chemical reactions in the body. Growth hormone, corticotropin, and thyrotropin act to increase the blood glucose level. Insulin is the only hormone that lowers blood glucose.

Insulin is also secreted in response to an increase in amino acid concentration. Insulin promotes the uptake of amino acids by skeletal muscle, increases protein synthesis, accelerates lipid synthesis, and inhibits lipolysis and gluconeogenesis.

ABNORMAL FUNCTIONING

Insulin-dependent Diabetes Mellitus

In IDDM, symptoms of a lack of insulin secretion usually occurs abruptly. The loss of beta cell secretion of insulin actually occurs over a period of time, but is not manifested until a considerable number of beta cells have been destroyed. When there is insufficient insulin to facilitate the movement of glucose into cells, blood glucose increases. When the blood glucose reaches levels above 180 mg/100 mL, (considered the renal threshold for glucose, which may be elevated in elderly persons), the glucose is spilled out into the urine, taking water and electrolytes with it. In an attempt to meet the cellular needs for glucose for producing energy, the body begins to break down fat and muscle tissue. Adi-

pose tissue breaks down into free fatty acids, resulting in the formation of ketone bodies that, unchecked, produce the medical emergency of ketoacidosis. Breakdown of protein stores increases the plasma concentration of amino acids and speeds gluconeogenesis. In order to survive, people with IDDM require treatment with exogenous insulin.

Noninsulin-dependent Diabetes Mellitus

In NIDDM, essentially the same process as in IDDM occurs but to a lesser extent. The severity of the process is dependent on the degree of insulin insufficiency. The advent of the radioimmunoassay in the 1960s revealed that early in the course of NIDDM, obese people have higher levels of circulating insulin when compared with lean people who do not have diabetes. The insulin lack in NIDDM appears to be a relative deficiency as opposed to the absolute deficiency in IDDM. As time passes there is a decline in the secretion of endogenous insulin so that eventually the person with NIDDM may require exogenous sources of insulin.

Resistance to the effects of available insulin is believed to be responsible for the hyperglycemia of NIDDM, particularly in the obese individual. In NIDDM the hyperglycemia is often noted in a routine examination of blood or during a search for the cause of other problems, such as visual disturbances, slow healing of skin lesions, or urinary or vaginal infections. Often, the person is not symptomatic. Obesity, infection, or other body stresses such as myocardial infarction increase the body's need for insulin to balance the blood sugar, and the beta cells are unable to produce enough insulin to meet the increased demand. In these situations the individual with NIDDM may become symptomatic with polyuria, polyphasia, polydipsia, fatigue, and weight loss.

DIFFERENTIAL DIAGNOSIS

The diagnosis of diabetes mellitus is complicated by disagreement in what constitutes an abnormal blood glucose level. Consideration of blood glucose level must include whether the blood specimen was taken when the person was fasting or had recently eaten a meal. If an oral glucose tolerance test (OGTT) is done to establish diagnosis, the person must undergo 3 days of a 300-mg carbohydrate diet before the OGTT in order to secure a valid test. If the individual has elevated fasting blood glucose levels greater than 140 mg/dL, the OGTT confirms the diagnosis but does not provide any additional information. OGTT is not recommended for the elderly because of difficulties with standardization and there is no evidence that people diagnosed in this manner are at increased risk (Davidson, 1986). Postprandial glucose concentration levels increase with increasing age.

The difficulty in diabetes mellitus in the elderly is not so much one of differentiating it from another condition but rather one of deciding at what point increasing blood glucose is due to diabetes mellitus and not solely the aging process. Caution is warranted when one considers the impact the diagnosis of diabetes may have on individuals. It may be an additional disease added on top of other diseases with which the individual is coping. It may carry stigma to the individual; it may interfere with the right to drive a car; and it may affect health insurance availability and cost. The person may feel guilt for possibly passing on a pathologic condition to descendents and for certain individuals it is seen as a death warrant.

The qualitative diagnostic criteria for diabetes in adults are as follows:

Diabetes Mellitus
1. Unequivocal elevation of plasma glucose (≥ 200 mg/dL) and classic symptoms of diabetes, including polydipsia, polyuria, polyphagia, and weight loss
2. Fasting plasma glucose ≥ 140 mg/dL on two occasions

3. Fasting plasma glucose < 140 mg/dL and 2-hour plasma glucose ≥ 200 mg/dL with one intervening value ≥ 200 mg/dL after a 75-g glucose load OGTT

Impaired Glucose Tolerance
1. Fasting plasma glucose < 140 mg/dL and 2-hour plasma glucose ≥ 140 and < 200 mg/dL with one intervening value ≥ 200 mg/dL after a 75-g glucose load (American Diabetes Association position statement, 1990)

MANIFESTATIONS

The most easily measured manifestation of diabetes is an elevated blood glucose level, either in the fasting or fed state. If the blood glucose is elevated, then urine glucose will also indicate the presence of diabetes. In IDDM other manifestations are often the classic signs of polyuria, polyphagia, polydipsia, weight loss, and fatigue. Occasionally the first manifestations individuals with NIDDM become aware of may be recurrent urinary or vaginal infection or skin wounds that heal slowly.

In the elderly, the classic signs of polyuria, polydipsia, and polyphagia with weight loss are often blunted or ascribed to other causes (Messana and Beizer, 1991). The age-associated decrease in the sense of thirst may result in a lack of the complaint of polydipsia, and the polyuria may be ascribed to mechanical problems with urination, such as decreased control over bladder sphincters or an enlarged prostate.

Relevant baseline data to be established and documented are shown in Table 24–3.

TABLE 24–3 *Baseline Data*

Cardiovascular	Renal Function	Eyes	Skin	Blood Glucose
Fasting cholesterol and triglycerides	Urine culture and sensitivity	Blurring of vision	Breaks in skin	Fasting blood sugar Random blood glucose
ECG	Blood urea nitrogen	Evaluation of presence of cataracts, glaucoma	Callus formation	24-hour urine glucose
Evaluation of pulses bilaterally	Urine protein	Microaneurysms or proliferative retinopathy	Rashes	Glycosylated hemoglobin
Lying and standing blood pressure	Creatinine		Changes in oral mucosa	

PROGNOSIS

The actual death rate from diabetes is difficult to obtain since mortality statistics generally do not specify contributing causes of death. Considering the elderly as a group, diabetes ranked fifth as a cause of death in the age group between 65 and 74. In the age group between 75 and 84 diabetes ranked as the sixth leading cause of death, and in the age group of 85 plus, diabetes was the eighth cause of death (National Center for Health Statistics, 1983).

The most frequent cause of death for people with diabetes is myocardial infarction. Statistics vary greatly in statement of life expectancy for people with diabetes; however, all agree that duration of life is decreased.

Management

There is controversy about the management of the person with diabetes, primarily over "tight" versus "loose" control of the blood glucose level. This controversy can be confusing to patients making decisions about treatment in the face of divergent opinions and changing treatment regimes.

Current medical literature contains opinions supporting both views. The primary argument for tight control is that maintaining blood glucose levels at normal or near normal values may prevent or delay the onset of complications associated with diabetes. The research data are not conclusive. Supporters of tight control argue that time will bear them out and they will have done everything possible to prevent the advent of some complications.

Advocates of loose control propose that the data do not indicate that tight control of blood sugar leads to control of complications, and that it is not possible to justify risking serious hypoglycemia with possible injury and possible decreased intellectual function. In addition, those advocating loose control point out that there is stress associated with stringent dietary stipulations that seriously alter customary lifestyles. Nurses helping people cope with diabetes need to be prepared to assist these individuals in understanding the main points of each view because the client ultimately decides on the management.

For the population over 70 years of age, gains that may be made by tight control are offset by the psychological and physiologic effects of a stringent lifestyle. A grave concern is the potential cardiac stress on an already compromised heart that occurs in hypoglycemia.

The nature of diabetes treatment requires that the individual be well versed in self-management and the final judge as to tight or loose control. Main concerns of the nurse are (1) assessing level of understanding, (2) ascertaining learning readiness, (3) determining learning goals, (4) implementing an effective teaching program, and (5) conducting repeated evaluation of learning. It should be emphasized that the evaluation needs to be based on actual unprompted statements as well as demonstration of required psychomotor skills of self-monitoring of blood glucose, urine testing for ketones, and insulin administration. Additional areas of required education for sound self-management include understanding onset, peak, and duration of oral hypoglycemic agents, recognition and treatment of hypoglycemic reactions, care during illness, care for feet, and dietary guidelines.

MONITORING

BLOOD GLUCOSE TESTING

Technology now provides several methods of measuring blood glucose level. The choice of method depends on what information is sought. Some methods require venous blood specimens analyzed by laboratory personnel and some can be done by nurses and patients.

If one wants to know the current blood glucose level immediately, then a capillary specimen can be tested with one of a variety of blood glucose measuring methods, using either visually read strips or a glucose meter. Most color charts are in the blue to green color range. Individuals who have alterations in their ability to distinguish color due to color blindness or aging usually have difficulty in the blue-green range. It is prudent to determine the individual's ability to accurately distinguish colors. There are glucose meters on the market that require that a drop of capillary blood on a strip is inserted into the meter or a drop of blood is placed directly on a designated spot on the meter and after precise timing a digital readout is displayed. Developing technology is decreasing the amount of interaction with glucose meters and hence decreasing the potential for human error.

Glycosylated Hemoglobin A1$_c$ Long-term control can be measured by a glycosolated hemoglobin, which requires sending a venous blood specimen to the laboratory for analysis. A glycosylated hemoglobin level, normally between 4% and 7%, determines the amount of hemoglobin that has become glycosylated and is a reflection of the average blood glucose level for the past 120 days or the life of a red blood cell (Guthrie, 1988). Fructosamine measures the glycosylation of albumin and reflects the blood glucose control over the preceding 7 to 10 days (Guthrie, 1988). Both glycosylated hemoglobin and albumin provide data about the average blood glucose level over time. The tests are costly and must be done by laboratory personnel; however, these may be the methods of choice in determining long-term control and may prove more useful and less costly when compared with the cost of doing self-monitored blood glucose (SMBG) four times a day when no changes in daily insulin doses are planned. In the elderly person with stable NIDDM, monthly fasting blood glucose measurements are probably sufficient to monitor control and the need to adjust therapy (Messana and Beizer, 1991).

URINE TESTING

People with diabetes need to understand enough about the pathology to appreciate how blood glucose level is reflected in urine testing. A person whose understanding goes only as far as knowing that his blood glucose level is elevated may see little value in testing urine.

Although urine testing has a place in monitoring, results of urine testing may not correlate closely with current blood glucose levels, due to renal and neurologic changes. For *individuals with NIDDM not treated with insulin* urine testing has been found to be as effective as self-monitoring of blood glucose levels when glycosylated hemoglobin levels and fasting plasma glucose levels were compared (Allen et al, 1990).

If urine testing is used to estimate blood glucose levels, it is imperative that the test be done carefully. Emptying the bladder and then collecting the next voided urine specimen within 30 minutes improves the validity of urine testing, reflecting the current blood glucose level. A first voided urine may give more useful data on overall glucose control.

Various methods of urine testing have merits and drawbacks. Choices are dipsticks and tablets on which drops of urine are placed. Timing during actual testing is crucial for accurate results, i.e., if instructions state that the dipstick is to be inserted into urine for 2 seconds, removed, and the color compared with the color chart after 30 seconds, the timing should be done with a clock or watch where seconds are easily counted. On plastic dipsticks the chemically impregnated paper is on only one side of the plastic strip. If the dipstick is read through the plastic, no color change will be noted. To avoid affecting results, portions of the paper to be read should not be touched. Larger forms of the dipsticks are available for people with alterations in vision or manual dexterity.

Tablets used for testing should be poured into the lid of the bottle and from there to the paper or test tube. This will avoid altering test results and skin damage if fingers are wet.

Collection of a 24-hour urine specimen provides data for determining control over a day. This information coupled with results of second voided urine specimens during the day aids in determining time and extent of glucosuria.

Urine Testing for Ketones Testing urine for the presence of acetone or ketones should be done every 4 hours when the person is ill or when urine or blood glucose level testing reveals elevated blood glucose levels. Testing for ketones is necessary during illness, no matter what treatment regimen the individual uses, i.e., diet, exercise, oral sulfonylureas or insulin.

RECORD KEEPING

Keeping a record of monitoring of blood glucose or urine is necessary for decision making regarding treatment, especially at times when blood glucose level control is erratic, i.e., during illness or overeating (Fig. 24–1).

NUTRITIONAL CONTROL OF BLOOD GLUCOSE

The basis of treatment of every type of diabetes is diet. For older persons consideration needs to be given to special needs such as fixed income, difficulty with shopping and preparing food, lifelong eating habits, and functional disabilities such as ease of chewing raw vegetables for those individuals who have dentures.

WEEK STARTING MONDAY: _June 1_

DAY	TIME	INSULIN OR ORAL DRUG	BLOOD GLUCOSE TEST				URINE KETONE TEST	NOTES
			BEFORE BREAKFAST	BEFORE LUNCH	BEFORE DINNER	BEDTIME		
MON	7 AM	glyburide	180	190	180	200		
TUE	7 AM	glyburide	240	245	286	243	7Am neg 11 Am 1+ 5 pm 1+ 10 pm 1+	feel tired, a little nauseated
WED	8 AM	glyburide	230	232	218	270	7Am neg 11 Am 1+ 5 pm 1+ 10 pm 1+	vomited vomited drinking liquids feeling better
THUR	8 AM	glyburide	200	174	170	180	7 neg 11 Am neg	feeling OK
FRI								
SAT								
SUN								

FIGURE 24–1 Record-keeping form.

GOALS OF DIET MANAGEMENT

1. Achieve and maintain ideal body weight (based on age-adjusted weight tables)
2. Avoid wide swings of blood glucose levels
3. Avoid concentrated carbohydrates
4. Increase complex carbohydrates and fiber
5. Keep blood cholesterol under 200 mg
6. Consume adequate vitamins and minerals
7. Eat a variety of foods daily

Consultation with a dietitian is useful, particularly if frequent follow-up and support groups are available. If a dietitian is not available, dietary management is of such importance that the nurse needs to develop expertise in this area. A useful guideline is to carefully evaluate the person's current diet and food preferences and suggest as few changes as possible (see Chapter 12).

MEAL PLANS

The following are general dietary approaches. The so-called *free diet* is one with no restrictions so long as the person is not overweight or underweight, has no elevated blood fats, hypertension, or excessive elevations in blood glucose. Next in order is a meal plan called *sugar free*, with the only restriction being omission of concentrated refined sugar and items that contain concentrated sugar.

The *exchange system* provides a useful means of attaining the goals of diet treatment. In this system food is divided into six groups:

milk products, vegetables A and B, fruit, breads, fats, and meat. Designated portions of foods within each group contain about the same amount of carbohydrate, protein, and fat. Therefore, foods within each of the groups can be exchanged for any other food within that food group. Each individual receives a prescription for the number of exchanges in each food group that will provide adequate nutrition and result in weight maintenance, loss, or gain as the individual's needs dictate. In determining the diet prescription the need for saturated fat and/or sodium restriction is also considered. The exchange system is designed to provide flexibility in meal plans by allowing the individual variety and ease in eating. One knows which and how many exchanges he is allowed each day and at each meal and chooses foods that meet the exchange allowances. Local chapters of the American Dietetic Association and American Diabetes Association can provide materials on the exchange system.

The most stringent meal plan requires *actual weighing or measuring and recording of all food and fluid consumed.* This prevents any error of estimation in portion size and calls attention to the importance of diet. Following this most rigid plan for a period of time is a way to learn portions and reestablish appropriate eating choices and habits.

Protein recommendations in the diabetic diet have changed over the past few years. When it was thought best to avoid carbohydrates, protein and the accompanying fat was then emphasized. There is some evidence that decreasing the amount of dietary protein to 0.8 g/kg of body weight is correlated with a delay in the onset of kidney disease (Schafer, 1989).

Obesity   Obesity is the primary management problem in NIDDM. Obesity is complex and requires an investment of time on the part of the nurse, dietitian, and patient to gain insight into each individual's eating patterns. Weight reduction of as little as 10 to 15 pounds can result in improved glycemic control in those who are obese. Weight reduction must be monitored carefully because older individuals who are minimally overweight may experience profound weight loss on a restricted diet (Morley and Kaiser, 1990).

Establishing an attitude of acceptance of the person that is not contingent on his size is paramount. Investigation has shown that obese people may be caught in a cycle of feeling low personal worth because of obesity. This feeling leads to depression relieved by overeating that in turn leads to greater obesity. After the nurse has shown acceptance of the obese person, an accurate dietary assessment can be obtained to determine eating patterns as well as diet components that help to reveal behavior modification needs. For example, once it has been established that the person is accepted regardless of size, the question "When and on what foods do you overeat?" may be asked.

After current patterns and eating styles are documented, plans can be made for teaching nutritional content and calories of various foods. Involving the individual in the analysis and planning of eating and then providing ongoing support are associated with successful compliance. Frequent dietary consultation emphasizes weight loss as treatment. Involvement in organizations with the goal of lifelong weight control has shown positive results in achieving and maintaining ideal body weight.

HYPOGLYCEMIC AGENTS

ORAL HYPOGLYCEMIC AGENTS

The oral sulfonylurea drugs have been the primary treatment for elderly individuals with NIDDM when treatment with diet and/or exercise do not control blood glucose levels. Introduced in the 1950s with tolbutamide, there are now six sulfonylurea drugs available. See Table 24–4 for a description of the characteristics of the sulfonylurea drugs.

The oral sulfonylurea drugs are usually well tolerated, with prolonged hypoglycemia the only significant side effect. Drug interactions with sulfonylureas do occur, with the result being either an increase or decrease in the effectiveness. Because the elderly may be on several maintenance medications, it is prudent to verify if any potential for drug interactions exist. Clinically significant interactions involving sulfonylurea drugs are as follows (Messana and Beizer, 1991):

Decreased Hypoglycemic Effect
  Beta-adrenergic blockers
  Corticosteroids
  Epinephrine
  Rifampin
  Thiazide diuretics

TABLE 24–4 *Oral Hypoglycemic Agents Available in the United States*

Drug	Half-life (hr)	Duration (hr)	Dosage Range
FIRST-GENERATION SULFONYLUREAS			
Acetohexamide (Dymelor)	5–8	12–24	0.25–1.5 g[*]
Chlorpropamide (Diabinese)	30–36	60	0.1–0.5 g[†]
Tolazamide (Tolinase)	7	10–14	0.1–1 g
Tolbutamide (Orinase)	4–6	6–12	0.5–3 g[‡]
SECOND-GENERATION SULFONYLUREAS			
Glyburide (Micronase, Diabeta)	10	up to 24	15–30 mg[*]
Glipizide (Glucotrol)	2.1–2.6	up to 24	2.5–40 mg[*]

[*]Divided or single dose.
[†]Single dose.
[‡]Divided doses.

Increased or Prolonged Hypoglycemic Effect
Beta-adrenergic blockers
Clofibrate
Ethanol (acutely)
Monoamine oxidase inhibitors
Salicylates
Sulfonamides

It is generally believed that chlorpropamide is not a prudent choice of hypoglycemic agent for the elderly due to the long half-life, with concomitant danger of prolonged hypoglycemia and also the increased risk for developing the syndrome of inappropriate antidiuretic hormone secretion.

INSULIN

When the blood glucose level is not controlled by diet, exercise, and oral sulfonylurea agents, insulin is the next layer of treatment. There are more than 40 forms of insulin available and all fall into three general types based on duration of action: short, intermediate, and long acting. See Table 24–5 for a description of the onset, peak, and duration of the various types of insulin.

Generally, diabetes in elderly individuals can be adequately controlled with one or two daily doses of an intermediate-acting insulin. Rarely is it necessary to include a short-acting insulin except in acute situations.

Basic to safe administration of insulin is the understanding that exogenous insulin is absorbed at a predetermined rate, as opposed to the action of endogenous insulin, which is secreted on a second-to-second basis as determined by the fluctuating blood glucose. Knowledge of onset, peak, and duration of actions of the particular insulin underlines the requirement of regularly spaced meals and snacks and regular exercise in order to avoid hypoglycemia.

Site Rotation Rotation of the site into which insulin is injected is important to ensure similarity of absorption on a day-to-day basis. Goals include (1) giving every injection 1 inch from other injection sites, (2) reusing a specific site only once every 6 weeks, (3) changing major sites, arms, legs, abdomen, as infrequently as possible because insulin is absorbed at different rates in different major sites. The most rapid absorption occurs in the abdomen, with the slowest absorption occurring when insulin is injected into the legs and arms. Insulin, injected into areas that will be exercised, is absorbed even more rapidly (Bantle, 1990). One convenient system for rotation of injection sites is illustrated in Figure 24–2.

Insulin Injection The objective in administering insulin subcutaneously is to place the insulin in the potential space between adipose

TABLE 24–5   *Approximate Action of Various Types of Insulin*

Type	Preparation	Onset (hr)	Peak (hr)	Duration (hr)
Rapid-acting	Crystalline zinc insulin (regular)	$\frac{1}{2}$–1	2–4	8
		$\frac{1}{2}$–1	2–4	14
Intermediate-acting	Isophane insulin injection (NPH)	2	6–12	20–30
	Lente	2	6–12	24–28
Long-acting	Ultralente	7	18–24	36+

Actual times of onset, peak, and duration vary greatly in individuals according to their present activity and circulatory status.

and muscle tissue. Pinching up the skin and inserting the needle at a 90 degree angle to the pinch and a 45 degree angle to the extremity or abdomen is generally believed to achieve the objective. It is thought desirable to maintain the pinch throughout the injection with one hand, while aspirating with the little finger of the hand holding the syringe. Some people

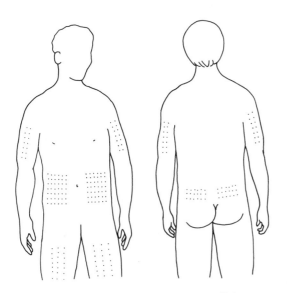

FIGURE 24–2 Insulin injection sites. Inject one hand's width from any joint. Make sites 1 inch apart. When using the thighs, begin at the knee and use one row per week. After sites on one leg are used, move to the other leg. If you use this pattern, each site will be used once every 6 weeks.

may lack the manual dexterity needed for this technique. Some health professionals are currently advocating the pinch method only for use in abdominal sites, and stretching the skin and inserting the needle at a 90 degree angle to the skin for arm and leg sites. The rationale for this technique is that this approach theoretically results in more consistent placement of the insulin using a $\frac{1}{2}$-inch needle and it is simpler.

Massage of the site is seldom recommended as it may accelerate the absorption of insulin and cause increased tissue damage.

Teaching Insulin Administration   Self-injection of insulin can constitute a seemingly overwhelming obstacle. It is the authors' experience that after an initial session of about 1 hour, using an audiovisual guide that the individual takes with him, most people can safely manage self-injection with the nurse conducting follow-up by telephone, daily if necessary, until the insulin dose and comfort with administration are established. This is coupled with clinic visits or employing home visits for evaluation and further teaching until the person can manage safely and confidently.

Insulin Administration Equipment   Insulin syringes are now available in a variety of volumes: 30, 50, and 100 units. Needles are as small as 28 gauge. There is evidence that outpatients may safely reuse disposable syringes for up to 2 months. After each injection the syringe and attached needle can be replaced in the packet and kept in the refrigerator. When the needle becomes dull it is replaced with a new disposable syringe. Cleaning the site in preparation for injection with soap and water or alcohol is easily done; however, infections from not cleaning the skin have not been demonstrated. Pen-type injectors, devices that hold prefilled insulin cartridges, are convenient, easy to use, and small.

COMBINATION SULFONYLUREA AND INSULIN THERAPY

Currently there is some interest in combination therapy when control of hyperglycemia is difficult to achieve. Over time people with NIDDM show a decline in insulin production, which is added to the problem of insulin resistance. Rationale for combination therapy is that the oral sulfonylurea drugs stimulate beta cell insulin secretion and exert various extrapancreatic effects and adequate amounts of insulin are provided by injection (Lebovits, 1990). Effects of combination therapy are not clearly understood and most studies have been done on middle-aged rather than elderly people. Improvements in glycemic control must be weighed against risks of polypharmacy, increased cost, and increased hypoglycemia (Messana and Beizer, 1991). Combination therapy is generally thought to be a hazardous choice for elderly people with diabetes.

EXERCISE

Exercise in elderly people with diabetes has not received much attention. What is known has been extrapolated from studies of younger and nondiabetic individuals. It has been established that with acute exercise, there is a marked increase in glucose uptake and use despite a decline in plasma insulin concentration. In diabetes, there is a breakdown in the usually precise balance between glucose delivery and use necessary to maintain stable blood glucose concentrations during acute exercise. In situations of insufficient insulin or untreated diabetes mellitus, glucose production by the liver can be greater than muscle uptake and use, resulting in hyperglycemia (Schwartz, 1990). It is recommended that individuals not exercise unless the blood glucose level is below 240 mg/dL.

Potential benefits associated with endurance exercise training includes improvement of blood glucose and lipid levels, decreased

blood pressure, weight loss, with preferential reduction in central and intra-abdominal adiposity, increased strength, flexibility, and bone mineral content, reduced stress and anxiety, and improvement in depression and psychomotor reaction time. Diminished cardiac reserve and functional disabilities may limit the ability to exercise in elderly individuals. Risks associated with exercise, musculoskeletal injuries, sudden cardiac arrest, and hypoglycemia, can be minimized by monitoring blood glucose level control, preexercise stretching and warm up, postexercise cool down, and avoiding excessive joint trauma (Graham, 1991). Careful examination of feet and footwear, regularity, and moderation are significant considerations.

Exercise plans can begin with active range of motion while sitting, walking increasing distances, and exercising in water. As stamina increases and no risk factors evolve, the strenuousness of the exercise can be increased.

Short-term Problems

HYPOGLYCEMIA

A main hazard of the treatment of diabetes with insulin and oral hypoglycemic agents is hypoglycemia. This occurs when the blood glucose level drops below 50 mg/dL in spite of the body's counterregulatory mechanisms. Hypoglycemia can cause damage to the neurons of the cerebral cortex. Results of lack of adequate glucose to the cerebral cortex can cause physical injury if, for example, the person loses consciousness and falls down. Brain cells in general do not require insulin to use glucose; however, they have very little ability to store glucose.

Hypoglycemia can develop whenever the three-way balance of diet, exercise, and hypoglycemic agents is disrupted. Some precipitating factors are decreased food intake, delayed food intake, additional exercise, or an erroneously large dose of insulin or sulfonylurea. Every person taking hypoglycemic agents, sulfonylureas, or insulin must be able to recognize the signs and symptoms of hypoglycemia (usually shakiness, diaphoresis, blurred thoughts) and know the correct action to take.

Hypoglycemia is potentially a serious complication, because of its effects on the cerebral cortex, resulting in slowed thinking at a time when rapid, correct action is crucial to reversing the hypoglycemia. In addition, complications from diabetes may result in damage to the autonomic nervous system, which in turn may prevent the individual from quickly becoming aware of the signs and symptoms of hypoglycemia. The elderly person may have physiologic changes caused by aging and perhaps other chronic diseases that confuse the interpretation of the signs and symptoms of hypoglycemia.

The rapidity with which a hypoglycemic reaction occurs depends on many factors, but it is primarily related to the rapidity of action of the specific hypoglycemic agent. Regular insulin usually causes rapid onset of hypoglycemia, whereas the prolonged-action insulins cause slower onset of signs and symptoms. When the cause of the hypoglycemic reaction is a sulfonylurea, the onset of signs and symptoms is slow and easily mistaken for some other cause of change in level of consciousness. When hypoglycemia occurs during sleep, patients may experience nightmares and find damp bedclothes and more than the usual disarrangement of their bedclothes. Aging and alteration in neurologic functioning may blunt the neurologic response to hypoglycemia, resulting in the elderly person being unaware of hypoglycemia.

TREATMENT OF HYPOGLYCEMIA

Clearly the objective of treating hypoglycemia is to rapidly restore blood glucose to normal ranges, without overshooting and causing hyperglycemia. Availability of blood glucose level testing with a fingerstick blood sample and immediate reading of results has simplified verification of blood glucose levels should doubts exist as to the cause of the signs and symptoms. Treatment of hypoglycemia in conscious patients consists of ingestion of 10 g of rapidly absorbed carbohydrate: two sugar cubes, two to three small pieces of hard candy, or 4 oz of juice or sugared soda. If there is no diminution of signs and symptoms in 5 minutes, the same dose of carbohydrate is repeated. When the symptoms abate, the individual needs to have the next scheduled meal or snack early to prevent a return of the hypoglycemia.

If the person is unconscious and near health professionals, 10 to 50 g of 50% glucose is administered intravenously. Glucagon can be administered intramuscularly to the unconscious person, although raising the blood glucose by this method is slower than by the intravenous route. When the cause of the hypoglycemia is a sulfonylurea, the person usually requires hospi-

talization for close monitoring and continuous intravenous glucose because of the long duration of action of the oral agents.

After the hypoglycemic episode has been treated, it is important for the individual to retrace the events that led up to the incident to detect anything that could have caused the hypoglycemia. Prevention of hypoglycemia is preferable to treating it, and this can be accomplished through careful education of patients regarding the balance of food intake, exercise, and hypoglycemic agents, even spacing of food intake and exercise, and signs and symptoms of hypoglycemia. Diabetic individuals who are taking insulin should have as part of their daily meal plan three regular meals, a midafternoon snack, and a bedtime snack.

All diabetic individuals should wear a bracelet or necklace that identifies their diabetic state. In addition, all diabetic individuals who take insulin should carry a source of rapidly absorbed carbohydrate to take for immediate treatment in the event of hypoglycemia. Diabetic individuals need to (1) inform family, friends, and coworkers of their condition, (2) explain signs and symptoms of hypoglycemia, and (3) explain the appropriate treatment in the event the diabetic individual is unable to help him- or herself.

If there is any doubt as to the cause of hypoglycemic-like signs and symptoms in a person taking insulin or sulfonylureas, treatment for hypoglycemia should be administered without delay. If the signs and symptoms are from hypoglycemia, the symptoms will quickly abate and if symptoms are caused by something else, the small amount of carbohydrate will have done no harm.

HYPERGLYCEMIC HYPEROSMOLAR NONKETOTIC SYNDROME

Hyperglycemic hyperosmolar nonketotic syndrome (HHNS) is a metabolic disturbance that usually occurs in people who have NIDDM and are over 60 years of age. In the majority of patients there is a history of some concurrent illness or stressful event such as an upper respiratory illness, gastrointestinal disturbance, cerebrovascular accident, or myocardial infarction, during which the individual has become hyperglycemic and volume depleted. The prodromal period is usually days or weeks, longer than that of diabetic ketoacidosis.

The pathogenesis of HHNS is poorly understood and the mortality is high, (Wachtel, 1987).

Several factors contribute to the predisposition of the elderly to develop HHNS:

1. An age-related reduction in the kidney's ability to concentrate the urine, allowing the loss of more water as the body is obligated to the excretion of an osmotic load
2. A decrease of glomerular filtration rate and kidney mass with aging
3. Elderly persons have a lower total body content with which to buffer changes in osmolarity
4. Elderly persons have a decreased sense of or response to thirst
5. Physical disability, sedation, restraints, confusion, and isolation may compromise a person's ability to seek and ingest necessary water (Matz, 1989)

Blood glucose levels in HHNS are higher than 500 mg/dL, serum osmolarity is greater than 330 mOsm/kg, serum and urine ketones are absent, arterial pH is greater than 7.3, and plasma HCO_3 is greater than 20 mEq/L. Generally, there are a variety of neurologic signs, such as hemisensory deficits and hemiparesis and focal seizures, that can evoke the most common misdiagnosis—that of cerebral vascular accident. The major differences between diabetic ketoacidosis and HHNS are the advanced age and absence of blood and urine ketones in HHNS.

Treatment of HHNS is aimed at careful correction of the extreme volume depletion and the hyperosmolar state, and then detecting and treating the underlying illness. Surveillance of all potential causes of volume depletion in the elderly person with NIDDM will work toward early detection and hence more successful treatment of HHNS.

INTERCURRENT ILLNESS

When an individual who has diabetes develops an intercurrent illness such as gastrointestinal flu or an upper respiratory infection, the body has an increased need for insulin. Infection results in insulin resistance and hormonal actions that increase blood glucose levels. Individuals who normally control their blood glucose with diet and exercise may find that their blood glucose increases dramatically during an illness. Frequent assessment of blood glucose levels with SMBG and urine ketones will alert the individual and caregivers to situations requiring support by health care professionals. See guidelines for diabetic individuals during an intercurrent illness (see box below).

Long-term Problems

Long-term physiologic problems associated with diabetes in the elderly are large vessel disease, small vessel disease, and neuropathy.

Guidelines for the Diabetic Individual during Intercurrent Illness

1. Test blood glucose level and urine ketones every 4 hours. Record results
2. Take the usual AM dose of oral sulfonylurea or long-acting insulin
3. Maintain 24-hour fluid intake to at least 750 mL or $1\frac{1}{2}$ quarts
4. Eat a 24-hour total of 150 g of carbohydrate in the form of broth, crackers, or milk
5. Call health professional if any of the following occur:
   a. Altered sensorium
   b. All blood glucose levels are elevated over 240 mg/dL
   c. Urine tests show acetone
   d. Unable to continue fluid intake
   e. Unable to ingest 150 g of carbohydrate
   f. Thirst and frequent urination

From Rocci ML, Vlassis PH, Abrams WG. Geriatric clinical pharmacology. Geriatr Cardiol 1986; 4:54; with permission.

Clearly, elderly people have changes in their blood vessels and nerves related to normal aging and may have changes related to other disease processes. Since there is an incomplete understanding of how the diabetic changes occur, and care is mostly supportive, the nurse plays an important role in helping people adapt to the alterations in their blood vessels and nerves.

MACROVASCULAR COMPLICATIONS

Macrovascular complications are a major cause of the development of other chronic diseases in individuals with diabetes (Hernandez, 1989). The incidence of atherosclerosis and arteriosclerosis is increased in patients with diabetes. Diabetic individuals have angina at an earlier age than do nondiabetic individuals. Coronary heart disease accounts for half of the deaths among adults with NIDDM, and the incidence of hypertension increases with the duration of diabetes and the person's age. In the older person with NIDDM, there is a positive correlation between increased systolic hypertension and both peripheral vascular disease and cerebral vascular disease. Whether NIDDM is a cause of the systolic hypertension or whether the hypertension is simply reflecting changes in the vessels is not clear. Arteriosclerosis and atherosclerosis with resultant heart disease and hypertension are accelerated in people who have diabetes (see Chapters 23 and 28). There are initial data supporting a relationship among hyperinsulinemia, hypertension, hyperlipidemia, and progressive glucose intolerance (Kaplan, 1991).

TREATMENT OF LARGE VESSEL DISEASE

Blood pressure measurements can be taken at each appointment. The reader is referred to Chapter 28 for a comprehensive review of accurate blood pressure measurement and management of hypertension. Buerger-Allen exercises will maximize the remaining circulation of the legs (see box). Smoking and diabetes interacting with the increased risk of cardiovascular disease, hyperlipidemia, and hypertension produce up to an 11-fold increased likelihood of death by cardiovascular disease (Haire-Joshu, 1991).

Buerger-Allen Exercises

1. Elevate feet above the level of the heart, i.e., elevate them on one pillow until feet blanch—2 minutes
2. Dangle feet below the level of the heart until feet turn rubor—3 minutes
3. Lie with feet level with the heart—5 minutes
4. Repeat these steps five times and do the exercises three times daily

---

MICROVASCULAR COMPLICATIONS

Microvascular disease as it affects circulation to large blood vessels, hyperglycemia, hyperlipidemia, and perhaps an altered immune response are facets in the pathogenesis of macrovascular disease in diabetic patients (Hernandez, 1989).

Treatment of small vessel problems is essentially the same as for nondiabetic patients, control of triglycerides, weight, and blood pressure, except that the beta-adrenergic blocking agents are usually excluded. These agents can impair counterregulatory responses and blunt the sympathetic reflex response to hypoglycemia, so that the diabetic individual may not be aware of a hypoglycemic reaction until the hypoglycemia is severe or prolonged.

TREATMENT OF MICROVASCULAR DISEASE

Research supports poor glycemic control as a cause of the microvascular changes in both IDDM and NIDDM (Forrester, 1987; Tooke, 1987). In diabetes, the first change in the small blood vessels is a thickening of the basement membrane. While thickening of the basement membrane is occurring in every capillary in the body, the effects of the changes are first noted in the eyes and kidneys.

DIABETIC RETINOPATHY

Diabetic changes in eyes can be divided into two major groups: nonproliferative and proliferative retinopathy. Identical types of lesions may occur in patients with IDDM and NIDDM.

In *nonproliferative retinopathy,* more prevalent in NIDDM, three basic pathologic processes occur: (1) increased retinal vascular permeability, (2) structural alteration of the retinal capillaries, and (3) retinal capillary obliteration. Nonproliferative retinopathy may progress very slowly, with little interference in vision (Fig. 24–3).

Proliferative retinopathy, more prevalent in IDDM, is a growth of fibrovascular tissue on the inner surface of the retina and is thought to be caused by retina ischemia (Fig. 24–4). Newly formed vessels develop in the area between the retinal and vitreous gel. Fibrous tissue is associated with the new vessels and this tends to cause tension on the retina, resulting in hemorrhage into the vitreous gel and in retinal distor-

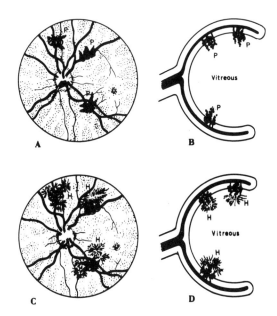

FIGURE 24–4 Proliferative retinopathy is the more severe form of the disease. *A,* Vessels (P) have sprouted from the existing ones, proliferating into the vitreous. *B,* Cross-section of the eye shows the same new vessels growing into the vitreous. *C,* Hemorrhages that commonly develop surround the new or proliferating vessels. *D,* Cross-section shows hemorrhages (H) leaking into the vitreous from proliferating vessels. (From Association for Education and Rehabilitation of the Blind and Visually Impaired. Blindness Annual, 1969. Alexandria, VA; with permission.)

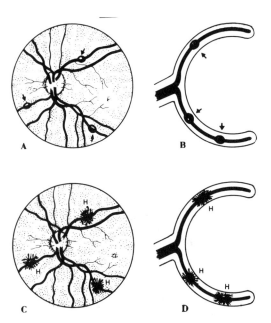

FIGURE 24–3 In the milder or nonproliferative form of diabetic retinopathy, the blood vessel damage is contained within the retina. *A,* Damage first occurs in the walls of the retinal capillaries. Arrows point to areas in the capillary wall that balloon out, forming aneurysms. *B,* Cross-section of the eye also shows aneurysms. *C,* The walls of the aneurysms are weak, and blood can easily flow through them. *D,* The cross-section shows hemorrhages contained within the retina. (From Association for Education and Rehabilitation of the Blind and Visually Impaired. Blindness Annual, 1969. Alexandria, VA; with permission.)

tion and detachment (Fig. 24–5). Early detection of proliferative retinopathy allows treatment with laser photocoagulation to stop the proliferation of new blood vessels. Vitrectomy is done to remove blood when a hemorrhage occurs. Diabetic individuals over 30 years of age with diagnosis of diabetes of at least 5 years duration should have eye examinations by an opthalmologist yearly.

VISUAL IMPAIRMENT

In addition to the retinopathies associated with diabetes, cataracts are common in patients who have diabetes. The changes in the lens are identical to cataracts associated with aging; however, the incidence is increased and the changes occur at an earlier age in diabetic individuals.

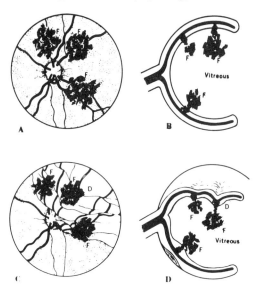

FIGURE 24-5 Hemorrhages into the vitreous that accompany proliferative diabetic retinopathy are often replaced by fibrous or scar tissue that forms in the vitreous. *A*, Ophthalmoscopic view shows this fibrous tissue (F). *B*, Cross-section depicts the same process with fibrous tissue forming in the vitreous. *C*, Traction from the fibrous tissue has pulled on the retina and caused a detachment (D). *D*, Cross-sectional sketch of the retinal detachment shows the fibrous tissue pulling the retina into the vitreous. (From Association for Education and Rehabilitation of the Blind and Visually Impaired. Blindness Annual, 1969. Alexandria, VA; with permission.)

When vision loss is partial, there are a number of devices that allow the individual to remain independent, such as insulin needle guides that fit over the vial of insulin, and small magnifying lenses that can be attached to the insulin syringe. Systems for self-monitoring of blood glucose have incorporated brightly colored, large bold print digital readouts. Instructions are prepared with bold, large print. Rehabilitation programs directed toward compensating for vision loss have been shown to have beneficial effects, both in diabetes control and psychological parameters, particularly when instituted early in the course of vision loss (Bernbaum et al, 1988).

When vision loss is complete, the diabetic person requires daily contact with someone who can carry out monitoring, examine the feet, and set up oral hypoglycemic drugs, or draw up insulin. Though not the most desirable procedure, insulin can be drawn up by someone else before it is needed and kept under refrigeration. The diabetic individual then removes the syringe from the refrigerator a few minutes before injecting to allow the insulin to reach room temperature, gently rotates the syringe to distribute any suspension that has precipitated out, and then injects the insulin.

NEPHROPATHY

In 1988 diabetes ranked as the most prevalent cause of end-stage renal disease (Friedman, 1989). Thickening of the capillary basement membrane in the kidney eventually impairs renal function. Concentration of the thickening in one or several areas in the glomerulus is termed Kimmelstiel-Wilson disease or nodular glomerulosclerosis. As the accumulation occurs throughout the glomerulus and causes glomerulosclerosis, renal function is compromised (Davidson, 1986). Intermittent proteinuria is the first clinical evidence of renal complication and may progress within 1 to 3 years to persistent proteinuria and a subsequent decline in renal function as measured by decreasing creatinine clearance. The decline in renal function progresses to renal failure about 5 years after the appearance of persistent proteinuria. At this stage frank hypertension is almost always present.

Early treatment of nephropathy is directed to keeping blood glucose and blood pressure within normal ranges. Low protein diets are under investigation as treatment for early nephropathy (Schafer, 1989). Currently at least 20% to 25% of all people who begin renal dialysis have diabetes. Other organ involvement makes dialysis difficult for diabetic individuals and thus renal transplantation is often a next step for diabetic individuals who have renal failure. These treatments would be unusual in the elderly.

NEUROPATHY

Neuropathies associated with diabetes are probably the most common long-term complication in diabetic individuals. The problem of defining diabetic neuropathy has made estimating incidence ineffectual. Evidence supporting a metabolic cause for the neurologic dysfunction is strong; however, the specific biochemical lesions leading to morphologic changes have not been established. Causation appears to be multifactorial, involving hyperglycemia inhibiting the uptake of myoinositol and increasing the polyol pathway. The polyol pathway can independently decrease nerve myoinositol, which leads to a decrease in sodium potassium ATPase activity that eventually leads to a decrease in nerve function (Green et al, 1985).

In general, diabetic neuropathies cause a slowing of nerve conduction and loss of deep tendon reflexes. The diabetic peripheral neuropathies can be divided into peripheral and autonomic. The peripheral neuropathies are more common and can be described as being symmetrical, of slow, progressive onset, and of a stocking-glove distribution on the feet and hands. The symptoms are burning sensations, tingling, numbness, and pain, particularly in the feet. Weakness and atrophy of distal muscles of the hands and feet can occur. Lack of sensation results in injuries of which the patient is unaware (Davidson, 1986).

Autonomic nervous system involvement is manifested in a wide variety of dysfunctions (Funnell and McNitt, 1986). Absence of sweating of the feet, atrophy of the skin, and malformations of the toenails are common. Postural hypotension and nocturnal diarrhea are frequent. Gastric atony is not common, but creates major problems of management because of uneven absorption of meals. Neurologic complications of diabetes generally, but not exclusively, occur in persons in older age groups who may have neuropathies from other causes in addition to typical age-related neurologic changes.

COMBINED NEUROLOGIC AND VASCULAR PROBLEMS

Sexual Impotence Sexual impotence in all diabetic men over 40 years of age has been estimated between 8% and 50% (Pfeifer, 1988). This high incidence of sexual impotence is believed to have a vascular and neurologic basis. Psychogenic factors are well established as causes of sexual dysfunction, and drug and alcohol abuse are also associated with impotence. Generally, the investigation of impotence begins by ruling out any other endocrine cause. Efforts are made to get the blood glucose level under strict control. Additional treatment modalities include psychological counseling to determine causes, relieve anxiety, and examine alternative methods of sexual expression. The specific male sexual dysfunctions are inability to achieve and/or maintain erection and pre-

mature ejaculation. Surgical implantations to simulate penile erection are available.

Approximately 30% of diabetic women report sexual dysfunction. The specific dysfunctions ranged from desire disorders, sexual avoidance, lack of lubrication, problems reaching orgasm, sexual dissatisfaction, and dyspareunia (Schreiner-Engel, 1988). Discerning causes of sexual dysfunction in diabetic women is complicated by the frequent occurrence of urinary and vaginal infections.

Foot Problems The feet of diabetic patients merit special attention. The incidence of amputations of the lower extremities of diabtetic patients is 15 times greater than nondiabetic patients at a cost of about $500 million each year not including rehabilitation (Bild et al, 1989). The foot problems have a basis in vascular and neurologic changes resulting from diabetes. The *angiopathies* lead to decreased circulation and to atrophic skin changes, so that injuries to the feet are slower to heal, more readily infected, and more difficult to reach with systemic antibiotics. Concomitantly, the *neuropathies* result in decreased sensation and muscle atrophy, with changes in pressure points on the feet (Fig. 24–6). Without pain to alert the person to injury and to remind him or her to protect and treat the injured area, there is continued trauma and healing is slowed.

Preventative care of feet is imperative. A complicating factor is that people assign importance to sensation and if sensation is decreased one tends to pay little attention to measures of prevention. Diminished eyesight and obesity may interfere with a careful daily examination of the feet. Podiatrists and physical therapists can assist patients when muscle atrophy from a neurologic cause or malalignment of bones has occurred. Shoes with extra depth and padding, custom-made to evenly distribute body weight, can relieve and prevent further problems. During clinic visits, home visits, or hospitalization, health care professionals can emphasize the importance of deliberate attention to the condition of feet through careful, consistent inspection of the feet and toenails. See the box on p. 471 for a summary of care for feet.

Evaluation

The importance of periodic evaluation of self-care with uncued verbalization of information

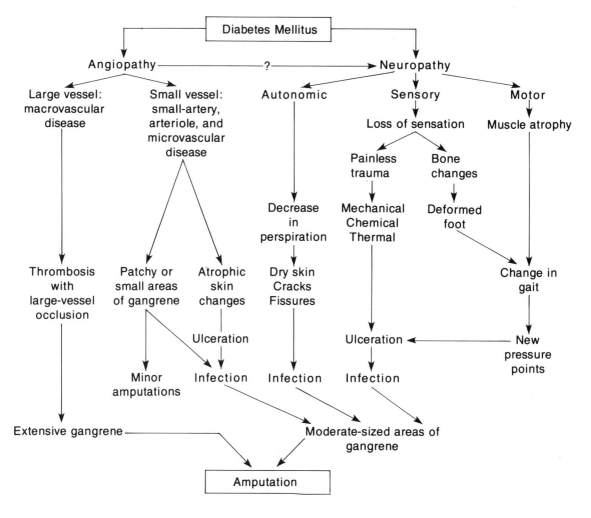

FIGURE 24–6 Pathogenesis of diabetic foot lesions. (From Levin ME, O'Neal LW, eds. The diabetic foot, 4th ed. St. Louis: C. V. Mosby, 1988; with permission.)

and demonstration of psychomotor skills cannot be overemphasized. Evaluation of diabetes control is dependent on the criteria set by care providers.

Helping the older person cope with diabetes is complex. Perhaps the strongest support can be offered by being interested and available, either at clinic appointments, by telephone between visits, or in 24-hour care facilities. Asking "What concerns you the most today?" works toward clarifying current personal stresses and short-term goals. A realistic consideration of the elderly person seems to justify the following goals:

1. Absence of hypoglycemia
2. Absence of acidosis
3. Attainment and maintenance of ideal body weight
4. Absence of ketonuria
5. Absence of symptoms of polyuria, polyphagia, and polydipsia
6. Absence of infections of the mouth, urinary tract, vagina, and feet
7. Absence of atrophy, scarring, or hypertrophy at injection sites

A flow sheet for routine visits aids in evaluating these goals (see box on p. 472).

Foot-care Guidelines for the Patient or for People Responsible for the Diabetic Person

1. Inspect feet daily for blisters, breaks in skin, calluses, and bruises
2. Wash with mild soap testing temperature of water with elbow. Rub callus or soft corns gently with a pumice stone
3. Lubricate with any lanolin-type cream, giving attention to calluses
4. Inspect the insides of shoes for foreign objects, nails coming through the bottom of the shoe, or wrinkles in soles or lining of shoes before putting them on
5. Avoid stockings with holes or mended places
6. Avoid placement of feet near any heat source, i.e., stove, fireplace, or heating pad
7. Always wear shoes or slippers to avoid injury
8. Break in new shoes gradually
9. Avoid any constricting garments, i.e., garters, tight girdles, and tight shoes. Apply panty hose carefully to ensure evenly distributed pressure
10. Cut toenails following contour of toes—have someone else assist if unable to reach easily or if vision is impaired

---

Nursing Diagnosis and Management of High-risk Areas in Daily Living

Many elderly persons are able to deal with the diagnosis of diabetes and incorporate the symptoms and adaptations required by the diabetic regimen into their lives. They are able to manage the changes required in daily living without becoming overly frustrated. However, a significant number have major problems accepting the diagnosis and its implications or learning and integrating diabetic health care into their lifestyles. There are times and circumstances that make it difficult, if not impossible, to participate in either the learning or implementation of diabetic health care.

Because diabetes is a metabolic condition with widespread effects on blood vessels and nerves, there are multiple dysfunctions that interfere with the ability to manage daily living. Older people vary in the rate and degree with which these dysfunctions appear and the ways in which their lives are disrupted.

The diabetic regimen places new demands on individuals (and caregivers) to

Acquire and use new knowledge and skills

Become conscious of and purposeful in eating and meal planning

Be aware of subtle physical cues and act on the inferences drawn

Spend time on self-monitoring, medicating, and foot care

Spend money on medications, supplies, and health care

Live with some level of knowledge about the high risk of future complications related to diabetes

The literature is filled with the prerequisite knowledge, skills, routines, and eating patterns that the older person with diabetes must learn. Strategies for teaching the patient and/or the caregiver are also available, as these are standard protocols for nursing treatment. It is not cost-effective to merely expose an older person to knowledge and skills or even to require evidence of short-term learning. Ongoing monitoring for confirmation of long-term compliance, while important, is insufficient.

The skill in nursing diagnosis and treatment for the elderly diabetic individual comes in diagnosing the person's current willingness and

---

Checklist for Routine Visit

Data to be evaluated at every routine review of the individual's diabetic status

Mentation or behavioral change

Polyuria

Polydipsia

Polyphagia

Hypoglycemic episodes

Vagina: burning, itching, drainage

Urine: burning, itching, frequency, urgency, nocturia, dipstick for protein urine

Vision: blurry, any change

Skin: any breaks in skin or oral mucosa

Feet: calluses, blisters, malformation in toes, pain, vibratory sense, lack of sensation

Insulin injection sites: hypertrophy, atrophy

Weight

Blood pressure

Insulin or sulfonylurea dosage schedule

Presence of identifying bracelet or medallion on person

Possession of source of rapidly absorbed sugar if person takes insulin

Glycosylated hemoglobin, cholesterol/triglycerides value every 4 months

Yearly ophthalmology examination

---

living and internal and external resources of chronically ill elderly people are vulnerable to change. It follows then that their willingness and capacity to engage in self-care may be variable, unpredictable, and often out of their control. Similarly, difficulties in managing daily living can vary in both predictable and unpredictable ways. The nurse's expertise in predicting areas of daily living at risk and strategies for their management is an important external resource for older people with diabetes and their primary caregivers.

Alteration in health maintenance is the most comprehensive nursing diagnosis for problems that occur when daily living with diabetes is threatened by changes in internal and external resources. This diagnosis can be related to a number of components. Among them are noncompliance because of the complexity and chronicity of the care regimen and potential for impaired skin integrity related to diminished sensitivity of the feet, with a reduced capacity for managing foot care (Carpenito, 1989, 1991).

POTENTIAL FOR ALTERED HEALTH MAINTENANCE RELATED TO NONCOMPLIANCE WITH A COMPLEX DIABETIC HEALTH CARE REGIMEN

Compliance with the diabetic treatment regimen is a significant problem even after over 20 years of research on the subject (Anderson, 1990). Living with diabetes imposes major demands on the daily living of both the older patient and significant others. Internal and external resources may be seriously challenged as the necessary alterations in daily living are adapted from a former freer lifestyle. Various factors influence the degree to which individuals adhere to the treatment program. These present risks for successful health maintenance.

RISK FACTORS

Times of High Risk   One of the predictably high-risk times for noncompliance is the period immediately following the diagnosis. Often the diagnosis is made while the individual is being treated for a more acute problem, e.g., fracture, surgical procedure, or while being seen for a routine examination. Diabetes, with its complex care modalities, added to the original problem can be so overwhelming that the elderly

capacity for engaging in self-care. Subsequent to diagnosis, treatment must be administered with the same sensitivity, expertise, and precision used in addressing the knowledge and skill deficits or pathology. Given the dysfunctions and lack of internal or external resources often experienced by older people, nurses are responsible for diagnosing the barriers to effective self-care and daily living.

Ongoing diagnosis and treatment adjustment are required with each contact, as daily person feels overburdened with losses. Diabetes represents a loss of:

Body integrity
Physical abilities
Hope of "ever being cured"

Loss is followed by the normal grieving process, which must begin before healing is accomplished. During this grieving time the person is still expected to begin a new regimen of self-care that is complicated and demanding. The added burden of this new diagnosis may hinder adherence to the program at the precise time when there is an urgent need to learn and change.

Another high-risk time for noncompliance is when new manifestations of diabetes appear. The grief response is duplicated and adherence may again be compromised. Other personal losses may also generate a grieving response. Episodes of intercurrent illness, i.e., infections, exacerbations of chronic conditions, or injuries may lower the person's energy level and subsequently alter his adherence to diabetic health care.

Other Risk Factors The desire or ability to participate in learning or implementing self-care is also diminished by:

Cognitive impairment caused by high blood glucose, disease, or delirium
Physical disabilities, i.e., loss of or altered vision or hearing, chronic pain, and diminished tactile sensation
Depression, a frequent problem in older people, causing decreased interest in self-care
Health care beliefs that do not include preventive care of medication administration
Chronic disease affecting function, i.e., arthritis, hypertension, or cardiovascular disease with drug therapies that may cause interactions with hypoglycemic agents
Perceived health status and expectations being ascribed to aging rather than to disease, causing failure to report symptoms
Alcohol or other substance abuse
Diminished external resources related to physical assistance, finances, transportation, nutrition, and safety
Amount of behavioral change necessary to comply with the diabetic health regimen (Anderson, 1990)
Relationship with the health care professional (Anderson, 1990)

Additional demands on coping mechanisms
Chronicity of the diabetic condition with complex treatment programs
Having major caregiving responsibilities for others, leaving little energy for personal needs
Living alone or with others who choose not to be involved

SIGNS AND SYMPTOMS

Elderly people may report that they "can't follow all the instructions given" or that they "just don't feel up to doing all the things necessary" to comply with the regimen. They may have adapted to the symptoms of uncontrolled diabetes and attribute the effects of hyperglycemia to aging. Remarks such as "I don't feel enough better to go through all this work" may be expressed. Health care and laboratory appointments may be broken and the patient might admit to not doing the blood glucose testing or keeping accurate records. They may complain that the blurry vision is still a problem. In subsequent contacts, the following are signs of the individual's noncompliance with diabetic health care activities:

Continued high blood glucose levels
Hypoglycemic reactions
Failure to have scheduled laboratory work done
Failure to keep follow-up appointments
Increased hemoglobin A_{1c} levels
Weight gain
Exacerbations of diabetic symptoms
Inability to demonstrate proper administration of medication or correct dosage, selection of unsuitable foods, inappropriate skin care, and no beneficial exercises
Not wearing diabetes identification
Evidence of body odor

PROGNOSTIC VARIABLES

A poor prognosis for compliance with the diabetic regimen is associated with elderly diabetic patients who:

Fail to move through the grieving process
Do not hear or see adequately to comprehend the information necessary for self-care and have no support system
Have impaired cognitive ability
Have chronic disease affecting the mobility and dexterity necessary for self-care

Are experiencing fatigue because of providing care for others

Had a premorbid personality of apathy and dependence

Have concurrent or intercurrent illnesses

COMPLICATIONS

Failure to comply with diabetic monitoring, meal planning, medications, and personal hygiene on a daily basis can be expected to result in exacerbation of the high-risk pathology and complications associated with diabetes. If the patient does not return for follow-up appointments he can "get lost in the system" and complications can occur.

TREATMENT

Successful treatment for the nursing diagnosis of noncompliance depends on the patient's and/or the caregiver's level of commitment to long-term management. Assessment of the patient's cognitive and emotional status is of paramount importance. Data regarding the priority level the patient assigns to diabetic health care are also important. Regimen complexity, amount of behavioral change necessary, and the period of time over which the behavior must be performed are all aspects of treatment that can affect compliance (Anderson, 1990). A trusting relationship with a health care provider who will actively listen to the patient and probe for underlying reasons for noncompliance can be the key to management.

Nursing strategies for dealing with noncompliance in participation in diabetic health care activities include the following:

Assess patient's mental status to determine whether noncompliance is due to short-term memory loss, emotional stress, or depression related to the diabetes

Assess the level of literacy, i.e., the ability to read and write

Assess the patient's physical abilities to see the printed material and blood glucose monitoring device, read prescription containers, remove bottle caps and manipulate the insulin syringe and give the injection

Provide large, boldly printed instructions on white or yellow paper for those people with vision problems

Seek assistance from a responsible resource

person to keep blood glucose under control while the patient is learning

Assess health care beliefs about diabetes and correct any misconceptions

Provide information for resource material, i.e., Diabetes Supply Club, Meals on Wheels, local or national Diabetes Association, and the Community Services for the Blind

Sensitively question the patient about the priority level of diabetic care in his life

Use personal, financial, environmental, and social resources available to maintain compliance at a healthy level

Explain the regimen so that all treatments show association and have meaning in the patient's daily living routine. Keep the treatment regimen at the simplest level possible and hold teaching sessions to 15 to 20 minutes each. Older people take longer to learn new material, requiring follow-up with printed information

Determine what area of the regimen is the most difficult for the patient (e.g., stopping smoking, losing weight, administering insulin, controlling diet, shopping for food, preparing food, or self-monitoring of blood glucose). Modify the program if possible to show an understanding of the difficulty being experienced

Provide a medical alert identification tag along with an explanation of why it is important

Involve the patient in meal planning, taking into consideration his likes and dislikes

Provide recipes that encourage variety to prevent boredom from eating the same foods just because they are "quick and easy"

Provide a telephone number for triage care. This gives the patient a sense of acceptance and access to immediate answers. Many hospitals sponsor 24-hour telephone information services staffed by nurses

Provide flow sheets for record keeping

Negotiate a contract for problem areas, i.e., weight loss or maintenance, providing ideas for nonfood rewards that the patient can give himself

Set up an exercise program that is agreeable, possible, and safe, e.g., walking around the block, house, or in a mall a specified number of times. In a long-term care facility a walking club can be instituted that meets on a regular basis and walks as a group. This creates a social outlet and a sense of belonging. Sitting exercises can be designed for those unable to walk (Norstrom, 1988). The activity department in nursing homes is often the resource for the exercise program. Nurses should instruct the leaders on safe aerobic exercise and signs and symptoms of hyperglycemia and hypoglycemia

Phone the patient to inquire about how he is doing. This shows interest and gives encouragement

Stress the importance of preventive care, i.e., foot care, regularly scheduled visits to various professional specialists (podiatrist, ophthalmologist, and dentist) for evaluation

Teach the patient and a support person (caregiver) the skills of home-monitoring of blood glucose, signs and symptoms of hypoglycemia and hyperglycemia and the treatment for each

Emphasize the importance of close attention to blood glucose levels during times of acute illness or surgery

Provide audio or video tapes to allow the patient to have consistent repetition of instructions while at home in an unstressed environment

Recommend the least complicated blood glucose monitoring device

Use a positive approach about the regimen. The elderly person may experience many losses and take on a negative approach to challenges

Reevaluate patient goals and management strategies regularly so the patient does not feel neglected

EVALUATION

Outcome criteria with which to evaluate the older patient's compliance are for the patient to

Report a lifestyle that is improved or maintained at its previous level as evidenced by increased involvement in self-care or management on a daily basis

Participate in care decisions

Report improved sense of well-being and self-esteem

Accept diabetes-related pathology without assuming he failed to be effective in care

State the benefits and risks involved in following the treatment plan and enter into a contract to set mutual goals

Remain free of hyperglycemic/hypoglycemic symptoms

Success is a powerful reinforcer; therefore, goals have a motivational function when achievement is possible.

POTENTIAL FOR IMPAIRED SKIN INTEGRITY RELATED TO DIMINISHED SENSITIVITY

Approximately half of the nontraumatic amputations in the United States occur in people with diabetes. Estimations are made that over half the amputations in individuals with diabetes are preventable (Bild et al, 1989). Improved foot care is a most important factor. Management of the diabetic foot may be conducted by the individual, a significant other, or by professional nurses either in the community or institutional setting. Foot care is an area in which nurses can have great impact for the person with diabetes. Foot ulcers and deformities due to diabetes that result in lower extremity amputations might have been prevented if professional health care providers had instituted prophylactic measures.

RISK FACTORS

Two major risk factors leading to foot problems for people with diabetes are peripheral vascular disease and peripheral neuropathy. Preventive measures provide enhancement of quality of life and decreased treatment costs. Several other risk factors have an additional bearing on the development of foot lesions in the older person with diabetes. These include the following:

Smoking

Obesity

Hyperglycemia

Hyperlipidemia

Decreased vision or physical ability to see and care for his or her own feet or lack of another to provide this service

Dry skin caused by autonomic neuropathy and nonsweating feet

Loss of the protective sensation (pain) due to diminished sensory response

Cognitive impairment affecting memory and judgment

Corns, calluses, and ingrown toenails

Decreased immune response to infectious processes

Trauma

SIGNS AND SYMPTOMS

Indicators that skin integrity of the feet may be an actual or potential problem include the following:

Elderly individuals reporting that the "heating pad must be set on high in order to keep my feet warm" or that "I don't get around as well anymore because of leg cramps"

Complaints of severe calf pain during walking that disappear when at rest

Heavy calluses, corns, bunions, and ingrown or jagged toenails

Reported use of corn removal plasters or ingrown toenail remedies

Wearing constricting stockings and/or ill-fitting shoes

Open areas on legs or feet that are not healing

Foot drop

Extremely sensitive feet and legs or decreased sensation and proprioception

Little or no hair growth on the legs

Unclean, dry feet with interdigital fissuring

Hammertoes

Foot blanching on elevation and dependent rubor

Atrophic leg skin changes

PROGNOSTIC VARIABLES

Early recognition of problems fosters a favorable prognosis for incorporating foot care into daily living. When patients experience the deteriorating effects of aging, they are not able to independently monitor their feet. A caregiver may become necessary, either in the home or through a long-term care facility.

COMPLICATIONS

Ulceration, infection, and amputation are high-risk complications associated with lack of diabetic foot care. Deterioration in the quality of the individual's life, loss of independence, and pain are further problems that can occur as a result of disregarding foot care.

TREATMENT

Prevention is the key to healthy diabetic feet. Education of the patient regarding the importance of daily monitoring and regular comprehensive screening by a professional are two major components of preventive treatment.

Daily inspection of the feet should be as routine as blood testing (Brand and Coleman, 1990). If the patient cannot accomplish this independently, assistance must be provided by the family or others. Nursing treatment for diabetic foot care for the older person includes the following:

Ask how the person has been caring for his feet at home. This will provide information about whether or not a podiatrist has been involved.

Check the patient's mobility by requesting that he walk away and return, noting any disruption in gait pattern that may affect weight distribution on the feet

Assess the feet for edema, signs of skin irritation, hydration, cleanliness, increased temperature, tenderness, or discoloration. Inspect toenails for fungal infections, growth pattern (ingrown, thickened, jagged, or overgrown), and color. Palpate for pedal pulses and capillary refill time. Inspect for corns, calluses, hammertoes, bunions, hair growth on toes, and tenderness on plantar surface

Test the feet for sensory response to warmth, cold, and pain

Vibratory and positional sense should also be checked along with reflexes. This examination will indicate the presence of neuropathy

Shoes should be carefully fitted and made of leather or fabric, with wide toes and extra depth. Vinyl and plastic do not adapt to relieve pressure. The "5-hour shoe change" (Brand and Coleman, 1990) is a good rule of thumb for the elderly person with diabetes. This entails wearing a pair of shoes only 5 hours at a time. Specially made shoes are expensive so athletic running shoes have been used and shown to be successful in reducing the size of plantar calluses (Soulier, 1986)

Inspect the patient's shoes both inside and out for worn spots that indicate abnormal pressure areas. Feel the inside of the shoes for hard seams or tears. Note how the shoe fits. Friction occurs when shoes are too loose, causing blister formation. Stockings should be of soft absorbent fabric. Pressure areas can be caused by stockings that are too tight (causing constriction) or too loose (resulting in wrinkles). Warn the patient or caregiver to examine the inside of the shoes before putting them on to be certain they are free of foreign objects

Stress the avoidance of walking barefooted and

the importance of wearing slippers when getting out of bed at night

Warn the patient of the dangers of using chemicals or razors to remove corns or calluses. Suggest using a pumice stone, a little each day, for callus removal. Calluses and hard, brittle toenails can be softened with warm wet washcloths

The skin of dry, nonsweating feet needs water and the treatment is to provide moisture without causing maceration (Brand and Coleman, 1990). Daily foot soaks for 15 to 20 minutes (warm not hot water) provide the water the skin needs to prevent drying and cracking, which leads to infection. Blot dry and dry between the toes with a hairdryer on cool temperature. Apply mineral oil or moisturizing cream (except between the toes) to prevent evaporation of the moisture (Brand and Coleman,1990; Sims et al, 1988)

Feet with infected wounds should not be soaked (Brand and Coleman, 1990)

Use mirrors to visualize the soles of the feet

Trim nails following the contour of the toes

Advise the regular services of a podiatrist for nail trimming when the nails are extremely thick

Explain to the patient that calluses can be the cause of foot ulceration by creating pressure and damaging the underlying tissue

In the nursing home setting, nursing assistants are the caregivers who are in a prime position to assess the feet as they dress and undress the patient. This calls for special instruction given by the professional nurse

EVALUATION

The elderly person will show no evidence of breaks in skin integrity on the feet. If living independently he will demonstrate proper foot care procedures. If living dependently either in the community or in a long-term care setting, the caregivers will demonstrate knowledge of daily diabetic foot care and report early signs of problems.

Nursing management of older persons who have diabetes requires skillful ongoing assessment of the current status of self care abilities or those of the caregiver. Because effective management of diabetes requires daily attention, changes in compliance with the regimens can have serious consequences. The prevalence of diabetes in the nursing home population mandates education of all levels of staff to prevent complications and hospitalization.

Resource List

American Diabetes Association
Washington, DC Area Affiliate, Inc.
1660 Duke Street
Alexandria, VA 22314
(703) 549–1500

Diabetes Supply Club
3510 NE 57th Ave
Portland, OR 97213
Portland (503) 287–9303
Oregon (800) DSC–CLUB
Outside Oregon (800) 358–2525

References and Other Readings

Allen B, DeLong E, Feussner J. Impact of glucose self-monitoring on non-insulin-treated patients with type II diabetes mellitus. Diabetes Care 1990; 13:1044.

American Diabetes Association WA NEWS. 1991; 5.

American Diabetes Association position statement: Office guide to diagnosis and classification of diabetes mellitus and other categories of glucose intolerance. Diabetes Care 1990; 13(suppl 1):3.

Anderson LA. Health-care communication and selected psychosocial correlates of adherence in diabetes management. Diabetes Care 1990; 13(suppl 2):66.

Andres R. Aging and diabetes. Med Clin North Am 1971; 55:835.

Bantle J. Injection site rotation. Practical Diabetology 1990; 9:1.

Bernbaum M, Albert S, Duckro P. Psychosocial profiles in patients with visual impairment due to diabetic retinopathy. Diabetes Care 1988; 11:551.

Bild D, Selby J, Sinnock P, et al. Lower-extremity amputation in people with diabetes: epidemiology and prevention. Diabetes Care 1989; 12:24.

Brand P, Coleman W. The diabetic foot. In Rifkin H, Porte D Jr, eds. Ellenberg and Rifkin's Diabetes Mellitus. New York: Elsevier, 1990:792.

Carpenito L. Nursing diagnosis: application to clinical practice, 3rd ed. New York: Lippincott, 1989.

Carpenito L. Nursing care plans and documentation: nursing diagnosis and collaborative problems. New York: Lippincott, 1991.

Christensen M, Funnell M, Ehrlichd M, et al. How to care for the diabetic foot. Am J Nurs 1991; 91:50.

Davidson M. Diabetes mellitus: diagnosis and treatment, 2nd ed. New York: Wiley, 1986.

Dellasega C. Self-care for the elderly diabetic. J Gerontol Nurs 1990; 16:16.

Forrester J. Mechanisms of new vessel formation in the retina. Diabetes Medicine 1987; 4:189.

Friedman E. Diabetic nephropathy. Diabetes Spectrum 1989; 2:86.

Funnell M, McNitt P. Autonomic neuropathy: diabetics' hidden foe. Am J Nurs 1986; 86:266.

Genuth S. Insulin use in NIDDM. Diabetes Care 1990; 13:1240.

Graham C. Exercise and aging: implications for persons with diabetes. Diabetes Educator 1991; 17:189.

Green D, Lattimer S, Ulbrecht J, et al. Glucose induced alterations in nerve metabolism, current perspective on the pathogenesis of diabetic neuropathy and future directions for research and therapy. Diabetes Care 1985; 8:290.

Guthrie D, Hinnen D, DeShetler E. Diabetes education: a core curriculum for diabetes educators. Chicago: American Association of Diabetes Educators, 1988.

Haire-Joshu D. Smoking, cessation and the diabetes health care team. Diabetes Educator 1991; 17:54.

Hernandez C. The pathophysiology of diabetes mellitus: an update. Diabetes Educator 1989; 15:162.

Hirsch I, McGill J. Role of insulin in management of surgical patients with diabetes mellitus. Diabetes Care 1990; 13:980.

Holler H, Pastors J. Nutrition guidelines and meal planning: a step by step process. Diabetes Spectrum 1991; 14:58.

Jackson R. Mechanisms of age-related glucose intolerance. Diabetes Care 1990; 13(suppl 2):9.

Kaplan N. Hyperinsulinemia and diabetes and hypertension. Clinical Diabetes 1991; 9:1.

Kumanyika S, Ewart C. Theoretical and baseline considerations for the diet and weight control of diabetes among blacks. Diabetes Care 1990; 13:1154.

Leahy J. Natural history of B-cell dysfunction in NIDDM. Diabetes Care 1990; 13:992.

Lebovits H, Pasmanter R. Combination insulin sulfonylurea therapy. Diabetes Care 1990; 13:667.

Levin M. Diabetic foot lesions: pathogenesis and management. Journal of Enterostomal Therapy 1990; 7:29.

Lima J. Lessening the risk: preventive diabetes foot care. Caring 1988; 7:42.

Madsbad S. Classification of diabetes in older adults. Diabetes Care 1990; 13(suppl 2):93.

Matz R. Summary and comment. Spectrum 1989; 2:3.

Messana I, Beizer J. Diabetes in the elderly, practical considerations. Practical Diabetology 1991; 10:4.

Minaher K. What diabetologists should know about elderly patients. Diabetes Care 1990; 13(suppl 2).

Morley J, Kaiser F. Unique aspects of diabetes mellitus in the elderly. Clinical Geriatric Medicine 1990; 6:693.

Mykkanen L, Laakso M, Uusitupa M, et al. Prevalence of diabetes and impaired glucose tolerance in elderly subjects and their association with obesity and family history of diabetes. Diabetes Care 1990; 13:1099.

National Center for Health Statistics. Advanced report, final mortality statistics 1980. Monthly Vital Statistic Report, vol 32, no. 4 suppl. Hyattsville, MD, PHS, August 1983, DHHS Publ 83-1120.

Nelson R. The OGTT. Diabetes Spectrum 1990; 2:219.

Newman D, Smith D. Geriatric care plans. Springhouse, PA: Springhouse, 1991.

Norstrom J. Get fit while you sit: exercise and fitness options for diabetics. Caring 1988; 7:52.

Permutt M. Genetics of NIDDM. Diabetes Care 1990; 13:1150.

Permutt M, Elbein S. Insulin gene in diabetes: analysis through RFLP. Diabetes Care 1990; 13:364.

Pfeifer M. Diabetic sexual dysfunction. Clinical Diabetes 1988; 6:97.

Podolsky S. The diabetic foot. In: Gambert SR, ed. Diabetes mellitus in the elderly: a practical guide. New York: Raven Press, 1990:87.

Porte D, Kahn S. What geriatricians should know about diabetes mellitus. Diabetes Care 1990; 13(suppl 2):47.

Reaven G, Thompson L, Nahum D, et al. Relationship between hyperglycemia and cognitive function in older NIDDM patients. Diabetes Care 1990; 13:16.

Schafer R. Implementation of low-protein diets for treatment of person with early diabetic nephropathy. Diabetes Educator 1989; 15:231.

Schreiner-Engel P. Diagnosing and treating the sexual problems of diabetic women. Clinical Diabetes 1988; 6:121.

Schwartz R. Exercise training in treatment of diabetes mellitus in elderly patients. Diabetes Care 1990; 13(suppl 2):77.

Selam J, Charles M. Devices for insulin administration. Diabetes Care 1990; 13:955.

Sims D, Cavanagh P, Ulbrecht J. Risk factors in the diabetic foot: recognition and management. Physical Therapy 1988; 68:1887.

Soulier S. The use of running shoes in the prevention of plantar diabetic ulcers. Journal of the American Podiatrist Association 1986; 76:395.

Tonino R. What should health-care providers in long-term nursing care facilities know about diabetes? Diabetes Care 1990; 13(suppl 2):55.

Tooke J. The microcirculation in diabetes. Diabetes Medicine 1987; 44:189.

Turner R, Holman R. Insulin use in NIDDM: rationale based on pathophysiology of disease. Diabetes Care 1990; 13:1011.

25
Gastrointestinal Problems

MARGARET HEITKEMPER   DORIS CARNEVALI

There are no clear-cut gastrointestinal disease entities that can be attributed directly to the aging process. There are several, however, that show a higher incidence in the elderly. In addition, other gastrointestinal disorders may have a greater impact on the elderly person's general physical and social well-being.

Little research has been done on the effects of aging on the main portions of the gastrointestinal tract. Systemic changes in the functions of digestion and absorption of nutrients seem to be more affected by changes in the cardiovascular and neurologic systems than in the gastrointestinal tract itself. Arteriosclerosis and other circulatory problems may result in reduced splanchnic blood flow and decreased absorption from the small intestine. Degenerative changes in the nervous system may decrease the motility of the esophagus, stomach, small intestine, and colon and thus increase or decrease transit time through the tract. Long-term pathology such as diabetes mellitus has been associated with peripheral neuropathy and may influence motility of the gastrointestinal tract, predisposing the person to gastric reflux and fecal incontinence.

Esophagus

ESOPHAGEAL MOTILITY ALTERATIONS

With increasing age, changes in esophageal motility begin to occur. Age-related changes include amplitude of contractions, increased resting pressure, and increased numbers of disordered contractions (Brandt, 1984).

This less effective functioning is thought to be related to degenerative changes in the smooth muscle that lines the lower two thirds of the esophagus. Neurogenic, humoral, and vascular changes may also contribute to decreased esophageal motility. Persons with accompanying diabetes mellitus, parkinsonism, brain stem infarct, or Raynaud's disease are more likely to experience abnormal esophageal motility. Hypothyroidism and hyperthyroidism may also produce changes in smooth and skeletal muscle function and result in altered esophageal motor function. Decreased esophageal peristalsis may be partially responsible for the long periods of time necessary for elderly persons to comfortably consume a sizeable meal or the necessity of several small meals to obtain adequate nutrition in the elderly population.

For many individuals changes in esophageal motility are subclinical and are only detected by radiographic or manometric studies. Esophageal motility disorders are considered when an individual complains of aspiration, nasal regurgitation, or dysphagia (Saladin, 1989).

However, some people do experience episodes of substernal pain and difficulty in swallowing. The substernal discomfort, produced by altered contractions of the esophagus, can be confused with the pain of angina—an occasional person experiencing pressure and radiation to the left chest wall from the substernal

479

discomfort. The representing symptoms may be confusing to both the patient and the nurse because the patient may have both coronary artery disease and esophageal dysfunction.

Esophageal motility disorders are generally characterized by intermittent rather than progressive symptoms. The person complains of inability to handle liquids as well as solids. Further, certain acidic foods such as citrus juices or tomato paste may cause problems; they are thought to stimulate abnormal esophageal motility as well as to affect the lower esophageal sphincter (LES).

REFLUX

Gastroesophageal reflux is a common problem in the elderly. Reflux of acid, depending on the amount and frequency, can pose an inherent danger to the esophageal mucosa and the lungs. Gastroesophageal reflux has been associated with hiatal hernia, increased intra-abdominal pressure, hormones, and certain foods. While reflux may occur due to a number of factors and diseases (e.g., scleroderma), hiatal hernia is one of the more common causes in the elderly.

The resting pressure of the LES has been shown to decrease with advancing age. Hiatal hernia frequently is seen in elderly persons with lowered LES pressure. However, a number of persons also will have symptomatic sphincter incompetence without hiatal hernia.

HIATAL HERNIA

DESCRIPTION

A hiatal hernia is the protrusion of the stomach into the thoracic cage through an opening in the diaphragm.

ETIOLOGIC FACTORS

Even under normal conditions the esophagus is not rigidly attached to the diaphragm as it enters the hiatal ring. Thus, even young individuals can exhibit herniation of the stomach through the hiatal ring of the diaphragm during increased abdominal pressure, such as in forceful vomiting or Valsalva maneuvers. Hiatal hernias in the aged may be the result of degenerative changes in the already weak supporting system. Individuals with lumbar kyphosis in which there is a widening of the diaphragm are also at risk for hiatal hernia. As a result the tran-

sient herniation may be exaggerated and more frequent.

HIGH-RISK POPULATION

The elderly are at high risk for hiatal hernias. The incidence may be as high as 40% to 60% in persons over age 60. Men aged 50 to 70 are at highest risk.

DYNAMICS

There are two common types of hiatal hernia. The parahiatal *rolling* type is a hernia through the diaphragm near the esophageal hiatus. With this type of hernia, the LES barrier mechanism remains intact. Complications include ulceration of the hernia and stricture.

The second type is the *sliding* hernia. This is the more common type. Here the fundic portion of the stomach slides directly through both the membranous and muscular openings of the diaphragm so that the gastroesophageal junction is above the diaphragm. In the sliding type the LES is patulous and incompetent, and reflux esophagitis and esophageal stricture tend to be more common. Pain may be described as a lump, pressure, or burning at the level of the xiphoid process, or as a severe vise-like pain. It may be referred to the epigastrium, along both costal margins, and to the back, upper thorax, or arms. It can be precipitated or made worse by bending, reclining, coughing, overeating, or exertion that increases intra-abdominal pressure. Walking about tends to bring relief, often abruptly.

SIGNS AND SYMPTOMS

The symptoms of alterations in esophageal motility or LES pressure are extremely variable. Frequently there are no symptoms. Distress when present can be severe or mild, intermittent or constant. Complaints, when they occur, will be of heartburn, sour stomach, or epigastric distress following the eating of certain types of foods. Symptoms tend to occur with a recumbent position. Recurrent episodes of pneumonia, bronchiectasis, or intractable cough may be indicators of esophageal reflux or obstruction with pulmonary aspiration.

DIFFERENTIAL DIAGNOSIS

Not only can esophageal hernias mimic angina and pulmonary distress, large esophageal hernias can also cause difficulty in swallowing. However, difficulty in swallowing may also be a primary symptom of esophageal cancer.

COMPLICATIONS

Esophageal reflux is the primary complication of hiatal hernia and incompetent LES. *Pulmonary problems* result from nighttime regurgitation of gastric contents or saliva into the respiratory tract. Elderly persons may be particularly prone to pulmonary aspiration owing to a diminished cough reflex. Also, because of the symptoms of episodic cough that generally interrupt the person's sleep, nighttime - aspirations may mimic congestive heart failure.

Esophageal reflux of gastric contents can lead to esophagitis. The acidic gastric juice corrodes the mucosal cells that line the esophagus. The esophagitis, in turn, is responsible for the sensations of substernal pain or heartburn. This pain of esophagitis may mimic angina pain. However, esophageal pain is generally associated with eating and with a recumbent position, whereas angina is related to exertion. Further, with esophagitis there are no blood pressure or heart rate changes. Where the patient has difficulty in differentiating the pain in terms of concurrent activities, the nurse will want to take a careful history of symptoms and associated activities.

Less common complications of hiatal hernia include *ulceration* of the fundic portion of the stomach, stricture, and hernia incarceration. These are serious complications in the older person and generally are accompanied by acute pain or symptoms of obstruction.

MEDICAL MANAGEMENT

Medical management of hiatal hernias usually is conservative. Surgery does not always correct the situation and relieve the symptoms, so that it tends to be reserved for use if medical measures fail and symptoms are severe or when complications such as bleeding or ulceration arise.

Antacids frequently are used for the relief of heartburn or esophagitis. They work through two avenues. First, they neutralize the acidity of the gastric juices and, therefore, decrease the corrosive effect of the reflux. Second, the alkalinization stimulates a release of gastrin (a gastrointestinal hormone) from the stomach; this acts to increase the resting pressure of the LES and blocks or minimizes the reflux of gastric juices. Side effects of prolonged antacid therapy are given in Table 25–1. One way to minimize side effects is to take the antacids in response to symptoms rather than on a regu-

TABLE 25–1 *Side Effects of Prolonged Antacid Therapy*

Antacid Ingredient	Possible Problems
Calcium carbonate Alkets, Camalox, Alka-2, Titralac, Tums, Dicarbosil	Gastric acid rebound, hypercalcemia, constipation, and decreased renal function; safe for low-dose occasional relief
Sodium bicarbonate* Soda Mint, Alka-Seltzer	Sodium overload. In large dose may produce systemic alkalosis, increase stomach pH, and increase acid output
Magnesium Milk of Magnesia, Chooz	Diarrhea. Use with caution in those with renal disease
Aluminum Amphojel, Basaljel	Constipation, phosphate depletion
Magnesium and aluminum hydroxide Maalox, Mylanta, Gelusil, Aludrox, Di-Gel, WinGel	Phosphate depletion syndrome, low sodium content. Can cause diarrhea or constipation

*Many pharmaceutical firms are reformulating their antacids to reduce the sodium content, so it would be wise to read the labels for sodium content rather than rely on previous information. It must be printed on the label if the antacid contains more than 0.2 mEq of sodium per dosage unit.

larly scheduled basis. Gaviscon, or other antacids containing sodium bicarbonate, have been found useful for esophageal reflux. These tablets taken after meals help to remove food particles that may be trapped as a result of the herniation. The antacid portion again neutralizes the gastric contents.

Another form of management is to ascertain whether particular foods cause greater difficulties (Saladin, 1989). Low fat or skim milk should be used to relieve heartburn rather than high fat whole milk. Chocolate, tea, ethanol, cola, and caffeine have also been found to reduce the LES resting pressure and, therefore, should be limited or avoided. Reducing the amount of animal fat or saturated fats in the diet has been found to be particularly useful. Elimination of alcohol is also beneficial. Smaller, more frequent feedings have been found to be helpful. Walking about after eating effectively uses

gravity to empty the esophagus and fundus. Lying down after eating is to be avoided.

The increased risk of reflux in the recumbent position can be decreased by elevating the head of the bed on blocks or bricks for sleep and rest. Drugs commonly used in the elderly patient such as theophylline, beta-adrenergic agonists, alpha-adrenergic antagonists, dopamine, diazepam, and calcium channel blocking agents increase the problem of reflux (Cattau and Castel, 1982).

Table 25–2 summarizes the problems, signs and symptoms, and nursing management in hiatal hernia.

Stomach

Little is known at this time about the effect of aging on the stomach. The age-related decrease

TABLE 25–2   *Summary of Hiatal Hernia*

Problem	Assessment	Nursing Care
Motility disorder	Episodic substernal discomfort	Feed slowly—never rush the individual
	Difficulty swallowing liquids rather than solids	Give thick liquids; soak liquids up with bread, toast, crackers, or cookies
	Complaints of difficulty taking medications	Increase neural stimulation; give frozen or very cold liquids; mix medication with ice cream or sherbert
Esophageal reflux	Complaints of heartburn; pain or epigastric distress after eating; in very impaired elderly, there is confusion, agitation, increased motor activity, rubbing epigastric or lower abdomen following a meal or during a meal, belching following a meal	Keep head of bed elevated on 4- to 6"-blocks after eating; could roll up head of bed 45°; encourage not to lie down following a meal for 45 min to 1 hr and to walk about following eating; encourage low fat diet, decrease in cholesterol, avoidance of chocolate, cola, coffee, alcohol; watch for side effects of antacids and anticholinergics that may be used (see Table 25–3); encourage to avoid large meals that result in increased abdominal pressure; discourage eructation and air swallowing; make sure dentures fit
Nocturnal aspiration	Intractable cough, recurrent pneumonia	No eating 1–2 hr before bedtime; no fluids before bedtime; head of bed slightly elevated at 30°; encourage to sleep on side at night
Herniation (sliding or rolling)	May be palpable	Avoid conditions that increase abdominal pressure such as tight-fitting clothing, corsets; encourage to avoid heavy lifting or straining and to reduce weight if obese

in hydrochloric acid may be the result of gastric cell loss, as in gastric atrophy or chronic atrophic gastritis. Functionally, the relative decrease in stomach acidity could reduce the solubility of acidic drugs such as aspirin (Hanan, 1978). It also is thought to hamper the absorption of iron and calcium. A decrease in hydrochloric acid may leave the elderly person more vulnerable to gastroenteritis secondary to ingestion of contaminated food. Because there is little evidence of changes in the stomach related to normal aging, it becomes important to view the older person's gastric complaints as presenting the likelihood of pathology. Therefore, gastric complaints merit investigation because they are likely to be genuine health problems.

CHRONIC ATROPHIC GASTRITIS

DESCRIPTION

Chronic atrophic gastritis, as the name implies, is an inflammatory phenomenon in which the mucosa becomes thinned, gray or greenish-gray, and abnormally smooth, with hemorrhagic patches. It is usually distributed irregularly, but the entire stomach may be involved. Superficial gastritis is said to occur in 50% of people after the fourth decade (Saladin, 1989).

ETIOLOGIC FACTORS

The etiologic factors of chronic atrophic gastritis are not known. However, the disease is associated with aging. It has been found to occur with gastric ulcer, recurrent gastritis, pernicious anemia, and iron deficiency anemia. Dietary patterns, such as use of alcohol, tobacco, or coffee, and nutritional deficiencies have been suggested as contributors, but the linkage is inconclusive. It may also be an autoimmune disorder since some individuals with type A gastritis have circulating parietal cell antibodies that are directed against the gastric mucosa. The presence of parietal cell antibodies increases with age. These antibodies have been associated with the development of pernicious anemia. However, not all individuals with parietal cell antibodies develop pernicious anemia. Drugs that cause damage directly to gastric mucosal cells such as aspirin, alcohol, and Butazolidin (phenylbutazone) may also be a factor. Corticosteroids may also be potentially destructive to the gastric mucosal barrier, although the exact mechanism has not been determined. Another potential factor in the development of gastritis and peptic ulcers, particularly type B gastritis, which affects the antrum, is *Helicobacter pylori*. *H pylori* has been isolated in the stomachs of individuals with gastritis; however, it is not known whether the organism causes gastritis or invades the area secondary to the inflammation. There is an age-related increase in the population of gastric *H pylori* (Perez-Perez et al, 1988). In this type of gastritis, bismuth and amoxicillin are used to eradicate the organism.

HIGH-RISK POPULATION

Gastric atrophy and chronic atrophic gastritis have been determined to increase with advancing age.

DYNAMICS

The entire stomach wall is involved in the cellular changes. The mucosa is thin with hemorrhagic patches, the submucosal vessels are visible as red or blue ramifications, and the folds are diminished in size and number. All layers are atrophied. As the severity or degree of atrophic gastritis increases there is a concurrent decrease in chief and parietal (pepsin and hydrochloric acid-secreting) cells. These cells are replaced by goblet cells and fibrous tissue. With the loss of parietal cells there is a decrease in acid output and intrinsic factor secretion. There is disappearance of glandular cells and increase in fibrous tissue. The course is persistent or recurrent with alternate erosions, hemorrhage, and healing.

SIGNS AND SYMPTOMS

The evaluation of symptoms is often difficult. Chronic atrophic gastritis can be demonstrated to exist without symptoms. Symptoms, when they do exist, are varied and vague, nor can their type and severity be correlated with the severity of the gastritis. The most frequent symptoms are loss of appetite, vague epigastric pain, belching, feeling of fullness, nausea, and vomiting.

COMPLICATIONS

Hypochromic microcytic anemia and iron deficiency anemia are both associated with atrophic gastritis. Anemia is a potential complication of chronic atrophic gastritis. In addition, intrinsic factor may be decreased as a result of either cell loss or decreased stomach acidity. Since intrinsic factor is responsible for the absorption of vitamin B_{12} in the terminal ileum, patients with advanced chronic atrophic gastritis may develop a vitamin B_{12} deficiency that may border on pernicious anemia; however, progression to a full-blown state of pernicious anemia is rare. The risk of vitamin deficiency is slightly greater in women than men. Atrophic gastritis has also been associated with a higher than normal risk of gastric carcinoma.

MEDICAL MANAGEMENT

Symptoms may be relieved by the use of a bland diet, small feedings, and antacids, antisecretory and antispasmodic drugs. This does not treat the underlying pathology but can make the person more comfortable. Patients are monitored at regular intervals for the presence of gastric carcinoma.

EVALUATION

Evaluation criteria concern management of symptoms, control of associated anemia, and the person's ability to manage and obtain satisfaction from the diet.

ULCERS

Both gastric and duodenal ulcers occur in the elderly, with gastric ulcers being the more common. The incidence of peptic ulcers necessitating hospitalization or surgery over the past 20 years have decreased in all age groups except the elderly (Shamburek and Farrar, 1990; Kurata and Corboy, 1988). In particular there has been a marked increase in the number of women over 65 with gastric ulcers (Kurata et al, 1985). Deaths among the elderly from peptic ulcers are increasing, while deaths from stomach malignancies are decreasing.

ETIOLOGIC FACTORS

Ulcer disease in the elderly may be a continuation of a chronic problem that originated in the fourth, fifth, or sixth decades. Ulcers are seen to be related to stress in the elderly, as complications of other diseases and trauma. Drug-induced ulcers are also common among the elderly who take many more drugs than younger persons. Alcohol consumption and smoking may also predispose to ulcer development. Regardless of the etiology, the consequences of gastrointestinal bleeding are much more severe in the elderly.

HIGH-RISK POPULATION

Any elderly person experiencing a major body insult, whether medical or psychogenic, is at risk of ulcer development, particularly if a pre-existent atrophic gastritis is present. Some events known to have precipitated peptic ulcers include fractures, pneumonia, and admission to a nursing home—conditions and circumstances that initially may seem quite unrelated to peptic ulcers. Persons who have had strokes or who have chronic obstructive pulmonary disease are at greater risk of peptic ulcers because of attendant rehabilitation and social stresses associated with these illnesses.

Those on ulcerogenic drugs such as aspirin, reserpine, tolbutamide, phenylbutazone, colchicine, corticotropin, or adrenal cortical steroids also need to be observed for peptic ulcers. In a study of patients over 65 years old, 40% admitted for upper gastrointestinal bleeding and 30% admitted for perforation were taking anti-inflammatory drugs (Watson et al, 1985).

SIGNS AND SYMPTOMS

Peptic ulcer disease in the elderly presents differently from the symptoms in younger patients. Epigastric pain is not a prominent feature. More frequently the outstanding symptoms in elderly people include poorly localized pain, decreased appetite, decreased general energy level, melena, weight loss, vomiting, and anemia. Systemic responses to blood loss and anemia may be the dominant indicators. For example, dyspnea secondary to blood loss and anemia-induced heart failure may be a presenting symptom (Saladin, 1989).

The usual symptom of bleeding is not a cardinal symptom of ulcer disease in the elderly. It is more common to see sudden onset of hemorrhagic bleeding resulting from the perforation of an ulcer rather than minor or occult bleeding episodes. Ulcer development in the elderly is an insidious process that may be diagnosed only by upper gastrointestinal roentgenography studies. Before roentgenography, astute and sensitive nursing observations that are attendant to changes in normal eating patterns, energy levels, and body weight status may be the only clues of gastric pathology.

DIFFERENTIAL DIAGNOSIS

Duodenal ulcers are ten times more common than gastric ulcers in the general population. Duodenal ulcers occur primarily in the young and middle-aged adult, whereas gastric ulcers are more common in the elderly person, particularly those with drug-induced ulcer disease. It becomes important, therefore, that differential diagnosis be made between gastric ulcers and gastric carcinoma lesions. Symptoms are similar. The malignancies have been known to occur more commonly in men.

Medical philosophies of therapy vary. Some physicians believe that because the prognosis is so guarded for stomach malignancies, if there is a possibility that the disease is benign, conservative treatment should be tried for a few weeks. Gastric ulcers improve or disappear in 4 to 6 weeks with adequate treatment. Smoking delays the healing of gastric and duodenal ulcers.

Ulcers, like many other physical illness syndromes in the elderly, may present as depression. A careful history of eating patterns, stress, drugs, ulcer risk factors, and signs and symptoms becomes important.

COMPLICATIONS

Complications accompanying peptic ulcer disease are of particular importance in the elderly person because of the high risk involved in emergency surgical procedures. Bleeding is the most significant complication of peptic ulcers. Other complications include obstruction and perforation, both of which have a high mortality in the elderly age group.

Fluid dynamics involved in treatment of the complications create risks in themselves. Excessive or overly rapid flow of blood transfusions may precipitate congestive heart failure in the older person, while sudden loss of blood volume through hemorrhage increases the risk of stroke or central nervous system cell death resulting from hypoxia.

MEDICAL MANAGEMENT

Conservative management of gastric and duodenal ulcer disease in the elderly person is preferred because any type of surgical procedure poses many risks. However, surgical procedures are required for those patients who cannot be managed medically and in those in whom gastric cancer is suspected. Elective surgery (i.e., gastrectomy) may be performed to reduce the mortality associated with emergency surgical management.

Some of the earlier strategies in conservative management are now open to question. Half-and-half or whole milk, once a standard treatment, has been found to cause a rebound acid output as well as to increase blood cholesterol levels, which may be particularly counterproductive in an older person. Low fat or skim milk is preferable.

Agents known to increase hydrochloric acid production should be avoided. These include alcohol; caffeine-containing beverages such as coffee and colas; spices such as curry, pepper, and mustard; and tobacco. Antacids play an important role in the symptomatic relief of peptic ulcer pain. They neutralize gastric juice and thus reduce irritation and further ulceration; however, they appear to have little role in the actual healing process. Although there is no debate about their usefulness, they can create some problems for the user, particularly the older person. The nurse can consider these in terms of the presenting problem of the patient—low sodium diet, tendency toward diarrhea or constipation, edema, or renal disease. Some antacids increase secretion of acid. Besides these problems, aluminum hydroxide gels and antacids with calcium and magnesium bind antibiotics such as tetracycline. The absorption of other drugs such as pseudoephrine are improved by the increase in gastric pH produced by antacids.

The advent of histamine (H_2) blockers (e.g., cimetidine and ranitidine) has markedly altered the course of ulcer therapy. H_2 receptor blockers decrease acid secretion by preventing the stimulation of parietal cells. These drugs promote healing of an ulcer. However, they are also used prophylactically in persons at risk for ulcer formation. A small percentage of people have the side effects of confusion and sexual impotence. Because these drugs are cleared by the kidney, adequate renal function is important. In patients over 50 years of age the half-life of these drugs is increased. Because antacids may delay the absorption of cimetidine in fasting patients, they should be administered 1 hour apart. Another drug that promotes ulcer healing is sucralfate, a nonsystemic agent that has a protective effect on irritated mucosa. This drug has a specific advantage for persons with liver disease in that it is nonabsorbable.

Antacids decrease the absorption of tetracycline and ferrous sulfate, as well as some acidic drugs such as isoniazid, penicillin, sulfonamides, and salicylates. Antacids should not be given concurrently with enteric coated tablets. In an alkaline environment the acid-resistant coating is broken down and the drug is released in the stomach rather than the intestine. This can result in gastric irritation as well as alteration in drug absorption.

Anticholinergics are given occasionally to decrease acid output. Anticholinergics (e.g., Belap and Pro-Banthine) and synthetic anticholinergics (e.g., Bentyl and Valpin) generally are given three to four times per day, before meals and at bedtime. They help to reduce acidity and hypermotility. However, they should be ad-

ministered cautiously to the older person. Long-term anticholinergic administration can result in a variety of serious side effects. The nurse and the patient should be alert to the signs and symptoms listed in Table 25–3.

Small Intestine

The functions of the small intestine of digestion and absorption of nutrients tend not to be affected by aging despite some ultrastructural changes, e.g., flattening of the intestinal villi. However, pathology such as inflammation and infection can result in functional changes.

MALABSORPTION

Malabsorption in the elderly is most likely the result of pathology, previous bowel resection,

---

TABLE 25–3   *Side Effects of Anticholinergic Medications*

Mouth	Dryness owing to reduced salivation may make swallowing difficult and increase dental diseases
	Dryness of the respiratory tract is particularly critical for the patient with chronic lung disease
Skin	Dry, hot, red because of decreased sweating and vasodilation
	Interference with normal cooling mechanisms may predispose the elderly to hyperpyrexia, with resultant dehydration in warm weather or hot climates
Eyes	Possible photophobia resulting from widely dilated pupils
	Vision blurred owing to paralysis of accommodation
	Crowding of iris and ciliary muscle into angle of eye chamber may raise intraocular pressure by interfering with draining of the aqueous humor
	These drugs are contraindicated in patients with narrow angle glaucoma
	Caution in all elderly patients owing to the increased incidence of acute, and prevalence of chronic, glaucoma
Urinary tract	Urine retention may occur as a result of loss of bladder tone
	Elderly men with prostatic hypertrophy are particularly at risk
Heart	Due to loss of vagal control, side effects of prolonged tachycardia episodes may include coronary insufficiency, chest pain, and cardiac decompensation (CHF) in patients with a history of heart disease
Constipation	Result of reduced tone and motility of gastrointestinal musculature
	Particularly at risk is the elderly patient with decreased physical exercise, decreased food volume consumption, and low-residue dietary pattern
Central nervous system	Anticholinergic psychosis
	Confusion, disorientation, belligerence, paranoia-type delusions, dizziness, delirium
	Particularly at risk is the elderly patient who may be receiving anticholinergic medication for psychiatric conditions, e.g., depression

or inadequate nutritional intake secondary to decreased financial resources or limited mobility rather than age per se. Changes in the stomach (gastritis) and exocrine pancreas can also result in absorption problems. Malabsorption may be detected by blood chemistry, hematology (e.g., anemia), and physical manifestations (see Chapter 12 on Nutrition).

INFLAMMATORY BOWEL DISEASE

Colitis in the elderly may result from inflammatory bowel disease or from ischemia (Texter et al, 1983; Brandt et al, 1981). Crohn's disease and ulcerative colitis were once thought to occur only in young adults. However, inflammatory bowel disease has a bimodal distribution, with a second smaller peak occurring in the 60 to 70 age group (Harper et al, 1986). Ten percent or more of patients with Crohn's disease have their first attack after the age of 60. When it occurs in the older population the mortality is higher. Recurrent bouts of diarrhea and intestinal bleeding are particularly debilitating in the older person. Because inflammatory bowel disease is considered unusual in the older person, diagnosis may be delayed.

ETIOLOGY

The etiology of inflammatory bowel disease in any age group is unknown. Idiopathic inflammatory bowel disease is responsible for approximately 5% to 10% of the inflammatory bowel disease noted in persons over 65 years of age.

SIGNS AND SYMPTOMS

Inflammatory bowel disease manifests in periods of diarrhea, which may be bloody, particularly if the colon is involved. Abdominal cramping, if present, tends to be more diffuse than in younger persons. Because of the individual's age, such symptoms may be mistaken for diverticulitis or infectious diarrhea, which may delay diagnosis and treatment.

COMPLICATIONS

Recurrent or prolonged bouts of diarrhea can produce significant reductions in circulating fluids as well as electrolyte imbalances (e.g., water deficit, hypokalemia), both of which are particularly hazardous in the elderly. A minority of older persons develop fulminating inflammatory bowel disease. Acute and chronic bowel obstruction can also be complications of inflammatory bowel disease.

TREATMENT

Treatment for inflammatory bowel disease in the elderly is much the same as for the young, except that about 50% of the elderly require surgery and thus the morbidity and mortality is considerably higher. Conservative management includes steroid therapy such as prednisone, use of sulfasalazine (Azulfidine), and possibly immunosuppressive treatment. Corticosteroids may exacerbate problems with osteoporosis and diabetes.

ISCHEMIC BOWEL DISEASE

Age-related alterations in the blood supply to the small and large intestine can result in ischemic bowel disease. Occlusive disease can result from thrombus formation or emboli. Therefore, patients with atrial fibrillation, myocardial infarction, and rheumatic valvular heart disease would be at risk. This type of occlusion is generally acute and the patient experiences cramping pain followed by more generalized abdominal discomfort. With decreased perfusion to the gastrointestinal tract there is loss of function that may be acute or chronic. In addition, the presence of vasospasm may exaggerate or increase the size of the ischemic lesion.

Colon

DIVERTICULOSIS

DESCRIPTION

Diverticulosis is the herniation or sacculation of the mucosa. They occur at specific anatomic locations, such as the points of penetrations of the muscle wall by nutrient arteries. This begins to develop at about age 50, with sacculations increasing in number and size with age. They are located predominantly in the sigmoid portion of the left colon.

ETIOLOGIC FACTORS

This is a disease of aging, with atrophy of the musculature in the intestinal wall seen as a contributing factor. Because of its geographic distribution in western countries where refined foods are used, diet is thought to be a factor. The refined, low residue foods are thought to alter the colonic motility, with higher intraluminal pressures in the colon created as a result of sustained muscular contractions. In time, such abnormally high pressures may lead to the outpouching of the mucosa. Aging results in a decrease in elasticity of the intestinal wall. This also predisposes to the development of the diverticuli. Constipation, obesity, and emotional tension have also been suggested as contributors.

HIGH-RISK POPULATION

The risk of diverticulosis increases with age (40% of people over age 70 are estimated to have diverticulosis), obesity, constipation, presence of hiatal hernia, history of diet high in refined, low residue foods, and emotional tension.

SIGNS AND SYMPTOMS

The majority of persons with diverticulosis are asymptomatic. This is because the diverticuli themselves do not interfere with the normal function of the colon. Symptoms, when they occur, may be due to the increased motor activity of the sigmoid colon and factors that enhance it. They may take the form of pain in the lower abdomen, occurring or increasing in severity at a definite interval after meals or following emotional disturbance, being relieved or temporarily abolished by a bowel movement. Diverticulosis may also result in slight rectal bleeding.

DIFFERENTIAL DIAGNOSIS

Careful investigation to rule out other lesions causing rectal bleeding must precede the diagnosis of diverticulosis. Fiberoptic sigmoidoscopy can be used for direct visualization of the diverticuli opening. However, diagnosis is generally made by barium enema studies.

COMPLICATIONS

Diverticulitis occurs in a few persons with diverticulosis, more commonly among men. It is precipitated by obesity, eating irritating foods, or alcohol. Severe coughing or straining at stool may also contribute to the development of inflammation. A small perforation of a diverticulum and the associated peridiverticulitis causes the symptoms of left lower quadrant pain, chills, fever, constipation or diarrhea, nausea and vomiting, and gross blood in the feces. Diverticulitis is also associated with leukocytosis.

Because of the close approximation of the diverticuli to the nutrient arteries, arterial bleeding can occur. Most of these episodes stop spontaneously. Serious complications include major bleeding, perforation, peritonitis, abscess formation, fistulae, and obstruction.

MEDICAL MANAGEMENT

Eating is an important part of the life of elderly people. Much of their lives focuses on food and activities around food. It is used as rewards and in social activities. Nurses in their daily questioning of patients ask about food and liquid intake and related area (bowels), so it should come as no surprise when patients remark about these same areas. An accurate dietary history is the beginning of effective diverticulosis management.

Diverticulosis is managed by use of a nonspicy diet, weight reduction if the individual is obese, management of constipation, and administration of an iron supplement if anemia occurs. The role of fiber supplementation in the prevention of diverticuli formation remains to be proven. Although fiber and in particular, bran, are often recommended for prevention of complications, the efficacy of this treatment still remains questionable. Because it is thought that dry, hard feces may precipitate the inflammation, fiber supplementation that increases fecal water as well as keeping the stool soft may be helpful. Fiber also has positive effects on constipation and symptoms of irritable bowel syndrome, which often occur in the patient with diverticulosis. If hypermotility is a problem, anticholinergic drugs may be used. (See Table 25–3 for important side effects in the elderly.) Harsh laxatives should be avoided in managing this type of constipation.

HEMORRHOIDS

DESCRIPTION

Hemorrhoids are swollen or dilated superior hemorrhoidal plexus veins that can be located internally or externally. Those located externally are covered by skin, whereas internal hemorrhoids are covered by mucous membranes.

ETIOLOGIC FACTORS

Hemorrhoids are caused or aggravated by factors that increase intra-abdominal pressure or partial obstruction of venous return, e.g., constipation and straining to defecate, portal hypertension, and congestive failure.

HIGH RISK

Usually hemorrhoids have developed at a younger age, particularly among persons who have had occupations that required long periods of standing, e.g., barbers, dentists, surgeons, and scrub nurses. They also tend to occur in women who have had one or more pregnancies. Persons with a history of constipation, congestive heart failure, and portal hypertension also are at higher risk.

SIGNS AND SYMPTOMS

Clinical manifestations include perianal itching and pain. Bleeding may also occur. Typically it is seen as bright streaking on the surface of the stool; however, it may be more extensive than this. Pain is usually the result of thrombosis of external hemorrhoids and increases with defecation.

COMPLICATIONS

Thrombus formation and strangulation of the blood vessels are the most common complications. Both are accompanied by severe pain. Some individuals find that certain foods such as fresh pineapple, mangos, and certain nuts also increase irritation and pain. Anemia is a risk associated with extensive or ongoing bleeding.

DIFFERENTIAL DIAGNOSIS

Rectal bleeding should always be taken seriously in the older age group and checked out medically. One source of anemia could be rectal bleeding.

Rectal bleeding is one of the earliest signs of rectal or colon cancer. Cancer of the colon is common in the older population. Bright bleeding can also occur with rectal polyps.

MEDICAL MANAGEMENT

Management of hemorrhoids usually is conservative. Surgery is used only if there is disabling pain, bleeding sufficient to cause anemia, or severe anal itching. Hemorrhoids may recur following surgery.

Day-to-day management of hemorrhoids involves stool softeners or bulk-forming agents to control constipation and reduce straining. Pain and pruritus usually can be controlled by soaking in warm water in the tub or sitz bath several times a day, washing the area after bowel movements, and application of anorectal preparations. These ointments or creams usually contain an anesthetic agent and emollients. Some also include corticosteroids. Topical preparations are more effective than suppositories because the suppository moves into the upper rectum and does not deposit the medication in the area requiring treatment. Prolapsed hemorrhoids sometimes can be pushed manually back into the rectum to provide relief. Symptomatic relief during acutely painful episodes may be provided by decreasing the amount of time spent standing and by elevating the feet and legs when sitting or lying in bed.

EVALUATION

Criteria for evaluation of response to management include the person's ability to participate in control of constipation, hygiene measures, and use of the topical medication. Ultimate evaluation is the relief of symptoms and control of associated anemia.

DIARRHEA

Diarrhea can be a more serious problem in the person over 70 than it is in the younger age group. It is a particular risk for those who already have a precarious fluid and electrolyte balance because of other conditions or drug treatment that fosters imbalance in electrolytes and dehydration.

DESCRIPTION

Diarrhea is the frequent passage of unformed stools, a result of increased bowel motility or interference with the normal absorption of water and nutrients from the bowel. Because of the great variability in the definition of the term diarrhea, it is important to have the patient describe his definition of diarrhea.

ETIOLOGIC FACTORS

The older person, the same as a younger person, is subject to intestinal infections and food poisoning that cause diarrhea. Diarrhea also is associated with irritable bowel syndrome and diverticulitis. Diarrhea may also be a symptom of inflammatory bowel disease (see earlier section). Malignancy will change bowel habits, including diarrhea. Emotions and stress, anticipation of an event, or concern about a problem can cause diarrhea. Fecal impaction should be considered a cause of diarrhea when there is history of constipation. This can be checked easily by doing a rectal examination.

Medication-incurred diarrhea is a more frequent cause of diarrhea in the over-60 age group. Drugs that produce diarrhea (in addition to laxatives taken for this purpose) include the following:

- Broad-spectrum antibiotics (by altering the normal bowel flora)—ampicillin, clindamycin, lincomycin, tetracycline, neomycin, and cephalexin (Kefiex)
- Guanethidine (Ismelin) (can cause profound diarrhea)
- Colchicine
- Ferrous sulfate
- Antituberculin
- Magnesium-containing antacids—Gelusil M, Kolantyl Gel, Maalox, Mylanta, Riopan, Amphojel

Drug-induced diarrhea tends to be mild. It may begin acute or may be chronic. Abdominal cramping and fever usually are not present. The exception is the patient on broad-spectrum antibiotics who develops staphylococcal enterocolitis where fever, severe diarrhea, and crampy abdominal pain are present. This situation should be called to the physician's attention promptly.

DYNAMICS

The mechanism of diarrhea can be classified as osmotic, secretory, or mixed. Under normal conditions the stool content of water and electrolytes (Na and K) remain relatively constant despite dietary intake. The type of diarrhea that occurs affects the nature of electrolyte balance and it is especially important, with the elderly, to predict the nature of losses that are occurring and replace them.

Secretory diarrhea results from an excessive stimulation or irritation of the intestinal mucosa. As a result, an excessive secretion of electrolytes occurs—especially sodium. The increased luminal Na content cannot be totally conserved by the colon and, as a result, Na is lost in the feces. Water will follow the Na and move out of the mucosa into the lumen. The

result is a high risk of dehydration. The stool pH is usually neutral, approximately 7.

Secretory diarrhea results from either exogenous sources such as enteric infections or endogenous secretagogues such as deconjugated bile salts. Neoplasms may cause secretory diarrhea also. In the elderly person who has undergone gastric or intestinal resection surgery, secretory diarrhea may occur as a result of intestinal stasis with subsequent bacterial overgrowth. Decreased peristalsis of the small intestine associated with diabetic neuropathy may also lead to bacterial overgrowth and secretory diarrhea (Sodeman, 1989).

Osmotic diarrhea occurs when unabsorbed intestinal solute draws water into the intestinal lumen. The presence of solute also holds water in the lumen, and diarrhea occurs when the solute and water load exceeds the absorptive capacity of the colon. Sorbitol, a substance food in sugar-free gums and candies, acts as an osmotic cathartic and can produce diarrhea. Fructose, which is found in many carbonated beverages, is also only partially absorbed and thus acts as an osmotic cathartic.

Gastric surgery can precipitate osmotic diarrhea through rapid gastric emptying. The hyperosmotic chyme dumped into the duodenum draws water into the lumen. Laxatives such as lactulose and sorbitol, which are nonabsorbable, increase the solute content in the lumen, as do antacids that contain magnesium.

Osmotic diarrhea differs from secretory diarrhea in that it causes potassium loss (in excess of sodium). For patients on potassium-losing diuretics this places them at high and early risk of hypokalemia. Also, in contrast to secretory diarrhea, osmotic diarrhea causes the stool to be acidic as a result of fermentation of unabsorbed solute. Both forms of diarrhea cause water loss and dehydration.

SIGNS AND SYMPTOMS

The person will have stools that are more frequent and more liquid than normal. Diarrhea may or may not be associated with cramping or fever, depending on the cause. Onset may be sudden or slow. Green or yellow–green may imply intense diarrhea with very rapid transit through the small intestine. Mucus is an indicator of an inflammatory process in the colon. Bleeding may occur, as in diverticulitis.

Data should be gathered on usual bowel and dietary patterns; onset of diarrhea; frequency and consistency of stools; associated symptoms; stress; what food was eaten; and any changes of eating, activities, or medication taking, including over-the-counter drugs.

COMPLICATIONS

In the elderly person with diarrhea, the complication of highest risk is electrolyte imbalance (Na^+ and K^+) and saline depletion. Symptoms of saline depletion should be noted. They include furrowed brown tongue, sunken cheeks, loss of skin turgor, orthostatic hypotension, increased hematocrit with stable hemoglobin, flat neck veins, and thirst. With electrolyte imbalance, lassitude is an important added feature.

Of particular importance is the risk of hypokalemia. It is very common but may go unrecognized because the symptoms are apathy, malaise, lassitude, cardiac arrhythmias, profound weakness, and even general paralysis. When the individual is on diuretics, or has a history of low potassium values, the nurse needs to be alert to both the risks and the insidious presenting symptoms. It is validated by a low serum potassium level. Agate (1986) suggests that it is wise to suspect hypokalemia in any older person showing lassitude, weakness, or prostration when there is also doubt about hydration. The hypokalemia is treatable but, when missed, is quickly fatal.

MEDICAL MANAGEMENT

The management of diarrhea depends on the cause. Discontinuation of medications causing diarrhea usually results in a return to normal within 1 to 3 days. Where there is any indication of possible impaction, a rectal examination should be done before suggesting the use of any antidiarrheal medications. Maintaining fluid intake during and following diarrhea as well as replacing lost fluids and electrolytes is crucial. A nonirritating diet is important until the symptoms subside.

If the diarrhea is a response to lactase deficiency, as may occur following gastric resections, the treatment is to avoid milk and milk products.

Categories of drugs used to treat diarrhea are adsorbents, demulcents, intestinal flora modifiers, and astringents. In addition, fluid and electrolytes are administered to replace diarrheal fluids and ions. Systematically acting antidiarrheals are derivatives of either opium or belladonna. Table 25–4 lists actions of various drugs. It is wise to remember, however, that undertreatment is better than overtreatment with drugs.

TABLE 25–4 *Pharmacologic Treatment of Diarrhea*

Drugs	Reactions
SYSTEMIC	
Opiates	Decrease hyperperistaltic movement. Intestinal contents slow, allowing absorption of water and electrolyte. CNS depressants
LOCAL	
Adsorbents Aluminum hydroxide Activated charcoal Kaolin Bismuth subsalts Magnesium trisillicate Pectin Cholestyramine Psyllium Lactobacillus Methylcellulose	Frequently found in nonprescription drugs. Adsorption is not a specific action; it can also adsorb other drugs given at the same time
Anticholinergics Belladonna	Decrease intestinal tone. Usually require prescription. Do not give to people with glaucoma. Stop if blurred vision, vertigo, rapid pulse, or eye pain develops

Risks of additional fluid loss because of the temperature of the environment is important in those who are dehydrated. High temperatures can occur daily in warm climates or during summer months. Problems can also occur in winter when rooms are kept at high temperatures and low humidity. Orthostatic hypotension due to saline depletion may also be a problem that jeopardizes the person's safety.

Because of the precarious fluid imbalance in the elderly, electrolytes should be drawn to accurately judge the status of the patient. Sodium and potassium may need to be replaced intravenously during the diarrhea. Diarrhea caused by food poisoning will run its course in several days. This may be too long for a patient to go without medical attention. Fluids and calories need to be maintained during the course of the diarrhea.

The nurse should treat diarrhea in an older patient as a potential emergency. This includes carefully monitoring the person, consulting with the physician, and initiating supportive therapies to prevent complications. A return to normal bowel flora is the aim of treatment once diarrhea has stopped, and this can be achieved by giving fermented dairy products, i.e., buttermilk or yogurt.

Some people have irritable bowel syndrome, which is characterized by alternating periods of constipation and diarrhea. It is essential for management to begin with identification and elimination of foods that tend to irritate the bowel. These individuals frequently benefit from the addition of bran to the diet. Bran slows down intestinal transit in those with diarrhea and facilitates stool passage in persons with constipation. Gas-producing foods can be particularly irritating.

CONSTIPATION

Constipation is one of the most common complaints of older people and a problem nurses spend considerable time resolving. Constipation can be acute or chronic (intermittent or constant). It has been estimated that 15% to 30% of people over age 60 take one or more laxatives each week. However, the idea that all old people have or will have constipation as a result of "wearing out" of the gastrointestinal tract in the course of normal aging is not valid.

DESCRIPTION

Constipation is viewed as an alteration from the individual's normal bowel pattern. There is a decrease in the number of bowel movements. Feces usually are firm and dry and accumulate in the descending colon. Evacuation is difficult. Stool weights normally decrease with age beginning around the sixth decade.

Not everyone has a bowel movement every day, nor should this be expected. People establish their own bowel functioning patterns of frequency and times of day. The range of normal frequency of bowel movements is from three times a day to three times a week. In the United States most individuals have one to two bowel movements per day.

Normal fecal matter consists mainly of water, bacteria, undigested cellulose, mucus, cell debris from the turnover of the intestinal epithelium, bile pigments, and small amounts of salt. Primarily it is the lower bowel that functions in storing and controlling the release of fecal material. It also has secretory and absorption functions that are of primary interest in the aged population. Mucus is secreted primarily by the goblet cells to lubricate the feces. Its volume is increased by drugs or any other condition that stimulates the parasympathetic nerves and is decreased by stimulation of the sympathetic nerves. Absorption within the lower bowel is the active transport of sodium with the resultant reabsorption of water. Fecal material left in the bowel for long periods of time will reabsorb almost all the water, resulting in hard dry pellets of fecal material, or constipation.

ETIOLOGIC FACTORS

Contrary to common opinion, constipation in the elderly is not related to the wearing out of the gastrointestinal system, although Palmer coined the term *presbycolon*, which would indicate age-related changes (Palmer, 1976).

In the elderly the term *presbycolon* has been used to mean constipation and complications of colon gas and impaction. It includes three forms of constipation: hypertonic, hypotonic, and "habit" constipation. All are found in the elderly.

Hypotonic constipation shows soft putty-like stool in the rectum on digital examination. The colon is full of feces and impactions are common in this form of constipation (Palmer,

1976). This type of hypotonic constipation is due to a decrease in intestinal motility, both the segmental contraction and the contractions that accomplish mass movement. The aim of treatment in this type of constipation is to stimulate motility. Motility abnormalities may occur as a result of diabetes, hypokalemia, antiparkinsonism therapy, and oral iron therapy (Sodeman, 1989).

Constipation caused by *hypertonicity* of the bowel is characterized by hard, dry stools and, in some cases, lower abdominal pain (Williams and Dickey, 1969). The phenomenon is a result of an increase in activity of the segmental-type muscle contractions, which mix bowel contents, but not of the propulsive-type bowel contractions, resulting in decreased transit and increased reabsorption of water.

Habit constipation is due primarily to eating habits that include a diet devoid of bulk (cellulose) or consciously or unconsciously ignoring or preventing the urge to defecate.

General factors that contribute to constipation include the following:

- Neglecting to respond to the defecation urge. Irregular bowel habits develop after a long period of time, inhibiting normal reflexes—if defecation does not occur when these reflexes are excited they become progressively weaker
- Diet—inadequate bulk and fluids. Excessive ingestion of foods that harden stools, e.g., processed cheese
- Chronic enema or laxative patterns
- Environmental changes: Changes in daily biologic patterns—eating, sleeping, time of bowel and bladder evacuation, lack of privacy for bowel movements
- Atony or hypertonicity of the colon, hypertonicity of the ileocecal valve
- Dentition: Loss of teeth or chewing power, creating difficulties for eating high fiber foods
- Neurologic degeneration
- Painful anorectal disorders
- Mental stress, depression, feelings of inadequacy or insecurity (Sklar, 1972), short attention span in cognitively impaired elderly
- Drugs: Aspirin, anticholinergic drugs, aluminum hydroxide or calcium carbonate antacids, opiates (e.g., codeine, morphine), mineral oil, tranquilizers
- Loss of abdominal muscle tone

Constipation also can occur with pathology. Acute constipation may be the presenting symptom for acute intestinal obstruction. The possibility of underlying local pathology always exists. Change in bowel movements and bleeding are symptoms of malignancy. In addition, central nervous system pathology such as organic brain diseases, particularly those with frontal lobe deterioration and perceptual motor disturbances, involving body image will also contribute to constipation.

HIGH-RISK POPULATION

Individuals on bed rest who take medications that are known to cause constipation (e.g., anticholinergics, opiates, barbiturates), those who reduce fluids or bulk in their diet, those who develop central nervous system disease or local lesions causing pain, or those who become depressed are at risk of developing constipation.

DYNAMICS

Factors that increase the dehydration of the stool, slow the transit time, or interfere with the usual pattern of reflexes contribute to delayed defecation, production of drier stools, and subsequent difficulty in evacuation.

The presence of fecal material in the rectum alone is not sufficient to initiate the defecation reflex. It must be an amount large enough to exceed the individual threshold of the stimulus. Defecation is a special reflex initiated by mass movement of fecal material into the rectum. The defecation reflex is mediated by the internal nerve plexus. It can be inhibited voluntarily by contraction of the external anal sphincter. Defecation occurs by relaxation of the internal and external anal sphincter, increased peristaltic activity of the sigmoid colon, and contraction of the abdominal muscles. This causes an increase in intra-abdominal pressure, which is transmitted to the contents of the large intestine and assists in the elimination of feces. Distention of the stomach by food, particularly the first meal of the day, initiates contractions of the rectum and frequently a desire to defecate (gastrocolic reflex).

The prolonged use of laxatives can produce anatomic changes in the colon. Removal of the colon was indicated in a study of 12 chronic users of laxatives of 30 to 40 years' duration (American Pharmaceutical Association Handbook, 1977). It was found that there was loss of intrinsic innervation, atrophy of smooth muscle coats, and pigmentation of the colon (*melanosis coli* due to anthracene laxatives such as cascara). The cathartic colon can be diagnosed by barium enema radiography. This is shortening and loss of haustration. In addition, chronic laxative use can result in electrolyte imbalances, in particular potassium. In patients with short-term memory deficits there are risks of overmedicating due to the inability to remember to take medications. The prolonged stimulation of the neurons by the irritant laxatives results in cell death.

SIGNS AND SYMPTOMS

The most frequent indication of constipation is the complaint of the person and his attendant concern. Data are needed on what the person considers to be normal bowel movement in terms of frequency and consistency, what the usual patterns of defecation are, and any changes in activity, diet, medication, mood, or pain. The stool should also be observed for size, consistency, mucus, and blood. Unless the nurse regularly checks on bowel movements in some way, she will be unaware of constipation until symptoms of fecal impaction occur. There is a need to check in a way that does not focus on bowel movements as the expected daily behavior because this leads the person into thinking that he is constipated when he may not be.

Assessment areas include decreased appetite, increased restlessness, frequently noted trips to the bathroom, complaints of nausea, increased irritability, headache, abdominal cramping, increasingly active gas pattern, abdominal palpation, absence of bowel movement for a longer time period than the individual's usual pattern, abdominal distention, and urinary incontinence.

DIFFERENTIAL DIAGNOSIS

It is important to differentiate between the types of constipation—hypotonic, hypertonic, and habit. The treatment for each of these types differs. The wrong form of management will precipitate side effects and produce confounding symptoms that will obscure the original problem. One will, in effect, then be treating a condition they produced rather than the primary problem. An elderly person is likely to

have several other attendant problems and cannot afford the physiologic and psychic stress in terms of energy expenditure on an iatrogenic condition.

Medications should always be considered as a potential cause of constipation. Knowledge of drugs is essential. Each nurse who cares for older persons should have a list available of medications that have constipation as a side effect. In clinics, offices, or institutions a list could be posted in a convenient area.

COMPLICATIONS

Aside from the discomfort and accompanying anxiety the individual experiences with constipation, a major complication is fecal impaction following prolonged accumulation of feces. The complications of constipation more frequently are the effect of the treatment rather than the original constipation.

MEDICAL MANAGEMENT

Treatment of constipation should not be taken lightly. It is a serious problem and older persons themselves take it seriously. As indicated in differential diagnosis, it is important to take a careful history to find out not only the nature of the problem but also what the individual usually does to relieve the problem. Their own strategies may be very simple and something they can tolerate. If what they use has potential dangers, this becomes an opportunity to introduce change, although the likelihood of change being accepted often is small. Successful therapy often involves trial and error.

Palmer (1976) warns that those who care primarily for geriatric patients err when their goal for the elderly is a return to normal by overcoming longstanding bad habits through educational programs. He believes that efforts should be directed toward relieving the constipation by any available tried means.

Anyone who is constipated wants relief as soon as possible. The first things that are considered usually are laxatives, enemas, and suppositories. The ideal laxative is not yet available. It would be one that was nonirritating, nontoxic, acted within a few hours, produced normal stool, and then allowed the bowel to return to normal activity. Currently available laxatives are classified by their action and include bulk formation, emollient, lubrication, stimulant, saline, and hyperosmotic (Table 25–5).

TABLE 25–5 *Laxatives*

Mechanism of Action/Examples	Action and Uses
Stimulants Castor oil (1–3 hr) Senokot Nature's Remedy Carter's Little Pills Cascara sagrada Dulcolax (bisacodyl) Feen-A-Mint Dorbane (danthron)	Prompt in action (6–8 hr) Peristaltic action increased by local irritation to the intestine or by selective action on the nerve complex of intestinal smooth muscle. Used before bowel surgery or radiographic examination. Limited to short-term use (1 week)
Bulk forming Metamucil Serutan Bran	Not useful in patients with hypomotility. Increases peristalsis by increasing bulk. Take 12 hours to 3 days to be effective. Should not be used with patients who have intestinal adhesions, stenosis, or difficulty swallowing because of danger of impaction or intestinal obstruction. Used cautiously in patients with active colitis. These drugs interact with salicylates and digitalis and other drugs. Take each dose with a full glass of water
Emollient/lubricant Colace Doxinate Mineral oil* (use the emulsion) Emulsified mineral oil† Agoral Petrogalar	Require 1–2 days to have an effect. Not to be used in patients with swallowing problems **Emollient:** useful with people who should not strain to defecate. Increases the wetting efficiency of intestinal water and forms oil and water emulsions. Prevents development of constipation, does not improve existing constipation. Used in fecal impactions **Lubricant:** softens fecal contents by coating. Useful in keeping stool soft to avoid straining. Long use of mineral oil can produce toxicity and side effects. Affects absorption of calcium, phosphates, and vitamins A and D. Do not take with meals because they delay gastric emptying
Saline laxatives Magnesium sulfate Fleets (sodium biphosphate, sodium phosphate) Phospho-Soda	Intestinal wall acts as semipermeable membrane to magnesium, sulfate, tartrate, phosphate, and citrate ions. Water is retained in the intestine, causing pressure, which increases intestinal motility. In poor renal function, magnesium is retained, which can depress CNS. Dehydration can occur with hypertonic solutions of saline cathartics Not to be used in patients with cardiovascular problems due to sodium
Other Milk of Magnesia (magnesium hydroxide and peppermint oil) Haley's MO (magnesium hydroxide and mineral oil)	

*Do not take mineral oil with other medication or with meals. Take 1 hour before bedtime to avoid reflux aspiration.
†Use of emulsion (Agoral or Petrogalar, Lactulose, Sorbitol) is preferred with the elderly.

The dosage of the laxative is important. One tablet for a young person may be too large a dose for an older person. Try different dosage levels for individuals. In the elderly, one cannot just give a laxative and not monitor the effects of this drug.

In selecting or recommending a laxative to older persons it is important to know the type of constipation they have. For example, it would be foolish to recommend a stool softener to an individual who already has soft stools. Caregivers need to be familiar not only with the person's bowel patterns but also with the mechanical and pharmacologic actions of the drugs in terms of both their therapeutic potential and the harm they can cause. Beyond this, there is a need to be aware of attitudes toward the use of laxatives and enemas and the way they influence observation and decision making in managing constipation. When this is resolved and any biases are detected, it can be easier for both the older person and the caregiver. Of all the laxatives available at this time, the bulking agents are the most useful (Sodeman, 1989). These can also contribute to reducing serum cholesterol by binding bile acids in the intestine.

Enemas are given to clean the bowel for a number of reasons, including constipation relief. The enema, properly done, is the nearest substitute for the ideal laxative. Improperly administered, an enema can produce electrolyte and fluid imbalance, hemorrhage, and spasm as well as local trauma if the nozzle is inadequately lubricated or improperly directed.

As with laxatives, the content of the enema produces the action. Soap suds act by irritating the colon; oils lubricate and soften feces.

The enema should be administered with the person lying on his side—preferably the left side. If the person sits on the toilet, only the rectum is cleaned of feces. Fluid should not be administered with force. Frequently 250 mL of solution is all that is necessary to empty the lower bowel.

Water is absorbed through the large bowel; therefore, accuracy of total fluid intake and output is important, particularly when more than one enema is necessary. When more than two enemas are given with return that is much less than the liquid given, accurate measurement should be made to determine the actual discrepancy. When multiple enemas are given, an isotonic saline solution should be used to avoid electrolyte imbalance.

Suppositories are useful in some instances. The two most commonly used suppositories are glycerine and Dulcolax. Glycerine suppositories are used with persons who require lubrication and digital stimulation as a means of eliminating stool. Dulcolax suppositories are used in persons who require added neural stimulation to the intestinal wall. Be aware that Dulcolax produces cramping and can cause problems to a debilitated person. (A mild oral agent such as danthron, one-half tablet, or milk of magnesia is preferable.) Suppositories are effective only if they are inserted correctly. They must be inserted above the internal sphincter.

Diet, fluids, and exercise are considerations that, hopefully, decrease constipation. Fiber in foods holds water and helps the stool to pass more rapidly. Exercise, particularly the isometric type, may improve sphincter and abdominal muscle tone and improve the efficiency with which the abdominal muscles assist in propulsion of stool out of the rectum.

EVALUATION

A bowel pattern can be established through a bowel program. Criteria for improvement, however, include not only improvement in bowel patterns but also participation of the older person in improving fluid intake, diet, and exercise patterns. Self-satisfaction with the efforts is important.

IMPACTION

A fecal impaction is a hard, compacted mass of fecal material in the rectum that the individual cannot expel.

ETIOLOGIC FACTORS

Impaction usually presents when the person has constipation. Therefore, factors contributing to constipation will increase the likelihood of impaction. These include decreased dietary intake, in particular decreased fiber, decreased physical exercise, depression, impaired sensation of rectal vault, inability to get to the toilet, and impaired cognitive function.

HIGH RISK

Individuals with hypotonic constipation, particularly those who are debilitated, immobilized, or have central nervous system lesions are at high risk.

SIGNS AND SYMPTOMS

The individual will report or will be known not to have had a normal bowel movement for several days; however, he may have some leakage of liquid stool and fecal incontinence. Rectal examination and a finding of hard stool in the rectum validates the diagnosis.

TREATMENT

The treatment of a fecal impaction involves manually removing the stool with or without prior oil enemas to soften it.

1. Explain the procedure. Ensure privacy.
2. Position the person on his side (left side) and drape.
3. Ask the person to breathe deeply, slowly, and quietly through the mouth during the procedure.
4. Lubricate the gloved finger with water-soluble gel.
5. Gently break up the impaction, being careful not to traumatize the wall of the rectum. Stop if the person complains of excessive pain.
6. Remove whatever fecal material can be freed from the mass.
7. Do not manipulate the impaction beyond the fatigue tolerance of the person. Allow a rest period during and following removal.
8. Administer a warm oil-retention enema. Allow expulsion of oil and feces.
9. Follow with a cleansing soap suds enema (do not administer more than two enemas in any 8-hour period).

For 3 days after the removal of the fecal impaction it would be appropriate to give a combination of stool softener and bowel stimulant.

Once the initial impaction has been eliminated, an assessment of why the individual developed an impaction is imperative. Then a program of preventive management needs to be undertaken to avoid or minimize future recurrences.

FECAL INCONTINENCE

Stool incontinence occurs in a small percentage of noninstitutionalized elderly persons. Brocklehurst (1951) identified 10% of the elderly patients in four general hospitals as incontinent and in a geriatric hospital the incidence rose to 20%. One third of the incontinent patients were found to have evidence of organic neurologic changes and another third were mentally confused (Geokas and Haverback, 1969).

Fecal incontinence can occur among those who are aware of it and embarrassed by it as well as among those who are not conscious of it because of confusion, disturbed consciousness, or brain damage. Inability to control audible release of flatus is probably even more common and can cause some individuals to alter their lifestyle.

Fecal incontinence can occur as a result of organic changes in neural innervation of the rectum, including decreased sensation of rectal filling, increased excitability of the rectal external sphincter, decreased anal muscle tone, or loss of cortical control (Geokas and Haverback, 1969; Percy et al, 1982). Local colorectal causes include inflammation, cancer of the rectum, prolapsed anus, and the semifluid quality of the stool. Some individuals are so debilitated as to be unable to control the sphincter against the defecation reflex. By far the most common cause of fecal incontinence is gross constipation with impaction in the anal canal and subsequent overflow (Agate, 1986). Laxative abuse can also result in fecal incontinence.

Management of constipation and elimination of mental confusion where it exists can be important ways of managing fecal incontinence. A rectal examination to determine the presence of impactions is important. Enemas may be needed for several days to give the person a fresh start. Where control is not possible, suppositories or Fleet enemas to time the defecation and reduce risk of accidents may be useful. The use of absorbent pads and waterproof panties may also be reassuring and allow more mobility. These should be used following discussion, explanation, and acceptance by the person involved. Careful consideration and attention to the integrity of the skin should be of paramount importance when using protective devices to avoid skin breakdown.

Nursing Diagnosis and Management of High-risk Areas in Daily Living

DAILY LIVING WITH EPIGASTRIC DISCOMFORT

Peptic ulcer disease, gastritis, and hiatal hernias are common chronic and often intractable conditions in the elderly whose symptoms require knowledgeable adjustments in daily living if they are to be controlled.

RISK FACTORS

Individuals at greater risk for being unsuccessful in managing daily living with the problems of peptic ulcers, gastritis, and hiatal hernia are those who

Do not understand the underlying mechanisms that are producing the symptoms and therefore cannot knowledgeably make adaptations in eating, medication taking, positioning, and activity to manage them

Are unwilling to modify these dimensions of their daily living in order to adapt to the presenting situation

Have gastric malignancies

SIGNS AND SYMPTOMS

Manifestations of ineffective management include reports of continued symptoms, and evidence of failure to use medications appropriately or to engage in regimens that could improve the situation.

PROGNOSTIC VARIABLES

Improvement in the ulcer and its manifestations are contingent on adherence to the medication regimen and the responsiveness of the lesion, and beyond that, eating appropriately.

Living effectively with hiatal hernia is contingent on intelligently following an eating, positional, and activity regimen to minimize reflux of gastric contents into the esophagus. Diabetic neuropathy and associated gastric retention create additional hazards.

Gastric malignancies carry a poor prognosis for maintaining comfort and well-being.

COMPLICATIONS

Failure to manage the conditions and their manifestations can interfere with nutrition, sleep, and the capacity for engaging in the routines and social activities of daily living. It can also result in expansion of the pathology to esophagitis and gastritis.

TREATMENT

Elderly persons and their caregivers need assistance in the following areas:

Understanding the role and therapeutic use of antacids and the antisecretory agents such as H_2-receptor blockers as well as their side effects

Understanding the dietary changes (types of food, times of eating, and amounts of food) needed to minimize problems associated with the condition

Finding acceptable ways to incorporate these alterations into current patterns of daily living

Understanding when and what type of physical activity contributes to control of the condition

Where position in sleeping is a factor, obtaining assistance in adjusting the bed for positional effect and comfort

EVALUATION

Evaluation is in patient comfort, symptom management, and satisfaction with the resultant quality of life.

DAILY LIVING WITH DIARRHEA

For some elderly people diarrhea is a regular or intermittent phenomenon that interferes with daily living. It creates discomfort in terms of cramping and anal inflammation. The need to have sudden, rapid access to a bathroom limits where people can go and what they can do—it may make them homebound. Fecal incontinence when diarrhea is intense or the sphincter is incompetent contributes to laundry problems, to say nothing of the person's self-image.

RISK FACTORS

Managing daily living with diarrhea becomes increasingly difficult with the following:

The severity and intensity of the diarrhea

Rectal sphincter incompetence

Increased distance of the bathroom from the normal living and sleeping space or from the car or other means of transportation

Lack of money for protective clothing

Lack of creative, positive caregivers or companions who find ways to engage in a preferred pattern of daily living even with the presence or risk of diarrhea

Diagnosis of irritable bowel syndrome, which in some patients is associated with recurrent bouts of diarrhea

SIGNS AND SYMPTOMS

Manifestations that daily living is not being managed effectively with diarrhea include the following:

Reports that cramping or diarrhea are making a formerly active person afraid or unable to engage in usual activities

Persistent sleep deprivation associated with discomfort or diarrhea

An inappropriate or undesirable weight loss pattern

An anal area that is inflamed or painful

Fluid intake that is less than output, plus signs of dehydration and electrolyte imbalances

Laboratory values in electrolytes and hematocrit that become increasingly or dangerously abnormal

Alternating constipation and diarrhea due to inappropriate use of medication

PROGNOSTIC VARIABLES

The ability to manage daily living with diarrhea is associated with the following:

The underlying pathophysiology that predicts the course of the disease and its trajectory

The premorbid personality—the drive to be active, to make adaptations, ego strength, and so on

The knowledge and desire to incorporate preventive and palliative measures into daily living

The presence of others who will plan activities, provide transportation that takes diarrhea into account as a realistic possibility

COMPLICATIONS

The complications of persistent or intermittent diarrhea in daily living include both pathophysiologic and psychosocial dimensions. Severe or persistent diarrhea can result in dehydration, saline depletion, hyponatremia, and hypokalemia. Fecal incontinence and anal excoriation may become progressively severe. Malnutrition may occur secondary to inadequate absorption of nutrients. In the psychosocial area, older persons' self-concept as competent adults with control over their lives may be threatened. Social activities may be curtailed; the person can become housebound and isolated.

TREATMENT

Management in daily living includes medication control, hydration activities, skin protection, control of pain, modification of the diet, and careful planning for activities.

Medication Some medications increase diarrhea (see earlier section on etiologic factors of diarrhea). These need to be recognized and avoided where possible. Some alleviate diarrhea, and these need to be used correctly (see previous section on management of diarrhea). As with all medications in the elderly, the idea "If a little is good, more is better" is to be avoided. Undermedicate and gradually increase the dose.

Food Gas-causing foods tend to exacerbate diarrhea. There are general categories of gas-causing foods; however, each individual tends to have idiosyncrasies, so gathering specific data is important before negotiating a diet plan. Bran is normally seen as a laxative, yet it can have an effect of slowing transit of food through the bowel. Gradual introduction of bran into the diet is advisable; then the results should be observed before more is added.

Fluid Conscious increasing of fluids, beyond coffee and tea consumption, becomes crucial. Reminders not to include coffee and tea in the calculations may be needed.

Skin When diarrhea is a regular pattern or a high risk, anal skin protection makes better sense than having to deal with tissue breakdown. Gentle thorough washing of the anal area after each bowel movement, followed by application of zinc oxide or another protective ointment can limit or delay inflammation. An anesthetic ointment may control discomfort where inflammation has occurred.

Protection New absorbent protective clothing is on the market. It is expensive but may make it possible for the person to engage in special activities and social events with greater confidence. Small pieces of sheeting over a piece of plastic can reduce the effort needed to change and launder sheets. The same may be used on chairs when there is loss of sphincter control.

Activities When the major barrier to participating in activities and social events is diarrhea, plans and advance arrangements can be made to locate the person close to bathrooms (e.g., carefully planned seating on a plane, in a restaurant, or at a picnic in a park). The length of the drive from home to the destination can be kept within the predicted interval between episodes. It can be scheduled during the time of the day when there is the least problem.

EVALUATION

Effectiveness of nursing intervention falls in the areas of judging hydration, electrolyte balance, skin integrity, and comfort and participation in valued activities.

DAILY LIVING TO PREVENT OR MANAGE CONSTIPATION

Many factors make constipation a frequent condition among elderly persons. Eating patterns with reduced fiber and fluids, a prescription or use of constipating medications, a less active lifestyle, and previous laxative or enema dependence contribute to this condition among the elderly. How this condition is prevented or managed is dependent to a great extent on patterns of daily living.

RISK FACTORS

Those who are at greatest risk of not preventing or managing constipation in daily living are those who

Prefer a low fiber and roughage diet or are unable to chew a high fiber diet (e.g., persons who are edentulous, have new dentures, whose teeth are in need of dental work, who have arthritic jaws)
Drink very few liquids
Take constipating drugs (see the previous section on constipation)
Are inactive or losing abdominal muscle tone
Ignore the urge to defecate at the time it occurs
Value laxative or enema use
Have constipating pathology or conditions, e.g., diverticulosis, irritable bowel syndrome, anorectal lesions, prolapsed uterus

SIGNS AND SYMPTOMS

The elderly person or caregivers report concern with (1) failure to have bowel movements, (2) difficulties associated with elimination, and (3) accompanying abdominal discomfort. One may observe consistent use of laxatives and enemas

and the reported valuing of their efficacy. Fecal material is dry and hard. Impactions occur.

PROGNOSTIC VARIABLES

Success in preventing or managing constipation is contingent on removing or addressing the causative factors when these rather than lifestyle are the major force (e.g., changing to nonconstipating drugs and treating lesions) and if necessary making lifestyle changes to minimize the constipating features (e.g., inactivity, inadequate roughage use, underhydration). Longer duration of constipation and growing physical disability increase the likelihood of not relieving the constipation.

COMPLICATIONS

Constipation has the pathologic consequences of fluid and electrolyte imbalances, impaction, and fecal incontinence. It can also become an area of preoccupation to the point of neglecting other important and positive areas in daily living.

TREATMENT

Nursing management is concerned with preventing the onset of constipation despite increasing risks associated with aging, as well as managing daily living to reduce existing constipation.

Prevention   Negotiate with the elderly person and primary caregiver about the elderly person's willingness to engage in and plan for the following:

Increasing the intake of nondiuretic liquids to 2000 mL daily (if not contraindicated by other pathology)
Continuing to include or beginning to increase fresh fruits and vegetables, whole grains, and bran in the diet in sufficient amounts
Participating in physical activity, some of which includes isometric exercises for abdominal muscle setting
Minimizing the use of over-the-counter constipating drugs and negotiating with the physician to limit the use of constipating drugs where this is possible

Giving high priority to defecating promptly when the urge is felt; failure to do so will mean the urge to defecate loses strength

Using laxatives, suppositories, or enemas as a last resort or temporary treatment

Treatment of Existing Constipation Treatment of existing constipation is determined by diagnosing the factors that are causing it and gathering data on past history of constipation as well as the strategies the older person has used to deal with it. The treatment for prevention is negotiated and incorporated into daily living as well as the temporary use of appropriate laxatives until other measures become effective.

EVALUATION

Response to treatment is judged on the extent to which the individual integrates the management strategies into daily living and the avoidance or improvement of the constipation itself.

DAILY LIVING WITH ENTERAL FEEDING

It has become increasingly common to support the nutrition of ailing older persons with oral nutrient-rich supplements or tube feedings. Thus, nurses in long-term care settings and caregivers in home settings are concerned with incorporating these support therapies into daily living in a safe, therapeutic, and positive way.

RISK FACTORS

Both age-related biologic changes and common pathophysiologic conditions create risks for ineffective daily living with tube feedings.

Aspiration Decreased gastric emptying rate with subsequent residual volume combined with an incompetent LES permits reflux of gastric contents into the esophagus. This, combined with the decreased gag reflex, heightens the risk of aspiration. Hiatal hernia increases the risk of aspiration, and diabetic neuropathy with the associated decrease in gastric emptying creates even greater risk of reflux and aspiration. Decreased resistance to infection and decreased mobility contribute to the risk of aspiration pneumonia.

The ongoing presence of a nasogastric tube that keeps the LES open also facilitates aspiration. Thus, it has been suggested that gastrostomy tubes may decrease the risk of aspiration.

Metabolic Abnormalities (Hypernatremia, Hyperchloremia, Acidosis, Azotemia, Hyperglycemia) The introduction of formula by nasogastric or gastrostomy/jejunostomy tube carries the risk of creating metabolic abnormalities. Of these the greatest risk is due to increasing glucose intolerance in the later years. Factors that increase the risk of metabolic abnormalities include normal age-related changes in glucose utilization, homeostasis of fluid balance, and decreased renal excretion of glucose. Coexisting central nervous system pathology that limits communication or masks the first signs of hyperglycemic or hyperosmolar coma increases the risk that it will become well established before it is recognized.

Risks of Ineffective Enteral Feeding There are higher risks to incorporating tube feedings effectively into daily living when the caregivers are not knowledgeable about the techniques, safeguards, and early manifestations of complications, and when it is difficult to obtain clinical laboratory services due to transportation problems or lack of accessibility of a laboratory.

SIGNS AND SYMPTOMS

With gastric retention, the older person may complain of fullness. Gastric distention in the epigastric region may be observed. Residual volumes may be greater than 100 mL.

Enteral feedings that result in aspiration may be recognized by the presence of glucose in tracheal aspirations. It can be confirmed by the use of blue dye added to tube feedings followed by monitoring for the presence of this blue coloring in respiratory secretions.

Metabolic changes are reflected first in subtle changes in mentation—withdrawal, confusion, then moving on to coma. Urinary glucose content is measured at regular intervals, particularly during the first week.

Changes in hydration can be noted in rapid weight gains or losses, edema, and imbalance in intake and output values.

Gastrointestinal responses may include diarrhea, abdominal cramping, and nausea.

Ineffective administration of the treatment may be reflected in failure to recognize any of the previously mentioned abnormalities, in giving the formula in a way that the older person reports as being uncomfortable, or in failure to maintain the formula in a safe microbial environment.

PROGNOSTIC VARIABLES

Effective incorporation of tube feeding into daily living is associated with a relatively intact lower esophageal sphincter, effective gastric emptying, and adequate renal function. It also depends on the expertise of the caregiver, or that of the older person when it is self-administered.

COMPLICATIONS

Pneumonia, iatrogenic infections due to improper control in the preparation of the formula or its storage at a temperature that promotes microbial growth, nasal tissue breakdown, coma, and death are the major complications of enteral feeding for elderly persons.

TREATMENT

The person should be positioned at greater than 45°, preferably upright, during the feeding and for 1 hour following feeding. The tube position should be checked before diet administration. Recurrent problems with aspiration may indicate the need for gastrostomy or jejunostomy to decrease the risk of aspiration.

Careful and regular nose and mouth care are imperative. The presence of a nasogastric tube increases mouth breathing. When possible, ice chips or hard candy to suck on will facilitate oral secretions. The nares is checked every day for bleeding, and water-soluble lubricant is used to prevent tissue injury. Nasogastric tubes are changed every 2 weeks, alternating nares.

Medications are evaluated to determine the appropriateness of mixing them with the tube-feeding diet. Medications are scheduled around tube feeding to maximize drug absorption.

When the person has complications associated with enteral nutrition, the cause of the problem is sought. For the person with diarrhea, the feeding is stopped, tube placement is checked, and feeding is withheld for several hours. When it is restarted, it is at a reduced concentration and a slower rate. However, attention needs to be given to the number of calories missed during this period. Antidiarrheal medications may be used, but with caution in the older person.

For patients on home tube feeding, the tube may be passed only at feeding time. This allows the person greater mobility and facilitates social interaction. The presence of a feeding tube is an outward sign of illness and loss of function.

EVALUATION

Enteral feedings in daily living may be evaluated on the basis of absence of complications, comfort with the administration, desired weight pattern, and degree of satisfaction with the quality of life that ensues.

DAILY LIVING WITH ENTERAL SUPPORT THERAPIES

Oral nutrient-rich supplements are used in older persons when their normal dietary intake is less than required for normal maintenance. These individuals have normal gastrointestinal function and are able to swallow.

Any oral supplement when used exclusively is likely to become boring. Taste adaptation to a particular supplement will result in decreased intake. Commercially prepared supplements such as Sustacal and Ensure come in multiple flavors and there are flavored additives that can be used. These formulas are lactose-free and may be better tolerated by individuals with lactose intolerance. Such products can be purchased at drugstores.

Oral supplements are best tolerated when served cold, or even over ice. Homemade nutritional supplements that are frequently used include milkshakes and eggnogs. Alternating oral supplements may result in the greatest effectiveness.

References and Other Readings

Agate J. Common symptoms and complaints. In: Rossman I, ed. Clinical geriatrics. 3rd ed. Philadelphia: JB Lippincott, 1986:138.

Alikhan T, et al. Effects of aging on the motor function of the esophagus and lower esophageal sphincter. In: van Trappen G, ed. Proceeding of the Fifth International Symposium on Gastro-Intestinal Motility, Leuven, Belgium, September 3–6, 1975. Ekelstraat: Belgium Typoff Press.

American Pharmaceutical Association. Handbook of

non-prescription drugs, 9th ed. Washington, DC: American Pharmaceutical Association, 1988.

Brandt L, Boley L, Goldberg L, Mitsudo S. Colitis in the elderly: a reappraisal. Am J Gastroenterol 1981; 76:239.

Brandt LJ. Gastrointestinal disorders of the elderly. New York: Raven Press, 1984.

Brocklehurst JC. Incontinence in old people. Edinburgh: E & S Livingston Ltd, 1951.

Castell DO, Harris LD. Hormonal control of gastroesophageal sphincter strength. N Engl J Med 1970; 282:886.

Cattau EL, Castel DO. Symptoms of esophageal dysfunction. Adv Intern Med 1982; 27:151.

Christensen J. The controls of gastrointestinal movements; some old and new views. N Engl J Med 1971; 285:85.

Foxworthy DM, Wilson JA. Crohn's disease in the elderly: prolonged delay in diagnosis. J Am Geriatr Soc 1984; 33:492.

Geokas M, Haverback B. The aging gastrointestinal tract. Am J Surg 1969; 117:881.

Hanan ZI. Geriatric medications—how the aged are hurt by drugs meant to help. RN 1978; 41:57.

Harper PC, McAuliffe TL, Buken WL. Crohn's disease in the elderly: a statistical comparison with younger patients matched for sex and duration of disease. Arch Intern Med 1986; 146:753.

Holt PR. The small intestine. Clin Gastroenterol 1985; 14:689.

Kurata JH, Corboy ED. Current peptic ulcer time trends: an epidemiological profile. J Clin Gastroenterol 1988; 10:259.

Kurata JH, Haile BM, Elashoff JD. Sex differences in peptic ulcer disease. Gastroenterology 1985; 88:96.

Lundegardh G, Adami H-O, Helmick C, Zack M, Merrik O. Stomach cancer after partial gastrec-

tomy for benign ulcer disease. N Engl J Med 1988; 319:195.

Palmer ED. "Presbycolon" problems in the nursing home. JAMA 1976; 235:1150.

Percy FP, et al. A neurogenic factor in faecal incontinence in the elderly. Age Ageing 1982; 11:175.

Perez-Perez GI, Dworkin BM, Chodos JE, Blaser MJ. *Campylobacter pylori* antibodies in humans. Ann Intern Med 1988; 109:11.

Rodman MJ, Smith DW. Clinical pharmacology in nursing, 2nd ed. Philadelphia: JB Lippincott, 1984.

Shamburek RD, Farrar JT. Disorders of the digestive system in the elderly. N Engl J Med 1990; 322:438.

Sklar M. Functional bowel distress and constipation in the aged. Geriatrics 1972; 27:79.

Sklar M. Gastrointestinal diseases in the aged. In: Working with older people, vol IV. Washington, DC: US Government Printing Office, 1974:124.

Smith CW, Evans P. Bowel motility. Geriatrics 1961; 16:189.

Sodeman WA, Saladin TA, Boyd WP. Geriatric gastroenterology. Philadelphia: WB Saunders, 1989.

Soergel KH, et al. Presbyesophagus: cineradiographic manifestations. Radiology 1964; 82:463.

Texter E, et al. The clinical features of inflammatory bowel disease in the after-50 patient. In: Texter EC, ed. The aging gut: pathophysiology, diagnosis, and management. New York: Masson Publishing, 1983.

Watson RJ, et al. Duodenal ulcer disease in the elderly: a retrospective study. Age Ageing 1985; 14:225.

Williams R, Dickey J. Physiology of colon and rectum. Am J Surg 1969; 117:849.

Zimmerman J, Gavish D, Rachnilewitz D. Early and later onset ulcerative colitis: distinct clinical features. J Clin Gastroenterol 1985; 7:492.

26
Genital Problems

DORIS CARNEVALI

Older persons are at high risk for a variety of problems in their genital tracts. Both men and women have higher risks for neoplastic disease in reproductive organs, benign and malignant. Infections are another major problem. Atrophy and loss of strength in supporting structures create additional difficulties for aging women.

As with many other health conditions to which the aged are subject, these problems tend to be chronic. They can have an ongoing impact on daily living and lifestyle. Therefore, they are areas for nursing assessment and management as a part of the health care of the older person. It may be an area of assessment that is neglected as both the older person and the nurse may be reluctant to talk about genital problems. However, there is successful treatment for some of the difficulties such as senile vaginal atrophy and yeast infections and ways to avoid unnecessary complications with others such as the combination of alcohol consumption and difficulty in voiding with the man who has benign prostatic hyperplasia. Therefore, nursing assessment of this area is as essential as any other.

Benign Prostatic Hypertrophy

Hyperplasia of the periurethral glands leads to prostatic enlargement. Since the gland surrounds the urethra, growth in that area may lead to the symptoms of urinary tract obstruc-

tion. If the growth is predominantly in the posterior region, the condition may produce no symptoms.

RISK FACTORS

Age is the major risk factor in the occurrence of benign prostatic hypertrophy, with the highest occurrence between 60 to 70 years of age. In the over-80 age group 90% have been found to have definite enlargement (Walsh, 1986).

SIGNS AND SYMPTOMS

Unless the enlargement encroaches on the urethra, the man is asymptomatic, the condition being known as a *silent prostatism. Obstructive prostatism* is evidenced by urinary frequency, reduced size and force of urinary stream, dribbling incontinence, hesitancy, and interruption of the stream during voiding. Nocturia and hematuria may also be present. *Obstruction with distant symptoms* occurs late and results from urinary stasis and retention with infection, back pressure, and altered renal function. Here the symptoms are those of uremia (see Chapter 31, Renal Failure: Acute and Chronic).

DIFFERENTIAL DIAGNOSIS

Benign prostatic hypertrophy has some signs and symptoms in common with neurogenic bladder, strictures, inflammatory disease, and prostatic malignancies. If the nurse is involved in a situation where she sees the patient more frequently than the physician and, therefore, is having a significant role in case finding, it will be important to take a careful history as a basis for consulting with the physician or making a referral.

One other area of differential diagnosis is associated with drug therapy. The man with only marginally obstructive prostatic disease can be thrown into retention with the administration of atropine-like drugs, tranquilizers, antihistamines, diuretics, or bronchodilators. The nurse who knows that a patient has benign prostatic hypertrophy should alert the prescribing physician to the situation if drugs of this nature are prescribed. When a patient is seen who is on these drugs and exhibiting retention symptoms, the drugs should be stopped if possible and voiding and residual urine evaluated.

COMPLICATIONS

Complications associated with benign prostatic hypertrophy include urinary obstruction, retention, stasis, infection, and uremia. Complications of prostatic surgery include retrograde ejaculation and excessive bleeding. Impotence is not usually a problem unless there were previous difficulties.

MEDICAL MANAGEMENT

Treatment tends to be conservative in the absence of progressive obstructive symptoms. Conservative management includes ascertaining that renal output is adequate and treating secondary symptoms such as infection. Estrogens, progestins, and flutamide have been tried to improve urinary flow. More studies are needed to evaluate their effectiveness (Walsh, 1986).

Surgical removal of a portion or all of the gland is indicated with clear symptoms of progressive obstruction, retention, hematuria, or recurrent infection. Surgery may be open prostatectomy using a perineal, suprapubic, or retropubic approach. Transurethral surgery is also widely used because open excision is not necessary and postoperative recovery generally is quicker. The choice of surgical technique depends on factors like the age and health of the patient, the size and location of the gland, and the training and skill of the physician.

Carcinoma of the Prostate

HIGH-RISK POPULATIONS

Cancer of the prostate is rare before age 50. The incidence increases with every decade after age 50. African American men have a very high risk for prostatic cancer (Bush, 1991).

SIGNS AND SYMPTOMS

Prostatic carcinoma often is asymptomatic, even with widespread metastasis; or there may be symptoms of obstruction. Symptoms associated with advanced cancer and metastasis include hematuria, hematospermia, back and leg pain (the spine and pelvis are sites of frequent metastasis), anemia (which may be extreme as bone marrow is replaced by tumor), elevated serum acid phosphatase, elevated serum alkaline phosphatase, and perineal pain.

DIFFERENTIAL DIAGNOSIS

Rectal examination is essential for detecting prostatic carcinoma. It should be done yearly for all men over age 50. The cancerous gland is hard and nodular. Finding a gland of this description is presumptive diagnosis of prostatic carcinoma. Positive diagnosis is assured by needle biopsy and radiologic examination of the urinary tract and skeleton, and laboratory studies. Prostatic acid phosphatase (PAP) is an adjunctive test. Elevation usually indicates metastatic disease. Rectal ultrasonography is also improving to the point where it is an adjunct in the work-up of susceptible lesions (Breschi, 1989). Serum alkaline phosphatase often increases with bone metastasis.

PROGNOSIS

Tumor virulence tends to be inversely related to age. A large percentage of men with prostatic cancer die from causes other than the cancer. Treatment causes morbidity so its advantages must be balanced against quality of life and life expectancy (Abrams and Berkow 1990).

COMPLICATIONS

The complications from the tumor include obstructive or metastatic pathology. Obstruction can lead to problems like infection or renal failure. Metastasis to the pelvis and spine is evidenced by low back pain and pathologic fractures at the site of metastasis.

The problems associated with estrogen therapy are an increased incidence of thrombi and emboli, nausea and vomiting, jaundice, and fluid retention. Mammary enlargement, testicular atrophy, and decreased libido may also occur. If the patient lives long enough, he can also become resistant to estrogen therapy. The patient should be informed of the potential side effects before therapy is started.

MEDICAL MANAGEMENT

Treatment and prognosis is currently in a state of flux (Breschi, 1989). Treatment modalities include radical surgery, radiation, hormonal therapy, or nontreatment, depending on the age and health status of the person. Obstruction is relieved by transurethral resection and this may need to be repeated as the tumor progresses.

Vaginitis

All elderly women are considered at high risk for atrophic vaginitis unless they are on estrogen replacement. It is the leading cause of postmenopausal bleeding.

The woman may complain of dyspareunia and bleeding following douching or coitus. The epithelium loses the normal rugal folds and becomes friable and vulnerable to infection.

Treatment consists of local application of estrogen creams or suppositories on a once-nightly basis for 1 to 2 weeks (Glowacki, 1989). Response is excellent, with reestablishment of rugal folds and recovery. Where infection is also present, antibiotic creams may be applied concurrently.

Where the woman has difficulty using the applicator for topical creams, the following method may be useful (Reid, 1985):

1. Place about 1 inch of cream on the index finger (with or without a finger cot).
2. Lie on your back or stand with one leg on a chair, then insert the finger into the vagina and gently massage the cream onto the vaginal mucosa.
3. Do the treatment at bedtime to minimize leakage and maximize absorption.

4. Refrain from sexual intercourse on the nights when the cream is applied.

In the presence of specific pathogens such as *Trichomonas* or *Candida* other medications are used.

Femstat, 2% cream	3 days at bedtime
Monistat, 3DS-suppositories or cream	3 days at bedtime. External cream twice a day 7 to 10 days
Myclex G, 500 mg	1 day at bedtime
Nizeral, 200 mg	Twice a day (orally) for 5 to 7 days

Metronidazole therapy, 2 g as a single dose (Glowacki, 1989) is used to treat trichomoniasis.

Use of systemic antibiotics places the elderly woman at great risk for occurrence of candidal vaginal infections. Diabetics too are at higher risk for vaginal infections.

No diseases should be ruled out merely because they seem unlikely. Genital herpes was diagnosed in a 90-year-old woman by nurses in the Iowa Veterans home. Older persons like anyone else deserve accurate diagnosis and treatment. Acquired immunodeficiency syndrome is another disease reported in older women and overlooked by physicians (McCormick, 1991).

Nursing Diagnosis and Management of High-risk Areas in Daily Living with Genital Problems

Because sexuality and reproductivity are not seen as important factors in the daily life of the elderly, age-related changes and pathology in the genitalia are often ignored or tolerated, much to the detriment of quality of life.

Older persons may be quite reluctant to talk about problems they are having in these areas. Observant, sensitive nurses with knowledge of the risks and manifestations can help older persons to recognize and discuss the problems as well as realize that these dysfunctions do not need to be merely tolerated—that there often is treatment available.

When the dysfunction cannot be remedied, nursing can become involved in managing daily living with the greatest comfort and least disruption for both the older person and those who share his or her daily living.

DAILY LIVING WITH PROSTATIC DISEASE

The potential for prostatic problems should be assumed with all men in the older age population. Since the man may be asymptomatic initially with either benign prostatic hypertrophy or cancer, nursing responsibilities include increasing the older man's awareness of prostatic problems and their management.

Men with only marginally obstructive disease can be thrown into urinary retention with the administration of these drugs: atropine-like drugs, tranquilizers, antihistamines, bronchodilators and alcohol consumption. Any man on these drugs and exhibiting retention symptoms should be evaluated for residual urine, and the drugs should be stopped if possible.

At times nurses are in a better position to gather information about symptoms of nocturia frequency or dribbling—problems that the man may feel are too insignificant to report to a physician, particularly one who does not have time to listen. The man with treatable prostatic hypertrophy may be spared the rejection and isolation that can occur with prostate-related incontinence, if the disease is diagnosed and treated. Nurses can play an important role in case finding.

Other problems such as daily living with incontinence, increased fluid intake, and metastatic pain can be found in Chapters 22 and 29 (see also Carnevali and Reiner, 1990).

DAILY LIVING WITH VAGINITIS

Given the reality of age-related changes in the female genitalia with the increased friability and vulnerability to infections, daily living for older women needs to include consideration for both the natural status and pathologic risks. It is not a topic most older women are likely to discuss voluntarily unless signs and symptoms concern them. Nurses can make sure to include this high-risk area for daily living in their history taking and assessments.

Once data are gathered, nurses can share information as appropriate about normal aging of the tissues of the genitalia, and the signs and symptoms that can arise merely from normal age-related changes: friability, bleeding, vulnerability to infection. Beyond that, nursing intervention involves helping older women to consider activities in daily living that need to be managed in particular ways to minimize risk of trauma or infection.

PERINEAL CARE

A clean, dry perineum is basic to preventing growth of pathogens. The perineum of the obese person may be subject to maceration and fissure and may be impossible to keep dry. A small fan or a portable hair dryer may be helpful in coping with this problem, but its use may prove to be an uncompromising task for someone with limited mobility. The need to keep the perineum dry is a strong case against tight-fitting pants and failure to change damp sanitary napkins. Cotton panties are advised, as is going without them when the patient finds this acceptable. It is an advantage that many elderly women prefer dresses and garters instead of synthetic slacks and pantyhose that only increase moisture problems. The cause for incontinency or dribbling should be remedied whenever possible, or bacterial vaginitis may be inevitable.

Perineal care is often neglected or assigned to the least trained personnel in care settings. The woman who is doing self-care may neglect it entirely or use an incorrect technique. Auto-infection becomes a real possibility. Not all persons are aware of the anatomic relationship of the rectum, vagina, and urethra and a mirror or drawings may help the elder person visualize what her nurse is describing. Patients should be taught to wipe and cleanse the perineum always from the front to the back of the area. Without this knowledge, even the most alert patient may suffer from autoinfection.

LAUNDRY

Elderly women living at home may need help with laundering to effectively rid their clothing of pathogenic organisms. Someone who does her own laundry may rinse her garments by hand, failing to destroy pathogens with the simple measure of hot water laundry.

DOUCHES

Douching is a common habit of many older women and its use probably should be discouraged. However, the nurse may not be able to interrupt a lifetime habit; then her actions may best be directed as altering or modifying the methods of douching. Vinegar and saline douche are supported by several experts as safe and useful for giving a feeling of cleanliness. Overuse of douche, however, dilutes the normal vaginal flora and may increase leukorrheic (abnormal vaginal discharge) symptoms by irritating the thin, atrophic membrane. Soda douche should not be used since it is alkaline and the woman already has the problem of a higher vaginal pH. Technique is problematic, particularly when self-douching is practiced. Delicate vaginal membrane may be damaged, or the unknowing patient may substitute contaminated equipment such as an enema tip. A douche of potassium sorbate is useful after coitus for reducing recurrent *Candida* infection. The pharmacy can prepare a concentrate of this douche from a stock supply of potassium sorbate powder. The concentrate is prepared in a solution of 10 g/30 mL. One ounce of this concentrate is then used per quart of water.

OVER-THE-COUNTER TREATMENTS

Over-the-counter sprays and deodorants may be tried by the elderly woman who is attempting to combat problems such as odor or pruritus. She may find it difficult to abandon these remedies unless her nurse can help her find suitable treatment for the underlying cause of her discomfort. Most elderly women are familiar with cornstarch dusting of the perineum and this can follow adequate perineal cleansing. However, medical diagnosis and treatment is necessary for persistent discomfort.

SEXUAL ACTIVITY

Dyspareunia is common with vaginitis. Relief of symptoms (as estrogen for atrophic vaginitis) is paramount to comfort. K-Y jelly may be used as a lubricant with coitus after pathogenic organisms are treated. It is especially important that the woman find relief for her vaginal symptoms or she may abandon sexual intercourse. This is an unfortunate circumstance that need not occur.

Intercourse should be avoided or condoms should be used during active treatment of any infectious vaginitis. The sexual partner should be checked for possible surface infection when an infectious vaginitis persists. Treatment should be matter-of-fact and supportive so that the woman does not feel embarrassed and reluctant about seeking help.

FOREIGN BODIES

Vaginal discharge with a confused patient should be investigated for the possibility of a foreign body. After the foreign body is removed, gentle physiologic saline irrigation is useful for washing out any retained particles (as toilet paper) from the vagina.

CHECKING pH

pH readings could be a nursing measure routinely used with vaginal infection. These readings should be helpful in differential diagnosis as well as in noting vaginal changes that may support pathogens. For example, pH readings would be beneficial if the woman was being maintained on estrogens; susceptibility to *Candida* infection could be projected by a drop in pH from the estrogenic replacement. Susceptibility to bacterial vaginitis could be predicted by a higher pH. Nurses could monitor the effectiveness of acid douches with pH readings. pH could be checked at the completion of douching and an hour or so later. If permanent pH benefit could not be demonstrated, it would seem reasonable to suggest alternate therapy.

LABORATORY TESTS

Nurses should advocate the use of correct laboratory procedure for diagnosis of vaginitis. Treatment of candidiasis without potassium hydroxide (KOH) smear or fungal culture should be questioned. Saline smear should be used to diagnose *Trichomonas* infection, and culture should be used to identify the specific organism of bacterial vaginitis.

EVALUATION

When a problem area has been identified, then evaluation would be contingent on relief of symptoms (i.e., Does pruritus persist? Is there vaginal and vulvar soreness? Has the excessive discharge been eliminated?). The nurse should base her evaluation on verbal reporting and examination results. Looking at the discharge or taking a pH reading has more merit than simply recording absence of subjective complaint.

Evaluation should also include an assessment of daily hygiene. The nurse should know whether the patient is doing good perineal care, whether douching is used, and the adequacy of the procedure. The nurse in a care facility should occasionally assist with the patient's bath and with toileting to assess hygiene. The nurse in the community should be able to get clues from the patient's environment. The home health care nurse who establishes good rapport with the person will eventually get an opportunity to assess something as personal as perineal care.

References and Other Readings

Abrams W, Berkow R. The Merck Manual of Geriatrics. Rahway, NJ: Merck Sharp & Dohme Research Laboratories, 1990.

Breschi L. Common lower urinary tract problems in the elderly. In: Reichel W, ed. Clinical aspects of aging, 3rd ed. Baltimore: Williams & Wilkins, 1989:264.

Bush JP. Non-neoplastic and neoplastic disorders of the male reproductive system. In: Patrick M et al. (eds.). Medical surgical nursing-pathophysiological concepts, 2nd ed. Philadelphia: JB Lippincott, 1991.

Carnevali D, Reiner A. The cancer experience: nursing diagnosis and management. Philadelphia: JB Lippincott, 1990.

Glowacki G. Geriatric gynecology. In: Reichel W, ed. Clinical aspects of aging, 3rd ed. Baltimore: Williams & Wilkins, 1989:283.

Grayhack JT, Keeler TC. Carcinoma of the prostate: hormonal therapy. Cancer, 1987; 1(suppl 3): 589.

Libman E, Fichten CS. Prostatectomy and sexual function. Urology 1987; 29:467.

McCormick W. Lecture: Primary management for gerontological nurse practitioners. University of Washington, August 1991.

Walsh PC. Benign prostatic hyperplasia. In: Harrison JH, Gittes RF, Perlmutter AD, et al, eds. Campbell's urology, 5th ed. vol 2. Philadelphia: WB Saunders, 1986:1248.

27
Hearing Loss

DENISE RENTON DAVIGNON

Hearing loss is one of the most common disabilities in the United States. The prevalence of hearing loss in the elderly for the most important frequencies was 36% in the Framingham Heart Study (Moscicki et al, 1985). Figures from the National Health Interview Survey, conducted in 1989 are lower (Adams and Benson, 1990). According to data from this survey 28.5% (8.372 million) of the elderly have a hearing loss, 4.268 million of those are aged 65 to 74 and 4.104 million aged 75 years or older.

Data on the prevalence of hearing loss in elderly nursing home residents varies widely from 23% to 82%. Based on data from the US National Health Interview Survey (1982) the American Speech-Language and Hearing Association has stated "the prevalence of hearing loss in nursing home residents has been reported in the range between 48–82% of the elderly in long term care facilities." In the National Nursing Home Survey (1985) 23% of those 65 years and over were found to have a hearing loss. The larger figures in the 23% to 82% prevalence range are more reflective of this author's experience in the nursing home setting. The next National Nursing Home Survey is planned for 1993 or 1994. There will be a National Hospice and Home Care Survey in 1994, which will provide data on hearing loss in these populations of the elderly.

The major cause of hearing loss for older adults is usually of the sensorineural type and is called *presbycusis*. Tinnitus may accompany the hearing loss. These problems are not usually amenable to medical or surgical intervention. Other hearing rehabilitation modalities are available to the elderly. Nurses can play a key role in screening and referring older persons with hearing loss and in helping them identify and choose from among the various hearing assistance measures currently available.

Hearing loss is common in the elderly and should not be overlooked or ignored. For the elderly who often face multisystem changes with age, it is important to consider therapeutic options that reduce the dysfunctional impact of hearing loss, even when full restoration is not possible. The removal of cerumen impactions, or the use of hearing aids or other rehabilitative measures may not restore full hearing abilities, but they can improve communication and overall quality of the individual's life (Mulrow et al, 1990). A bibliography is included at the end of the chapter that lists basic resources to review when counseling the hearing impaired elder and selected national organizations related to hearing impairment.

The author gratefully acknowledges Doctors James H. Donaldson, Thomas S. Rees, and Barbara E. Weinstein for their time and suggestions for the content of this chapter.

510

Aging Changes, Hearing Loss, and Problems of the Ear

The aging process affects all portions of the physiologic structures involved in the pathways of hearing. Aging changes of the ear are discussed in Chapter 8. Hearing loss may be one of three types: conduction, sensorineural, or mixed (both conduction and sensorineural) (Fig. 27–1). Interference with the external or middle ear pathway for hearing is referred to as a conductive hearing loss. Problems in the inner ear (organ of Corti), eighth cranial nerve, or brain portions (brain stem auditory pathways and auditory cortex) of the hearing pathway cause a sensorineural hearing loss (Fig. 27–2). Interference with hearing pathways in the external or middle ear and the inner ear (and brain pathways) results in a mixed hearing loss. It is possible that elderly who have a hearing loss may experience a continuous loss at least into the ninth decade (Keay and Murray, 1988).

EXTERNAL EAR

In the external ear there is a decrease in the number and activity of the cerumen glands located in the distal half of the ear canal. The se-baceous glands and epithelium of the external ear canal atrophy and may cause the skin to atrophy and dry. While the elderly do not have an increased incidence of external ear infections, there may be more pain and tenderness in the ear canal when a disease is present.

PROBLEMS OF THE EXTERNAL EAR

Cerumen impactions are common in the elderly and often result in an insidious conduction hearing loss. The impactions may occur because of an increased dryness and adherency of the cerumen to canal walls. Other causes include hairy external ear canals, primarily found in elderly men, which prevents the normal extrusion of cerumen and benign bony growths (osteophytes, lateral osteomas) that narrow the external auditory canal. The latter cause is less common than the others. Cerumen removal requires a careful and slow separation of the cerumen from the skin to prevent pain or bloody discharge. Several drops of oil (Cerumenex, Debrox) can be used for several days to soften dry, hard cerumen followed by irrigation of the ear canal with water at body temperature. The canal should not be irrigated if there is a history of a tympanic membrane perforation or if the tympanic drum has not been visualized and

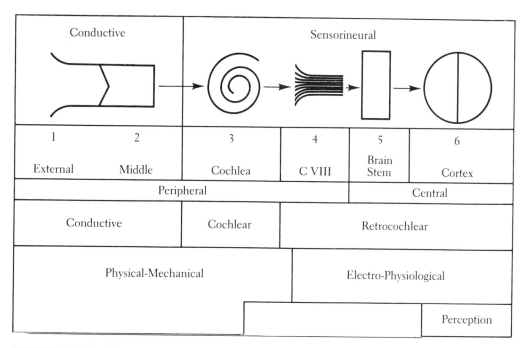

FIGURE 27–1   Schematic diagram for classifying auditory function and dysfunction. (From Snyder J. Office audiometry. J Fam Pract 1984; 19:535. Reprinted by permission of Appleton & Lange, Inc.)

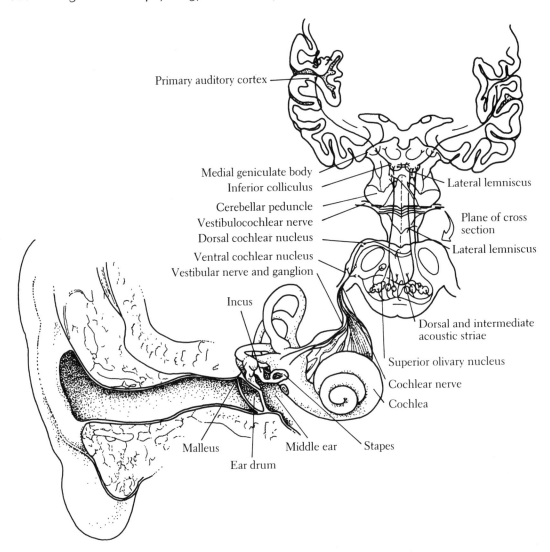

FIGURE 27–2 Sensorineural apparatus of the inner ear. (From Weinstein BE. Geriatric hearing loss: Myths, realities, resources for the physician. Geriatrics 1989; 44:42; with permission.)

found to be intact and showing no evidence of infection or unusual atrophy. Curretage and suctioning are other methods of removal but require more skill.

External otitis may be caused by bacterial or fungal infections. Cultures should be obtained and the ear treated with the appropriate ear drops (i.e., Vesol). Malignant otitis externa begins as an infection of the ear canal. It is uncommon but life-threatening and affects mainly elderly individuals with poorly controlled diabetes. The infecting organism is usually *Pseudomonas aeruginosa*. The infection spreads from the outer ear to the soft tissues below the temporal bone, then invades the

temporal bone. An osteomyelitis of the temporal bone develops. The infection goes on to invade the meninges. There is a high mortality, usually caused by meningitis, which led to the use of the adjective *malignant*. Symptoms include rapidly evolving pain in the ear, with or without purulent discharge, swelling of the parotid gland, and paralysis of the 6th to 12th nerves. Treatment consists of intravenous antibiotics and surgical debridement.

Elderly people with diabetes should be aware of and avoid activities that put them at risk for malignant otitis externa. Swimming in pools and using hot tubs or jacuzzis increases the risk of introducing water containing infectious organisms such as *Pseudomonas* in the ear. Sharp objects used to clear or relieve itching of the ear canal may cause sites of infection by traumatizing tissue in the canal. Surgical instruments should not be used to remove cerumen impaction because they also may traumatize tissue.

Pruritis in the external canal may be associated with or without dry skin. Preventative measures include avoiding moisture, trauma, and the use of defatting agents such as rubbing alcohol. Emollients are helpful because they act as an epidermal seal to reduce dryness associated with moisture loss from the skin.

The distal half of the external canal can also be the site of dermatoses, infected sebaceous cysts, and furunculosis. These infections should be treated early with the appropriate medicated topical cream such as an antibiotic or steroid, depending on the problem.

Though malignancies are rare in the external auditory canal, any increased granulation tissue or bloody otorrhea should be evaluated with a biopsy. The majority of carcinomas are squamous cell. Others include basal cell carcinomas and ceruminomas (adenomas, pleomorphic adenomas, adenoid cystic carcinomas, adenocarcinoma). Symptoms of malignancy include chronic otalgia that may be associated with otorrhea, facial nerve paralysis, vertigo, and hearing loss.

MIDDLE EAR

The ossicular articulations of the middle ear develop arthritic changes with age. The joint capsules show hyalinization and calcification, and there is calcification of the articular cartilage. However, despite these observations there appears to be little conductive hearing loss associated with these changes (Rees and Duckert, 1990). The tympanic membrane may develop atrophic or sclerotic changes, which do not usually cause significant loss of hearing (Yoder, 1989). Hearing loss that is moderate to severe will occur with tympanic membrane retraction or malfunction of the ossicular chain.

PROBLEMS OF THE MIDDLE EAR

Serous effusions are usually caused by viral upper respiratory infections (otitis media with serous effusion) or by sudden changes in barometric pressure that occur with flying or diving (otitic barotrauma). The effusion occurs when the eustachian tube cannot equalize the air pressure in the middle ear with that of the outside air. Air is completely or partly absorbed into the blood and serous fluid accumulates in its place. Symptoms may include a fullness and popping sensation in the ear, with a mild conduction hearing loss. There also may be pain.

Secretory otitis media occurring bilaterally may develop following a common cold, allergic rhinitis, or sinus disease. The mucosa secrete large amounts of an amber, mucoid, or grayish fluid, possibly because of a primary allergic response rather than as a result of a negative barometric pressure in the inner ear (as with otic barotrauma). It can produce a moderate-to-severe painless, conductive hearing loss. Secretory otitis media occuring unilaterally is rare (unless there is a history of middle ear disease) and in the elderly may be associated with nasopharyngeal carcinoma. Secretory otitis media is usually treated with decongestants and antibiotics. Myringotomy, aspiration, or middle ear ventilation tubes may be necessary to permit drainage of the excess fluid. Chronic otitis media with perforation of the tympanic membrane can occur as the result of acute otitis media, trauma, or otomastoiditis. In addition to the infection, bleeding or vertigo may occur. Perforations may close spontaneously following local therapy. Small perforations without middle ear complications may be patched using tissue paper, temporalis fascia, or sclera from tissue banks. Patches may be effective in closing the perforation and restoring hearing. Larger perforations may need to be treated with a tympanoplasty or myringoplasty.

Ossicular fixation refers to a fixation of the malleus, incus, or both. Fixation of these tiny bones can immobilize the tympanic membrane and result in conductive hearing loss. Diagnostic measures include audiologic testing and tympanometry, which measures impedance of the middle ear and stapedius response. Ossicular fixation is treated surgically. Amplification with a hearing aid is an alternative to surgical treatment.

Otosclerosis refers to the formation of spongy bone in the capsule of the labyrinth of the ear. This often leads to fixation of the stapes footplate to the oval window, resulting in a conductive hearing loss. In addition, this process may produce a sensorineural component to the hearing loss by affecting parts of the labyrinth and otic capsule. The etiology is not known; there may be genetic link, and vitamin deficiency and otitis media may contribute to the development of otosclerosis. Progressive loss of hearing is the most noticeable symptom, though tinnitus may be an early symptom. It is thought to affect approximately 10% of the population and while onset of the disease usually occurs in young adulthood, it may go unrecognized until secondary presbycusis occurs in the later years and hearing loss becomes pronounced. The patient's medical history that includes progressive hearing loss and tinnitus and otologic and audiologic examinations leads to a diagnosis. Treatment may consist of surgery, the use of a hearing aid, or both. Surgical treatment consists of freeing the stapes or performing a stapedectomy, which involves removal of the stapes and replacing it with a grafted body tissue attached to a plastic tube or a stainless steel wire. There have been excellent results for patients over 70 with profound mixed type hearing loss treated with stapedectomy (Yoder, 1989).

INNER EAR

After the fourth or fifth decade of life the auditory system functions less efficiently, due to degeneration of sensory and neural elements. Chapter 8 discusses changes in the inner ear as they relate to the complex functioning of the hearing pathway.

PROBLEMS OF THE INNER EAR

Presbycusis is a progressive, often bilaterally symmetric, perceptive hearing loss occurring with age. There are no known preventative measures for presbycusis. Presbycusis is considered to be a complex disorder because in addition to a diminished perception of pure tones, there can be a loss of speech processing and discrimination as well (Welsh, 1985).

PRESBYCUSIS

Presbycusis is usually characterized by an impaired sensitivity to tones in the higher frequencies that is greater and more severe than in low frequency tones. There are different kinds of presbycusis, each believed to have a different structural origin in the inner ear and each resulting in different functional impairment. While individuals do not typically fit any one type of presbycusis, audiometric results may more closely resemble one of the types (Fig. 27–3). Sensory presbycusis is caused by a degeneration of hair cells in the organ of Corti.

Audiograms show a sharp increase in hearing loss for high frequencies. Sensitivity for tones within the normal range for speech are better preserved. Neural presbycusis is due to degeneration of nerve fibers and affects on transmission of neurally coded information used in analyzing speech patterns. The functional impairment of this type of presbycusis is a reduction in speech discrimination abilities, beyond that which might be predicted from pure tone audiographic testing. Strial (metabolic) presbycusis is due to a slowly progressive atrophy of the stria vascularis. Strial cell atrophy affects the fluid in the scala media. This fluid transforms the mechanical sound wave to a neural signal. The effect on hearing is a reduction in sensitivity to all frequencies and a more uniform hearing loss than other types of presbycusis. There is essentially little change in speech discrimination since the neuronal population is well preserved. When pure tone hearing thresholds become elevated beyond 50 dB speech discrimination does decline (Rees and Duckert, 1990). Cochlear conductive (mechanical) presbycusis is thought to be caused by dysfunction of the vibratory motion of the basilar membrane in the cochlea. This results in a hearing loss across all frequencies at a magnitude that increases linearly from lower to higher frequencies. "Whether or not this type of presbycusis actually exists is controversial" (Rees and Duckert, 1990). A number of degenerative patterns of the basilar membrane have been identified. Yet there is no definite histopathologic correlate to cochlear presbycusis.

An important clinical aspect of presbycusis in the elderly is the evaluation of continuing factors: (1) true age phenomena, (2) the results of acoustic trauma and noise-induced hearing loss, and (3) results of undiagnosed cochlear lesions that may have nothing to do with age (e.g., lesions caused by arteriosclerosis, cholesterol metabolism, diet, or nutrition).

The true age phenomena (changes) have been discussed here and in Chapter 8. Hearing loss that is caused by acoustic trauma and noise may occur in conjunction with normal presbycusis. At risk for acoustic trauma are those with prolonged exposure to noise-intense environments such as industry, military, aircraft, music (loud band performances), and hunting. In some older people reduced cerebral function may cause a central nervous system auditory pathway lesion and a resulting loss of vocal sounds. This is evident as a phonemic regres-

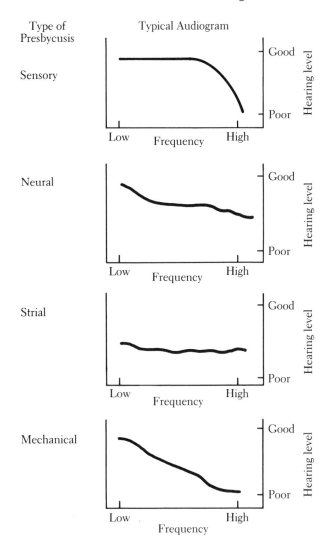

Type of Presbycusis — Typical Audiogram

Sensory

Neural

Strial

Mechanical

FIGURE 27-3 Audiogram results associated with types of presbycusis. (Adapted from Whitbourne SK. The aging body. Physiological changes and psychosocial consequences. New York: Springer-Verlag, 1985.)

sion where hearing for speech is much worse than the pure tone audiogram might suggest. This individual is likely to have greater difficulty with speech in a noisy background. Fluctuating pure tone and speech discrimination score values may suggest complicating metabolic, vascular, or central nervous system problems, and a one-time audiogram would not be reflective of the true diagnosis. Other conditions such as diabetes, arteriosclerosis, hypertension, and thyroid disease can result in an intermittent cellular hypoxia (Goodhill, 1986). The hypoxia can cause fluctuating cochlear hearing levels, which when superimposed on a preexisting mild presbycusis, result in what appears to be a more severe presbycusis. Individuals with presbycusis should, therefore, be reexamined periodically.

Ototoxicity, which results in a bilateral hearing loss, may be mistaken for presbycusis. Such ototoxicities may result from high doses of salicylates or aminoglycoside antibiotics. High doses of ethacrinic acid and furosemide (Lasix) may be ototoxic. A list of some of the drugs that can cause ototoxicity is contained in Table 27-1. The hearing impairment may be reversible for aspirin, ethacrynic acid, and furosemide. The other drugs produce an irreversible hearing loss. Ototoxic drugs are thought to cause a loss of hair cells in the cochlea and vestibular end organs. Elderly individuals with impaired renal function are at greater risk for hav-

TABLE 27–1   Some Drugs That Can Be Ototoxic in the Elderly

Aspirin	Kanamycin
Chloroquine	Mechlorethamine
Cisplatin	Neomycin
Dibekacin	Quinidine
Dihydrostreptomycin	Quinine
Erythromycin	Reserpine
Ethacrynic acid	Sisomicin
Furosemide	Streptomycin
Gentamicin	Tobramycin
Hydroxychloroquine	Vancomycin
Indomethacin	

From Committee on Hearing, Bioacoustics, and Biomechanics. Speech understanding and aging. Washington, DC: National Research Council, 1987.

ing ototoxic effects from these drugs because small doses can create high blood levels.

TINNITUS

Tinnitus is the perception of a sound that has no source in the environment. It can be a disturbing continuous sound or an occasional annoyance. Individual descriptions of the type of sound vary. It may be described as a ringing, humming, hissing, or clicking. In some cases the individual hears a single sound while in others two, three, or more sounds are heard. Since the noise is produced within the body it is not heard by others except when there is a vascular origin (bruit) and then it may be audible by stethoscope. Tinnitus can be a symptom of hearing loss or of a more serious medical condition. To rule out these more serious conditions, it is imperative that a complete evaluation of the tinnitus be conducted. Unilateral tinnitus may be the first symptom of a tumor of the internal auditory meatus or of the cerebellopontine angle. Unilateral or bilateral tinnitus can be the first symptom of the beginning of otosclerosis.

In certain situations everyone may experience a "normal" tinnitus. These are internal body sounds that become apparent when an individual is in an environment that has very few

or no background noises. In such an environment internal visceral sounds (breathing, cardiac contractility, and vascular flow), usually masked by environmental sounds, can be heard. Tinnitus becomes a symptom when internally heard sounds become louder than environmental sounds.

The etiology of tinnitus is unclear but may be related to a number of pathologic conditions in the ear, the eighth cranial nerve, the brain stem auditory pathways, and the auditory cortex. A recent study has suggested origination in the cochlea, with possible additional involvement of central pathways (Dauman and Cazals, 1989).

Tinnitus can be a source of suffering and disability. Its severity can be assessed only through the report of the person experiencing it. Loudness and severity or annoyance are the two primary factors assessed. Goodhill discusses several descriptors of tinnitus which may be useful clinically to understand and more accurately describe the problem (Table 27–2).

MANAGEMENT OF TINNITUS

When tinnitus is thought to result from a specific lesion or disorder of the ear (tinnitus auriem) or from a cerebrovascular or other intracranial lesion (tinnitus cranii) therapy is directed at the underlying problem, with medical or surgical treatment specific for that problem. The tinnitus may resolve once the underlying problem is corrected. If there is no specific problem found to be associated with the tinnitus or if the symptom persists despite adequate otologic or other medical treatment, then treatment would focus on converting a decompensated tinnitus to a compensated tinnitus. As described in Table 27–2 a decompensated tinnitus is a tinnitus reported as a major ear complaint by the individual. A compensated tinnitus is a tinnitus that is not complained of by the individual but is acknowledged during the interview for a medical history. There are a number of possible approaches to consider when the treatment goal is conversion.

Patient information and education is a significant aspect of treatment. It is known that those with uncompensated tinnitus are often anxious and frightened by the constant noise that they live with. The disturbing reality of continuous noise without obvious cause is distressing. The individual should be given infor-

TABLE 27–2   *Adjectives Useful in Clinical Descriptions and Assessment of Tinnitus*

Subjective tinnitus	Auditory sensation of a sound (ringing, humming, whistling, roaring, clicking) or any other sensation of tones or noise
Objective tinnitus (bruit)	A tone or sound that can be heard by the examiner (the physician) as well as the patient
Ear tinnitus	Usually accompanied by hearing loss (conductive and/or sensorineural). Can be unilateral (as associated with cerumen impaction, otitis media, tympanic membrane perforation), or bilateral (symmetrical bilateral otosclerosis). If bilateral it can resemble nonlocalized head tinnitus
Head tinnitus (tinnitus cranii)	Nonlocalized subjective sensation of a sound that is usually diffuse in the head and has a nonspecific quality. Usually due to vascular disease (extracranial or intracranial vascular lesions, anemia, polycythemia, hypertension or hypotension may play etiologic roles)
Compensated tinnitus	Individual does not complain of the tinnitus but will acknowledge its presence when interviewed for the medical history
Decompensated tinnitus	Individual reports the tinnitus as a major ear complaint

Adapted from Goodhill V. Deafness, tinnitus and dizziness in the aged. In: Rossman I, ed. Clinical geriatrics, 3rd ed. Philadelphia: JB Lippincott, 1986:416.

mation about the findings of the diagnostic work-up and outcomes from the otologist, ENT physician, and generalists who have evaluated the individual. The information is used to help the individual understand possible causes of tinnitus and inform him what has been done to rule out those causes. Common patient fears about the tinnitus are that they may be going deaf, having a stroke, have a brain tumor, or are at the beginning of serious mental illness. While the remote possibility exists for some of these concerns, they are not a reality for most (Goodhill, 1986). Information about the nature of tinnitus should cover what the tinnitus represents, that it is real and that it is not an illusion, delusion, or hallucination (Goodhill, 1986).

Uncompensated tinnitus may be helped by methods that create a masking effect on the tinnitus. Masking refers to the decreased awareness of the tinnitus that results from the production of another sound or sounds in the environment. Tinnitus may be relieved by the use of a hearing aid, if one is required due to hearing loss. Rarely, a hearing aid will accentuate tinnitus rather than mask it (Goodhill, 1986). Amplification of all sounds may mask the tinnitus. At quiet times, such as bedtime, tinnitus will become more apparent. Radios, a loud clock, or any other device that produces a

sound may be used to mask the tinnitus. Masking devices that produce sounds or electrical stimulation and are worn by the patient are an option for those who are more severely or continuously bothered by tinnitus. The tinnitus may also be relieved for several hours after removal of the device.

Depression has been associated with tinnitus. Current early research in the area demonstrates success in relieving tinnitus with the use of antidepressants. Those with the most severe tinnitus may have the best response to such treatment (Sullivan et al, 1991).

Biofeedback and stress management training may be helpful in reducing the tension created by living with tinnitus. For those who do not have access to such training, there is at least one book on relaxation and stress reduction available in book stores that approaches this problem (Davis et al, 1988).

NURSING ASSESSMENT OF THE EAR

Ear assessments should be completed on all older persons as treatment and rehabilitation can affect the older adult's quality of life (Mulrow et al, 1990). Nursing assessment of the ear and hearing loss may be completed during a comprehensive nursing history and physical examination or done separately. In either situation information should be obtained about the individual's medical history as it relates to the ear and hearing before the physical examination and hearing testing.

HEALTH HISTORY OF THE EAR

The nurse should ask questions about the ears; have there been any earaches, tinnitus, vertigo, discharge, infection, or mastoiditis? In addition, ask questions about hearing. How does the elderly person rate his own hearing: good, fair, or poor? Does he hear better in one ear or another, or both equally? More direct questions about specific hearing difficulties should follow. Does he have problems hearing in groups, hearing sounds at a distance, hearing on the telephone, hearing soft voices, or hearing in noisy public places? Direct questions will often identify a hearing loss not detected on physical examination (Rees, 1990). If the elderly person is unable to give a history because of cognitive dysfunction or a communication impairment, for example, then the nurse can review the person's medical chart and talk with relatives or caretakers to gather any known information. The health and medical history of other body systems may reveal problems that can contribute to hearing loss (Weinstein, 1989). For example, is there a history of vascular disease (hypertension, cerebrovascular arteriosclerosis, strokes), metabolic disease (diabetes mellitus, renal disease, hypothyroidism, hyperlipoproteinemia), or infections (herpes zoster)? The occupational history can reveal exposure to loud noises for a prolonged time, contributing to a noise-induced hearing loss. Evaluation of the elderly person's current medications and drug history is important in evaluation of hearing loss related to ototoxicity.

PHYSICAL EXAMINATION OF THE EAR

A physical examination of the ear should begin with an inspection for discharge or inflammation. The nurse should ask about ear pain. If it is present move the auricle up and down, press the tragus, and press firmly just behind the ear. Acute otitis externa may be present if there is pain with movement of the auricle or tragus. Otitis media would be suspected with tenderness elicited behind the ear. Further inspection of the ear canal and drum requires the use of an otoscope. Position of the patient and correct, safe use of the otoscope are important to re-

member on examination (Bates, 1991). The patient's head should be tipped to the opposite side of the ear being examined and the patient instructed not to move the head. The auricle is then gently pulled upward, back, and slightly out. The speculum of the otoscope is inserted in the canal. The otoscope may be held with the handle pointing either up or down. The safest position is with the handle held up and the fourth and fifth finger of the hand grasping the otoscope placed firmly against the head of the patient. This positioning is referred to as anchoring because it stabilizes the position of the otoscope and thereby avoids injury to the canal should the patient move his head.

The view of the canal and drum may be wholly or partly obstructed by cerumen. The cerumen may appear as flaky yellow, sticky brown, or hard and very dark. Inspect the ear canal for discharge, foreign bodies, redness, or swelling. A nonmalignant overgrowth called an osteoma may appear as a nontender nodular swelling covered with normal skin that is deep in the canal. It may obstruct the view of the drum. Acute otitis externa presents a swollen, narrowed, moist, pale, and tender canal. If the otitis externa is chronic, the skin will appear thickened and red and will be itchy. The tympanic membrane (TM) should be inspected for color and contour. Acute purulent otitis media can cause the TM to become red and bulge (Bates, 1991). A serous effusion would be suspected with an amber colored TM. If the short process and handle are unusually prominent the TM may be retracted. The speculum should be moved gently to view as much of the drum as possible while looking for any perforations. A perforation will appear as an oval hole through which a dark shadow may be seen. Anterior and inferior borders of the TM may be obscured by the canal.

SCREENING EXAMINATIONS FOR HEARING LOSS

There are a number of methods to choose from when screening for hearing loss in the elderly. Free field (live) voice testing (the whisper test), the Rinne test, and the Weber test have been used in general clinical practice. No special equipment is needed for free field voice testing. A tuning fork is required for the Weber and Rinne tests. Self assessment questionnaires have been developed (Gutnick et al, 1989; Schow and Nerbonne, 1977; Lichtenstein et al,

1988; Weinstein, 1989). One is specific for use in the nursing home (Schow and Nerbonne 1977). The audiometer may be used. It is a specialized piece of equipment and more suited for office examinations. The audioscope is a more recently developed portable screening tool that is combined with an otoscope (Bienvue et al, 1985; Frank and Peterson, 1987; Lichtenstein et al, 1988).

Controversy exists over the reliability and usefulness of the whisper, Weber, and Rinne tests (Rees and Duckert, 1990; Browning, 1989). Criticisms include that the method of test administration and interpretation can vary widely. As Rees (1990) notes, physical diagnosis textbooks are inconsistent in their recommended approaches to auditory screening evaluations. The American Speech-Language and Hearing Association recently concluded from their studies that screening guidelines are inappropriate at this time in part because of unresolved issues (such as the age after which elder screening should occur). Their report is due to be published as this text goes to press. Until screening guidelines are established, the nurse may choose from among the several methods to screen for hearing loss. The current trend, however, is the use of the Hearing Handicap Inventory for the Elderly Screening Version (HHIES) and the audioscope because they are valid, reliable, simple, and inexpensive.

AUDIOMETERS AND AUDIOSCOPES

Audiometers and audioscopes are preferred forms of screening because they are more sensitive and yield data that are more objectively interpreted (Rees, 1990). Audiometers are more frequently used in office settings and are available in portable models. Learning to use one and interpret results is relatively easy. The use of audiometers is discussed by Snyder (1984). The audioscope is a handheld portable version of the audiometer. It is called an audioscope because it is housed within an otoscope (Fig. 27–4). It is considered a reliable and valid tool (Bienvue et al, 1985; Frank and Peterson, 1987; Lichtenstein et al, 1988). In many settings, however, these types of tools may not be available or familiar to the nurse. Questionnaires, free field voice testing, the Weber and the Rinne tests are alternatives for screening when they are administered and interpreted with an understanding of their limitations (Browning, 1989).

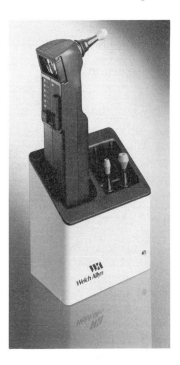

FIGURE 27–4 The audioscope: a screening audiometer housed within an otoscope. Has four frequencies (500, 1000, 2000, and 4000 Hz) and three intensity levels (20, 25, and 40 dB HL). (Photograph courtesy of Welch-Allyn, Inc., Skaneateles Falls, NY.)

QUESTIONNAIRE

The Hearing Handicap Inventory for the Elderly (HHIE) is designed for use with noninstitutionalized elderly and is considered both valid and reliable (Lichtenstein et al, 1988; Weinstein, 1989). There are 25 items that assess emotional and social reaction to the hearing loss. The scoring helps to determine the degree of impact or handicap on the individual's life as a result of the hearing loss. There is a shortened 10 item screening version (HHIES) (Table 27–3). In the nursing home setting the Nursing Home Hearing Handicap Index (NHHHI) could be used (Gutnick et al, 1989; Schow and Nerbonne 1977). This self-assessment survey consists of 10 items and also measures the social and emotional handicap caused by hearing loss. The validity and reliability of the NHHHI has not been well established (Gutnick et al, 1989). Nurses in nursing homes may achieve more accurate screening results by using the HHIE or its shortened form, HHIE-S (Weinstein; personal communication, 1991). Since both tests require appropriate re-

TABLE 27–3   ***Hearing Handicap Inventory for the Elderly Screening Version***

Does a hearing problem cause you to feel embarrassed when you meet new people?

Does a hearing problem cause you to feel frustrated when talking to members of your family?

Do you have difficulty hearing when someone speaks in a whisper?

Do you feel handicapped by a hearing problem?

Does a hearing problem cause you difficulty when visiting friends, relatives, or neighbors?

Does a hearing problem cause you to attend religious services less often than you would like?

Does a hearing problem cause you to have arguments with family members?

Does a hearing problem cause you difficulty when listening to television or radio?

Do you feel that any difficulty with your hearing limits or hampers your personal or social life?

Does a hearing problem cause you difficulty when in a restaurant with relatives or friends?

Scale: 0 = no; 2 = sometimes; 4 = yes.
Score interpretations: 0 to 8 points = no or slight handicap; 10 to 22 points = moderate handicap; 24 to 40 points = severe handicap.
From Ventry I, Weinstein B. Identification of elderly people with hearing problems. Rockville, MD: ASHA. July 1983, p. 37; with permission.

sponses to be accurate, testing of mental status should be completed before administration of either the NHHHI or the HHIE. There are a number of short mental status examinations that may be used (see Chapter 16).

FREE FIELD VOICE TESTING

The free field voice test is a rough quantitative test for hearing loss that is easily administered. One ear is tested at a time while the patient or examiner occludes the other ear with a finger. The occluding finger may be moved back and forth rapidly but gently to mask sound and prevent the untested ear from doing the work of the ear being tested. This maneuver is particularly useful when there is a difference in auditory acuity on the two sides. The examiner should be at a distance of 1 or 2 feet from the

patient. To prevent the patient from reading your lips have them close their eyes or place your hand in front of your mouth so they are unable to see your lips. Or you may stand behind the patient at the same distance. After fully exhaling your breath to minimize the intensity of your voice whisper words with two equally accented syllables such as "nine-four" or "countdown." If before the examination the patient reports that they hear but that they do not understand you may also test acuity with words that contain high frequency sounds such as *f*, *s*, and *th*, which are more easily misunderstood in the patient who has a speech discrimination problem. Examples of such words are "thin, fin, and sin." A false-negative test result can occur with the free field voice test when there is a high frequency loss. Therefore, patients who report a hearing loss but demonstrate no hearing deficit with free field voice testing should be referred.

WEBER AND RINNE TESTS

When hearing is diminished the Weber and Rinne tests may be used to distinguish between a conduction loss and a sensorineural loss (Bates, 1991). The tests should be conducted in a quiet room and require the use of a tuning fork with a frequency that falls within the range of human speech (300 to 3000 Hz). The 512-Hz tuning fork is the most frequently used and is possibly the most reliable and valid (Snyder, 1984). Browning's study (1989) suggested the 256-Hz tuning fork is superior in detecting airbone gaps irrespective of magnitude. Frequencies are inscribed on the tuning fork.

The Weber tests for lateralization of sound to one or the other ear. To perform the test set the fork into light vibration by stroking up the outside of the tines on the tuning fork with your thumb and index finger or gently tap the tines with a reflex hammer. Place the vibrating fork firmly on top of the patient's head or in the mid forehead. Ask the patient if he hears the sound and if so where he hears it, on one or both sides. The sound should be heard in the midline or equally in both ears. If the sound is heard unilaterally it can indicate either a conduction loss or a sensorineural loss. If the loss is due to a conduction problem, the patient will hear sound better in the impaired ear because the conduction impairment of this ear will block room noise and the vibrations of the tuning fork through the bone will be detected better than normal. If the loss is of a unilateral sensorineural type, sound will be heard in the good ear because sound will not travel well in the impaired inner ear, cochlea, or nerve whether transmitted by air or bone.

The Rinne test compares air conduction and bone conduction. The lightly vibrating tuning fork should be placed on the mastoid bone behind the ear at the level of the ear canal. The patient is asked if he can hear the sound and then instructed to report when the sound stops. When the patient indicates the sound has stopped the tuning fork is quickly moved to the front of the ear close to the ear canal without touching the ear with the U shape of the fork facing forward to maximize sound. The patient is again asked if he can hear the sound. Normally the patient will hear the sound in the air after he has stopped hearing the sound through the bone; air conduction is about twice as long as bone conduction (air conduction > bone conduction or a positive Rinne result). When a sensorineural loss is present the normal pattern (positive Rinne) prevails. However, in a conduction loss, sound will be heard as long (the sound in front of the ear stops immediately after first hearing it) or longer (no sound is heard in front of the ear) through the bone than it is through the air.

AUDIOLOGIC EVALUATION

When hearing loss has been identified and a complete otologic examination performed to rule out the existence of problems that may be helped by medical management, patients should be referred for a thorough audiologic examination. The purpose of the evaluation is to develop an individualized rehabilitation program. Experts in the field of audiology stress the need for an individualized approach in rehabilitation. They cite the variability in impairment of the different characteristics of hearing loss from one person to the next (Matkin and Hodgson, 1982). When differences in the psychosocial, physical, and financial needs between individuals are also considered, the heterogeneity of the population of hearing impaired elders is even more apparent.

Patients who are thought to be in need of an audiologic examination and a hearing aid should be counseled about their options in choosing an individual who can provide them with these services. Hearing aid dealers are individuals licensed by the state to dispense hearing aids. Licensure requirements vary from state to state, with some states requiring that a hearing aid dealer only be at least 18 years of age and pass a state licensing examination. Consequently, the skill and training in evaluation of hearing impairment and fitting of hearing aids may differ considerably from one dealer to the next. There is no guarantee of a standard skill level in evaluation. Some dealers may be more oriented toward sales. Clinical audiologists are university educated professionals, holding a master's degree or a doctoral degree. Clinical audiologists are trained in the area of nonmedical management of hearing loss, including hearing aid amplification, rehabilitation therapies, assistive listening devices, or a combination of rehabilitative approaches. Most audiologists sell aids from a variety of manufacturers. Those who do not will refer their patients to a hearing aid dealer. The audiologist will check the aid during the trial purchase period. While the hearing aid dealer may offer more competitive prices on standard models of hearing aids, the audiologist is by training better prepared to provide a comprehensive plan of treatment for hearing loss beyond the evaluation and selection of hearing aids.

The audiologic examination includes obtaining a pure tone audiogram, detailed speech audiometry, and evaluation of loudness tolerance. These tests help evaluate hearing function at the various anatomic levels of the hearing pathway (Kane et al, 1989). Standard tests help evaluate the peripheral pathway, and binaural tests are for brain stem evaluation and difficult speech tests for cortical problems. The standard tests include pure tone audiometry, which assesses the intensity (measured in decibels) at which sound of increasing frequencies are heard. This sound threshold is assessed for both air conduction, using ear phones, and bone conduction, using an oscillator placed behind the ear. The results are graphed as relative loss of decibels at different frequencies. The difference in the results from air conduction and bone conduction is referred to as the air-bone gap. Hearing loss in air conduction alone would indicate a conduction loss. A similar amount of loss in air and bone conduction suggests a sensorineural loss. This pattern is often found in age-related hearing loss as hearing is normal for the low frequencies but shows impairment in the higher frequencies. A loss in sensitivity for bone conduction with a greater loss for air conduction represents a mixed loss (Rees and Duckert, 1990).

Speech audiometry examinations involve presenting two syllable words and determining the softest level at which 50% of the words can be identified. The results should agree within ± 10 dB of the pure tone average of 500, 1000, and 2000 Hz. Results are a reliability check on pure tone thresholds. Age-related hearing loss is often manifested by a reduction of speech understanding in addition to hearing sensitivity loss. Speech discrimination evaluations test the clarity or intelligibility of speech. In this examination, 25 to 50 monosyllabic words are presented at comfortably loud levels. It is scored by determining the percentage of correct responses. This test is important in determining the degree of functional impairment or communication handicap associated with the hearing loss. It also provides additional diagnostic information. Higher speech discrimination scores are associated with hearing aid success because of decreased distortion in the auditory system. Speech discrimination scores that are consistent with pure tone testing suggest a cochlear lesion. Scores that are poorer than what pure tone loss would suggest would indicate neural involvement. The presence of poor speech discrimination in the face of minimal hearing loss is referred to as phonemic regression.

Binaural testing assesses integrative functions of the brain stem. Binaural interaction allows localization of sound and extraction of signals from a noisy environment (Kane et al, 1989). Loudness comparison testing assesses the individual's ability to balance intensity of sound from both ears. Lateralization tests the ability to fuse sounds from both ears, while masking level differences assesses the ability to pick out specific sounds from a background of noise. Monotic graded tasks present difficult sounds such as noise background, filtered sound, and time compressed speech; dichotic tasks simultaneously present sense and nonsense speech, which the individual is asked to repeat.

REHABILITATION FOR HEARING LOSS

There are only a small fraction of individuals with hearing losses who have medically treatable problems. Presbycusis, the sensorineural loss common in the elderly, is not treatable

through medical intervention. Instead the hearing loss of presbycusis is managed by rehabilitative methods, with the goal of improving communication. The hearing aid is the most common device used for rehabilitation. Other devices include amplifiers, telephones that will transmit written messages, and light systems that are connected to door bells or fire alarms. The National Information Center on Deafness (NICD) has a list of assistive listening devices centers across the United States that display technical devices and aids such as these. Speech reading classes are often recommended for learning how to more fully develop the skills of observing a speaker's lip, face, and body movements. Auditory training includes special listening sessions for amplification device users and helps the individual adjust to amplified sound.

HEARING AIDS

Hearing aids are miniature loud speaker systems that increase the intensity of sound and deliver it to the ear with as little distortion as possible. There are a number of basic styles of hearing aids (Fig. 27–5). The major differences among them are cost, size, ease of handling, and acoustic characteristics. The behind the ear (BTE) aid has the battery, amplifier, and receiver in a small curved case that fits behind the ear. A small plastic tube from the case to an ear mold in the canal transmits sound. The eye glasses hearing aids have the aid components in the temple piece on one side of the frame and a small plastic tube is connected to a mold in the ear. In the ear aids (ITE) contain all the compo-

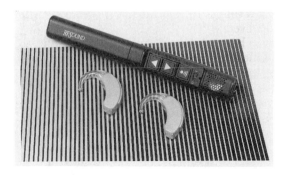

FIGURE 27–5   Personal hearing systems. (Photo courtesy of ReSound Corporation, Redwood City, CA 94063.)

nents in an ear mold unit that fits in the bowl of the external ear. In the canal aids (ITC) also contain all the components in an ear mold, but this mold fits in the external canal. The body aid contains all the components in a rectangular case the size of a shirt pocket. A wire from the case to an ear mold transmits sound.

The BTE aid is more visible but may be easier for some to manipulate the volume controls because of its larger size and location. The eye glasses aid is not commonly selected because one cannot be used without the other. The ITE models are cosmetically appealing and are inserted with relative ease. They are preferred by many. The ITC models are very appealing to some because their location in the external canal make them fairly obscure. These aids are very small and more difficult to insert and adjust. This type would be a poor choice for someone with arthritic fingers or other problems that affect fine motor control and dexterity. Body hearing aids are bulky and highly visible. They are the best choice for those with profound hearing loss and those who may have difficulty manipulating the smaller units. Individuals who may be unable to use any of the various hearing aids, cannot afford to buy one, or are reluctant or unable to be evaluated or fitted for a hearing aid may benefit from a simple amplifier with a head set. These may be purchased at electronic stores.

Use of Hearing Aids Hearing aids function to amplify sound. All sounds will be amplified for the hearing aid user. The hearing aid will not correct distortion of sound or improve difficulties with processing. The hearing aid user must be counseled to understand the limitations of the aid and ideally receive instruction in how to use it. The elderly person should know that the quality of restored hearing that is achieved with a hearing aid will be different from hearing the way he was used to. Since all sounds are amplified, background noises may be louder and intrusive on other sounds. A period of time will be needed for the elderly person to get used to hearing all sounds at the same intensity and to learn to "tune in," selectively, to the sounds that are most important to hear at different times. As with any assistive device there are skills to be learned. Often hearing aid users will initially use the aids in environments where background sounds are minimal. Gradually, as they become accus-

tomed to hearing all sounds of a greater volume, they will wear it for longer times in situations with more background noises.

There are books written by older persons who have had to adapt to a loss of hearing and the use of hearing aids. They can be instructional as well as motivational (Himber, 1989; Combs, 1989). They also include information on local and national organizations that directly or indirectly may be of help to the hearing impaired. Such books offer the advantages of reinforcing teaching or counseling, having much information in one text rather than in multiple pamphlets or handout materials, and a personal perspective of the problem of hearing loss.

All professionals who provide care to hearing aid users should know how to assist them in inserting their ear molds and adjusting the volume control to a comfortable level. Older persons who benefit from the use of their aid but who may be temporarily unable to manage it themselves will be encountered in all health care settings. General maintenance measures are easy to remember and important to know. The ear mold should be cleaned regularly by sponging with soap and water to remove cerumen accumulation. A toothpick can be used to clean the small aperture if it becomes clogged with wax. Batteries should be checked regularly. The usual life is about 5 to 6 weeks although they may last a little longer if the hearing aid is turned off when not in use. Ear molds should be inserted so that they fit comfortably and snugly. The hearing aid will squeal if there is a loose fit. Because changes on the cartilage of the ear continue to occur with aging and may change the shape of the external ear and canal, ear molds should be reevaluated periodically and a new one made if necessary. The life of a hearing aid unit will vary from 5 to 10 years. If a hearing aid is more than 5 years old and has been repaired once it may be more cost effective to replace it rather than repairing it again if it malfunctions (Himber, 1989).

ASSISTIVE LISTENING DEVICES

There are a number of technological mechanisms now available for use in homes and in institutions. They help link hearing impaired individuals to the world of sound by enhancing sound transmission or replacing sound with visual (lights) or written communication. They may be used independent of or in conjunction with hearing aids.

An Induction Loop is used in small institutional rooms. The listener needs to have a hearing aid with a T coil or may rent or purchase a special receiver. A loop of wire circles the room and is attached to the amplifier's speaker. The loop is either permanent or portable and enables the listener to hear the speaker more clearly by reducing background noise.

An FM system can be used in large auditoriums or in smaller spaces where there is other noise or multiple conversations such as restaurants, cars, or buses. It is a wireless amplification system that transmits sounds from the speakers microphone on an FM system radio wave. The speaker wears a microphone and transmitter and the listener wears a receiver. It is used in situations where one person speaks at a time or there is a single speaker.

The infrared system is also wireless and converts television sound waves into infrared waves. A microphone is fastened to the television speaker. Velcro can be used so it can be easily removed for use on other televisions. A transmitter is plugged into the wall socket. A lightweight cordless head set is worn by the listener and can be used without hearing aids. The device allows the hearing impaired listener to receive amplification of sound while nonhearing impaired individuals listen at the normal volume. There is also clearer reception of the sound. There are different units available at different prices, from $100 to $350 or more. Some allow far more freedom of movement in a room while still getting good reception while others may allow less movement but improved clarity. These systems are light sensitive; bright sunlight and fluorescent lights can interfere with sound transmission.

TELECOMMUNICATIONS DEVICES

There are several ways to allow the hearing impaired better access to the use of a telephone. Telephone amplifiers amplify the voice of the caller and may be used by those with hearing aids who find aid amplification is not sufficient for telephone use. They may also be used by those who do not wear a hearing aid. There are several types of telephone amplification systems. The portable type straps onto the telephone receiver. Another type has a unit that is placed near and is plugged into the telephone. The built-in type has an amplifier in the hand-

set of the telephone and may be adjusted for regular use when amplification is not needed. There are also cordless telephones with built-in amplification systems. Electronic stores carry some of these amplifiers, including the built-in type. Telephone companies carry the built-in type. AT&T has a Special Needs Center that will assist hearing impaired customers with obtaining amplification devices for the telephone (see list of organizations). In at least one state (Washington) amplifiers are available at no charge.

Telecommunication devices for the deaf (TDD) is a telephone system that displays a typed message on a screen that is attached to a unit that is either permanent or portable. Both the caller and receiver need a unit. Some TDDs have printers. There are a variety of models. The National Technical Institute for the Deaf is a good source for information. Telecommunications for the Deaf produces an informational and trouble-shooting pamphlet.

A telecaption decoder is a unit (caption decoder) that is attached to the television set. Many new television models have built-in telecaption decoders. The telecaption decoder provides the television user with a written narrative at the bottom of the television screen. The printed narrative often enhances understanding of the spoken words on the television. There are some national network news programs that transmit their programs closed captioned; television program guides identify these.

ALERT AND SIGNAL SYSTEMS

There are a variety of devices that use lights or create vibrations for in-home use. Telephones, doorbells, smoke alarms, alarm clocks, and cooking timers can be altered for severe or profoundly impaired persons. They may be purchased at electronic or supply stores or from national companies (Himber, 1989).

HEARING DOGS

Dogs who are professionally trained are another resource for hearing impaired individuals. Dogs are trained in a number of locations throughout the states (Himber, 1989). They are taught to identify common sounds of everyday living, find their owners, and lead them to the sound. Some charitable organizations may provide financial assistance in obtaining a dog.

Nursing Diagnosis and Management of High-risk Areas in Daily Living

The most obvious nursing diagnosis associated with a hearing impaired elder is that of impaired interpersonal communications. Other areas that may be affected by hearing loss include mobility (in the community), general health, coping (tension, negativism), emotional status (depression, paranoia), social isolation and cognitive function (inattention, confusion). Safety and reduced auditory cues (telephone, doorbells, alarms) may also be problem areas.

DAILY LIVING WITH IMPAIRED INTERPERSONAL COMMUNICATION: HEARING LOSS

Hearing loss in the elderly is often a gradual process. Persons may state they can hear but they do not understand. Some may deny the extent to which hearing loss has affected their ability to communicate with others (Himber, 1989). Others may recognize their problem but lack the knowledge or resources to seek evaluation and obtain the information or equipment that might improve communication. Hearing loss may be considered inevitable with advanced age; a loss for which there is no real help.

RISK FACTORS

Anyone experiencing a loss of hearing will have some difficulties with interpersonal communications. The elderly persons at risk for having their loss greatly affect daily living include those who

Are employed
Are involved in community service
Have a lifelong pattern of involvement in social activities
Provide care or support to others

SIGNS AND SYMPTOMS

Persons with hearing loss may deny the significance of their loss when it is mild (Himber, 1989). They will adapt to difficulties with hearing in subtle ways. The impairment is often noticeable to those who are in frequent close con-

tact. The person may ask for others to repeat what they have said or may misinterpret what has been said. He will state that people mumble or do not speak clearly. Sometimes the hearing impaired person develops skills in lip reading and in observing general expression. Such skills will be useless when using the telephone, trying to hear someone in another room, or when listening to someone whose face or lips are not visible or are distorted because his back is turned, he is too far away, has a moustache, or is chewing gum. In these situations the person will ask for others to repeat themselves more often, claim that there are other distracting noises preventing him from hearing, and sometimes respond out of context to what has been said. Occasionally hearing-impaired persons do not respond at all if they are unaware they have been spoken to.

When in large groups where hearing is more difficult, the person may appear less talkative than usual. He may look either distracted or somewhat less animated. His expression may be intense and serious as he copes with the situation by "tuning out" or by increasing his concentration and vigilance for nonverbal cues to understand conversation. Often hearing impaired elders will seat themselves close to and in front of a speaker. They may arrange to be with someone who is aware of their loss and helps them by summarizing conversation or alerts them to changes in topics.

Some hearing impaired elderly may withdraw partially or completely from usual activities involving verbal communication that become too difficult to participate in and therefore are less enjoyable or productive. They may also withdraw to avoid situations that expose the hearing loss. They may avoid other people because they are frustrated or depressed.

PROGNOSTIC VARIABLES

The degree of handicap that the hearing impaired person feels may strongly contribute to how successful he is in living with the hearing loss. Early onset of hearing loss and a perception that it interferes greatly with one's life are thought to increase the likelihood of feeling handicapped (Hinchcliff, 1983). Negative attitudes of others about the hearing loss stigmatize the individual. If the hearing impaired elder is frequently exposed to people who contribute to a sense of stigma he may cope with the problem by "hiding" from others. Such behavior will often create major, unfavorable changes in daily living. Mobility in the community, general health, emotional status, and cognitive function can be adversely affected (Hinchcliff, 1983; Lichtenstein et al, 1988).

COMPLICATIONS

Depression, isolation, paranoia, and cognitive impairment have been associated with hearing loss in the elderly. The depression may be related to a strong feeling of being handicapped and, in very active people, the amount of interference the hearing loss causes in their usual outward going lifestyle. For those who are already isolated, hearing loss will intensify isolation. Hearing impairment may be a risk factor for having cognitive dysfunction and dementia (Uhlmann et al, 1989). Correction of the hearing impairment would not prevent the dementia but could improve or ameliorate symptoms. As discussed in prognostic variables, general health and mobility may also be affected by hearing loss. Personal safety may be threatened, especially if the individual is living alone and has moderate-to-severe hearing loss.

TREATMENT

Improving Communication There are a number of basic techniques that can be learned by hearing impaired individuals and those who are communicating with them that will minimize the effects of hearing loss on the interaction.

Techniques for Communicating with Hearing-impaired Persons

Choose a speaking location with good light; avoid positioning that places a bright light or the sun's glare behind you (both cause problems with seeing the speaker)

Select an area that has sound-absorbing qualities such as carpets, drapes, and doors

Get the person's attention

Use touch to gain attention

Face the person every time you speak

Use a normal speaking voice; shouting causes word distortion and is uncomfortable if the person is already receiving amplified sound with an aid

Maintain voice intensity to the end of the sentence; dropping voice level at the end of the sentence causes straining to hear and missed words

Use normal expression while speaking; exaggerated enunciation distorts facial features and can be distractive and lessen understanding

Lower the pitch of the voice

Speak in an even, moderate-to-slow pace (talking rapidly in haste or excitement makes sounds run together, causes distortion, and makes lip reading more difficult)

Repeat some of the words of a missed phrase or sentence (this may help in central processing of the full message)

Use different words when repeating a missed phrase or sentence (the sounds of different words may be frequencies that can be heard more easily)

Gesture and point to objects to reinforce the spoken message

Make sentences convey complete thoughts (if parts of the sentence are missed the individual may still understand what is said)

Speak more slowly when talking on the telephone (without visual contact for lip reading or seeing gestures the individual may need a slower pace to hear and process sounds)

EVALUATION

The general goal (outcome) of management in impaired communication due to hearing loss is to maintain or restore usual or preferred activities of daily living that require verbal communication. Evaluation of a plan of care will assess attainment of this goal.

Specific goals that quantify outcomes and are based on the patient's preferred lifestyle should be established. For example, "attends three activities of choice each week"; "reports good verbal communication"; "reports understanding verbal communication 90% of the time."

If there are other problems related to hearing loss such as decreased mobility in the community, threatened safety, poor general health, or depression, the outcomes for management of these problems would be evaluated also. Outcomes of care for these problems may include the following:

1. Devices that replace or enhance the sound of alarm systems are in place
2. The individual reports no loss of mobility in outside activities

Organizations

American Speech-Language Hearing
   Association
10801 Rockville Pike
Rockville, MD 20852
(301) 897-5700

American Telephone and Telegraph
Special Needs Center
1-800-233-1222

American Tinnitus Association
PO Box 5
Portland, Oregon 97207

Hearing Dog Program
American Humane Association
9725 East Hampden Ave, Department HD
Denver, CO 80231

National Hearing Aid Society
20361 Middle Belt Rd
Livonia MI 48142
(1-800-521-5247 to request a consumer
   education kit)

National Information Center on Deafness,
Information and Research
Gallaudet University
800 Florida Ave, NE
Washington, DC 20002
(202) 651-5051

National Technical Institute for the Deaf
Division of Public Affairs, Dept. C
One Lomb Memorial Dr, PO Box 9887
Rochester, NY 14623-0087
(716) 475-6400

Nationwide Flashing Signal Systems
8120 Fenton St
Silver Spring, MD 20910
(301) 589-6671

Self Help for Hard of Hearing People, Inc.
7800 Wisconsin Ave
Bethesda, MD 20814
(301) 657-2248
(Local chapters, pamphlets, bimonthly newsletter)

Telecommunications for the Deaf
814 Thayer Ave
Silver Spring, MD, 20910
(301) 589-3006

---

3. Hearing aids or other listening devices are available, maintained, and used with some degree of success
4. There is improvement in general health as evidenced by self-report, fewer health problems, and improved management of existing health problems
5. There is a general feeling of well-being and absence of clinical symptoms of depression
6. Communication techniques are understood and used with some degree of success

References and Other Readings

Adams PF, Benson V. Current estimates from the National Health Interview Survey, 1989. National Center for Health Statistics. Vital Health Stat 10(176), 1990.

Bates B. A guide to physical examination and history taking, 5th ed. Philadelphia: JB Lippincott, 1991.
Bienvue GR, Michael PL, Chaffinch JC, Zeigler J. The audioscope: a clinical tool for otoscopic and audiometric examination. Ear and Hearing 1985; 6:251.
Browning GG. Clinical role of informal tests of hearing. J Laryngol Otol 1989; 103:7.
Dauman R, Cazals Y. Auditory frequency selectivity and tinnitus. Arch Otolaryngol 1989; 246:252.
DeGowin EL, DeGowin RL. Bedside diagnostic examination, 5th ed. New York: Macmillan, 1987.
Frank T, Peterson DR. Accuracy of a 40 dB HL audioscope and audiometer screening for adults. Ear and Hearing 1987; 8:180.
Goodhill V. Deafness, tinnitus and dizziness in the aged. In: Rossman I, ed. Clinical geriatrics, 3rd ed. Philadelphia: JB Lippincott, 1986.
Gutnick H, Zillmer E, Philput C. Measurement and prediction of hearing loss in a nursing home. Ear and Hearing 1989; 10:361.

Hinchcliffe R, ed. Hearing and balance in the elderly. New York: Churchill Livingstone, 1983.

Kane RL, Ouslander JG, Abrass IB, eds. Essentials of clinical geriatrics, 2nd ed. New York: McGraw-Hill Information Services, 1989.

Keay DG, Murray JAM. Hearing loss in the elderly. A 17-year longitudinal study. Clin Otolaryngol 1988; 13:31.

Lichtenstein MJ, et al. Validation of screening tools for identifying hearing impaired elderly in primary care. JAMA 1988; 259:2875.

Matkin ND, Hodgson WR. Amplification and the elderly patient. Otolaryngol Clin North Am 1982; 15:371.

Meisami E. Aging of the nervous system: sensory changes. In: Timiras PS, ed. Physiological basis of geriatrics. New York: Macmillan, 1988.

Moscicki E, Elkins E, Baum H, McNamara PM. Hearing loss in the elderly: an epidemiologic study of the Framingham heart study cohort. Ear and Hearing 1985; 6:184.

Mueller HG, Geoffry VC. Communication disorders and aging: assessment and management. Washington, DC: Gallaudet University Press, 1987.

Mulrow C, Aguilar C, Endicott J, et al. Quality of life changes and hearing impairment. Ann Intern Med 1990; 113:188.

National Center for Health Statistics, Hing E, Sekscenski E, Strahan G. The National Nursing Home Survey 1985 summary for the United States. Vital and Health Statistics, Series 13, No 97. DHHS Pub No (PHS) 89-1758 Public Health Service. Washington, DC: US Government Printing Office, 1989.

Rees TS, Duckert LG. Auditory and vestibular dysfunction in aging. In: Hazzard WR, et al, eds. Principles of geriatric medicine and gerontology, 2nd ed. New York: McGraw-Hill, 1990.

Schow R, Nerbonne M. Assessment of hearing handicap by nursing home residents and staff.

Journal of the Academy of Rehabilitation Audiology 1977; 10:2.

Sever JC Jr, Harry DC, Rittenhouse TS: Using a self assessment questionnaire to identify probable hearing loss among older adults. Perceptual Motor Skills 1989; 69:511.

Snyder J. Office audiometry. J Fam Pract 1984; 19:535.

Sullivan MD, et al. Univesity of Washington measurements of tinnitus severity. Unpublished abstract of the 14th Midwinter Research Meeting: Association for Research in Otolaryngology. St. Petersburg, FL, February 1991.

Uhlmann R, Larson E, Rees T, et al. Relationship of hearing impairment to dementia and cognitive dysfunction in older adults. JAMA 1989; 261:1916.

Voeks S, Gallagher C, Langer E, et al. Hearing loss in the nursing home. J Am Geriatr Soc 1990; 38:141.

Weinstein BE. Geriatric hearing loss: myths, realities, resources for physicians. Geriatrics 1989; 44:42.

Welsh J. Central presbycusis. Laryngoscope 1985; 95:128.

Whitbourne SK. The aging body: physiological changes and psychosocial consequences. New York: Springer-Verlag, 1985.

Yoder MG. Geriatric ear, nose and throat problems. In: Reichel W, ed. Clinical aspects of aging, 3rd ed. Baltimore: Williams & Wilkins, 1989.

PATIENT EDUCATION MATERIALS

Combs A. Hearing loss help. Santa Marie, CA: Alpenglow Press, 1989.

Davis M, et al. Relaxation and stress reduction workbook, 3rd ed. Oakland, CA: New Harbinger Publishing Corp., 1988.

Himber C. How to survive hearing loss. Washington, DC: Gallaudet University Press, 1989.

28
Hypertension

NANCY ROBEN

Health care professionals have become aware of the prevalence of hypertension and its significance as a health problem in our growing elderly population. The National Health and Nutrition Examination Survey (NHANES II) found 63% of individuals between the ages of 65 and 74 years to have diastolic or systolic hypertension (>140/90 mm Hg). Until recently there was reluctance to treat elderly patients with hypertension. Controlled studies have now shown that therapy reduces the cardiovascular morbidity and mortality in the elderly population with both systolic and diastolic hypertension.

Pathophysiology and Medical Management

DESCRIPTION

Because criteria to define hypertension vary, the reported prevalence of hypertension in the elderly depends on the definition. The National High Blood Pressure Education Program Coordinating Committee says an average systolic blood pressure greater than or equal to 160 mm Hg and/or average diastolic pressure greater than or equal to 90 mm Hg on three consecutive visits constitutes the diagnosis of hypertension in the elderly. Isolated systolic hypertension (ISH) is a blood pressure in the 140 to160 mm Hg range when diastolic blood pres-

sure is less than 90 mm Hg. In the Systolic Hypertension in the Elderly pilot study, ISH occurred predominantly in the older patients, increasing from 6% of those aged 60 to 69 to 18% of those 80 years and older. It also tended to occur more frequently in women after menopause and in African Americans.

Elderly persons with systolic–diastolic hypertension may represent those who have survived with hypertension over the years. Certain individuals with isolated hypertension may develop diastolic hypertension over time. Diastolic hypertension alone is least common. Either of these last two situations may be secondary to another cause, often renovascular disease. Whatever the pattern of hypertension, there is increased risk of cardiovascular morbidity and mortality.

ETIOLOGIC FACTORS

Usually hypertension is classified arbitrarily as primary or secondary. Primary hypertension has no known or readily identifiable causes. Its multifactorial genesis is not well understood. A primary mechanism is presumed to be an increase in peripheral resistance in the systemic circulation resulting from vasoconstriction of the very small arterioles. In most people with high blood pressure the mechanism that causes this marked narrowing of the lumen of the arterioles is obscure.

AGE-RELATED CHANGES

In the older population age-related physiologic changes must be considered. It is also assumed that the atherosclerotic processes contribute to the elevated arterial pressure by a number of changes that promote progressive decrease in the distensibility of the aorta and its various branches.

Aortic Rigidity   As the aortic wall becomes more rigid there is a steeper slope of pressure increase per milliliter of blood injected into the large arterioles. The pulse generated during systole is transmitted to the arterial tree relatively unchanged. Hence, wide pulse pressure occurs, often giving a disproportionate increase in systolic pressure.

Decreased Baroreceptor Sensitivity   There may also be a decrease in baroreceptor sensitivity that reduces the potential to buffer wider swings in arterial blood pressure. Baroreceptors are stretch receptors located in the walls of the heart and blood vessels, particularly in the aortic arch. They are thought to be stimulated by distention of the structures where they are located. Impulses generated by baroreceptors result in vasodilation, a decrease in blood pressure, slowing of the heart rate, and a decrease in cardiac output.

Decreased Lumen in Arterioles   The atherosclerotic processes also occur in precapillary arterioles, contributing to the decreased lumen capacity. Vascular resistance is increased, adding to the total peripheral resistance.

Reduced Glomerular Filtration   The kidney undergoes a reduction in glomerular filtration and renal blood flow that may contribute to sodium retention. High sodium intake in the elderly then could lead to volume expansion and play a role in the genesis of hypertension.

Changes in the Renin–Angiotensin System
The renin–angiotensin system has been studied extensively as a possible factor in essential hypertension. It is thought that plasma renin activity decreases with age. Its importance is not now known as a contributing cause of hypertension in the elderly.

Hormonal Changes   Some studies have shown an age-related increase in plasma nor-epinephrine levels, suggesting the possibility of sympathetic nervous system overactivity. To what extent this proposed increased sympathetic activity may be considered a factor related to hypertension in the elderly is unclear.

Cardiovascular Changes   Cardiac output and stroke volume diminish with age. Elevated systolic blood pressure serves to increase left ventricular afterload and cardiac workload.

LIFESTYLE

Some observers believe that lifelong patterns of coping with social and environmental stress may contribute to the complex phenomenon of hypertension. However, studies in certain native populations where the pace of life appears to be relaxed have shown a prevalence of hypertension. Urban living alone does not seem to be an important factor, at least in the United States where hypertension is considerably more prevalent among African Americans living in the rural South and in large cities.

GENETIC FACTORS

It has been recognized that hypertension and hypertensive cardiovascular complications as well as atherosclerotic complications tend to occur in families. This link with heredity is helpful in establishing a diagnosis of essential hypertension.

SMOKING

A positive correlation between cigarette smoking and sustained hypertension has not been demonstrated. However, smoking is known to aggravate atherosclerosis. In combination with hypertension it greatly increases the risk of atherosclerotic complications, particularly coronary artery disease. Reduction of blood pressure may not be helpful in preventing coronary events when multiple risk factors including tobacco use are ongoing. In the elderly population its impact on the development of hypertension or its control is considered to be slight.

ALCOHOL

Many researchers have concluded that the consumption of six drinks per day or more is a definite factor in increasing blood pressure. Klatsky et al (1977) showed that the relationship between alcohol use and blood pressure may be strongest for those over 60. Alcohol consumption is thought to be responsible for as much as 11% of hypertension in men (Mc-Mahon, 1986). Short-term studies have indicated that abstinence in heavy drinking hypertensive patients may lower the blood pressure by an average of 13 mm Hg systole and 15 mm Hg diastole.

DIET

A comprehensive analysis of the relationships of 17 nutrients to the blood pressure profile of subjects from 18 to 74 years of age was done using a data base on the National Center for Health Statistics, known as Health and Nutrition Survey I (McCarron et al, 1984). It was noted that higher intakes of calcium, potassium, and sodium were associated with lower mean systolic pressure. Further studies have not validated any causative relationships implied in this study. However, low protein intake and concomitant potassium deficiency are a common problem in the elderly.

The evidence for the role of salt in the development of hypertension is indeed controversial. No one has shown that the level of sodium intake is a major etiologic factor for hypertension in the elderly. However, in a population where salt is an acquired taste learned at a very early age by flavoring infant foods, one wonders what implications there might be in considering the pathogenesis of hypertension in the aging adults of this society.

Studies of the use of salt by older persons are not available. It might be predicted, however, that there could be an increase in salting of food because taste buds involved in perceiving sweet and salty flavors are among those that show the greatest decrease with age. It is estimated that almost 64% of taste buds have been found to be lost by age 75. Research has also shown that it then requires greater intensity of stimulation to allow the older person with fewer taste buds to experience the taste sensation. It would seem reasonable to think that older adults who have grown up enjoying salt in their food might add more to achieve the same taste experience. Exploration of usual and preferred patterns in salt preference and intake in the older person would be an important nursing assessment item, particularly in the patient with any degree of renal failure.

OTHER PATHOLOGY

Hypertension is considered to be secondary if its occurrence can be clearly attributed to an underlying disease. Secondary causes include adrenal medullary tumor and states of excessive mineralocorticoid secretion such as Cushing's disease or aldosteronoma. These conditions tend to be even less common in the elderly.

Isolated systolic hypertension may present itself as a manifestation of severe anemia, Paget's disease, thyrotoxicosis, and aortic regurgitation. These conditions may be present in the elderly person and may contribute to the presence of systolic hypertension.

When diastolic hypertension occurs after the age of 60, renovascular hypertension must be suspected. Its prevalence is less than 1% and may occur when an atherosclerotic lesion in a renal artery becomes the site of a thrombotic or embolic process.

Hypertension occurring as a side effect of another therapy is seen with increasing frequency. The most common offenders include nonsteroidal anti-inflammatory agents, which are frequently used by the elderly. Chronic estrogen therapy may be associated with elevated blood pressure in some elderly women. Testosterone therapy can lead to fluid retention and aggravate elevated pressures. Chronic use of nasal decongestants or appetite suppressants (other causes of hypertension) is less common in the elderly.

EPIDEMIOLOGIC FACTORS

The consensus of longitudinal studies in population groups indicates that blood pressure increases with age. Diastolic blood pressure increases with age up to the fifth decade and then declines. Systolic blood pressure, on the other hand, tends to increase linearly with age, with no apparent leveling off. When systolic pressure increases more rapidly than diastolic pressure, a widened pulse pressure occurs giving rise to isolated systolic hypertension; this is commonly found in the United States and other western industrialized countries. The same pattern is not found in primitive societies where weight does not increase with age and salt intake is minimal.

Epidemiologic studies in other cultures, as in the Gilbert Islands and New Guinea, seem to show that hypertension is not prevalent; nor does the blood pressure increase with age. Some investigators believe that a low salt intake may account for this virtual absence of hypertension in these more primitive societies. Additional observations have been made in Japan. In a northeast province, where salt intake approximated 30 g/d, the incidence of severe hypertension and stroke was found to be very high (Sasaki, 1964).

Some epidemiologic, laboratory, and clinical studies indicate that dietary sodium, potassium, and calcium intake are potentially important in the etiology of essential hypertension and probably contribute to population differences. Sodium intake may increase the likelihood of developing hypertension among susceptible individuals, whereas potassium intake may have a protective effect. The relationships of the various nutrients to the development or maintenance of hypertension in the elderly remains unclear.

HIGH-RISK POPULATIONS OR SITUATIONS

Which individuals in the above 65- to 70-age group will develop hypertension? No one knows. Perhaps the majority of elderly persons who have managed to survive to this age group will never develop significant diastolic or systolic hypertension. Multiple studies have demonstrated the increased risks of cardiovascular morbidity and mortality associated with untreated hypertension in the elderly.

Hypertension in elderly persons may presume two *common* situations. One represents early onset of hypertension where the patient has managed to progress to older age despite the condition. The second is late onset in which there is a relatively recent elevation occurring at an older age. Aged patients with recent blood pressure elevation may reflect a history of lability during the course of a lifetime, gradually progressing with age to a sustained hypertension. In other patients a sudden onset of elevated blood pressure may be an indication of renovascular hypertension secondary to rapidly progressing atherosclerotic disease.

DYNAMICS

Blood pressure is simply the lateral force exerted against the walls of the arteries as blood flows from the heart. The pressure in the aorta and other large arteries increases to a peak value (systolic pressure) during each heart cycle and decreases to a minimum value (diastolic pressure). This arterial pressure is the product of two forces: cardiac output and peripheral resistance. Most of the peripheral resistance occurs in the arterioles and is governed by the contraction of their walls.

The caliber of the arterioles and arteries is under both nervous and chemical control. This is an important concept to have in mind when considering the antihypertensive drugs and how they are presumed to be effective. Nervous impulses from reflex centers in the brain may constrict or dilate the vessels. Chemical substances may alter the size of blood vessels either by acting directly in the vessels or by stimulating sensory receptors and, thus, initiating reflex control.

In general, increases in cardiac output increase the systolic pressure, whereas increases in peripheral resistance increase the diastolic pressure. An important cause of the increase in systolic pressure is decreased distensibility of the arteries (atherosclerotic process) as their walls become increasingly rigid. At the same level of cardiac output, the systolic pressure is higher in the elderly person because there is less increase in the volume of the arterial system during systole to accommodate the same amount of blood because of loss of vascular elasticity.

Cardiac work is more closely related to systolic blood pressure than to mean or diastolic blood pressure. Hence, systolic hypertension increases the workload of the left ventricle. Workload is one of the major factors determining myocardial oxygen demands. Thus, in the older person with isolated systolic hypertension, the workload of the left ventricle is increased at a time when the oxygen supply through the coronary arteries is likely to be compromised by atherosclerotic processes.

Health care providers who are assuming major responsibility in the care of elderly hypertensive individuals need an understanding of the hemodynamic relationships. Hypertension is indeed a different disease process in the older person than in the younger adult.

DIFFERENTIAL DIAGNOSIS

An accurate diagnosis of hypertension in itself is contingent on obtaining a precise and valid blood pressure reading. It is particularly important in the older age group so that potent and potentially hazardous treatment methods are not recommended needlessly. The American Heart Association (1980) has outlined a method that establishes greater reliability and uniformity in obtaining blood pressure readings. In elderly persons *special precautions* need consideration when taking the blood pressure:

1. The cuff must fit snugly and provide uniform compression of the extremity. Hemiplegic patients should have the cuff applied to the *unaffected* extremity.
2. The width of the cuff should be 20% greater than the diameter of the limb on which it is used. Use a smaller width cuff on thin or emaciated patients.
3. The lower edge of the cuff should be 1 inch above the bell of the stethoscope.
4. The patient should be positioned quietly for a few minutes before taking the recording. The artery over which the blood pressure is being recorded should be located at heart level.
5. The systolic blood pressure should be first determined by the palpatory method. This is done by taking the radial or popliteal pulse if the lower extremity is being used when the cuff is being inflated. The cuff should then be inflated to approximately 20 to 30 mm Hg above the pressure at which the pulse disappears. Occasionally the usual sounds heard over the brachial artery when the cuff pressure is high disappear as the pressure is reduced and then reappear at a lower level—this is called an auscultatory gap. Because this gap may cover a range of 40 mm Hg, one can seriously underestimate the diastolic pressure unless its presence is excluded by first palpating for disappearance of the radial pulse as the cuff pressure is raised.
6. When blood pressure sounds are difficult to hear, elevating the extremity above heart level or asking the patient to make a fist and then release it will frequently increase the audibility of the diastolic sound.
7. If successive readings are to be taken, the cuff should be deflated completely between determinations to permit venous return to occur.

Blood pressure measurement should begin after 3 to 5 minutes of rest and be taken in at least two positions—lying or sitting *and* standing. This will help in detecting postural changes that may be more common in elderly persons. Preferably the older person should stand for 2 to 3 minutes before measuring the blood pressure. In the active older person, *the standing blood pressure* determination should be used for defining pretreatment level or end point of therapy. Postural changes in blood pressure are commonly noted in persons with significant atherosclerotic disease, dehydration, or blood loss. It will also be an important observation when patients are taking antihypertensive agents to minimize potential complications of therapy. Postural decreases in blood pressure of greater than 20 mm Hg may need special protection, i.e., elastic hose. This may be especially true in patients with exceptionally high supine readings. Slower response of baroreceptors may indicate the need to make postural changes slowly and in stages.

Some observers have noted a dramatic difference in blood pressure measurement by conventional indirect method and intra-arterial method. A "pseudohypertension" in the elderly may be explained by the difficulty an air-filled bladder of a sphygmomanometer may have in compressing a stiff brachial artery.

Blood pressure fluctuates in response to changes in emotion, physical activity, or wakefulness. This "lability" may occur to a greater degree in the elderly where there are baroreceptor reflex changes that no longer can help to stabilize the blood pressure. It is imperative, therefore, to obtain several baseline readings in the older person with newly elevated or recently noted blood pressure elevation. Blood pressure should be taken in both upper extremities with differences noted, particularly if either extremity has sustained injury or incurred disablement from stroke. These baseline readings can be done on subsequent clinic visits, or consecutive days in a residence, clinic, or perhaps more accurately at home. Some patients might take their own blood pressure but this ability should be carefully evaluated when blood pressure values may be *critical* to differentiate presence or absence of elevated blood pressure. It is important to remember that the blood pressure often is responsive to emotional and environmental changes. Stress, apprehensions, or uncomfortable sensory environments have a high risk of increasing systolic blood pressure. These factors may be maximized in the medical facility setting.

Elderly patients with irregular heart rates present special problems in obtaining accurate blood pressure readings. In atrial fibrillation, the strength of each beat varies considerably. During early cuff deflation, only a few strong beats are heard, becoming more numerous as the cuff is further deflated. Often an estimate must be made by repeated determinations.

Persons with extremely slow irregular rhythms also present difficulties in obtaining accurate blood pressure readings. In this situation both stroke volume and blood pressure vary from one cardiac cycle to the next. The systolic blood pressure is related directly to the duration of the preceding pulse cycle and the stroke volume, whereas the pulse pressure is related inversely to the duration of the pulse cycle. Therefore, a long pulse cycle results in a decrease in the diastolic pressure of that cycle and causes an increase in systolic pressure of the next one.

Falsely high blood pressure readings often are obtained in obese individuals when the standard size bladder and technique are used. This can be minimized by using a cuff with a wider bladder width or using the standard cuff on the forearm and ascultating the blood pressure over the radial artery.

Occasionally, older people will have blood pressure readings that do not seem to have an easily determined diastolic sound. In fact, there may be no differentiation between systolic and diastolic sounds with the clear tapping sound all the way down to 0 mm Hg. These individuals have extensive atherosclerotic disease including the brachial artery or arteries. In this situation, one may have to rely on systolic blood pressure reading as the only marker of blood pressure and control.

The measurement of blood pressure in the elderly must be done carefully to minimize the pitfalls in what seems to be a very common nursing task. Often, blood pressure measurement is assigned to a paraprofessional. Health care professionals must take responsibility for ensuring that a correct procedure is followed so that needless treatment measures are not imposed on the elderly.

Extensive laboratory testing of the elderly hypertensive patient to differentiate secondary causes of the blood pressure elevation is generally not recommended. In view of the rarity of many of the specific recognizable causes of elevated blood pressure, coupled with both the cost in dollars and the small but real risk to the elderly patient of certain diagnostic procedures, it is recommended that more complex work-up be reserved for the severely elevated blood pressure that perhaps occurs suddenly and is not responsive to the usual treatment modalities.

MANIFESTATIONS

Despite the wealth of symptoms ascribed to hypertension by many authors and health care providers, there is no characteristic sign, symptom, or syndrome. The blood pressure is simply elevated. It has been referred to as a "silent disease." For example, headaches frequently do not accompany even severely elevated pressures. Many patients actually feel well and the elevation is casually noted when the patient seeks health care for a minor problem such as an upper respiratory infection.

In the elderly, associated processes of cerebral vascular atherosclerosis may be suggested by unsteady gait, memory deficits, transient ischemic attacks, and strokes. In addition, a history of substernal pain aggravated by exercise or emotion and relieved by rest may suggest coronary artery disease. These signs and symptoms should suggest the possible sequences of ongoing arterial disease known to be aggravated by hypertension.

COMPLICATIONS

In previous sections some of the complications of hypertension have been referred to. One of the major challenges to the geriatric health care provider is to *identify* elderly patients with sustained blood pressure levels in the range of 90+ mm Hg diastolic and/or 160+ mm Hg systolic. The evaluation should then be directed toward ascertaining damage to target organs (e.g., brain, heart, retina, kidney) to estimate the biologic significance of the hypertension. Other cardiovascular risk factors (including obesity, smoking, elevated lipids and blood glucose) need to be identified.

Concomitant associated problems such as congestive heart failure must be considered. In the Framingham study (Kannel et al, 1972) it was found that in 75% of patients with congestive heart failure in the age range from 30 to 62 years, the dominant etiologic precursor was hypertension. It is known that older hypertensive patients' risk of cardiovascular complications and death are from two to five times that of normotensive persons.

Another important finding from the Framingham study was that increased cardiovascular mortality and morbidity were associated with both systolic and diastolic blood pressure elevation. Women with normal diastolic blood pressure but borderline or definitely hypertensive systolic pressure have a risk 50% above the standard. With these findings in mind, the disproportionate increase in systolic pressure seen in aging must be looked at with concern.

Data from the Framingham study show that there are certain cardiovascular risk factors that *appear* to be important considerations in the geriatric age group. Little can be done to alter age, sex, or heredity factors. The most controllable of these risk factors was believed to be hypertension (Castelli, 1976).

In the Chicago stroke study (Shekelle et al, 1974) patient characteristics related to stroke in a population of noninstitutionalized persons 65 to 74 years of age were examined. In both black and white persons, it was found that hypertension was significantly associated with increased risk of stroke. Applying the data from this study, the investigators concluded that 25% or more of the total incidence of stroke in persons 65 to 74 years of age may be attributable to hypertension.

These studies are difficult to ignore when considering the elderly patient with hypertension. Multiple epidemiologic studies have clearly demonstrated the increased risks of hypertension in this age group. The European Working Party on High Blood Pressure in the Elderly Study was designed to examine the benefit of treatment in patients over 60 years of age with moderate hypertension. Fewer deaths were noted in the treated group until 80 years of age (Amery et al, 1985).

When the workload of the heart becomes too great in pumping blood against the elevated peripheral resistance/pressure, the heart (especially the left ventricle) may become enlarged and act as a reservoir for abnormal amounts of blood because it is then an inefficient pump. Pressure backs up into the lungs and symptoms of congestive failure can occur. As the heart muscle increases in size, the blood supply (coronary arteries) to the heart itself becomes inadequate and symptoms of coronary insufficiency with chest pain may occur. Myocardial infarction could become a part of this sequelae or its logical consequence. This is a very simplified explanation of a complication of hypertension frequently referred to as **hypertensive heart disease.** It can occur when sustained hypertension, often in combination with atherosclerosis, is ignored or poorly controlled.

In addition to the complications of the elevated blood pressure, there must be concern regarding complications of therapy. Special considerations are crucial when patients on antihypertensive agents are moved along the health care continuum. The following case synopses illustrate some of these potential complications of therapy.

Mr. B, aged 72, was admitted to a hospital surgical unit for a repair of an inguinal hernia. He has had hypertension for several years. He has been taking a diuretic and methyldopa 250 mg three times a day. His blood pressure on admission was 170/95 mm Hg. The morning after admission he collapsed on the floor and hit his head while trying to get out of bed.

This particular example illustrates frequent complications of drug treatment when the patient is taken from the home setting. When, in the more organized hospital setting, the patient encounters more or less stress and better dietary sodium observation combined with bed rest and less exercise, the hypotensive episodes can be common. To help prevent these episodes, the blood pressure should be routinely monitored in both lying and sitting positions, even though the patient is both ambulatory and well.

Mrs. A, aged 82, is no longer able to live alone in her home. Her relatives arranged for her to go to a nursing home. Her admission orders included her antihypertensive drugs and a low sodium diet that had been prescribed but poorly adhered to at home. Five days after admission she collapses after leaving the dining room.

The alert health care provider might have questioned whether the antihypertensive drugs had actually been taken before nursing home admission and what the normal dietary patterns had been.

The Mr. B in the earlier example had a successful hernia repair. His antihypertensive medications were never reinstituted postoperatively because the blood pressure continued to be about 150 to 160/80 to 90 mm Hg. Two weeks after the hospital discharge he was seen in the outpatient clinic in a follow-up visit. His incision was well healed. His blood pressure was 200/104 mm Hg.

This is a frequent finding in outpatient settings. Patients do not restart their antihypertensive medicines and the blood pressure goes back up. When patients are discharged from hospitals, health care providers must review the *total* plan of care with the patient and family.

When stroke or myocardial infarction occurs in the hypertensive patient, the blood pressure occasionally returns to normotensive levels post-hospital. Why this occurs is unclear. Care must be taken to follow the blood pressure of these patients. The nurse must be alert to reestablishment of hypertensive levels, if they should recur.

There is an increased potential for drug problems in the geriatric population when multiple drugs are taken or more potent drugs are used. If malnutrition or liver or kidney impairment are factors, there is an even greater danger. Acute episodic illness, as common to any age group, may pose additional hazards for the elderly patient who is taking antihypertensive agents. Older patients are more sensitive to volume depletion and sympathetic inhibition. Impaired cardiovascular reflexes make them susceptible to hypotension. Hypotensive episodes should be anticipated then and drug dosages may need to be tapered. Patients, families, and health care providers all need to be alerted to these risks.

The elderly person is also vulnerable to the side effects of the antihypertensive agents that the younger patient experiences. Impotence and decreased libido may be of great concern to the sexually active older person. This is when patient–health care provider rapport is critical. Is sexual activity important to this patient or his partner? It is important to ascertain whether changes in sexual lifestyle have occurred.

In addition, reserpine and methyldopa may promote or contribute to an underlying depression. If cerebral vascular atherosclerotic disease is present in the elderly, these and other potent antihypertensive agents may further compromise the psychologic equilibrium by increasing symptoms of depression and decreasing mentation.

Frequently observed side effects of diuretics include hyperglycemia, hypokalemia, hyperuricemia, and/or acute gout and muscle cramps. Older patients who are taking concurrent digitalis preparations will need to have their potassium monitored periodically or hypokalemia can lead to arrhythmias and death. Potassium-rich foods (see listing in Chapter 12, Nutrition) that should be eaten regularly may not be adequate,

readily available, or economically practical. Potassium salts (substitute salt) may be helpful. Symptoms of hypokalemia include neuromuscular disturbances (weakness and paresthesias) and cardiac abnormalities (arrhythmias, increased sensitivity to digitalis, and ECG changes). Potassium may be depleted severely before symptoms occur.

When potassium replacement drugs or potassium-sparing diuretics are used, hyperkalemia will need to be recognized, particularly in patients with renal disease. In these patients even use of salt substitutes will be dangerous since there will be decreased renal excretion of potassium. Symptoms of hyperkalemia include the same neuromuscular manifestations as hypokalemia.

When hypertension in elderly patients no longer responds to the usual treatment program or the drug treatment becomes more difficult, an underlying cause should be suspected, i.e., renovascular disease. As the health care provider gains more experience in the care of the elderly hypertensive population, it becomes more apparent that each patient's situation must be evaluated individually as to the significance of the hypertension. There are no clear guidelines. The risks of treatment in certain circumstances may be in fact greater than the goals of therapy.

PROGNOSIS

Data from multiple studies (Veterans Administration Study, Hypertension Detection and Follow-up Program, the Australian Trial and the European Working Party on High Blood Pressure in the Elderly) indicate that elderly patients with diastolic blood pressures of 90 mm Hg or greater will benefit from antihypertensive therapy. Care must be exercised so that the risks of treatment will not outweigh the goals of therapy in elderly patients.

A double-blind placebo-controlled trial, the Systolic Hypertension in the Elderly Program (SHEP) sponsored by the National Heart, Lung and Blood Institute and the National Institute on Aging has recently been completed. Data from this study has demonstrated significant efficacy of active antihypertensive drug treatment in preventing strokes in persons aged 60 years and older with isolated systolic hypertension. Favorable findings also were demonstrated in lower incidence of major cardiac and cardiovascular events (SHEP Cooperative Research Group, 1991).

PREVENTION AND MANAGEMENT

Hypertension is indeed a common condition in the population. One key to the prevention of dangerous hypertension in the elderly is emphasis on treatment and detection at an earlier age. Hypertension is simply and inexpensively determined. It has been recommended by the Joint National Committee on Detection, Evaluation, and Treatment of High Blood Pressure (1988) that all persons without regular contact with medical care should have their blood pressure measured every 2 years. Persons with blood pressure between 140 and 190 mm Hg systolic over 90 to 104 mm Hg diastolic on the first occasion should be checked again within 2 months.

CRITERIA FOR MEDICAL MANAGEMENT REGIMENS

Multiple factors need to be considered in every geriatric patient before initiating therapy.

1. What are the pretreatment blood pressures in both the supine and standing positions and what will be the target range of blood pressure reduction?
2. What is the total health status of the individual?
3. Are there other complicated social and economic problems?
4. Is there a history of congestive heart failure or cerebrovascular attack?
5. Might a major reduction in blood pressure immobilize this patient by reducing cerebral blood flow and decreasing mentation?
6. What alterations in lifestyle will the treatment program impose on the patient and family?
7. What will be the patient participation in the program?
8. Are there other risk factors present?

NURSING MANAGEMENT OF LIFESTYLE

In developing the plan of care, attention should be directed toward gradual reduction in blood pressure to the *individual* patient's goal level by using the *least potent* therapeutic measures. This goal level needs to be established by the appropriate health care provider *and* the patient or family. Initial efforts should stress and include the following:

- Maintenance of general healthful living
- Development of a weight control program when appropriate to within 15% of ideal body weight
- Limitation on sodium intake (no table salt)
- Promotion of adequate rest and exercise
- Generation of interest in activities that increase relaxation and socialization
- Moderation of alcohol intake to 1 to 2 ounces per day

Diet It is probably unreasonable to subject the elderly hypertensive person to diets that are severely restricted in sodium. Restriction to a 5-g sodium diet could allow use of a modest amount of salt for cooking purposes. This amount of dietary restriction is well below the estimated range of 8 to 14 g of sodium a day per person consumed in the United States. It would reduce use of salt at the table and limit salty foods such as bacon and sausage and snacks such as crackers, pretzels, and potato chips. The availability of modern diuretic drugs has made the strict low sodium diet an archaic form of treatment. More efforts may need to be placed on sodium restriction, however, if drug therapy is to be avoided.

There are no clear guidelines regarding the lowering of blood lipids of people already over age 70. It is recommended that elderly people with hypertension have their cholesterol (including HDL fraction) measured. Perhaps little can be done to remedy a lifetime of dietary intake of lipids. A well-balanced diet is perhaps the only reasonable goal. It should include adequate intake of calcium and potassium.

BEHAVIOR MODIFICATION

There has been an increasing interest in using behavioral treatment in controlled studies with hypertensive subjects. These modalities include traditional psychotherapy, biofeedback, relaxation training and meditation, assertiveness training, and systematic desensitization techniques. Behavioral interventions that elicit the relaxation response may be an important adjunct of drug therapy. So far, none of these studies has been done with a geriatric population.

PATIENT EDUCATION

Elderly persons need to be involved in the formulation of their treatment programs so there will be integration into the lifestyle at home or in the institution. What does the patient understand hypertension to be? Why is it being treated? Is it cured or controlled? Elderly persons need simple informative answers to these questions initially. They need to understand that hypertension does not mean being "too nervous." It is to be controlled because of the damage that has been shown to occur to the small blood vessels of the heart, kidneys, brain, and eye. Lastly, they need to understand that hypertension can be controlled by remaining on the treatment program and under regular supervision by their health care provider.

Most individuals with hypertension are asymptomatic. It is difficult for asymptomatic patients to take medicines and change lifestyles. Good nurse–patient relationships have been found to facilitate and motivate patients to stay with treatment regimens. The long-term "routine" care of hypertensive elderly persons offers little challenge to busy physicians who must use their time for diagnosis and treatment of complex medical problems.

A wealth of excellent educational materials for the hypertensive patient are available from the American Heart Association and the National Heart, Lung and Blood Institute Educational Program Information Center in Bethesda, Maryland (see box below). Nurses need to become familiar with these resources so that patient education can be individually tailored. Some sources of patient education materials are listed at the conclusion of this chapter.

Basic information can be given to the person by use of various media, but my experience has led me to believe that effective patient education requires a person-to-person approach to adapt the basic information to the person's needs. After that point, it may be appropriate to consider forms of group care and education. In the elderly population this may or may not be an appropriate adjunct to individualized care by a consistent health care provider or team.

Certain elderly patients will be able to take their own blood pressure. However, evidence of a hearing loss must be assessed. In addition, many elderly patients have blood pressures that are difficult to obtain, even by health care providers. This should be carefully evaluated, with thought given to how this may be helpful to the individual patient. Patients can be taught by slipping the already wrapped cuff on the arm. The stethoscope (if not a model that is sewn into the cuff) can be used with two flat elastic bands that hold it in place. It must be kept in mind that elderly persons may have significant atherosclerotic disease and may, therefore, have wide swings of pressure, depending on the time of the day and the particular lying or sitting position in which the readings are taken.

Basic to the accuracy of the reading is the assumption that the blood pressure equipment is functioning properly. Patients and health care personnel must know how to maintain the equipment. Aneroid manometers should be checked every 6 months with a Y-connector hooked to a mercury manometer of known accuracy. If the difference is greater than ± 5 mm Hg, it should be recalibrated by the manufacturer or authorized service center.

Mishandling of equipment may produce inaccuracies that are invisible at zero but apparent along the 0 to 300 mm Hg range. Tubing and cuff should be inspected regularly for leaks. This can be done by inflation to 200 mm Hg and closing the valve. Pressure should remain stable.

More expensive mercury manometers require less care, especially if they are wall mounted, and are usually considered to be more accurate. The service manuals that come with this equipment are helpful and should be referred to for proper maintenance on a yearly basis. This is a frequently ignored item, especially in busy medical care facilities.

Elderly persons may wish to purchase the less expensive aneroid manometers. They should be directed toward purchase of equipment that can be serviced easily. The least expensive stethoscope will be adequate for most

---

Patient Education Materials

GENERAL SOURCES

American Heart Association
National Center
7320 Greenville Avenue
Dallas, TX 75231

National Heart, Lung and Blood Institute
Cardiovascular Disease Education
   Programs Information Center
4733 Bethesda Ave., Suite 530
Bethesda, MD 20814
(301) 951-3260

situations when the purpose is only for taking of the blood pressure. The total investment in this equipment would be $60 to $125, an inexpensive adjunct to encourage patient participation.

PHARMACOLOGIC MANAGEMENT

When the decision has been made to lower the blood pressure, nonpharmacologic therapies should be tried for 3 to 6 months. These may include weight loss in the obese, appropriate regular aerobic exercise, restriction of dietary sodium to 5 g/d and reduction of alcohol consumption to less than 1 to 2 ounces per day. The overall effectiveness of nonpharmacologic measures has been shown to be at least as effective in 60- to 75-year-old patients as in a younger population (Stuart et al, 1989).

The data on potassium and/or calcium supplementation are not yet convincing but may be important in certain subsets of elderly hypertensive patients. Since cigarette smoking contributes to accelerated atherosclerotic processes, avoidance of tobacco may be reasonable in certain circumstances.

When nondrug therapies have not been helpful and systolic blood pressure remains greater than 180 mm Hg and/or diastolic blood pressure greater than 100 mm Hg and endorgan damage is present, antihypertensive drug therapy may be indicated. All commonly used agents have been documented as effective and safe in the elderly population when *carefully administered.* Drugs should be started with small doses (one half usual dose) of the selected drug and given at least 1 month before deciding that its full effect has been attained. Studies have found that elderly patients complied better than younger patients with antihypertensive regimens. It may be best to use simple regimens of long-acting or once per day medication that treat as many conditions as possible. Cost of drugs and monitoring may be an important issue. Side effects need to be identified by questioning the patient and appropriate laboratory testing done one to two times per year or when changes in therapy or patient condition occur. Careful blood pressure measurement in sitting and standing positions are imperative in the evaluation of hypotension and end points of therapy.

None of the antihypertensive drugs is without hazard. Diuretics have been used for over 30 years and have been included in many trials (ISH and S-DHTN) in the elderly, including the European Working Party on High Blood Pressure in the Elderly and the current study of ISH (SHEP, 1991). Diuretics in small doses are effective and generally well tolerated in the elderly but their metabolic effects have been controversial. When used they should be started at a very low dose and monitored closely to avoid dehydration, electrolyte disarray, or orthostatic hypotension. If there are no contraindications a potassium-sparing diuretic can be used. Elevated blood sugar and/or cholesterol and gout may also be complications. Diuretics may be helpful when congestive heart failure is present. When renal insufficiency is present, loop diuretics such as furosemide should be considered. Diuretics in general are thought to work by decreasing peripheral resistance. Because diuretics potentiate the antihypertensive action of other blood pressure lowering agents, they can be left as part of a multiple drug therapy program when other agents are added and when monotherapy is unsuccessful in bringing the blood pressure to the goal of therapy. When left ventricular hypertrophy is present, patients probably should not take a diuretic alone, because other antihypertensive medications may be more successful in reversing the hypertrophy. A study by LaCroix et al (1990) showed that long-term use of thiazides was helpful in reducing the incidence of hip fractures.

Calcium channel antagonists are often used as a first-line agent in treating hypertension in the elderly. They vary in their modes of action, but all lower arterial blood pressure by reducing total peripheral resistance. They may affect electrolyte status or worsen peripheral vascular disease. Constipation is a dose-dependent side effect. Nifedipine is a good choice in patients with a relative bradycardia since it does not prolong AV conduction time. Verapamil and diltiazem should not be used in patients with AV block, sick sinus syndrome, or impaired left ventricular function and may interact adversely with beta-blockers, digoxin, and antiarrhythmic drugs.

Beta-adrenergic antagonists may be selectively used in older patients who do not have peripheral vascular disease, congestive heart failure, obstructive lung disease, diabetes mellitus, or bradyarrhythmias. They may be very effective when hypertension is complicated by angina. Elderly patients are often very sensitive to side effects, i.e., sleep disorders, depression, fatigue, and bradycardia.

Peripheral alpha-blockers must also be used selectively in older patients. They tend to induce or worsen orthostatic hypotension. They do have favorable effects on the symptoms of prostate obstruction and hyperlipidemia.

Angiotensin-converting enzyme inhibitors can be effective in some elderly patients. Recent evidence indicates angiotensin-converting enzyme inhibitors may improve survival in patients with congestive heart failure and may retard the progression of renal disease in diabetic patients. However, they have been known to precipitate proteinuria and renal failure in patients with underlying renal insufficiency or renal artery stenosis and dehydration. Coughing may be a frequent side effect.

Peripheral vasodilators such as minoxidil and hydralazine have not been extensively tested. They have limited use at present in the elderly but may be useful in the setting of heart failure.

Centrally acting alpha$_2$-agonist agents such as methyldopa, clonidine, and guanabenz are generally not preferred in the elderly because they cause significant central nervous system side effects. They act by decreasing sympathetic outflow and thereby reduce blood pressure. The choice of antihypertensive therapy in the elderly must consider quality of life issues, concomitant medical problems and medications, and altered physiology of the elderly.

There are multiple combination tablets of the antihypertensive drugs available that may simplify drug taking after maintenance blood pressure levels are achieved. It must be kept in mind, however, that these combination tablets are difficult to modify to the individual patient's need because changes in doses affect all constituents of the combination tablet. If cost is a consideration, the combination tablets are often proportionately more expensive and may not contain a sufficient diuretic component.

In summary, all of these drugs will need to be initiated in very low dosages with the aim of drug therapy at a *gradual* reduction in blood pressure. Postural hypotension is a potentially greater problem in the elderly than in the middle-aged hypertensive patient. Dose levels that may be safe and effective in the younger patient may be excessive in the elderly. Symptoms of postural hypotension may occur when a sudden and excessive reduction in pressure occurs in a patient with atheromatous inelastic arteries. Dizziness, fainting, impaired vision, and inability to walk properly may then occur and actually mimic stereotypes associated with old age. The Medical Letter on Drugs and Therapeutics Drugs for Hypertension (1991) is a regularly updated resource that identifies current antihypertensive drugs, their dosages, and adverse effects in the treatment of chronic hypertension. Health care workers should be aware of the side effects and precautions of commonly used antihypertensive agents.

MANAGEMENT AND ASSESSMENT GUIDELINES

Health care providers must be conscientious and cautious in observation and approach to the elderly hypertensive patient or the therapeutic program may have disastrous consequences. Nurses with responsibility for long-term management and follow-up observation of these patients will need to monitor both subjective and objective data, using a management protocol appropriate to their skill level and clinical setting.

The assessment should include a focus on the following:

1. Patient and family participation in the treatment program
   a. Integration of patient and health care provider plan into the lifestyle
   b. Degree of impairment of quality of life and patient coping ability
2. Complications
   a. Hypertensive complications—symptoms of congestive heart failure, renal disease, stroke, hypertensive retinopathy, or resistance to a drug regimen previously effective
   b. Drug complications—*orthostatic hypotension,* age-related drug intolerances, side effects, drug interactions

Specific information regarding the antihypertensive drugs may be carried on 3 × 5 note cards in the pocket for ready reference by health care providers. Similar informational cards for patient use may also be helpful and increase patient independence in the treatment program.

A comprehensive follow-up program needs to include the monitoring of certain objective signs. Regular assessment should focus on the following:

1. Physical findings
   a. Blood pressure in lying, sitting, and stand-

ing positions—observe for symptoms of postural hypotension (refer to special precautions in taking the blood pressure). The standing blood pressure should be considered the end point of therapy

b. Pulse in lying, sitting, and standing positions—observe for changes in heart rate that may forecast heart failure

c. Heart sounds—gallops and/or murmurs, rate, and irregularities (a fourth heart sound is commonly heard in hypertensive patients and probably reflects decreased compliance of the left ventricle wall that in turn may be due to left ventricular hypertrophy)

d. Chest sounds—rales

e. Bruits—particularly carotid vessels (may help to explain depression symptoms)

f. Fundoscopic changes—papilledema, exudates, hemorrhages, or presence of nicking of vessels at arteriovenous crossings

g. Weight—pattern of changes or stability

h. Presence of peripheral edema

2. Laboratory determinations as indicated in the management protocol

a. Complete blood count, total cholesterol including HDL fraction and serum electrolytes, including serum creatinine or BUN

b. Urinalysis

3. Chest radiograph—note changes in cardiac size or silhouette

4. Electrocardiogram—note presence of left ventricular strain or hypertrophy indicated by voltage and/or ST-T changes (other changes in the ECG, such as heart blocks or ischemia, may indicate the presence of damage secondary to associated coronary artery disease)

These management suggestions as outlined only supplement the critical role of the health care provider in assessing the individual geriatric patient in the home, clinic, hospital, or long-term care facility.

EVALUATION

Reduction in life expectancy from hypertension is greater in the young patient. This must be kept in mind in setting the management goals and evaluating the outcomes. Hypertension in the elderly is a common disorder, extensively studied and poorly understood. Most important is the maintenance of the quality of life

and maximizing the ability of the patient and family to cope with the ramifications of *indicated and safe* treatment of a chronic health problem. This is, indeed, the challenge that nurses must assume.

Nursing Diagnosis and Management of High-risk Areas in Daily Living

Areas for nursing diagnosis in daily living tend to fall into two major areas: learning and integrating treatment regimens into daily living in effective and satisfying ways; and managing daily living with the symptoms or dysfunctions associated with the pathology.

Hypertension itself, being a silent disease, tends not to create dysfunctions disruptive to daily living. The areas for nursing diagnosis in hypertension then tend to fall into the first category—that of incorporating the treatment regimen into daily living. Optimal medical treatment of hypertension in the over-70 age group involves attempting to control the blood pressure by altering the lifestyle, i.e., moderating salt and sodium intake, managing weight, and incorporating exercise. Nursing assessment will determine the areas and degree of difficulty these proposed alterations will pose to the priorities and lifestyle of the elderly person. For example, a couple of ladies in one nurse's case load would report that "this week my blood pressure is going to be higher—my friends and I ate out on Tuesday, Wednesday, and Thursday." Following the diagnosis of high-risk areas, mutual planning can be initiated on the actions the elderly person *is willing and able to take* and on the best accommodations or strategies to use for optimal outcomes, given the circumstances.

The silent nature of the pathology presents another area for diagnosis and that is the potential for low motivation to take medications or follow the regimen when there are no symptoms. Every patient needs to be individually assessed as to the functional ability in his own setting. What does the person want to do? How can health care providers help with indicated medication regimens, minimize side effects, and encourage activities or exercise that maintain quality of life? Long-term nursing follow-up is essential when hypertension is asymptomatic and the impact of drugs on exercise tolerance and sexual function and the concomitant medical problems may alter the quality of life for an individual patient and those who share the daily living.

A third area for nursing diagnosis comes in living with the effects of diuretics or antihypertensive medications. Diagnosing the circumstances where diuresis would be inconvenient or incapacitating, or when the postural hypotension might be dangerous, the nurse can help the elderly person to plan strategies for timing the ingestion of the drug and actions to take to safely and satisfyingly cope with the drug effects.

For fuller treatment of nursing diagnosis and management of high-risk areas, see the section on inadequate motivation for incorporating diabetic self-care into daily living in Chapter 24, Diabetes, and the section on daily living with dietary alterations in Chapter 31, Chronic Renal Failure.

Many elderly persons may believe that having "hypertension" is a physical reflection of past social and environmental stressors. This illness belief system needs to be explored with the individual patient because it is often used to justify unwarranted social behavior and to assume various aspects of the sick role at a time in life when these people are already feeling "older," have other illnesses, and are growing more dependent. Studies of younger employed persons who were given a diagnosis of hypertension have shown more use of sick time. Perhaps this labeling effect may produce more discouragement, dependency, or illness behavior in the older patient as well.

References and Other Readings

American Heart Association. Recommendations for human blood pressure determination by sphygmomanometers. New York: AHA, 1980.

Amery A, Birkenhager W, Brixko P, et al. Mortality and morbidity results from the European Working Party on High Blood Pressure in the Elderly trial. Lancet 1985; 1:1349.

Castelli WP. CHD risk factors in the elderly. Hosp Pract, 1976.

Goldstein G, Materson BJ, Cushman WC, et al. Treatment of hypertension in the elderly II: cognitive and behavioral function: results of a Department of Veterans Affairs Cooperative Study. Hypertension 1990; 15:361.

Kannel WB, et al. Role of blood pressure in the development of congestive heart failure. N Engl J Med 1972; 287:781.

Klatsky A, et al. Alcohol consumption and blood pressure. N Engl J Med 1977; 296:1194.

LaCroix AZ, Wienpahl J, White LR, et al. Thiazide diuretic agents and the incidence of hip fractures. N Engl J Med 1990; 322:286.

Lepor H. Role of alpha-adrenergic blockers in the treatment of benign prostatic hyperplasia. Prostate 1990; 3(suppl):75.

MacMahon SW. Alcohol and hypertension: implications for prevention and treatment. Ann Intern Med 1986; 105:124.

McCarron D, et al. Blood pressure and nutrient intake in the United States. Science 1984; 224:1392.

Sasaki N. The relationship of salt intake to hypertension in the Japanese. Geriatrics 1964; 19:735.

Second National Health and Nutrition Examination Survey 1976-80. Series 1, No. 15. US Department of Health and Human Services, Publication PHS 81-1317.

Shekelle RB, Ostfeld AM, Klawans HL Jr. Hypertension and risk of stroke in an elderly population. Stroke 1974; 5:71.

SHEP Cooperative Research Group. Prevention of stroke by antihypertensive drug treatment in older persons with isolated systolic hypertension. JAMA 1991; 265:3255.

Stuart EM, Deckro JP, Mamish ME, Friedman R, Benson H. Nonpharmacological treatment of the elderly hypertensive patient. Circulation 1989; 80(suppl II):189.

RECOMMENDED MATERIALS

The 1988 Report of the Joint National Committee on Detection, Evaluation and Treatment of High Blood Pressure. NIH Publication No. 88-1088, May 1988.

Statement on Hypertension in the Elderly (Final report of the working group to revise the April 1980 Elderly Statement). JAMA 1986; 256:No. 1.

The Medical Letter Inc., 1000 Main Street, New Rochelle, NY 10801.

29
Incontinence and Urinary Problems

LYNN BERRY

Pathophysiology and Medical Management

Elderly people are at increased risk for urinary system problems. The effects of normal aging coupled with concurrent illness may disrupt the fragile balance that maintains continency or prevents infection. As with other health conditions facing older persons, urinary system problems can be acute or chronic and may affect activities of daily living or lifestyle. Nursing assessment and management are vital in addressing urinary conditions as part of the total health care of elderly persons.

Incontinence* Urinary incontinence may be defined as "any uncontrolled leakage of urine at any time" (Ouslander, 1981). Symptoms may range from occasional dribbling to complete loss of bladder control. Urinary incontinence is a complex problem with many possible causes. Thus, it becomes important to determine the etiology of the incontinence before planning successful treatment strategies.

*Guidelines for adult urinary incontinence are available from U.S. Public Health Service's Agency for Health Care Policy and Research (AHCPR). The free information includes a copy of the guidelines, a quick reference guide, and patient guide. Call 1–800–358–9295, or write AHCPR Publication Clearinghouse, P.O. Box 8547, Silver Springs, MD 20907.

HIGH-RISK POPULATIONS

Normal age changes do not result in incontinency but may predispose an elderly individual to its development. Older persons with chronic or acute illnesses affecting cognition, mobility, or neurologic function are at higher risk of developing incontinence. The prevalence is 1.5 to 2 times higher in women (Herzog and Fultz, 1990). Estimates of occurrence range from 15% to 30% in community elderly to 50% of institutionalized elders (NIH Consensus Development Conference, 1990).

DYNAMICS OF NORMAL VOIDING

The bladder consists of smooth muscle with the capacity to stretch as it fills, keeping intravesicle pressure relatively low until approximately 200 mL of urine is present. The stretch receptors from the detrusor (bladder muscle) send messages via cholinergic nerve fibers to the sacral micturition center of the spinal cord (S2–S4). When enough stimulation is received, the parasympathetic motor fibers are activated, resulting in detrusor contraction and emptying of the bladder. Sympathetic innervation (beta-adrenergic) relaxes the bladder as it fills as well as the bladder outlet during urination. Alpha-adrenergic stimulation contracts the internal sphincter in the proximal urethra and maintains continence against the increasing vesicle pressure. The external sphincter is a striated

543

muscle that is innervated via motor neurons and allows for voluntary interruption of voiding. The neurotransmitter at the sympathetic neuromuscular junction is norepinephrine. The parasympathetic neurotransmitter may involve more than just acetylcholine; other cotransmitters or those with an independent action have been suggested (Badlani and Smith, 1987). This entire micturition pathway can be thought of as a reflex arc that can be activated by the higher central nervous system centers in the brain stem and frontoparietal cortex. Without higher control, voluntary micturition cannot take place, and bladder emptying is less efficient due to loss of central nervous system mediated rhythmic detrusor muscle contractions during voiding. The cortical/brain stem involvement also allows for coordination of bladder contraction with sphincter relaxation. The normal bladder will protect itself from overdistention by activating the reflex arc at maximum tolerable fullness (500 to 700 mL). Accessory structures important to pathologic changes in micturition are the prostate gland in men and the pelvic floor musculature in women (Fig. 29–1) (Ouslander, 1981; Wein, 1986).

EFFECTS OF AGING

There is much to be learned about the normal age changes of the lower urinary tract. Research findings have shown no change in detrusor mass with aging. Aging bladder epithelium may show areas of undifferentiated cells only two layers deep scattered among normal transitional epithelium that is three to four layers deep. Bladder diverticula become more common with aging. The estrogen-dependent tissue of the urethra in women may become atrophic and friable after menopause, causing urinary frequency or dysuria.

There is an increased incidence of nocturia, which may be related to a decreased ability to concentrate urine, a change in the diurnal voiding pattern with aging, or increased circulating vascular volume with the supine position.

Two studies of subjects older than age 65 (Brocklehurst and Dillane, 1966; Andersen et al, 1978) suggest that uninhibited bladder contractions may occur more frequently with aging. Approximately half of the female subjects in the Brocklehurst and Dillane study without neurologic disease had a reduced bladder capacity (urge to void at <250 mL), resid-

ual urine of greater than 50 mL, and a late onset of the desire to urinate when the bladder was filled to capacity. The older male subjects in the study by Andersen et al had maximum and average flow rates lower than the control group of younger subjects.

Benign prostatic hypertrophy is also a common age change in men. Autopsy data have shown that 95% of men over age 80 have some hypertrophy, although not necessarily with any clinical symptoms.

PATHOPHYSIOLOGY OF INCONTINENCE

Urinary incontinence may be an acute or chronic condition. The incontinence may stem from a problem with the storage phase or the emptying phase (or both) of micturition.

The acronym **DIAPPERS** has been used to summarize the causes of acute incontinence (Resnick, 1990):

Delirium or confusional state
Infection, urinary
Atrophic urethritis or vaginitis
Pharmaceuticals
  Sedatives or hypnotics, especially long-acting agents
  Diuretics
  Anticholinergic agents
  Alpha-adrenoceptor agonists and antagonists
  Calcium channel blockers
  Vincristine
Psychological disorder, especially depression
Endocrine disorder (hypercalcemia or hyperglycemia)
Restricted mobility
Stool impaction

A careful history and examination should reveal the underlying etiology and ideally continency can be restored when the problem is resolved.

Chronic or established incontinence in the elderly can be divided into five main types, each of which has numerous etiologies (Table 29–1). In addition to those listed, Resnick (1990), in a study of 94 institutionalized elderly, identified another type that he termed "detrusor hyperactivity with impaired contractility." The symptoms of detrusor hyperactivity with impaired contractility are impaired emptying in combination with uninhibited bladder contractions. Incontinence in the elderly may have more than one cause and resto-

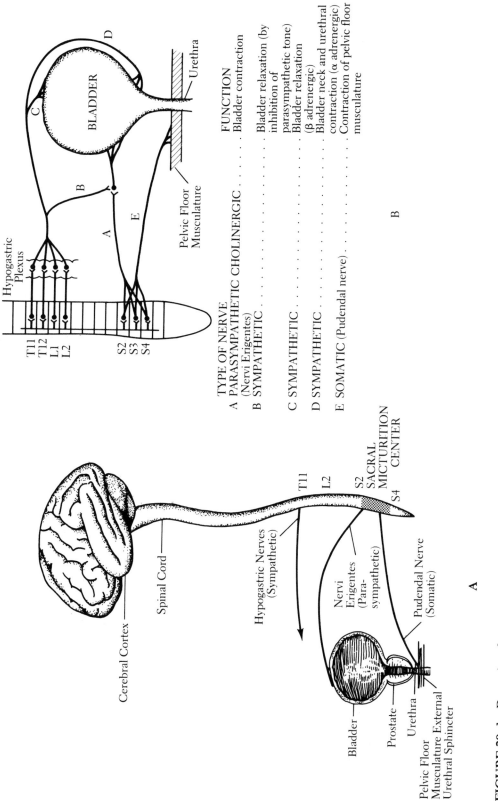

FIGURE 29–1 Dynamics of normal voiding. *A*, Structural components of normal micturition. *B*, Peripheral nerves involved in micturition. (From Kane RL, Ouslander JG, Abrass IB. Essentials of clinical geriatrics, 2nd ed. New York: McGraw-Hill, 1989; with permission.)

TABLE 29–1 *Types and Causes of Established Urinary Incontinence*

Type of Incontinence	Manifestations	Common Causes
Stress	Leakage of small amounts of urine with increases in intra-abdominal pressure (e.g., coughing or laughing)	Prolapse of pelvic structures in women Sphincter weakness or damage (e.g., postprostatectomy)
Urge	Leakage of urine from inability to delay voiding long enough to reach toilet after urge to void is perceived	Unstable bladder Disorders of the lower genitourinary tract such as tumors, stones, diverticula, atrophic urethritis or vaginitis, chronic cystitis, and mild outflow obstruction Disorders of the central nervous system such as stroke, dementia, parkinsonism, and multiple sclerosis, which cause bladder instability (detrusor hyperreflexia)
Overflow	Leakage of small amounts of urine Urinary stream often diminished Sensation of bladder fullness often impaired	Anatomic obstruction (prostate, urethral stricture), hypotonic or acontractile bladder (diabetes, spinal cord injury, anticholinergic drugs)
Functional	Physical inability or unwillingness to reach a toilet on time	Impaired mobility or cognitive function Inaccessible toilets or caregivers Psychological disorders such as depression, regression, anger, hostility
Total (incontinence of nonresistance)	Complete lack of control over voiding Concomitant fecal incontinence common	Sphincter damage Nerve damage (peripheral or spinal cord injury) Dementia (severe)*

*Incontinence may initially be nocturnal or intermittent but often becomes constant as cognitive impairment worsens.
Note: Stress, urge, and overflow incontinence can occur in various combinations in the elderly.
From Kane RL, Ouslander JG, Abrass IB. Essentials of clinical geriatrics, 2nd ed. New York: McGraw-Hill, 1989; with permission.

ration of even one or two factors may restore continency.

ASSESSMENT AND DIFFERENTIAL DIAGNOSES

The assessment of urinary incontinence may range from sophisticated urodynamic testing done by the urologist to bedside tests that can be performed by a nurse practitioner. Each elderly person's cognitive and functional status must be considered in the evaluation process. The core evaluation process is outlined in Figure 29–2 and in the box on p. 548, and consists of a history, physical examination, and laboratory tests (chemistry screen, BUN, creatinine, glucose, and urinalysis with culture). Selective referral to a urologist for more extensive evaluation (Table 29–2) can be based on these initial findings. If further evaluation is impractical or refused, bedside diagnostic tests (Table 29–3) can be helpful in the institutional or clinic setting.

As part of the assessment process, a 4- to 7-day bladder record is beneficial in identifying the frequency, amount, and time of day incontinence is occurring. The record can be filled

Core Evaluation

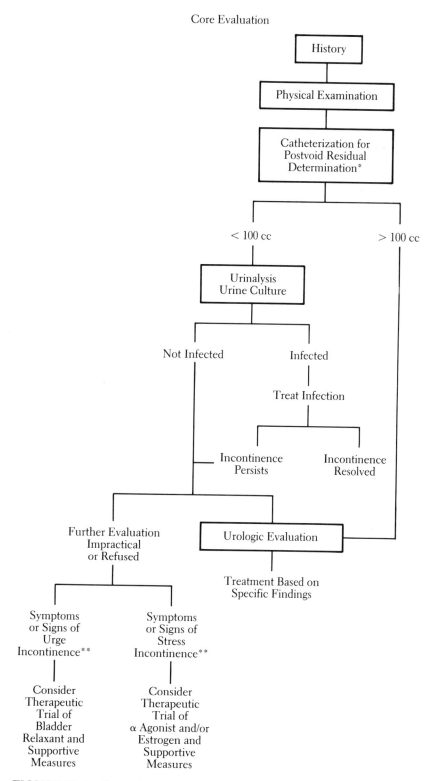

FIGURE 29–2 General paradigm for evaluation of established incontinence. If practical, other bedside diagnostic tests can be done at the time of catheterization. Results of bedside diagnostic tests can be helpful in making this therapeutic decision. (From Kane RL, Ouslander JG, Abrass IB. Essentials of clinical geriatrics. New York: McGraw-Hill, 1984; with permission.)

Evaluating Incontinence: Key Points in the History and Physical Examination

HISTORY

General medical history

    Current medical problems

    Medications

    Past genitourinary history (surgery, radiation, stones, recurrent infections, etc.)

Characteristics of incontinence

    Onset and duration

    Frequency, timing, and amount of leakage

    Sensation of bladder fullness/emptying

    Urgency versus stress versus both

    Associated symptoms (dysuria, hematuria, hesitancy)

    Concomitant fecal incontinence

Other information

    Current management of incontinence

    Location and accessibility of toilets

    Patient and caregivers' perceptions of the problem

    Patient and caregivers' expectations from evaluation and treatment

PHYSICAL EXAMINATION

Mental status

Mobility

Lumbosacral innervation

    Lower extremity motor/sensory/reflexes

    Perianal and genital sensation

    Bulbocavernosus reflex

Abdominal examination: bladder distention

Rectal examination

    Sphincter tone

    Fecal impaction

    Masses/prostate

Genital examination

    External abnormalities

    Perineal skin

    Vaginal mucosa

    Cystocele/urethrocele/rectocele

    Pelvic mass

From Kane RL, Ouslander JG, Abrass IB. Essentials of clinical geriatrics. New York: McGraw-Hill, 1984; with permission.

TABLE 29–2 *Urologic Procedures Used in the Evaluation of Incontinence*

Test	Purpose
Cystoscopy	Identify structural lesions of bladder and urethra
	Observe sphincter function
Urine flowmetry	Detect outflow obstruction or hypotonic bladder
Cystometrics	Identify bladder hyperactivity and hypoactivity
Urethral pressure profile	Detect sphincter weakness, hyperactivity, dyssynergy
Voiding cystourethrography	Observe dynamics of micturition and bladder and urethral anatomy
	Detect stress incontinence
Sphincter electromyography	Evaluate sacral innervation

From Kane RL, Ouslander JG, Abrass IB. Essentials of clinical geriatrics. New York: McGraw-Hill, 1984; with permission.

out by the patient or caregiver. An example of an easily used record is found in Figure 29–3.

COMPLICATIONS

Skin problems such as rashes or pressure sores develop more quickly in the incontinent person. Failure to diagnose overflow incontinence can lead to more acute problems of infection involving kidneys or bladder.

Studies of the psychosocial impact of urinary incontinence suggest that restriction of social and sexual activity is common. Ouslander and Abelson (1990) found that 60% to 70% of approximately 200 elderly outpatients with urinary incontinence felt that it was embarrassing, distressing, or inconvenient. The reaction to incontinence is variable, however, and the severity of the incontinence may not be directly correlated to the degree of social impairment (Wyman et al, 1990). Failure of the patient or family to effectively manage urinary incontinence may lead to the consideration of alternative living arrangements (Noelker, 1987).

PROGNOSIS

Success in treating incontinence depends on an accurate physical and mental assessment and the use of an effective therapy for the type(s) of incontinence identified. According to the National Institutes of Health Consensus Development Conference (1990), most cases of urinary incontinence can be cured or improved.

MEDICAL MANAGEMENT

The major methods of treating the different types of geriatric incontinence are outlined in Table 29–4. The assessment process may reveal several areas that can be addressed to improve continency, thus requiring a multidisciplinary approach to treatment.

Pharmacology Well-designed clinical studies of drugs used to treat urinary incontinence are limited. However, there are several medications that are commonly used for certain types of incontinence. These medications are outlined in Table 29–5. Further studies are also needed to evaluate the effectiveness of pharmacologic treatment in combination with other therapies.

Surgery Surgical intervention is most successfully used for stress incontinence. Common types of surgery are urethral suspension, urethral lengthening, and sphincter implants. Transurethral resection of the prostate is also beneficial in treating overflow incontinence caused by prostatic hypertrophy.

Electrical Stimulation The efficacy of neural stimulation continues to be studied. Stimulation of the sacral roots can produce a response at either the bladder to inhibit hyperreflexia or at the sphincter to improve contractility (Tanagho, 1990).

Intermittent Catheterization Intermittent catheterization is widely used to manage chronic urinary retention when urethral stricture or blockage is not a problem. The catheterization procedure can be taught to a caregiver if the patient does not have adequate manual dexterity. The procedure, found in Table 29–6, uses clean technique unless the patient is being cared for in an institution. Sterile technique is recommended in the hospital or nursing home

TABLE 29–3 *Bedside Diagnostic Tests Useful in Evaluating Incontinence*

Test	Information
WOMEN	
Postvoid residual	Residual >50 to 100 mL indicates urinary retention
With straight catheter still in place, slowly instill sterile water or saline at body temperature under 15 cm H_2O pressure*	Note onset of desire to void and/or any discomfort
	If 200 to 300 mL is instilled without leakage, unstable bladder is unlikely
	If leakage around catheter occurs at volumes <200 mL, unstable bladder is likely
	If there is difficulty instilling fluid under low pressure, bladder is probably poorly compliant
When patient senses bladder fullness, remove catheter and perform stress maneuvers (i.e., cough, strain) in supine and standing positions	If urine leaks coincident with stress maneuver, stress incontinence has been objectively demonstrated (unstable bladder cannot be ruled out)
	If uncontrolled urination begins after the stress maneuver ceases, unstable bladder may be present
If urine leaks with stress, place fingers in periurethral area (avoid directly compressing urethra), lift, and repeat stress maneuver (Boney or Marshall test)	If urinary leakage is prevented, patient may benefit from bladder neck suspension
MEN	
Observe urinary stream as patient voids voluntarily†	Slow interrupted stream with small volumes suggests outflow obstruction and/or bladder hypotonicity
Postvoid residual	Residual > 50 to 100 mL indicates urinary retention
With straight catheter still in place, slowly instill sterile water or saline at body temperature under 15 cm H_2O pressure*	Note onset of desire to void and/or any discomfort
	If 200 to 300 mL is instilled without leakage, unstable bladder is unlikely
	If leakage around the catheter occurs at volumes <200 mL, unstable bladder is likely
	If there is difficulty instilling fluid under low pressure, the bladder is probably poorly compliant

*This can be done by holding a container of fluid 10 to 15 cm above pubic symphysis.
†Urine flow can be measured with a timer and calibrated beaker. Flow rate < 10 mL/s suggests obstruction (or hypotonicity); > 26 mL/s makes obstruction unlikely.
From Kane RL, Ouslander JG, Abrass IB. Essentials of clinical geriatrics. New York: McGraw-Hill, 1984; with permission.

setting due to the increased pathogenicity of the environmental bacteria (Oliver, 1990).

Biofeedback Biofeedback for urinary incontinence provides a sensory reference (usually visual) of bladder pressure, abdominal pressure, and periurethral muscle pressure. The information can then help the individual learn to regain control of these muscles to facilitate urine stor-

age. In the case of urge incontinence, the goal is for the individual to be able to contract the periurethral muscle while relaxing the detrusor and abdominal muscles to prevent escape of urine. The goal of treating stress incontinence is selective contraction of periurethral muscles while keeping the abdominal muscles relaxed. Research has shown an improvement rate of 70% to 80% in ambulatory, cognitively intact

INCONTINENCE MONITORING RECORD

INSTRUCTIONS: EACH TIME THE PATIENT IS CHECKED:
1) Mark *one* of the circles in the BLADDER section at the hour closest to the time the patient is checked.
2) Make an X in the BOWEL section if the patient has had an incontinent or normal bowel movement.

◖ = Incontinent, small amount	⊘ = Dry	X = Incontinent BOWEL
● = Incontinent, large amount	△̸ = Voided correctly	X = Normal BOWEL

PATIENT NAME _____ ROOM # _____ DATE _____

	BLADDER				BOWEL			
	INCONTINENT OF URINE		DRY	VOIDED CORRECTLY	INCONTINENT X	NORMAL X	INITIALS	**COMMENTS**
12am	●	●	○	△ cc ____				
1	●	●	○	△ cc ____				
2	●	●	○	△ cc ____				
3	●	●	○	△ cc ____				
4	●	●	○	△ cc ____				
5	●	●	○	△ cc ____				
6	●	●	○	△ cc ____				
7	●	●	○	△ cc ____				
8	●	●	○	△ cc ____				
9	●	●	○	△ cc ____				
10	●	●	○	△ cc ____				
11	●	●	○	△ cc ____				
12pm	●	●	○	△ cc ____				
1	●	●	○	△ cc ____				
2	●	●	○	△ cc ____				
3	●	●	○	△ cc ____				
4	●	●	○	△ cc ____				
5	●	●	○	△ cc ____				
6	●	●	○	△ cc ____				
7	●	●	○	△ cc ____				
8	●	●	○	△ cc ____				
9	●	●	○	△ cc ____				
10	●	●	○	△ cc ____				
11	●	●	○	△ cc ____				

TOTALS:

FIGURE 29–3   Incontinence monitoring record. (From Greengold BA, Ouslander J. J Gerontol Nurs 1986; 12:31; with permission.)

TABLE 29–4   Primary Treatments for Different Types of Geriatric Urinary Incontinence

Type of Incontinence	Primary Treatments
Stress	Pelvic floor (Kegel) exercises
	α-Adrenergic agonists
	Estrogen
	Biofeedback, behavioral training
	Surgical bladder neck suspension
Urge	Bladder relaxants
	Estrogen (if vaginal atrophy is present)
	Training procedures (e.g., biofeedback, behavioral therapy)
	Surgical removal of obstructing or other irritating pathologic lesions
Overflow	Surgical removal of obstruction
	Intermittent catheterization (if practical)
	Indwelling catheterization
Functional	Behavioral therapies (e.g., habit training, scheduled toileting)
	Environmental manipulations
	Incontinence undergarments and pads
	External collection devices
	Bladder relaxants (selected patients)*
	Indwelling catheters (selected patients)

*Many patients with functional incontinence also have detrusor hyperreflexia, and some may benefit from bladder relaxant drug therapy.
From Kane RL, Ouslander JG, Abrass IB. Essentials of clinical geriatrics, 2nd ed. New York: McGraw-Hill, 1989; with permission.

subjects (Burgio and Engel, 1990). The technique requires some invasiveness (a vaginal and/or rectal probe and bladder catheter) for the patient and training in use for the clinician. A simpler system using electromyographic amplifiers has been developed and should allow biofeedback to become more accessible for home or clinic use (The Personal Perineometer, PerryMeter Systems, 242 Old Eagle School Road, Strafford, PA 19087, 1(800)537-3779).

URINARY TRACT INFECTION

Lower urinary tract infection (UTI) is one of the most common health problems in the elderly. It is the second highest cause of fever in older people.

RISK FACTORS

Age   The incidence of UTI increases with age in both men and women.

Urinary Stasis   Pooling of stagnant urine in the bladder as a result of obstruction or neurogenic factors is the major risk factor in producing UTIs.

Institutionalization   Older persons who live in their own homes are more mobile and active and have lower rates of UTI than those who live in institutional settings. In addition, there is greater risk of cross-infection in any congregate form of housing or health care setting.

Gender   Women are more susceptible to UTIs due to their shorter, straight urethras that are in close proximity to the anus. Hormonal changes and a decrease in vaginal defense mechanisms allow colonization of the vaginal introitus and subsequent colonization of the urethra and bladder (Mulholland, 1990).

Catheters and Instrumentation   There is a 1% to 10% rate of bacteriuria with instrumentation. Colonization of the urine after indwelling catheter placement is almost universal after 4 weeks.

Immobility   Immobility can lead to incomplete bladder emptying. The use of bedpans or urinals in the supine or semireclining position does not facilitate complete emptying. Immobility also results in increased calcium in the urine and a higher risk of stone formation.

DYNAMICS

The bladder mucosa normally has a low pH that exerts a natural bacteriostatic effect on in-

TABLE 29–5 *Pharmacologic Treatment for Incontinence*

Drug	Mechanism of Action	Potential Side Effects	Types of Incontinence
Propantheline bromide Imipramine	Anticholinergic: ↓ bladder contractility improved bladder capacity	Constipation Dry mouth Blurred vision Orthostatic hypotension ↑ intraocular pressure	Urge with unstable bladder Stress with unstable bladder
Oxybutynin chloride (Ditropan) Dicylomine hydrochloride Flavoxate hydrochloride (Urispas)	Musculotropic relaxant: ↓ uninhibited bladder contractions	Constipation Dry mouth Blurred vision Orthostatic hypotention ↑ intraocular pressure	Urge with unstable bladder Stress with unstable bladder
Terodiline (pending approval by the FDA)	Calcium antagonist Anticholinergic Local anesthetic effects	Dry mouth Blurred vision Tremor Nausea	Urge with unstable bladder Stress with unstable bladder
Pseudoephedrine Phenylpropanolamine	Alpha-adrenergic agonist: urethral sphincter contraction	Tachycardia Urinary retention ↑ blood pressure Headache	Stress with weak sphincter
Estradiol (systemic) Topical estrogen	Estrogens: ↑ sphincter tone in women	Endometrial cancer ↑ blood pressure Gallstones	Urge due to atrophic urethritis Stress
Bethanechol chloride (Urecholine) Cholinergic agonist: ↑ bladder contractions	Diarrhea Bradycardia	Bronchoconstriction Overflow due to atonic bladder	

vading organisms. Urinary retention dilutes this normal acidity, thus reducing its bacterisostatic effect. The urethral meatus is normally contaminated by some bowel flora. The outward flow of urine serves to prevent movement of bacteria up from the meatus to the bladder and kidney. Any change in this urine flow that reduces the outward direction will remove the natural barrier to the ascent of bacteria into the urinary tract.

SIGNS AND SYMPTOMS

A UTI in an elderly individual may present in a similar manner as in a younger person. Fever, hematuria, urgency, suprapubic discomfort,

frequency, and dysuria are all classic complaints of UTI. In the elderly, however, a fever may be low grade (99°F), absent, or masked by analgesics that are taken for other chronic illnesses. Older patients may also present with confusion, lethargy, delirium, anorexia, or acute urinary incontinence. Individuals with dementia may exhibit increased agitation that cannot be explained by other causes.

DIFFERENTIAL DIAGNOSIS

A distinction may be made between UTI and asymptomatic bacteriuria. The latter occurs with increasing frequency in aging persons. Studies have shown that approximately 15% of

TABLE 29–6   *Self-catheterization Patient Teaching Aid*

Women	Men
EQUIPMENT	
Lubricant, soap and water	Lubricant, soap and water
No. 14 French 6 inch or 16 inch catheter*	No. 14 French 16 inch regular or coude tip*

PROCEDURE

Women	Men
1. Identify the vagina and meatus with a mirror; feel the difference between the two openings	1. Wash hands with soap and water; lubricate catheter tip 1 to 2 inches
2. Wash hands with soap and water; lubricate catheter tip	2. Catheterize in a standing position
3. Sit on the toilet or stand with a foot on the toilet seat; spread labia with second and fourth fingers, identify meatus with middle finger	3. Grasp the penis just behind the glans and hold upward in an erect position; retract the foreskin if uncircumcised
4. Move the middle finger slightly above the meatus and guide the catheter tip inside	4. Insert the catheter slowly until slight resistance is met; take deep breaths, rotate the catheter slightly and continue to pass the catheter until urine begins to flow
5. Allow the catheter to drain completely and then remove	5. Lower the penis and catheter toward the toilet/receptacle and pass the catheter approximately 1 inch further
	6. Allow the catheter to drain completely and then remove; replace the foreskin to cover glans

Clean intermittent catheterization should be done on awakening, approximately every 4 hours during the day, and just before bedtime. Volumes at each catheterization should not exceed 400 mL. A foam rubber hair roller may be slipped over the catheter for persons with impaired manual dexterity to allow for a better grip.

CATHETER CARE

Catheters should be washed with soap and water, rinsed well, and outwardly dried with a paper towel. They can then be stored in a make-up case, plastic bag, or other pouch. Each catheter may be used for 2 to 3 weeks

*Plastic catheters may be more comfortable and easier to clean than red rubber catheters.

women and 0% to 3% of men aged 65 to 70 have bacteriuria as compared with 20% to 50% of women and 20% of men older than 80 years of age (Boscia and Kaye, 1988). Bacteriuria tends to reoccur after antibiotic therapy; thus, in the absence of symptoms or an etiology of obstruction or retention, there is little indication for ongoing treatment.

UTI is usually diagnosed on the basis of symptoms, a urine culture of greater than 100,000 organisms per milliliter, and pyuria. Persistent pyuria without significant bacteriu-ria is suspect for tuberculosis of the kidney or urolithiasis. Symptoms may occur with a lower organism count on culture, especially when the specimen is obtained via catheterization or if the patient produced a dilute urine. Most cultures isolate only one or two species of bacteria; more than three species may occur with a contaminated specimen or an indwelling catheter. To obtain an accurate urine sample from a patient with a long-term indwelling catheter, the old catheter should be removed and a new one inserted to collect the specimen. Catheters that have been in place for several weeks will be colonized with bacteria that may be different from the strain causing the present infection (Grahn et al, 1985).

Gram stain, which is 80% reliable, is used for immediate determination of bacterial type. The most frequent cause of UTI remains *Escherichia coli* (80%); however, *Proteus, Klebsiella, Enterobacter, Serratia,* and *Pseudomonas* may all be found in institutional settings or with an indwelling catheter.

PROGNOSIS

Prognosis is dependent on the severity of the infection, the baseline health status of the individual, and the prompt initiation of appropriate antibiotic therapy. Outcome can range from complete recovery to septicemia and death.

COMPLICATIONS

Urinary infections complicated by other pathology (such as obstruction) will not respond well to antimicrobial treatment until the underlying abnormality is recognized and corrected.

Side effects of antibiotic treatment must also be considered since many antibiotics interact with other medications a patient may be taking. Gastrointestinal upset, including pseudomembranous colitis caused by *Clostridium difficile* may also result from the use of antibiotic therapy.

MEDICAL MANAGEMENT

Treatment for a UTI is guided by data from urine cultures, organism drug sensitivity, and drug allergies of the patient. Antimicrobial therapy usually lasts from 1 to 2 weeks. Use of short-term antibiotic doses, a common treatment in younger women, can be effective in approximately 80% of community elderly with an uncomplicated UTI (Mulholland, 1990).

Oral suppressive therapy often is ordered when long-term treatment is needed. These drugs do not replace antibiotics but rather are used to prevent or at least reduce the frequency of acute attacks. The methenamine salts (Mandelamine, Hiprex) are commonly used medications that are safe and especially effective when residual urine is chronically present. They act by breaking urine down into organic acids and formaldehyde. The formaldehyde effectively suppresses the growth of many

urinary organisms without development of resistance. These drugs require an acid urine for effectiveness. Ascorbic acid (vitamin C) may be given to ensure the urine pH is less than 5.5. Nitrofurantoin or trimetheprim/sulfa may be used as urinary antiseptics when given in a single, low, every-other-day dose (Mulholland, 1990). Nitrofurantoin can have pulmonary side effects and should not be given with significantly impaired renal function (creatinine clearance < 40 mL/min).

Septic UTI requires a more aggressive approach for successful treatment. Blood cultures are done when there is rapid onset, marked fever, delirium, or prostration. Intravenous antibiotics and fluids are essential to treat the infection and maintain blood pressure and hydration. Duration of therapy will be guided by clinical response.

Nursing Diagnosis and Management of High-risk Areas in Daily Living with Lower Urinary Tract Problems

Lower urinary tract dysfunction is a common problem in old age. Many older persons believe it is part of the normal aging process or they may be reluctant to talk about problems that relate to bladder control. They may also fear that the only treatment available for urinary incontinence is surgery (Norton et al, 1988). A sensitive, knowledgeable approach can help the patient discuss these problems and recognize that in most cases, urinary tract difficulties need not be tolerated and that, in fact, treatment is available.

If urinary dysfunction cannot be remedied, nursing care may play a key factor in the management of an individual's daily routine. It can assist in maintaining the patient's level of comfort and dignity with minimum disruption to the activities of daily living.

DAILY LIVING TO PREVENT INCONTINENCE

The presence of urinary incontinence can be devastating to the quality of life. Therefore, managing daily living in such ways as to prevent, delay, or minimize incontinence is critical to the well-being of the older individual.

RISK FACTORS

The risk of acute or chronic incontinence may be increased by the following:

Constipation and fecal impaction
UTIs
Clothing that requires much time and manipulation for removal
Cognitive impairment
Use of diuretics, tranquilizers, sedatives, or medications with anticholinergic side effects
Inability to transfer oneself to the toilet
A view of incontinence as an expected part of aging
Immobility
Depression
Excessive use of alcohol or caffeine (which act as diuretics)

SIGNS AND SYMPTOMS

The reporting or observation of escape of urine at unplanned times is an indication that the activities of daily living are not preventing incontinence. There may be a reluctance to report the occurrence or a redefinition of what incontinence means. For example, if an individual is able to stay dry with the use of incontinent pads, an incontinent episode may come to mean that despite the pads, one's clothing became wet (Mitteness, 1987).

The data base needed to determine how daily living may be affecting continence includes information on the following:

Physical mobility, muscle tone, manual dexterity, balance, transfer capability, and vision
Attitude toward self: self-esteem, perception of aging
Mental status: orientation, ability to be aware of bladder cues, memory, interest and ability in learning, amount of sensory stimulation available
Medications being taken, particularly diuretics, sedatives, tranquilizers, and tricyclic antidepressants
Medical treatments: catheterization, surgery, intravenous fluids or prescribed fluid intake regimen, prescribed bed rest
Food, activity, sleep patterns, and bowel elimination
Fluid intake pattern, including amount and type of fluids ingested
Environment: location of toilet or commode,

use of urinal, distance of bathroom from normal daytime and sleeping areas, stairs to bathroom, lighting, effects on availability of bathroom because others use it
Social activities and personal support: presence or absence of others who care about the person, events, or activities in which the person wishes to participate

PROGNOSTIC VARIABLES

Urinary incontinence is less likely to occur if an older person is mobile and mentally alert. A motivated, informed individual who has received a thorough assessment for the cause of incontinence will be better able to participate in an appropriate treatment plan. A supportive environment with convenient toilet facilities will also enhance urinary control.

COMPLICATIONS

Incontinence that is unavoidable or that is allowed to become fully established may cause embarrassment and restrict one's ability to engage in usual social and sexual pursuits. It may become a major factor in the need to consider institutionalization.

TREATMENT

Organizing daily living in such a way as to reduce the risks of incontinence includes helping the older person or caregiver to do the following:

Understand the nature of continence and measures to maintain it, e.g., regular bowel elimination, fluid intake (35 mL/kg) taken more during the early hours of the day, early treatment for infections
Learn how to monitor patterns of urination and plan the accommodation needed in daily living to promote continence
Modify clothing to permit ease and speed of removal, given any handicaps the individual may have
Arrange the environment for safe efficient passage to and use of toilet facilities
Establish a sensory environment, social interaction program, and physical exercise activity to maintain emotional well-being.
Learn to establish food, fluid, and medication taking patterns that expedite continence, avoiding fluids that can cause irritation and

diuresis (caffeine, alcohol), and taking diuretics to fit into activity schedule

Know how to engage in pelvic floor exercises and carry them out as needed

EVALUATION

Effectiveness of nursing interventions can be measured in the degree of continence maintained.

DAILY LIVING WITH URINARY INCONTINENCE

There are times when urinary incontinence has become an established pattern. The degree of incontinence and its impact on daily living vary widely. Those with stress incontinence and living in the community often manage well without curtailing their social and daily activities. Where there is no urinary control, daily living can be altered drastically.

RISK FACTORS

Those at greatest risk for not managing daily living with incontinence are those who

Have no control over urinary flow

Have accompanying physical disability

Have cognitive deficits or psychiatric problems

Lack money for supplies and services

Experience recurrent UTIs

Do not wish to participate in an active treatment program

Have no primary caregiver to assist with treatments or maintain the hygiene of clothing and environment

SIGNS AND SYMPTOMS

Older persons are often reluctant to report incontinence and the effect it is having on their daily lives.

On direct questioning, some patients report incontinence that they feel they are managing effectively with frequent changing of small pads or incontinent briefs. These people continue their lives without overt disruption.

For those who are not managing their incontinence, one may observe urine stains on the clothing and an aura of urine odor.

Another area for manifestations of not managing daily living well is in the person's pattern of social interaction. Those who are aware of their incontinence can manifest signs and symptoms of increasing depression and social isolation. Primary caregivers also give evidence that management of daily living with incontinence is failing. Caregivers may report that they are (or are observed to be) fatigued, discouraged, angry, and socially isolated as well.

Failure to manage incontinence can also be seen in fluid intake far below what is needed for adequate hydration.

DIFFERENTIAL DIAGNOSIS

Identifying the type and etiology of incontinence is vital in choosing an appropriate nursing treatment. The physician and nurse must collaborate efforts to gather information that will achieve a differential diagnosis. It is crucial that a problem such as urinary retention is not overlooked as part of the incontinence evaluation.

PROGNOSIS

Effectiveness in managing daily living with incontinence is influenced by the degree and cause of the incontinence (amenability to treatment), motivation, physical and cognitive ability to participate in treatments, and the availability and consistency of personal support systems that maintain the person and the environment for daily living.

COMPLICATIONS

When incontinence is not managed well, the risk of becoming socially isolated and depressed may increase. Skin breakdown or excoriation may also be a problem.

TREATMENT

Nursing treatment regimens fall into two areas: those aimed at restoring continence and those that address the management of daily living when incontinence is present.

General nursing measures include ensuring adequate hydration (35 mL/kg) with nonirritating fluids and education regarding normal bladder function. Establishing realistic goals with the patient and family will help maintain a positive attitude regarding incontinence interventions. Table 29–7 offers guidelines for the use of the following nursing interventions.

TABLE 29-7   *Nursing Interventions for Incontinence*

Intervention	Description	Type of Incontinence
Pelvic floor exercises	Strengthening the pubococcygeus muscles by practicing daily contractions	Stress, urge
Bladder retraining	Gradual increase of toileting interval	Urge
Habit training	Fixed schedule for toileting, individualized to patient's pattern of voiding	Functional, urge
Environmental/functional modification	Careful modification of environment to meet a patient's toileting needs. Instruction/training to improve patient's functional status regarding toileting	Functional, urge
Contingency management/prompted voiding	Systematic reinforcement of appropriate voiding	Functional

Habit Training   Habit training is based on identifying a patient's individual pattern of incontinence. An incontinence monitoring record (Fig. 29–3) is kept by the patient or caregiver for 3 to 7 days and evaluated for the pattern and frequency of incontinency. A toileting schedule is then established that accommodates the patient's voiding pattern with the goal of preventing incontinent episodes.

Bladder Retraining   Bladder retraining is employed when a pattern of low volume frequency and urgency has become established. A baseline monitoring record is kept for 3 to 7 days. A toileting schedule is established as for habit training, but the time intervals between voidings are slowly increased until the patient is able to wait 3 to 4 hours between voidings. The patient must also be taught how to control the sensation of urgency so that micturition can be postponed. Deep breathing and abdominal relaxation are practiced when urgency occurs until the patient is able to use these techniques independently (Newman et al, 1991).

Continency Management and Prompted Voiding   The methods involved with these nursing interventions are based on behavior modification principles. The patient is asked on a regular schedule whether he or she is wet or dry and if he would like toileting assistance. Feedback is given on accuracy of wet or dry identification; positive verbal reinforcement is given for being dry and requesting toileting assistance. This type of intervention is especially effective when the patient has the cognition to recognize the need to urinate and the ability to initiate voiding when given assistance (Schnelle, 1990).

Environmental/Functional Modification
Careful assessment of a patient's functional abilities identifies the ability to transfer and maintain balance, manual dexterity, and ability to visualize and identify the bathroom. Nursing interventions include appropriate instruction or referral to a physical or occupational therapist to improve functional abilities. Environmental interventions may include improved lighting, rails around the toilet, a raised toilet seat, a sign or picture identifying the toilet, clothing that is easy to manipulate (Velcro closings, elastic waists), and shortened distance between bed or chair and toilet or commode.

Pelvic Floor Exercises (Kegel Exercises)
Pelvic floor muscle strengthening can be an effective treatment for stress and urge types of incontinence. The goal of the exercise is to strengthen the supporting musculature of the pelvic floor as well as the external sphincter that is under voluntary control. To instruct a patient in pelvic floor exercises the clinician must first help the patient identify the correct muscles (pubococcygeus). The most beneficial way is for the clinician to insert a gloved finger

into the vagina or rectum and ask the patient to squeeze around the finger while keeping the abdomen relaxed. An alternate method is to have the patient try to start and stop the flow of urine by contracting the pelvic floor, again keeping the abdomen relaxed. The patient is then instructed to hold the contraction for 10 seconds and relax for 60 seconds. Repetition should be slowly increased until 60 repetitions per day are reached. The exercises usually take several weeks to become effective. Some studies have suggested that the use of a perineometer for biofeedback may augment the ability to learn pelvic floor exercises (Burgio and Engel, 1990).

Managing Daily Living with Incontinence

When incontinence is a regular feature of daily living there are areas of nursing treatment that can maximize collection of urine and maintain optimal dignity and independence.

APPLIANCES   A variety of appliances are available for the management of urinary incontinence. There are two indications for the use of hygienic aids for prevention of wetting: when all other modes of treatment have failed or when treatment by other means is in progress and continence has not been regained. The decision to use these appliances must be made carefully so that an expectation of incontinency is not conveyed.

Bedside commodes or urinals can be beneficial when mobility is a problem. For men, condom catheters can be used and attached to a collection bag that allows an individual to be dressed and participate in activities without fear of accidents. Careful attention must be given to skin care so breakdown and infection can be avoided. A satisfactory external collection device for women continues to be explored.

Protective pads or briefs can be washable or disposable. Issues such as cost, comfort, fit, ease of use, absorption, and environmental impact can be explored by caregivers and patients in deciding which products are most beneficial.

SKIN CARE   Chronic incontinence requires meticulous skin care to prevent maceration and excoriation. Skin barriers can include Vaseline, Desitin, or incontinent care gels and creams available in drugstores. Gentle soaps must be used to prevent drying of the skin from frequent washing.

INDWELLING CATHETERS   An indwelling catheter is ordinarily the least desirable means of dealing with incontinence. However, there are situations in which it becomes necessary. Short-term use may be indicated to heal skin breakdown or in the final days of a terminal illness. Long-term use may be seen with inoperable prostate hyperplasia or urethral stricture.

Long-term catheterization results in polymicrobial bacteriuria after 30 days. Complications of catheter use include infection, urinary tract stones, vesicoureteral reflux, chronic tubulointerstitial nephritis, and renal failure. Men may experience additional periurethral complications such as epididymitis, scrotal and prostatic abscesses, and urethral fistulae (Warren, 1986). Patients with long-term indwelling catheters and their caregivers require information that promotes successful management. The following guidelines summarize current practice recommendations; however, further research is needed to clarify common care techniques.

1. Maintain a closed system as much as possible. Disconnection of the urine drainage bag has been associated with increased rates of UTIs (Platt et al, 1983).
2. Choose the smallest practical size catheter and balloon. A smaller lumen size should cause less pressure on periurethral tissues. The 30 mL balloon was originally developed to prevent hemorrhage after prostate or bladder surgery (Roe, 1989). The increased weight on the bladder outlet by a large balloon may cause bladder spasms and leakage.
3. Do not automatically increase lumen size when leakage or blockage occurs. When leakage is not caused by catheter obstruction, bladder spasms may be the cause. Reasons for the spasms can include infection, bowel impaction, a large balloon size, bladder calculi, or detrusor instability. The latter may respond to the same medications used to treat urge incontinence. Blockage from sediment may require catheter irrigation (a drawback due to a breach of the closed system). Adequate fluid intake may help dilute the sediment. Acidic urine slows the growth of bacteria such as the *Proteus* species, which may break down urea and encourage the precipitation of crystals (Bruce et al, 1974). Use of a pure silicone catheter may also decrease the development of catheter encrustations (Kunin et al, 1987).

4. Individualize frequency of catheter changes. A patient without problems of sediment and obstruction or frequent infections may require catheter changes every 8 weeks for a latex catheter or up to 12 weeks for a silicone catheter (Weiss, 1984).

5. Cleanse the meatal area daily with soap and water. Use of antiseptic solutions has been shown to be no more effective than soap and water in controlling bacteriuria (Burke et al, 1981).

6. Secure the catheter tubing to the thigh to prevent movement in and out of the urethra. In men this will also decrease pressure on the penoscrotal juncture (Fig. 29–4).

7. Common procedure for care of leg and overnight bags at home involves washing the bag when not in use with soapy water. The bag is then rinsed with plain water and soaked in a solution of one part white vinegar to four parts water or one part bleach to three parts water for 30 minutes. The bag is then emptied and the cap (disinfected by an alcohol soak) applied until use is required. This routine for bag care appears safe for nursing home residents if the bags are replaced on a weekly basis.

8. Prophylactic antibiotic therapy for bacteriuria is not indicated since it may predispose to infection from more resistant organisms (Boscia and Kaye, 1988). Use of methenamine preparations are not effective with catheter use as the constantly emptying bladder does not retain urine long enough to allow hydrolyzation to formaldehyde (Warren, 1986).

SUPPORT GROUPS   Older persons experiencing incontinency problems may find much assistance from support organizations. Help for Incontinent People has a quarterly newsletter and a resource guide of continence aids and services for those with urinary control problems. Inquiries can be made to Help for Incontinent People, Box 544, Union, SC 29379. The Simon Foundation also publishes a newsletter and offers a video cassette and book written for the incontinent person (Simon Foundation, Box 815, Wilmette, IL 60091, 1(800)237-4666).

CAREGIVER SUPPORT   Positive reinforcement is important for any caregiver trying to help an older person manage urinary incontinence. The nurse may need to evaluate the physical and emotional status of the family caring for the incontinent person. Need for physical assist-

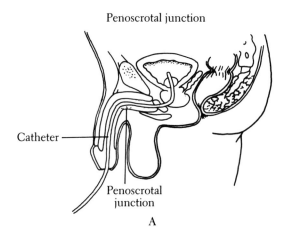

Penoscrotal junction

Catheter

Penoscrotal junction

A

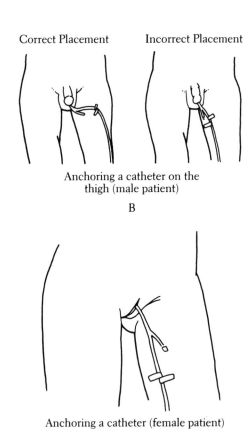

Correct Placement   Incorrect Placement

Anchoring a catheter on the thigh (male patient)

B

Anchoring a catheter (female patient)

C

FIGURE 29–4   Securing the catheter.

ance or respite in caregiving may become part of the nursing intervention. Caregivers in institutions also require support, encouragement, and education regarding reasons for incontinence. They must also be involved in the planning and evaluation of management interventions for their elderly patients.

EVALUATION

Effectiveness of nursing treatment is evaluated in terms of the person's observed and reported continence and the ability to participate in desired social interaction and activities of daily living. Where appropriate, the physical, emotional, and social status of caregivers also needs to be observed in response to nursing interventions.

DAILY LIVING AND URINARY TRACT INFECTION

The symptoms of urinary infection can be vague and may be overlooked without careful assessment. Mental status changes ranging from mild lethargy to delirium as well as nausea, vomiting, or agitation can indicate infection. Systematic examination can help rule out other causes of infection and increase the clinician's suspicion of UTI. Any change in voiding habits or elevation in temperature signals a need for further investigation. Dysuria, hematuria, onset or increase of incontinence are all symptoms that may suggest a UTI.

Once an infection has been identified and appropriate antibiotic therapy initiated, nursing measures should focus on supportive measures. Adequate hydration, rest, a safe environment and assistance with activities of daily living help to ensure recovery.

Nursing interventions should also include methods that help prevent recurrence of UTIs:

Adequate daily hydration (35 mL/kg)
Good perineal hygiene, especially for women
Signs and symptoms of UTI that should be reported to the health care provider
Alternatives (if possible) to indwelling catheters
Voiding after intercourse to "flush" the lower urinary tract
Toileting habits that foster complete bladder emptying, i.e., upright sitting position with feet supported for women, standing position for men
Avoidance of immobility

References and Other Readings

Andersen JT, Jacobsen O, Worm-Petersen J, Hald T. Bladder function in healthy elderly males. Scand J Urol Nephrol 1978; 12:123.

Badlani GH, Smith AD. Pharmacotherapy of voiding dysfunction in the elderly. Semin Urol 1987; 5:120.

Boscia JA, Kaye D. Asymptomatic bacteriuria in the elderly. Clin Geriatr Med 1988; 4:57.

Brocklehurst JC, Dillane JB. Studies of the female bladder in old age. Cystometrograms in 100 incontinent women. Gerontologica Clinica 1966; 8:306.

Bruce AW, Sira SS, Clark AG, Awad SA. The problem of catheter encrustation. Can Med Assoc J 1974; 111:238.

Burgio KL, Engel BT. Biofeedback-assisted behavioral training for elderly men and women. J Am Geriatr Soc 1990; 38:338.

Burke JP, Garibaldi RA, Butt MR, Jacobsen JA, Conti M, Alling DW. Prevention of catheter associated urinary tract infections. Am J Med 1981; 70:655.

Grahn D, Norman DC, White ML, Cantrell M, Yoshikawa T. Validity of urinary catheter specimen for diagnosis of urinary tract infection in the elderly. Arch Intern Med 1985; 145:1858.

Herzog AR, Fultz NH. Epidemiology of urinary incontinence: prevalence, incidence, and correlates in community populace. Urology 1990; 36:2.

Kunin CM, Chin QF, Chambers S. Formation of encrustations on indwelling urinary catheters in the elderly. A comparison of different types of catheter material in blockers and non-blockers. J Urol 1987; 138:899.

Mitteness LS. The management of urinary incontinence by community-living elderly. Gerontologist 1987; 27:185.

Mulholland SG. Urinary tract infection. Clin Geriatr Med 1990; 6:43.

National Institutes of Health Consensus Development Conference. Urinary incontinence in adults. J Am Geriatr Soc 1990; 38:265.

Newman DK, Lynch K, Smith DA, Cell P. Restoring urinary continence. Am J Nurs 1991; 19:28.

Nicolle LE, Brunka J, McIntyre M et al. Asymptomatic bacteriuria urinary antibody and survival in the institutionalized elderly. J Am Geriatr Soc 1992; 40:607.

Noelker LS. Incontinence in elderly cared for by family. Gerontologist 1987; 27:194.

Norton PA, MacDonald L, Sedgwick P, Stanton SL. Distress and delay associated with urinary incontinence, frequency and urgency in women. Br Med J 1988; 297:1187.

Oliver L. The neurogenic bladder. In: Jeter K, Faller N, Norton C, ed. Nursing for continence. Philadelphia: WB Saunders, 1990.

Ouslander JG. Urinary incontinence in the elderly. West J Med 1981; 135:482.

Ouslander JG, Abelson S. Perceptions of urinary incontinence among elderly outpatients. The Gerontologist 1990; 30:369.

Platt R, Polk BF, Murdock B, Rosner B. Reduction of mortality associated with nosocomial urinary tract infection. Lancet 1983; 1:893.

Resnick NM. Initial evaluation of the incontinent patient. J Am Geriatr Soc 1990; 38:311.

Roe BH. Study of information given by nurses for catheter care to patients and their carers. J Adv Nurs 1989; 14:203.

Schnelle JF. Treatment of urinary incontinence in nursing home patients by prompted voiding. J Am Geriatr Soc 1990; 38:356.

Tanagho EA. Electrical stimulation. J Am Geriatr Soc 1990; 38:352.

Warren JW. Catheters and catheter care. Clin Geriatr Med 1986; 2:857.

Wein J. Physiology of micturition. Clin Geriatr Med 1986; 2:689.

Weiss BD. Chronic indwelling bladder catheterization. Am Fam Physician 1984; 30:161.

Wyman JF, Harkins SW, Fantl JA. Psychosocial impact of urinary incontinence in the community-dwelling population. J Am Geriatr Soc 1990; 38:282.

30
Musculoskeletal Problems

RUTH CRAVEN   KRIS DIETSCH

Pathophysiology and Management

The effects of normal aging on the musculo-skeletal system and on mobility are pervasive. Some of the most common health problems of the elderly are associated with changes that occur in muscles, bones, and joints. The impact of these changes on the lifestyle and activities of daily living of the older person range from discomfort and decreased ability to perform physical activity to severe, chronic pain and complete immobility. Strength, speed, posture, body image, independence, and safety are all affected.

Aging alone does not need to limit mobility. While some signs and symptoms that occur are related to normal changes of aging, others are forerunners of treatable dysfunction where disability can be modified, delayed, or prevented by competent evaluation and appropriate therapy. Whether normal or dysfunctional, alterations are relatively common. The insidious onset and frequency of common symptoms may contribute to the willingness of the elderly to accept or minimize their dysfunction and discomfort as "normal" and delay diagnosis and management of potentially severe and treatable problems.

The normal changes of aging, in combination with disorders that may occur, have far-reaching implications for the elderly. The ability to move about freely, have confidence in movement, and maintain the desired lifestyle and pace contribute to a positive attitude toward aging.

GAIT AND MOBILITY

The ability of the older adult to maintain independence in a familiar environment hinges to a large extent on the efficiency of locomotion. Compromise in this critical function can seriously diminish essential coping resources, personal confidence, and initiative.

Although posture and movement in healthy aged persons cover a wide range of normal, a fairly typical pattern tends to emerge. With aging, posture tends to take on an attitude of general flexion. The lumbar spine tends to flatten causing the upper spine and head to tilt forward. Wedging of the vertebrae (Fig. 30–1) in the thoracic spine along with degenerative changes and thinning of the intervertebral disks results in kyphosis of the thoracic spine, which may vary in severity among individuals. Loss of flexibility and elasticity in the tendons and ligaments leads to a position of flexion in the joints of the long bones, i.e., elbows, wrists, hips, and knees.

Secondary to the postural changes with aging is a shift in the center of gravity. Upright posture and movement require a balanced center of gravity. The vertical gravity line is an imaginary line through which (if a string were

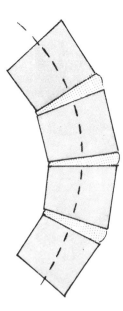

FIGURE 30–1 Wedging of the vertebrae. With thinning of the intervertebral disks, this causes a hunch-backed appearance.

attached and pulled upward) all the downward forces of gravity would be exactly balanced and the weight of the body centered (Vander et al, 1990). The usual line of gravity runs from the top of the head, bisecting the shoulders, trunk, the weight-bearing joints, and the base of support and slightly anterior to the sacrum (Fig. 30–2). The weight of the body is then centered in the torso where the downward forces of gravity are balanced. Because of the tendency for a flexed posture with the head tilted forward and in front of the usual line of the center of gravity, the older person is at increased risk for losing balance and having altered mobility.

In order to maintain gait and mobility, the older person must compensate for postural changes. Compensatory changes include flexion at the hip and knee joints and a wider based stance, which are attempts to rebalance the center of gravity. These changes lead to alterations in the walking gait: increased side-to-side sway; decreased extension and swing-through with each step; and a shuffling appearing gait as body weight is shifted from the ball of one foot to the ball of the other foot.

Balance depends on adequate input to the vestibular system through vestibulo-ocular (vision) or vestibulospinal (sensors in skin and joints) sources, proprioceptive abilities in the lower extremities, and sufficient muscle strength to allow upright posture. With aging, there is high risk for changes in all of these factors. The hair cells within the semicircular canals undergo degenerative changes, making the balance function less efficient. Visual input may be diminished due to aging changes in the eye, and input from spinal sources may be less efficient as a result of changes in nerve transmission time. Circulatory changes and decreased innervation in the lower extremities can lead to loss of proprioceptive acuity. Loss of muscle tone and bulk with aging contributes to decreased strength for maintaining balance and for the energy demands of mobility.

Data gathering on gait and mobility often begins with subjective data in which the nurse or physician talks with the older person about the pattern of mobility in relationship to the activities of daily living, preferred lifestyle, and home-neighborhood environment. Information is obtained on what activity can and cannot be accomplished.

Objective data can be obtained from observation during both informal and structured activities. In the home, clinic waiting room, senior citizen center, or nursing home corridor information can be collected about the following:

1. General posture: kyphosis, compensatory position of head and neck, flexion of extremities, contractures
2. Stance: distance between the feet when standing, toeing in or out
3. Gait: length of stride, height foot is lifted from the floor, shuffling
4. Normal speed in walking: does pace decrease progressively with distance?
5. Transfer activities: difficulty or ease in sitting down or standing? Note type of furniture selected to sit on
6. Balance and support provided by touching furniture, doorjambs, railings
7. Use of assistive devices: canes, crutches, walkers, skill in using devices, fit of the aid in relationship to size of the person
8. Stairs: ability to climb and descend stairs

Additionally, the nurse may direct the patient to engage in certain activities to observe other capabilities:

1. Standing independently, with eyes open and eyes closed; note balance and sway
2. Range of motion of head and neck, shoulders, elbows, wrists, hands, hips, knees, an-

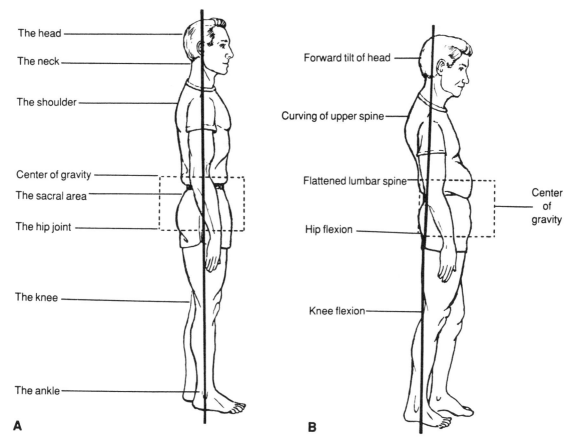

The head

The neck

The shoulder

Center of gravity

The sacral area

The hip joint

The knee

The ankle

A

Forward tilt of head

Curving of upper spine

Flattened lumbar spine

Hip flexion

Knee flexion

Center of gravity

B

FIGURE 30–2   Vertical gravity line and posture. A, Vertical gravity line and center of gravity. B, Postural changes with age. (From Craven, Hirnle. Fundamentals of nursing: Functional health approach. Philadelphia: J. B. Lippincott, 1992, p. 695.)

kles, and back. The height the foot can be raised in hip-knee flexion is important in assessing the ability to use public transportation and in agility and reaction time

3. Strength in lifting objects

Since disorders of the feet may be barriers to mobility, careful observation needs to be made for corns, calluses, leg or foot ulcers, flat arches, and bunions. The type of footwear selected for use can be a clue to foot difficulties. Soft-soled, nonsupportive slippers may be worn all day to avoid wearing shoes that may be painful or do not fit properly.

While disturbances in gait are easily noted, identifying the reason for the disability and the risk areas in daily living is essential. Only then can the nurse intervene appropriately in initiating referral for appropriate medical care, engaging in nursing management, or assisting the individual to develop better strategies for self-management.

FALLS

Falls in the elderly occur with great frequency, often with a considerable disruption in lifestyle. Injuries are the sixth leading cause of death over the age of 65, with the majority of deaths related to falls (Fig. 30–3). Among elderly persons living in the community, the annual occurrence of falls increases from 25% at 70 years of age to 35% over the age of 75. Women fall more often than men until age 75, after which the incidence of falls tends to equalize. The tendency for injury from falls in the elderly is associated to age-related changes along with the prevalence of clinical disease (Nelson and Amin, 1990).

Many elderly individuals realize that a fall may mean an end to their borderline independence and perhaps to their lifestyle. When an elderly person suffers trauma as a result of falling, hospitalization is usually required. Confinement to bed, even for short-to-moderate pe-

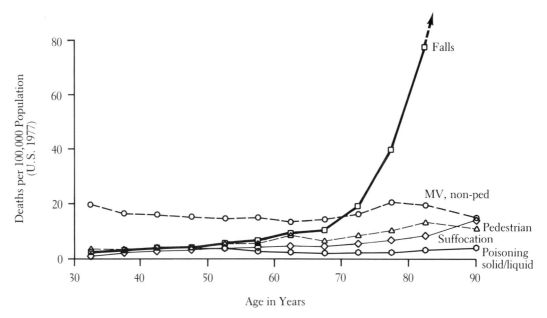

FIGURE 30–3   The distribution of deaths from accidents of different kinds in people from infancy to 80 years of age. Above 70 years of age, falls become the most common cause of accidental death. (From Baker SP, Harvey AM. Fall injuries in elderly. Clin Geriatr Med 1985; 1:502; with permission.)

riods of time, furthers bone demineralization, encourages stasis in the lungs and in peripheral circulation, causes trauma to the skin and soft tissue, and impairs cerebral oxygenation and orientation sufficiently to cause transient confusion or an increased alteration in existing cognitive problems. The cost of falls can be measured in physical suffering, mental suffering or impairment of cognitive function, number of days in the hospital, potential transfer to extended care facilities either on a temporary or permanent basis, and the disruption of what had been an independent, even if somewhat precarious, lifestyle (Craven and Bruno, 1986).

ETIOLOGIC FACTORS

Normal Changes of Aging   Changes that occur normally in aging contribute substantially to falls. Altered posture with a shift in center of gravity, decreased strength caused by muscle atrophy or deconditioning, slowed neurologic reaction time, and loss of visual acuity are contributors to a large number of falls. Impaired balance may be related to a variety of causes. Degenerative changes in the vestibular system and in the cerebellum predispose the elderly to a narrower range of balanced posture, with a loss or diminution of the ability to right

oneself when balance is challenged. Abnormalities of the walking gait related to structural and functional changes in the musculoskeletal, nervous, and cardiovascular systems may impair balance. These changes of aging contribute to the older person's propensity to fall.

Chronic Diseases   Chronic diseases also place the elderly at higher risk for falls. Many initially unexplained falls are later found to be the result of underlying pathology. Changes in vision resulting from cataracts, glaucoma, corneal opacities, macular degeneration, and retinopathy limit visual accuracy and lead to misplaced footing or failure to recognize hazards in the form of barriers, slippery floors, and uneven surfaces. Cerebral hypoxia, cardiac arrhythmias, vestibular disorders, syncope, and postural hypotension cause dizziness and inadequate perfusion to the brain that precipitate falls. Diabetes with concurrent peripheral neuropathy leads to diminished sensation and circulatory change, creating additional risk factors. Disorders such as Parkinson's or hemiplegia, with associated loss of balance, proprioception, muscle tone, and sensation and/or misperception of the environment, increase the risk for falls (see Chapters 20 and 21).

Medications Drugs can be precipitating factors in falls due to the number, types, and interactions. Antihypertensive drugs result in postural hypotension and sudden falls when an individual stands up quickly or has been standing in one position for a period of time. Sedatives, hypnotics, antidepressants, and tranquilizers interfere with balance and perceptions, resulting in decreased stability. Careful dosage titration and selection of drugs with a short plasma half-life may decrease untoward side effects. Diuretics, antihypertensives, and other drugs that change fluid and electrolyte balance can cause hypovolemia and arrhythmias and contribute to the risk of falling.

Alcohol Alcohol use is commonly related to falls among the elderly. Assessment of alcohol use of all elderly persons is necessary as it may be a previously undetermined problem. With this possibility in mind, careful history taking can reveal if alcohol is a problem.

Drop Attacks Increasing evidence supports a fairly high incidence of falls unrelated to specific causes. Falls in this category have been labeled *drop attacks* and are thought to be related to transient vertebrobasilar insufficiency or other diverse pathophysiologic mechanisms. In these situations, the individual describes a sudden loss of tone in the legs with an immediate fall. There is no corresponding loss of consciousness, identifiable neurologic deficit, or other symptoms. Some time may elapse before the individual can regain sufficient muscle tone to stand, and considerable assistance may be required.

Environmental Factors: In the Home Many factors in the immediate environment contribute to falls. They include the following:

- **Inadequate lighting**, particularly in stairwells and landings
- **Absence of railings** on stairs and grab bars in bathrooms
- **Slippery surfaces** in tubs and showers, on smooth surfaces with spills or throw rugs, failure to use nonskid wax
- **Obstructions** such as long extension or telephone cords, furniture in pathways, objects that are not picked up
- **Pets and small children** that can accidently cause tripping

Environmental Factors: Beyond the Home Hazards outside the home are similar to those in the home. The risk, though, is magnified by decreased familiarity. Steps, curbs, and uneven surfaces pose the greatest danger, along with wet, slippery surfaces. Buses, escalators, and building accesses are areas of high risk. Places with dim lighting or sudden changes in lighting can increase the danger of falls.

Clothing Clothing and shoes can contribute to falls. Loose-fitting and long robes may catch on furniture, doorknobs, or cooking utensils, causing a loss of balance or pulling an object into the path. Use of slippers such as heel-less scuffs or thongs, provide little stability, often fit poorly, and thereby increase the risk of falls. Shoes with either composite or plastic-type soles may contribute to falls by sticking to floor surfaces or slipping too easily. Shoes with leather soles or with an additional surface that adds some light friction are safer shoe soles for elderly persons.

COMPLICATIONS

Falls can cause both physical and psychological trauma. Bruises, lacerations, and fractures are the more obvious results of falls. The complications of immobilization that may result if the person chooses or is required to recover in bed from the effects of the fall can be much more dangerous than the fall itself. Less overt, but still significant, is the loss of confidence, courage, and independence that results from fear of recurrence of falls. Older persons may experience increased anxiety about their independence as a result of the loss in self-assurance and mobility following a fall.

The older person's family may have concern about the person returning home following hospitalization from a fall. The family's fear that the person may fall again and not be able to get assistance may influence the older person's sense of confidence and independence.

MEDICAL MANAGEMENT

Medical management is determined by the cause of the fall. Falls related to problems of cerebral perfusion may be managed by use of a cardiac pacemaker, antiarrhythmia drugs, improving circulatory volume, or use of elastic hose to minimize venous pooling. For specific disorders, such as Parkinson's disease, hemiplegia, or osteoarthritis, pharmacologic and physical therapy management may be the treatments of choice.

FRACTURES

Fractures are viewed as a major catastrophe to most elderly people. Without warning, lifestyle is disrupted and independence is threatened. Coping resources are compromised by the loss of mobility and self-care functions. Pain interferes with the ability to plan and concentrate. Reliable support systems are needed immediately to assist in short- and long-range planning. At best, the short-term result of a fracture is to be immobile for a few days; at worst, institutionalization for an indeterminate period in an unfamiliar environment may be necessary.

DESCRIPTION

Fractures in the elderly occur in areas of greatest stress such as the head and neck of the femur, the weight-bearing vertebral column, or the wrist. Bones already weakened by normal demineralization of the aging process are more prone to fracture. For older persons with osteoporosis, the tendency to fracture bones becomes great. Activities such as coughing, vomiting, or lifting can cause fractures in bones that are stressed by the activity.

ETIOLOGIC FACTORS

The major factors contributing to fractures in the elderly are loss of bone mass and falls. Chronic pathologic conditions such as alcoholism, osteoporosis, and metastatic disease affect bone density, again increasing the likelihood of fracture. Drugs such as corticosteroids used in the treatment of musculoskeletal disorders contribute to accelerated loss of bone mass. A relatively sedentary lifestyle over a lifetime contributes to the loss of bone mass as well.

HIGH RISK

Older women are at greater risk of fractures than older men by a ratio of 3:1 as are low-income white people. The largest number of fractures occur as a result of accidents in the home. Elderly people with alterations in mobility due to gait dysfunctions, chronic disorders of the joints or muscles, or cognitive impairments are at increased risk for accidents that may lead to fractures.

DYNAMICS

Bone cell density decreases and becomes less resilient with aging. Muscles, tendons, and cartilage decrease in elasticity. The combination of these changes increases the risk that fractures will occur. With a fracture, bleeding occurs within the bone and the surrounding tissue. As a result of the loss of tissue elasticity, the elderly may lose a considerable amount of blood, with accompanying loss of circulating fluid volume and altered perfusion of vital organs.

SIGNS AND SYMPTOMS

Pain and loss of function of the affected limb or area are the primary symptoms of fractures. Pain following a fracture is related to bleeding and swelling at the fracture site, causing pressure on nerve endings in the periosteum and surrounding soft tissue, and muscle spasms. Related pain behaviors in the elderly may include restlessness and confusion.

DIFFERENTIAL DIAGNOSIS

Differential diagnosis is to be made between soft tissue damage (sprain or strain) and an actual fracture. In any injury in which fracture is a possibility, radiographic studies are indicated. Occasionally initial roentgenographic films will not reveal a fracture. The patient may continue to complain of pain and or loss of function, and a fracture may be identified on a second film. Observe and listen attentively to the patient.

COMPLICATIONS

Locally the complications are related to interruption of the nerve and circulatory supply either in the surrounding soft tissue or to the bone itself. These can result in nonunion or malunion of the fracture and the need for further treatment.

The associated bed rest or physical immobilization required for fractures to heal contributes to the hazards of immobility in each body system. For the older person, the consequences of immobility and bed rest occur earlier and produce effects that last longer.

Thrombophlebitis and pulmonary emboli

are life-threatening complications of fractures caused by immobilization. They are less likely to occur presently than in the past because of improved surgical techniques, prophylactic medications, and early mobilization. Because of increased risks during the period of immobility, the older person's legs should be examined daily for evidence of phlebitis. Measurement of the diameter of the calf provides a baseline for comparison if signs of phlebitis develop. Daily assessment of the legs includes comparison of affected and unaffected leg change in diameter, tenderness, edema, and redness. Any complaint of tenderness should be investigated immediately. Homans' sign (pain in the calf on forced dorsiflexion of the foot) can be used as a reliable indicator of thrombophlebitis. (For a full discussion of thrombophlebitis, its diagnosis, management, and complications, see Chapter 23, Cardiovascular Problems.)

Pulmonary emboli can occur postfracture. This is a serious and often fatal complication. Shortness of breath, chest pain, hemoptysis, fever, restlessness, cough, and possibly, shock are signs and symptoms indicative of pulmonary emboli. Lung scans and pulmonary angiography may not reliably confirm the diagnosis. Medical treatment includes supporting ventilation and oxygenation and limiting further development of clots and emboli.

HIGH-RISK FRACTURE SITES

Hip The most common site of fracture in older people is the hip. Hip fractures occur in two main locations, involving the neck of the femur, referred to as the subcapsular or intracapsular region, and the intertrochanteric or extracapsular region. The shaft of the femur is a relatively uncommon site of fracture in the elderly. Owing to marginal circulation to and bone cell demineralization of the neck of the femur, fractures in this area carry greater risk of nonunion.

Characteristically, hip fractures result from falls. Frequently, a fracture seems unlikely in view of the minimal trauma incurred. Typically, the individual complains of pain in the hip or thigh, exhibits adduction, external rotation, and shortening, and is reluctant to move or bear weight on the affected extremity. If the fracture is impacted or undisplaced, the person may experience little discomfort and still be able to walk. *Minimal shortening of the leg may be the only evidence of injury.*

The elderly individual with a hip fracture, on occasion, may not be seen for treatment for 1 to 4 days, particularly if the person has fallen and has been unable to summon assistance. This delay in therapy can mean complications set in. Relatively minor problems with skin breakdown, poor nutrition, fluid imbalances, and joint stiffness can be intensified in a few days to cause arrhythmias, decubitus ulcers, and contractures.

Choice of treatment depends on (1) the location and severity of the fracture, (2) time elapsed since the initial injury, and (3) the general health of the individual. Major surgery using either internal fixation with a nail or a total hip prosthesis to stabilize the fracture is the treatment of choice. Use of a total hip prosthesis has made early ambulation a reality. Pinning or nailing of femoral neck fractures, while extremely satisfactory, can carry the risk of a second surgical procedure if problems caused by circulatory inadequacy or discomfort from pins develop. Depending on the type of fixation used, mobilization normally progresses soon after surgery, with assistance from physical therapy to increasing weight-bearing ambulation with a walker within a period of 4 to 6 weeks. If the patient has sufficient muscle strength, balance, and ability, mobility can continue to progress to use of a cane or to unassisted ambulation.

Occasionally, a fracture of the femoral head is stable without surgical intervention either because it is impacted into the acetabulum or shows only a hairline break. Bed rest ranging from a few days to a week is recommended to decrease muscle spasm and reduce pain. After the period of bed rest, ambulation with weight bearing to tolerance can be resumed.

Fractures of the hip are the most threatening to the elderly in terms of time required for healing, extent of treatment required, limitation of mobility, and the wide range of associated complications that occur. Hip fractures do not necessarily mean an end to independence. Attitudes and expectations of patients and health care professionals are gradually changing, with more positive outcomes anticipated and experienced. With this comes a more assertive approach by both nurses and patients to initiate and maintain the rehabilitative activities that will make return to normal activities a reality for as many patients as possible.

Wrist   Fracture of the wrist, typically a Colles' fracture, is an unfortunate result in many falls. The distal radius is frequently broken as the older person attempts to break a fall by landing on an outstretched hand. The fracture that results is described as a "dinner fork" deformity, with displacement of the wrist backward and toward the radius.

The goal of therapy is to restore joint function. This is accomplished by reducing the fracture through manipulation of bone fragments into alignment and immobilization, using a rigid plaster dressing or splint. Stability is difficult to achieve because of the many small bones in the wrist.

Following a wrist fracture, the patient must be alert to any change in circulation or nerve function in the lower arm and hand. The person should be taught to check for warmth, color, capillary refilling in the nail beds, and any abnormal sensation, including tingling, burning, and numbness, and to report these changes immediately. The weight of the cast can be a deterrent to movement of the shoulder in older people. To prevent this complication the person should be encouraged to resume activities that promote this movement, such as combing the hair. Raising the arm above the head several times each day will also prevent development of a stiff shoulder. To prevent dependent edema both before and after removal of the cast or splint, the arm and hand can be supported in a sling. While in place, the cast or splint provides a secure feeling that the fracture is healing and that additional damage cannot occur. When the device is removed, the joint usually feels weak and painful, and swelling may occur. Many patients have concern that they will damage the fracture site if they participate in activities. They may need reassurance that it is safe to resume activity. Light housework, folding laundry, setting the table, doing dishes, knitting, trimming grass with garden shears, or other typical activities of daily living are all activities that assist in regaining lost function.

Older persons who have had fractured wrists may find that it is common for some pain and stiffness to persist. Some persons relate these factors to changes in the weather.

Vertebrae   Compression fractures of the spine are relatively common in the elderly. Fractures of this type are sustained with minimal trauma, such as a jolt, coughing, vomiting, or even turning over in bed, in people with osteoporosis, metastatic disease, or those who have been on long-term steroids.

When seen for treatment, the patient's main complaint is localized in pain in the back. The amount of pain is a poor indicator of the extent or severity of damage; therefore, roentgenography is necessary to confirm the diagnosis. If multiple fractures have occurred, deformities of the back will be apparent, accompanied by loss of total body height. A more critical indicator of compression is the measurement of trunk height in relationship to total body height. The latter seems a justification for measurement of height and trunk height on routine examination as part of a patient's baseline data. If there has been a delay in seeking treatment, symptoms of abdominal distention with nausea, vomiting, and constipation may be present.

Since compression fractures seldom cause neurologic deficit, the treatment is directed at reduction of symptoms. Muscle spasms that cause back pain are alleviated by bed rest of 5 to 10 days. Mild analgesics are ordered for comfort. Rib belts and corset-type support provide bracing in the low thoracic and lumbar spine where the majority of these fractures occur. Braces, while helpful in providing support, are usually too restrictive for the older person and are soon discarded. The effect of these devices on limiting lung expansion is also a consideration in their use.

Following the initial period of immobilization, gradual resumption of activity is encouraged as soon as possible in order to minimize further demineralization of the bones and increased deconditioning of the muscles. The individual should be cautioned against extreme flexion or extension of the back.

MEDICAL MANAGEMENT

Early intervention to ensure proper alignment and stabilization of hip and wrist fractures is essential. When a general anesthetic is required, some delay in fixation may be indicated to evaluate existing chronic disorders that are aggravated by the situational stress of the fracture and the present risk factors to surgical intervention. For many older persons, a regional anesthetic block, such as spinal anesthesia, may be preferred.

Following surgery, attention is focused on relief of pain, prevention of infection, and avoidance of the complications of immobility.

Control of pain requires judicious use of analgesics to provide relief without compromising respiratory function, cognitive function, and the ability to begin physical therapy. Pain medication should not be withheld from the elderly, but should be administered under close monitoring by the nurse. A general rule for medication dosage in the elderly is to start with a lower dose than for a younger adult and to increase the dosage to relieve the patient's pain, observing for side effects.

Prophylactic antibiotics are ordered for 48 to 72 hours following hip surgery. Intravenous administration is used to provide the most effective treatment. Unless symptoms of wound infection develop, long-term therapy is not needed. The recentness of tetanus toxoid immunization must be considered if any open wound occurred at the time of fracture.

Anticoagulants Anticoagulants frequently are used as part of therapy to prevent thromboembolic complications following hip fractures. Acetylsalicylic acid, 5 to 10 grains (325 to 650 mg), may be given twice daily prophylactically to prevent thrombus in the acute phase following hip fracture. This regimen, which effectively decreases platelet aggregation without significantly increasing bleeding time, is often continued following discharge.

In high-risk patients, such as those with a history of thromboembolic disease or in whom extended immobilization is anticipated, prophylactic administration of short-term, low-dose heparin may be used. Heparin is standardized in terms of *units* rather than milligrams or milliliters. A typical dosage of "minidose" heparin is 5000 units every 12 hours. The suggested site of the subcutaneous administration is the abdomen. The usual laboratory tests to determine clotting time generally are not done with minidose heparin, since dosages of this size alter clotting time only minimally. Use of heparin continues until the amount of time out of bed is greater than that spent in bed or until hospital discharge.

If anticoagulant therapy is required following hospital discharge, warfarin (Coumadin) is used. Clotting times must be monitored carefully. Prothrombin time is the test of choice to determine the effectiveness of therapy. The patient needs to understand the importance of keeping appointments to have laboratory tests done and to monitor anticoagulation therapy. Written instructions including the date, time, and location of the appointment should be provided (see Chapter 10, Table 10-3 for adverse drug interactions). To ensure accuracy in dosing warfarin, a weekly pill dispenser can be used, the family can be taught the importance of reminding the patient, and follow-up as appropriate by phone calls or a visiting nurse can be initiated.

Both the patient and family need to know the implications anticoagulant therapy has for daily living. They should observe and report any unusual bleeding (e.g., from gums), bruising, or dark-colored stools. Due to the increased risk of bleeding, any individual on warfarin who falls or experiences any type of injury should be examined by a health care professional.

OSTEOPOROSIS

Osteoporosis, the most common metabolic bone disorder, is characterized by abnormally low bone mass for age, gender, and race. Osteoporosis affects over 20 million older Americans, 90% of whom are postmenopausal women, resulting in approximately 1.5 million fractures a year at a public health cost exceeding $3.8 billion (Gambrell, 1991). The human cost of disability and premature death due to osteoporotic fractures is inestimable.

ETIOLOGIC FACTORS

Estrogen deficiency is the major factor that leads to bone loss in postmenopausal women. However, not all postmenopausal women develop osteoporosis, suggesting additional factors. In fact, multiple biochemical factors have been identified in bone remodeling including (1) polypeptides (e.g., thyroid hormone, parathyroid hormone, interleukin-1, calcitonin, estrogens, progestogens, local growth factors), (2) agents that regulate bone mineralization, and (3) vitamin D metabolites that regulate calcium balance (Hahn, 1988). Abnormalities in the activity or quantity of one or all of these factors may contribute to bone loss.

Age, genetics, and lifestyle behaviors also contribute to bone loss, but the way these variables influence biochemical factors in the development of osteoporosis is not fully understood (Meier, 1990). In all likelihood, osteoporosis represents the accumulated effect of multiple etiologies acting on bone throughout the life span (Grisso and Attie, 1989). Osteoporosis can occur by itself (primary), or bone loss can be a secondary complication of various medical conditions and drugs.

Primary Osteoporosis Characteristics and proposed etiologies for two types of primary osteoporosis have been described (Riggs and Melton, 1986). Type I osteoporosis predominates in perimenopausal or postmenopausal women between the ages of 51 and 75 years old. The female to male ratio of type I osteoporosis is 6:1. Estrogen deficiency causes accelerated, short-term loss of trabecular bone, predisposing to vertebral and wrist fractures.

Type II osteoporosis occurs after age 75 in a female to male ratio of 2:1. Age-related defects in vitamin D synthesis, with subsequent decreases in calcium absorption, has been implicated as the causative factor. The gradual, long-term loss of cortical bone in type II osteoporosis predisposes to hip fracture. When type I and II osteoporosis occur simultaneously, the result is a biphasic pattern of bone loss (Zorowitz et al, 1990).

Secondary Osteoporosis A number of endocrine and gastrointestinal disorders, neoplasias, chronic illnesses, and drugs can lead to secondary bone loss. The most common causes are hypogonadism in men, early oophorectomy in women, gastrectomy, and pharmacologic doses of corticosteroids and thyroid hormones (Riggs and Melton, 1986). Alcohol abuse, cigarette smoking, and physical inactivity are also linked to bone loss. Several cross-sectional studies have shown that bed rest for at least 3 weeks within the preceding 5 years doubles the risk of osteoporotic fracture (Bauer, 1991).

RISK FACTORS

Major demographic factors associated with osteoporosis are increasing age, female sex, and white race. Women are at higher risk for osteoporosis than men because women have less bone mass at skeletal maturity, and female bone loss accelerates rapidly during the first 5 to 7 postmenopausal years (Meier, 1990). The relationship between race and bone loss is poorly understood, but white women are at higher risk for vertebral and hip fractures than Asian women (Hahn, 1988). Black and Hispanic women have the lowest fracture rates, possibly because these races achieve greater bone mass at skeletal maturity (Cummings et al, 1985).

While evidence is lacking for causative risk factors for osteoporosis, many factors are associated with osteoporotic fractures (Table 30–1). Unfortunately, there is no formula to reliably predict an individual's bone mass based on risk factors. In one study, risk factor analysis failed to predict 30% of women whose bone mass was actually low when measured by bone densitometry (Slemenda et al, 1990). Conversely, individuals can have multiple risk factors with normal bone density. Nonetheless, risk factors can be useful to identify lifestyle behaviors and dietary habits that are potentially correctable (Lindsay, 1988).

DYNAMICS

The continuous process of skeletal remodeling has been likened to rebuilding a brick wall. Sections of old, brittle bone are removed by osteoclasts, and new bone is laid down by osteoblasts. Normally, this cycle of resorption and formation results in complete bone remodeling in 4 to 5 months (Mundy, 1991).

When osteoporosis affects the aging adult, disturbances in osteoclast and osteoblast activity are superimposed on normal bone remodeling and the aging process. Bone loss accelerates during the early postmenopausal period because bone resorption exceeds bone formation. In other stages of osteoporosis, bone formation

---

TABLE 30–1 *Risk Factors for Osteoporotic Fractures*

Established	Proposed
Increasing age	Family history
Female sex	Early natural menopause
White race	Low calcium intake
Thinness	Sedentary lifestyle
Low bone mass	Caffeine intake
Bilateral oophorectomy	Moderate alcohol use
Chronic corticosteroid use	Thyroid supplements
>2 alcoholic drinks per day	High protein diet
Cigarette smoking	

Data from Lindsay R. Osteoporosis: an updated approach to prevention and management. Geriatrics 1989; 44:45.

slows because osteoblast activity is impaired. Impaired osteoblast activity is also an effect of aging seen universally in very old people (Mundy, 1991). The end result of osteoclast and osteoblast malfunction is bone loss.

If bone loss progresses, bone mass eventually falls below the critical fracture threshold. By age 60, for example, women may have lost one third of their peak bone mass, and the incidence of hip fracture doubles every 5 years thereafter (Gambrell, 1990). Although fracture risk increases with age, fracture activity is unpredictable in osteoporosis (Barzel, 1989). Vertebral fractures often occur in clusters, but years can elapse between these events and a wrist or hip fracture or another series of fractured vertebrae. During the fracture-free periods, loss of height and other overt signs of bone loss do not occur. This episodic fracture pattern gives the appearance that bone loss occurs in "spurts" (Mundy, 1991).

SIGNS AND SYMPTOMS

Osteoporosis is usually asymptomatic until a fracture occurs. The most common sites for osteoporotic fracture are the thoracic spine, femoral neck, and wrist. Other clinical features of osteoporosis are kyphosis and loss of height, muscular weakness, and back pain related to vertebral fractures.

DIAGNOSIS

Densitometry Early detection of bone loss is essential for the prevention of osteoporosis. Since risk factors have uncertain value in predicting bone mass, more clinicians are using bone densitometry to directly measure bone density in high-risk individuals (Tosteson et al, 1990). Dual-energy x-ray absorptiometry is the quickest and most reliable method to measure bone mass developed, thus far. X-rays are beamed through key fracture sites (e.g., spine and femur), and bone density information is fed to a computer resulting in near x-ray quality images. The procedure takes about 10 minutes, and radiation exposure is about one tenth the amount received from a conventional x-ray (Custis, 1990).

Densitometry is especially useful in guiding therapeutic decision-making. For example, a woman at high risk for osteoporosis, who is unsure about starting estrogen replacement, would greatly benefit from the additional information provided by a bone mass measurement

(Cummings et al, 1990). The use of densitometry for routine screening of osteoporosis is controversial. Opponents argue that available methods are too expensive and inconvenient to be practical for mass screening. Proponents contend that densitometry is necessary to predict fracture risk and that the risks of estrogen replacement are not justified unless a woman's bone density is low (Barden & Mazess, 1989; Slemenda et al, 1990).

Differential Diagnosis After bone loss has been established by densitometry in earlier stages or by x-ray in later stages, other metabolic bone diseases and secondary osteoporoses must be ruled out. A thorough history, physical examination, and selected laboratory tests are usually adequate to diagnose osteoporosis.

Normal serum concentrations of calcium, phosphorous, and alkaline phosphatase can usually distinguish primary osteoporosis from bone loss due to osteomalacia, multiple myeloma, metastatic carcinoma, and hyperparathyroidism (DeGowin and DeGowin, 1987). When laboratory tests suggest osteoporosis, it is also advisable to exclude hyperthyroidism with appropriate tests (Hahn, 1988). If necessary, biopsy of the iliac crest can distinguish osteoporosis from osteomalacia (Zorowitz et al, 1990).

COMPLICATIONS

Fractures are the most serious consequence of osteoporosis. Complications from severe kyphosis include pulmonary restriction, abdominal distention, and discomfort.

MEDICAL MANAGEMENT

Preventive Treatment With early detection, osteoporosis can be prevented. The goal of preventive treatment is to inhibit bone loss in people with decreasing bone density. Preventive strategies include risk factor reduction, calcium, exercise, and estrogen replacement.

Eliminating modifiable risk factors for osteoporosis is the first step in preventive treatment. Lifestyle behaviors like excessive alcohol use and cigarette smoking should be discouraged. Whenever possible, drugs that contribute to bone loss or cause falls should be reduced or eliminated.

There is little doubt that calcium deficiency contributes to bone loss and that gastrointestinal absorption of calcium decreases with age. However, studies about the efficacy of calcium supplementation on bone density have been conflicting (Riis et al, 1987; Dawson-Hughes et al, 1990), and there is no evidence that calcium supplementation, by itself, decreases the risk of osteoporotic fracture (Lindsay, 1988). Nonetheless, calcium is both safe and inexpensive and remains the most widely used treatment for osteoporosis (Riggs, 1990).

Current recommendations are 1000 mg of elemental calcium daily for premenopausal women and 1500 mg daily for postmenopausal women (Consensus Development Conference, 1987). Nonfat or low-fat milk is an excellent source of calcium and vitamin D. For individuals with lactose intolerance or those who prefer a supplement, calcium carbonate is inexpensive and easily absorbed. If calcium carbonate causes unpleasant gastrointestinal side effects (i.e., bloating, constipation, rebound hyperacidity), calcium citrate may be better tolerated.

Evidence is growing that moderate weight-bearing exercise not only prevents bone loss, but may even increase bone mass and reduce the risk of fracture. Several clinical trials have demonstrated slight increases in the bone density of exercising older women, both with calcium supplementation (Dalsky et al, 1988) and without supplementation (Smith et al, 1981). Data from a study of retired persons (n = 3110; mean age, 73) suggested that walking 1 mile at least three times a week is protective for fracture (Sorock et al, 1988). Although information is still lacking about the types, amount, and intensity of exercise required to prevent bone loss, the current recommendation for older adults is 30 to 60 minutes of walking at least three times a week (Grisso, 1989; Zorowitz et al, 1990).

Estrogen replacement therapy (ERT) is the most effective treatment available to prevent bone loss in women without endogenous estrogen. ERT reduces the risk of hip fracture by 50% in women who start estrogen within the first 5 postmenopausal years and who continue ERT for at least 5 years thereafter (Kiel et al, 1987). Unfortunately, there is controversy about who should start ERT and how long estrogen should be taken. The National Osteoporosis Foundation provides guidelines for ERT.

ERT may increase a woman's risk for uterine and breast cancer. Cycling estrogen with progestin is believed to reduce the risk of endometrial cancer to baseline, or below baseline, levels (Meier, 1990); however, progestin does cause light withdrawal bleeding for several days

---

Guide to Estrogen Replacement Therapy

Consider ERT to prevent bone loss in women at risk for osteoporosis, who have no contraindications, and who understand the benefits and risks

Start ERT as soon after menopause as possible and plan to continue it for at least 10 years

Prescribe low-dose ERT (e.g., 0.625 mg/d of conjugated estrogen on days 1 to 25, 10 mg/d of medroxyprogesterone on days 12 to 25, and nothing on days 26 to 31). Women who have had hysterectomies do not need progesterone replacement

Ensure frequent manual breast examinations, yearly mammography, and thorough evaluation of abnormal vaginal bleeding

Data from A physician's resource manual on osteoporosis. Washington, DC: National Osteoporosis Foundation, 1987.

---

a month in 60% of women over 65 years old (Gambrell, 1990). Results of studies are divided about the relationship of ERT and breast cancer, but taking estrogen for less than 10 years may decrease the risk (Wingo et al, 1987; Gambrell, 1991).

Available data suggest that the benefits of ERT outweigh its risks. For example, the risk of death from endometrial cancer while on ERT is approximately 1 in 20,000; comparatively, the death rate secondary to osteoporotic hip fracture is 1 in 60 for women 70 years of age and older (Gambrell, 1990).

Given the risks and benefits of estrogen replacement, a women may be uncertain about whether to start ERT. Bone densitometry can enhance decision-making, especially for the woman who would take estrogen only if she knew her bone density was low. Absolute contraindications for ERT include a personal history of breast cancer or thromboembolic disease, acute liver disease, or unexplained vaginal bleeding (Meier, 1990). Calcitonin injections have been used for women who cannot or will not take estrogen and for men with osteoporosis. Calcitonin suppresses bone resorption, but its effect on preventing osteoporosis may be minimal (Barzel, 1990).

Treatment of Established Osteoporosis

The goal of treatment for established osteoporosis is to increase bone mass. Therapies to increase bone mass are limited, but calcium and moderate weight-bearing exercise continue to be recommended. Some evidence suggests that estrogen slows bone loss and decreases the fracture risk even in established osteoporosis. However, estrogen cannot stimulate new bone formation, and critics contend that its risks are not justified after significant bone loss has occurred (Barzel, 1990).

Safe and effective drugs to increase bone mass have been limited. Fluoride increases bone mass, but adverse effects, especially lower extremity pain, have limited its usefulness, to date. There is also evidence that fluoride-induced cortical bone has decreased strength (Riggs et al, 1990). However, several therapeutic agents may increase the options for treating established osteoporosis in the future.

Etidronate, an antiresorption agent that inhibits osteoclasts, has increased vertebral bone mass and decreased the rate of new vertebral fractures in postmenopausal women (Storm et al, 1990; Watts et al, 1991). Based on 6 years of clinical trials at the Osteoporosis Prevention Center, etidronate has been a safe, effective, and relatively inexpensive (i.e, about $12 a month) treatment for osteoporosis when given cyclically (Riggs, 1990; Woodson and Carlson, 1991).

Coherence therapy is an experimental regimen that inhibits excess bone resorption while allowing normal bone formation. Coherence therapy uses cyclical administration of oral phosphorus, etidronate, calcium, and vitamin D. Preliminary data indicate that strong bone is formed, but the effect on fracture prevention is not yet known (Barzel, 1990). Other investigational agents that may prove beneficial for the treatment of osteoporosis include anabolic steroids, parathyroid hormone, vitamin D metabolites, and growth factors.

Few studies have been done on the treatment of osteoporosis in older men. Men should be carefully evaluated for secondary causes of osteoporosis, especially hypogonadism. If present, replacement of the deficient hormone may stabilize bone mass. If not, calcitonin injections may be helpful (Hahn, 1988). Calcium supplementation and moderate weight-bearing exercise may benefit male osteoporosis, but data to support this regimen are not available (Meier, 1990).

OSTEOARTHRITIS

Osteoarthritis, a degenerative disease of joint cartilage, is the most common type of arthritis among older adults. In most cases, the disease is asymptomatic or relatively mild, but osteoarthritis is also one of the leading causes of disability in persons over 65 years of age (Ettinger, 1990).

ETIOLOGIC FACTORS

Aging does not cause osteoarthritis. Changes that occur in aging cartilage and bone are not the same changes that occur in osteoarthritis (Hammerman, 1989). However, age-related changes in cartilage and/or joint mechanics may contribute to the development of osteoarthritis in the aging adult (Brandt, 1988).

There is increasing evidence that osteoarthritis is not a single disorder but a group of disorders with multiple causes. Osteoarthritis is classified as primary when there is no known cause and secondary when some predisposing factor is known.

Primary Osteoarthritis

The etiology of primary osteoarthritis is unknown. Generalized arthritis, a subtype of primary arthritis affecting three or more joints outside the spine, tends to be familial. The genetic predisposition to generalized arthritis suggests that systemic metabolic factors make cartilage more vulnerable to damage (Davis, 1988).

Secondary Osteoarthritis

Articular damage can develop from mechanical stress on joints and underlying medical disorders including metabolic and endocrine diseases (e.g., acromegaly, diabetes) and inflammatory arthritis (e.g., gout, rheumatoid arthritis).

RISK FACTORS

After the age of 60, approximately 25% of women and 15% of men report symptoms of osteoarthritis (Grob, 1989), but radiographic evidence of the disease is much higher in older populations. In the Framingham study, radiographic evidence of osteoarthritis was found in 85% of adults 75 to 79 years old (Sorensen, 1990). In addition to age, other risk factors for osteoarthritis include female sex, genetic disposition, congenital/developmental bone and joint disorders, inflammatory joint disease, mechanical stress, repetitive joint usage, joint trauma, and obesity (Hochberg, 1991).

Many congenital and mechanical risk factors for osteoarthritis are preventable or treatable. For example, early treatment of anatomic defects (e.g., congenital hip dislocation) can prevent the development of osteoarthritis. Occupational safety programs that help workers prevent joint injuries and repeated stress on joints may reduce the incidence of osteoarthritis. In addition, educational programs to prevent weight gain and encourage weight loss may decrease the incidence of osteoarthritis of the knee.

The effect of repetitive joint usage on normal joints is not clear, especially the types of usage that damage joints. In several studies of laborers and athletes, overuse of normal joints was associated with increased incidence of osteoarthritis of the knees and fingers (Peyron, 1991). Thus far, however, there are no data that vigorous exercise (e.g., walking, running, cycling) increases the risk of osteoarthritis in normal joints, although vigorous, repetitive exercise can increase damage in joints that are already damaged or otherwise abnormal (Gerber, 1990).

DYNAMICS

Despite its multiple etiologies, osteoarthritis leads to one final pathway: joint degeneration. Joint deterioration begins with thinning and loss of cartilage, often in areas of increased load. As articular cartilage erodes, bone proliferates at the joint margins and osteophytes (spurs) develop. In severe cases, cartilage loss leads to bone on bone contact at the joint. Local inflammation may occur in varying degrees; however, the pathogenesis of joint inflammation in osteoarthritis is unclear (Davis, 1988).

As joint deterioration progresses, increased stress is placed on supporting musculature. Muscles fatigue easily and may spasm in response to joint pain. Pain and disuse lead to muscle weakness that, in turn, contributes to increased joint pain.

Osteoarthritis usually affects one or two joints, but generalized osteoarthritis occurs in some middle-aged and older women. The joints most commonly affected in primary osteoarthritis are, in order of prevalence, the distal interphalangeals, proximal interphalangeals, knees, spine, feet, and hips (Davis, 1988). Secondary osteoarthritis can affect any joint.

SIGNS AND SYMPTOMS

Osteoarthritis has a gradual onset and slow progression. Morning stiffness that resolves in less than 30 minutes and stiffness after other periods of inactivity are common complaints. Joint pain is worsened by activity and relieved by rest. In later stages of the disease, joint pain may persist at rest also.

Signs of osteoarthritis include joint pain with movement, movement limitations, crepitus, and bony enlargements. Bony enlargements on the distal interphalangeals (Heberden's nodes) and proximal interphalangeals (Bouchard's nodes) are more frequently seen in women with primary osteoarthritis.

Inflammatory signs, if present, are usually mild. Joints may be tender but are seldom warm or red. Mild swelling may occur, especially small effusions of the knees. Characteristic radiographic findings include joint space narrowing, sclerosis of underlying subchondral bone, osteophytes, and bony cysts.

DIAGNOSIS

The diagnosis of osteoarthritis is based on clinical and radiographic findings (see box on p. 577). It should not be assumed, however, that joint pain in older persons with radiographic signs of osteoarthritis is due to osteoarthritis until other rheumatologic disorders are ruled out. For example, a person with radiographic evidence of osteoarthritis, but no symptoms of the disease, may develop acute gout or pseudogout following a stressful event like surgery. Attributing the joint pain to osteoarthritis would result in lack of treatment for the more acute arthritis (Senior Medical Review, 1989).

Synovial fluid analysis and selected laboratory studies can be helpful to distinguish osteoarthritis from rheumatoid arthritis, polymyalgia rheumatica, gout, and pseudogout. Noninflammatory synovial fluid, normal sedimentation rate, and negative rheumatoid factor are typical

---

Diagnosis of Osteoarthritis

Characteristic radiographic findings

Pain relieved by rest

Inflammation variable (usually mild or absent)

Normal laboratory findings

Data from Mongan E. Arthritis and osteoporosis. In: Kemp B, Brummel-Smith K, Ramsdell JW, eds. Geriatric rehabilitation. Boston: Little, Brown and Company, 1990, p. 91.

---

in osteoarthritis. Table 30–2 compares the clinical aspects of osteoarthritis and other arthritic disorders common in the elderly.

COMPLICATIONS

Neurologic and vascular complications can occur when severe osteoarthritis affects the spine. Neurovascular complications are not always treatable, but surgical procedures may correct complications if signs and symptoms are detected early.

Cervical Spondylitic Myelopathy Osteophyte formation on vertebral bodies can compress the posterior spinal cord and cause the serious disorder known as cervical spondylitic myelopathy. Early signs and symptoms include limited neck range of motion, pain radiating to the arms and back from head flexion or extension, brisk or very hyperactive tendon reflexes, and heaviness or numbness in the hands and feet. Late complications include spasticity, then weakness, of the extremities, difficulty walking, falls, and loss of sphincter control. Early recognition of the disorder and corrective surgery (e.g., stabilization procedures and procedures to decompress the spinal cord) may prevent eventual immobility and incontinence (Weins, 1990).

Vascular Syndromes When osteophytes form in the vertebral foramina, compression of the vertebrobasilar arteries can occur. Symptoms of basilar insufficiency may occur with cervical range of motion, including blurred or double vision, visual field defects, headache, syncope, and drop attacks (Sorensen, 1990). When osteoarthritis affects the lumbar spine, cord compression can result in leg pains, paresthesias, and a pseudoclaudication in which leg pain brought on by standing and walking is relieved by rest (Pottenger, 1990).

TABLE 30–2 *Clinical Features of Rheumatologic Diseases Common in the Elderly*

Finding	OA	RA	Gout	PG	PR
Gradual onset	+ + +	+ + +	0	+	+ + +
Joint pain	+ + + +	+ + + +	+ + + +	+ + + +	+
Joint swelling	+ + +	+ + + +	+ + + +	+ + + +	+
Symmetric pattern	+	+ + +	+	+	+ + + +
Muscle pain	+	+	+	+	+ + +
Radiographic abnormalities	+ + + +	+ + +	+	+ + +	0
Elevated sedimentation rate	+	+ + +	0	0	+
Positive rheumatoid factor	0	+ + +	0	0	+
Anemia	0	+	0	0	+ + +
Synovial fluid crystals	+	+	+ + +	+ + +	0

Abbreviations: OA, osteoarthritis; RA, rheumatoid arthritis; PG, pseudogout; PR, polymyalgia rheumatica.
Symbols: 0, does not occur; +, occasionally occurs; + +, frequently occurs; + + +, almost always occurs; + + + +, difficult to make diagnosis without it.
Adapted from Kane RL, Ouslander JG, Abrass IB. Immobility. Essentials of clinical geriatrics, 2nd ed. New York: McGraw-Hill, 1989:213.

MEDICAL MANAGEMENT

The goals of treatment for osteoarthritis are to protect joints, relieve pain, and preserve function. Joint protection, therapy, and medications to relieve pain and inflammation are the mainstays of medical treatment, but surgery is an option for the older adult if other measures fail to relieve symptoms.

Joint Protection and Therapy Joint-sparing activity adjustment and assistive devices to decrease loading on weight-bearing joints are frequently recommended. When osteoarthritis affects the spine, a cervical collar may be prescribed for several weeks to relive pain and muscle spasms. Cervical and lumbar symptoms that do not respond to simple rest may benefit from several days of continuous or intermittent traction (Grob, 1989). In addition to joint protection, physical therapy may also be prescribed to relieve pain and inflammation with modalities like heat (e.g., ultrasound, diathermy), cold, and therapeutic exercise.

Medications If joint-sparing measures fail to relieve symptoms, salicylates or other nonsteroidal anti-inflammatory drugs (NSAIDs) are commonly used to treat osteoarthritis (Table 30–3). Salicylates in moderate doses can relieve pain, but larger doses are required to reduce in-

TABLE 30–3 *Nonsteroidal Anti-inflammatory Drugs*

Class/Drug	Dose (mg)	Doses per Day
Acetylated salicylates		
Aspirin	600–1200	3–4
Nonacetylated salicylates		
Choline magnesium trisylate (Trilisate)	500–1000	2
Diflunisal (Dolobid)	500	2
Salsalate (Disalcid, Salflex)	1000–1500	2
Acetic acids		
Diclofenac (Voltaren)	50–75	2–3
Tolmetin (Tolectin)	300–400	3–4
Fenamates		
Meclofenamate (Meclomen)	50–100	3–4
Indole acetic acids		
Indomethacin (Indocin)	25–50	3–4
Sulindac (Clinoril)	150–200	2
Oxicams		
Piroxicam (Feldene)	10–20	1
Proprionic acids		
Fenoprofen (Nalfon)	600–800	3–4
Flurbiprofen (Ansaid)	100	2–3
Ibuprofen (Motrin, Rufen)	400–800	3–4
Ketoprofen (Orudis)	50–75	3–4
Naproxen (Naproxyn, Anaprox)	250–750	2
Pyranocarboxylic acids		
Etodolac (Lodine)	200–300	3–4

Adapted from Ettinger WH, Davis MA. Osteoarthritis. In: Hazzard WR, Andres R, Bierman EL, Blass JP, eds. Principles of geriatric medicine. New York: McGraw-Hill, 1990, p. 886.

flammation. Gastric irritation can be reduced by giving plain aspirin with food or using an enteric-coated product.

Older people are especially prone to salicylate toxicity even at therapeutic doses. Blood salicylate levels should be obtained whenever an older person presents with confusion, respiratory alkalosis, or pulmonary edema of unknown cause (Albrich and Bosker, 1990). Tinnitus is also an indication of salicylate toxicity, but it is not a reliable indicator in older adults with impaired hearing.

The newer NSAIDs are as effective as aspirin, but a number of factors can predispose older adults to side effects (e.g., age-related decreases in renal function and albumin levels and preexisting gastrointestinal, renal, and cardiovascular disorders). Evidence is growing that NSAIDs increase the risk of peptic ulcer and gastrointestinal hemorrhage in older adults (Griffin et al, 1988; Beard et al, 1987). In fact, NSAID-induced gastropathy accounts for over 70,000 hospitalizations and 7000 deaths a year in the United States (Fries, 1991). Accepted risk factors for NSAID-induced gastropathy include old age, dose, duration of use, treatment with combinations of NSAIDs, large ulcers, and a history of gastric ulcers (Zeidler, 1991). Other important side effects of NSAIDs are acute renal failure, increased congestive heart failure, altered mental status, and skin rashes.

Cautious use of NSAIDs in the elderly is essential. Recommendations for NSAID use in this population include the following:

1. *Make sure NSAIDs are needed.* Whenever possible, nonmedicinal and local therapies should be tried before relying on NSAIDs to treat osteoarthritis. Maximizing nonmedicinal treatments (e.g., braces/supports, canes, walkers, heat/cold, massage, exercise) and local therapies (e.g., topical analgesics, intra-articular steroid injections) may eliminate or reduce the need for NSAIDs, thereby decreasing the risk of adverse drug effects.

NSAIDs are indicated for mild-to-moderate pain caused by inflammation. If inflammation is absent, analgesic doses of acetaminophen or a salicylate that causes fewer gastric and renal side effects is appropriate (e.g., nonacetylated salicylates).

2. *Choose NSAIDs with the fewest gastrointestinal, renal, or cardiovascular side effects.* All older adults are at risk for gastrointestinal complications from NSAIDs, but factors like preexisting gastritis or peptic ulcer, alcohol and tobacco use, or female sex increase the risk. Select NSAIDs that cause less gastric irritation whenever possible (e.g., nonacetylated salicylates, etodolac), especially when there is a history of gastritis or ulcers. Coadministration of a synthetic prostaglandin (e.g., misoprostol) has been recommended for older adults at high risk for gastrointestinal complications.

Older adults are at increased risk for renal and cardiovascular complications from NSAIDs due to age-related declines in renal function or preexisting conditions (e.g., congestive heart failure, hypertension, diabetes, and diuretic use). Some data suggest that ibuprofen can cause rapid renal damage in the elderly, even at low doses, while sulindac and piroxicam may be "renal-sparing" (Murray et al, 1990; Whelton et al, 1990). Nonacetylated salicylates are also less likely to cause renal toxicity. Warn older adults about the risk for gastrointestinal bleeding and renal failure from over-the-counter ibuprofen (e.g., Advil, Nuprin).

3. *Avoid NSAID-drug interactions.* NSAIDs are highly protein-bound drugs that can increase the effect of coumarin-type anticoagulants, phenytoin, sulfonylurea-type oral hypoglycemic agents, and sulfonamides. Lithium levels can go up or down with NSAIDs. Renal failure has been reported from several NSAID–diuretic combinations, specifically ketoprofen with hydrochlorothiazide and indomethacin with triamterene. Ibuprofen, and possibly all NSAIDs, can interact with thiazide diuretics, beta-blockers, and angiotensin-converting enzyme inhibitors to decrease the antihypertensive effect of these drugs.

4. *Start with a low dose.* Begin NSAIDs at smaller doses and gradually titrate to the lowest effective dose. Whenever possible, reduce the dosage or the duration that NSAIDs are given.

5. *Find effective NSAIDs.* Patient response to individual NSAIDs is highly variable. If one NSAID is ineffective, NSAIDs from a different subclass may prove effective. Medication changes in the elderly require caution, however, and one NSAID should be given an adequate trial before switching drugs (e.g., 3 to 4 weeks at therapeutic doses), if feasible.

6. *Consider factors that influence NSAID compliance.* Simple scheduling and taking as few pills as possible are important considerations in the elderly. NSAIDs that require less frequent dosing may result in better compliance than NSAIDs that require more frequent dosing. Cost can also affect compliance. Aspirin and ibuprofen are the least expensive

NSAIDs; higher cost NSAIDs include piroxicam, sulindac, meclofenamate, and diflunisal.

7. *Monitor for NSAID side effects.* Patients can unknowingly combine NSAIDs by taking over-the-counter ibuprofen with their prescribed NSAID. To decrease the chance of adverse drug reactions from NSAID combinations, find out which over-the-counter drugs the older person is taking and warn against using NSAIDs in combination (Panush and Endo, 1988; Albrich and Bosker, 1990; Fries, 1991; Portenoy, 1990; Mazanec, 1991; Nesher et al, 1991).

Tell patients to stop taking NSAIDs and report symptoms if they feel weak or dizzy or develop vomiting, diarrhea, or loss of appetite. Closely monitor the older person for fluid retention, occult blood loss, and mental status changes. Recommended follow-up includes (a) creatinine, BUN, and potassium at 2 and 4 weeks, then every 1 to 3 months, (b) hemoglobin/hematocrit monthly for 3 months, then every 3 months or sooner if signs/symptoms indicate, and (c) endoscopic examination if there is new anemia, positive occult fecal blood (e.g., hemoccult), or persistent symptoms (4 weeks) despite therapy. Side effects are usually reversible when NSAIDs are stopped, and another NSAID can be tried when side effects resolve. Systemic steroids and narcotic analgesics are not recommended in the treatment of osteoarthritis.

Surgery Surgical treatment for arthritic joints is indicated for severe pain and disability that have not responded to joint protection, therapy, or medication. Debridement is used in early arthritis to smooth irregular joint surfaces and remove loose bodies and inflamed tissue. Joint fusion and osteotomy have been available for many years, but both procedures require prolonged immobility predisposing the older adult to numerous complications.

Total joint replacements can provide significant improvement in function and quality of life for older adults. Hip and knee replacements permit early mobility and provide sufficient joint strength and function for ordinary activities. The elderly person's general health and functional status, not age, should determine who is a candidate for joint replacement surgery. Hip and knee replacements are appropriate for older adults who, in otherwise satisfactory health, are losing the ability to walk (Ettinger, 1988). Other joint replacements (e.g.,

shoulder, elbow, wrist, metacarpophalangeal, and ankle) have, thus far, been less successful (Sculco, 1989).

Hip or knee replacement surgeries take 2 to 4 hours, and an uncomplicated hospital course is 7 to 10 days (Pottenger, 1990). Gait training is started on the second or third postoperative day, and the individual is advanced to independent ambulation with cane or walker by discharge. Rehabilitation includes daily range of motion, muscle strengthening exercises, and protected weight-bearing for 1 to 2 months. Typically, the older adult regains full strength and energy within 3 to 5 months after surgery (Harris and Sledge, 1990).

Complications in joint replacement surgery are relatively infrequent (e.g., approximately 5% for total hip arthroplasty), and most complications are correctable (Harris and Sledge, 1990). Major complications include deep vein thrombosis, infections, and mechanical failure of the prosthesis (Sculco, 1989). Prophylactic use of anticoagulants (e.g., low-dose warfarin) has greatly reduced the incidence of thromboembolism. Prophylactic antibiotics have effectively decreased the incidence of wound infections to less than 2% (Pottenger, 1990). Advances in artificial joint design and bone cement have reduced implant loosening to 3% after 11 years for artificial hips (Harris and Sledge, 1990). Research to develop improved bone cement and cementless implants for total joint replacement continues.

RHEUMATOID ARTHRITIS

Rheumatoid arthritis is a systemic disease of connective tissue that most commonly manifests as a joint disorder. Long-standing rheumatoid arthritis frequently leads to disabling joint deformities as well as extra-articular complications. Most older adults with rheumatoid arthritis have long-standing disease that began between the third and fifth decades (younger onset rheumatoid arthritis), but the disease can also develop after the age of 60 (elderly onset rheumatoid arthritis).

ETIOLOGIC FACTORS

The cause of rheumatoid arthritis is not known; however, the prevailing theory is that arthritogenic agents stimulate immune responses in genetically predisposed individuals (Sorensen, 1990). Substances under investigation as causative agents include viruses, connective-tissue proteins (e.g., collagen and proteoglycans), altered immunoglobulins, and rheumatoid factor (Harris, 1990). It is postulated that rheumatoid factor links with IgG, and the rheumatoid factor. The IgG complex activates a complement to initiate the inflammatory response in synovial tissue and other organ systems (Weins, 1990).

POPULATIONS AT RISK

The prevalence of rheumatoid arthritis increases with age due to carryover of younger onset cases and the development of new cases in this age group. Approximately 40% of all rheumatoid arthritis patients are over 60 years old, and of these, 10% to 20% have elderly onset disease (Grob, 1989; Nesher et al, 1991). Women are two to three times more likely to have rheumatoid arthritis than men, but no environmental or geographic risk factors have been identified for the disease (Nesher et al, 1991).

DYNAMICS

In joints affected by rheumatoid arthritis, synovial inflammation and connective tissue proliferation lead to synovial thickening (pannus). Pannus invades and erodes adjacent cartilage, underlying subchondral bone, ligaments, and tendons. As the disease progresses, joint deformities limit range of motion, and disuse leads to muscle atrophy and osteoporosis. In the later stages of rheumatoid arthritis, systemic manifestations can pose serious medical problems, including vascular, neurologic, ocular, pulmonary, and cardiac complications.

The course of the disease is highly variable. In most cases, rheumatoid arthritis is a chronic disease with periods of remissions and exacerbations. Less commonly, severe progression occurs without periods of remission. In rare cases, complete remission follows a short course of disease. Elderly onset rheumatoid arthritis often has a milder course and better outcomes than younger onset disease (Terkeltaub et al, 1983; Deal et al, 1985).

SIGNS AND SYMPTOMS

The onset of rheumatoid arthritis is usually gradual, but the presentation may be acute or subacute in the geriatric patient. Constitutional symptoms such as fatigue, anorexia, and low-grade fever can precede or accompany the onset of symptoms. Common complaints include painful, swollen joints and prolonged morning stiffness. Stiffness lasting longer than 30 minutes following periods of inactivity is common in rheumatoid arthritis.

Inflamed joints are swollen, warm, and tender. Joint involvement tends to be symmetrical and initially involves the proximal interphalangeals, metacarpophalangeals, and wrists. Proximal interphalangeals are characteristically spindle-shaped in acute rheumatoid arthritis due to joint swelling and muscle atrophy. Distal interphalangeals are less commonly affected.

Late joint complications include movement limitations of the knees and hips and characteristic joint deformities of the upper extremities, specifically (1) ulnar deviation of the wrists, (2) swan neck deformity (i.e., hyperextension of the proximal interphalangeals with fixed flexion of the distal interphalangeals, and (3) boutonnière deformity (i.e., flexion of the proximal interphalangeals with hyperextension of the distal interphalangeals. Subcutaneous rheumatoid nodules, if present, are usually seen around the elbow and proximal forearm. Rheumatoid nodules are asymptomatic, but skin breakdown can occur if a nodule occurs at the sacrum or other area exposed to pressure (Nesher et al, 1991).

Laboratory findings may include an elevated sedimentation rate, anemia, and positive rheumatoid factor. The presence of rheumatoid factor is not specific for rheumatoid arthritis, however, and may be absent in early disease (Weins, 1990). Radiographic findings include soft tissue swelling in early disease and, in later stages, joint space narrowing, bone erosions, and subluxations. Radiographic evidence of osteoporosis is frequently seen in advanced rheumatoid arthritis (Weins, 1990).

DIAGNOSIS

The diagnosis of rheumatoid arthritis is based on clinical findings. Diagnostic criteria for rheumatoid arthritis were developed by observing individuals with younger onset disease (see box on p. 582) and, in most cases, the clinical presentation is similar in younger onset and elderly onset rheumatoid arthritis. However, some clinical findings occur more frequently in elderly onset rheumatoid arthritis, including acute onset, large joint involvement (i.e., shoulders and hips), and pronounced constitutional

---

Diagnosis of Rheumatoid Arthritis

At least four of the following findings must be present

Morning stiffness*

Arthritis of three or more joints*

Hand-joint arthritis*

Symmetric involvement*

Rheumatoid nodules

Positive rheumatoid factor

Radiographic changes

*These findings must be present for at least 6 weeks. Data from Arnett FC. Revised criteria for the classification of rheumatoid arthritis. Bull Rheum Dis 1989; 38:2.

---

symptoms like fatigue, malaise, and fever (Terkeltaub et al, 1983; Deal et al, 1985). Findings that are less common in elderly onset disease are positive rheumatoid factor, bone erosions, and systemic complications (Sorensen, 1990; Nesher et al, 1991).

Because the clinical presentation of elderly onset rheumatoid arthritis can differ from younger onset disease, it may be necessary to observe the course over several months in order to exclude other arthritic disorders (e.g., polymyalgia rheumatica, polyarticular gout, pseudogout, carcinoma arthritis, osteoarthritis) and connective tissue diseases like systemic lupus erythematous and Sjögren's syndrome (Nesher et al, 1991). The clinical features of rheumatoid arthritis and other arthritic disorders common in the elderly are summarized in Table 30–2.

COMPLICATIONS

Numerous systemic complications can occur in rheumatoid arthritis, particularly in individuals with long-standing, severe disease. Rheumatoid vasculitis and bacterial infections are among the most prominent and serious complications of rheumatoid arthritis.

Vasculitis Inflammation of vessels often involves the skin and peripheral nervous system,

predisposing to dermal ulcers, gangrene of the fingertips and ends of toes, and neuropathies. Ocular complications from vasculitis (e.g., scleritis, episcleritis, or uveitis) cause painful, red eyes and, in the case of scleritis and uveitis, miotic pupils. Treatment includes oral steroids, steroid ophthalmic drops, and mydriatic drops for miotic pupils (Weins, 1990).

Cardiac and pulmonary complications can also result from vasculitis, specifically pericarditis and pleural effusions. The occurrence of heart and lung complications, although uncommon clinically, usually require treatment with high doses of prednisone (Nesher et al, 1991).

Infections Patients with rheumatoid arthritis are more susceptible to infections, possibly because of the disease process itself and from treatment with steroids and other drugs that suppress the immune system. Septic arthritis is an infrequent, but potentially fatal, complication of rheumatoid arthritis. Most cases occur in people over age 60, and mortality of 19% has been reported (Nesher et al, 1991). In most cases, the source of infection is staphylococci from the skin. Septic arthritis presents as an acute flare-up of arthritis in one or more joints with fever and elevated white cell counts.

Other Complications Rheumatoid arthritis frequently affects the cervical spine and can progress to subluxation and persistent neck pain. Subluxation can lead to neurologic deficits from cervical cord compression, including signs of spasticity, hyperactive reflexes, ataxia, hoarseness, difficulty swallowing, and pain or weakness in the arms (Weins, 1990). Minor trauma to the head or neck or extreme head positions can cause spinal cord injury or even sudden death. Patients with cervical involvement should avoid head and neck trauma and extreme head positions (e.g., hyperextension). Cervical collars are used for supportive treatment, and surgery to relieve cord compression is performed when there is severe subluxation and persistent pain (Nesher et al, 1991). Anemia, dry eyes and mouth, and carpal tunnel syndrome are other important complications of rheumatoid arthritis (Collo et al, 1991).

MEDICAL MANAGEMENT

The goals of treatment in rheumatoid arthritis are to control pain and inflammation and maintain joint function. Interventions include physical and occupational therapy, medications, and surgery.

Physical and Occupational Therapy To preserve joint and muscle function, individualized exercise programs with specific rest periods should be prescribed for all older adults with rheumatoid arthritis. Intermittent splinting can provide local rest when inflammation is acute, and cervical collars or short-term traction can decrease the pain and spasms associated with cervical spine involvement. Assistive devices for mobility and other activities of daily living are frequently recommended to protect joints and promote independence. Specialized shoes are indicated for painful foot deformities, and customized orthotics are sometimes recommended to maintain deranged joints.

Medications The traditional pharmacologic approach to rheumatoid arthritis has used sequential administration of single drugs. Salicylates and other NSAIDs have been first-line drugs. If NSAIDs fail to give relief, so-called disease-modifying drugs (DMARDs) are added to the drug regimen later in the disease (Table 30–4). Critics of this approach have argued, however, that sequential administration of single drugs is too slow and has failed to prevent disease progression and joint damage in rheumatoid arthritis (Kushner, 1989; Healey and Wilske, 1991).

The current trend is moving toward using DMARDs earlier in the course of disease and in combination. The rationale for early, aggressive treatment is to control inflammation before irreversible joint damage occurs (Wilske and Healey, 1989). Thus far, data indicate that DMARDs are as effective in older adults as younger people, but the adverse effects of these drugs warrant cautious use and close monitoring in the elderly. Older people are at higher risk for macular damage from hydroxychloroquine, skin rashes, and taste disturbances from penicillamine, and nausea and vomiting from sulfasalazine (Nesher et al, 1991).

Low doses of oral steroids are used to treat rheumatoid arthritis in selected situations. Prednisone therapy can enable severely dis-

TABLE 30–4 *Disease-modifying Antirheumatic Drugs*

Drug	Maintenance Dose	Adverse Effects
Gold (IM) solganal, myochrysine	50 mg once a week for 20 weeks, then tapered	Rash, oral ulcers, nephropathy, marrow depression, colitis
Gold (oral) auranofin (Ridaura)	3 mg twice a day	Same as above and diarrhea
Hydroxychloroquine (Plaquenil)	200 to 400 mg/day in divided doses	Macular damage, nausea, vomiting
D-penicillamine (Cuprimine, Depen)	250 to 750 mg/day in divided doses	Rash, nephropathy, marrow suppression, neuropathy, autoimmune manifestations
Sulfasalazine (Azulfidine)	1–3 g/day in divided doses	Rash, gastrointestinal symptoms, marrow suppression, hemolysis, hepatotoxicity
Methotrexate (Rheumatrex)	5–15 mg once a week	Oral ulcers, liver abnormalities, marrow suppression, pneumonitis
Azathioprine (Imuran)	50 to 150 mg/day in divided doses	Nausea, vomiting, liver toxicity, marrow suppression, infections, malignancy (?)
Cyclophosphamide (Cytoxan)	1–2 mg/kg/day	Nausea, cystitis, hematuria, marrow suppression, malignancy

Adapted from Nesher G, Moore TL, Zuckner J. Rheumatoid arthritis in the elderly. J Am Geriatr Soc 1991; 39:284.

abled patients to maintain ambulation, but the trade-off for enhanced mobility is the risk of steroid-induced osteoporosis and other complications (e.g., increased susceptibility to infection, peptic ulcer, and cataracts). Short-term, low-dose prednisone can benefit the person started on a DMARD until the drug takes effect or the older adult with prominent constitutional symptoms in elderly onset disease (Sorensen, 1990). Intra-articular steroid injections are used for acutely inflamed joints and are considered safe if not given more than once every 3 months in the same joint (Nesher et al, 1991).

Surgery   Surgical treatment of rheumatoid arthritis is indicated for pain and loss of function that have not responded to therapy and medications. The most common surgeries performed on older adults are carpal tunnel release, tendon repair, and joint replacement of the hips and knees. Most rheumatoid arthritis patients have good or excellent results from joint replacement surgery (Harris and Sledge, 1990), with significant improvements in function and quality of life (see Osteoarthritis Management for a review of joint replacement surgery).

NURSING ASSESSMENT OF CAPACITY FOR DAILY LIVING

Musculoskeletal problems can significantly limit an older person's capacity for activities of daily living (ADLs) and instrumental activities of daily living (IADLs). ADLs refer to self-care activities like bathing, hygiene, dressing, grooming, toileting, and feeding. Mobility and continence status are also considered ADL functions in many practice settings. IADLs include a range of activities that are generally required to live independently including using the telephone, shopping, housecleaning, using transportation, managing medications, and handling finances. Evaluation of an older adult's ADL and IADL status is an essential component of gerontologic nursing assessment.

Many tools are available to assess ADL and IADL status, but the nurse is cautioned to select a tool that is valid, reliable, and clinically practical (i.e., relevant to the practice setting, easy to administer in a reasonable length of time, and useful for monitoring functional

progress). Two instruments that meet these criteria are the Katz Index of ADL (Katz et al, 1963) and the Barthel Index (Mahoney and Barthel, 1965).

The Katz Index (see box on p. 585) uses direct observation of performance to rate independence or dependence in six ADLs: bathing, dressing, toileting, transferring, feeding, and continence. The Katz Index can be administered in about 5 minutes and is useful for acute, long-term care and in community settings.

The Barthel Index (see box on pp. 586–588) uses direct observation to rate the amount of assistance needed for 10 ADLs: bathing, dressing, toileting, transferring, feeding, hygiene/grooming, walking, using stairs, bladder control, and bowel continence. A score of 100 indicates complete independence in all ADLs. In one study (n = 269), Barthel scores between 41 and 60 predicted good potential for an intensive rehabilitation program, while scores less than 20 correlated with poor functional outcomes (Granger et al, 1987). The Barthel Index is most appropriate for use in rehabilitation and long-term care settings where direct observation of performance can be made (Kane and Kane, 1988).

The Philadelphia Geriatric Center Instrumental Activities of Daily Living Scale (Lawton and Brody, 1969) is a promising tool for assessing IADL function (see box on p. 589). The observer rates ability to use the telephone, shop, prepare food, do housekeeping and laundry, use transportation, take medications, and handle finances. Unfortunately, there are no instructions for summing the scores, and the tool may be more valid for assessing the functional status of women (Kane and Kane, 1988).

Nurses who assess older adults are encouraged to incorporate ADL and IADL assessment tools in all practice settings (i.e., hospitals, nursing homes, rehabilitation facilities, and home care). These tools provide for baseline and ongoing evaluation of the older adult's capacity for self-care and independent living; however, the following perspectives should be appreciated when performing functional assessments (Kane et al, 1989):

1. A functional assessment of a patient in an acute state is likely to be invalid (e.g., a patient transferred from a natural environment to the alien world of the hospital, particularly at a time of stress).

The Katz Index of Activities of Daily Living

1. *Bathing (sponge, shower, or tub)*
   - I: Receives no assistance (gets in and out of tub if tub is the usual means of bathing)
   - A: Receives assistance in bathing only one part of the body (such as the back or a leg)
   - D: Receives assistance in bathing more than one part of the body (or not bathed)
2. *Dressing*
   - I: Gets clothes and gets completely dressed without assistance
   - A: Gets clothes and gets dressed without assistance except in tying shoes
   - D: Receives assistance in getting clothes or in getting dressed or stays partly or completely undressed
3. *Toileting*
   - I: Goes to "toilet room," cleans self, and arranges clothes without assistance (may use object for support such as cane, walker, or wheelchair and may manage night bedpan or commode, emptying it in the morning)
   - A: Receives assistance in going to "toilet room" or in cleansing self or in arranging clothes after elimination or in use of night bedpan or commode
   - D: Does not go to room termed "toilet" for the elimination process
4. *Transfer*
   - I: Moves in and out of bed as well as in and out of chair without assistance (may be using object for support such as cane or walker)
   - A: Moves in and out of bed or chair with assistance
   - D: Does not get out of bed
5. *Continence*
   - I: Controls urination and bowel movement completely by self
   - A: Has occasional "accidents"
   - D: Supervision helps keep urine or bowel control; catheter is used, or is incontinent
6. *Feeding*
   - I: Feeds self without assistance
   - A: Feeds self except for getting assistance in cutting meat or buttering bread
   - D: Receives assistance in feeding or is fed partly or completely by using tubes or intravenous fluids

Abbreviations: I, independent; A, assistance; D, dependent.
From Katz S, Ford AB, Moskowitz RW, et al. Studies of illness in the aged: the index of ADL, a standardized measure of biological and psychosocial function. JAMA 1963; 185:914; with permission.

2. With functional scales, the patient's motivation and the environmental structure are important determinants of performance.
3. It is critical to distinguish what a patient can do under proper circumstances and what is actually done during the patient's daily life. For example, it is not realistic to expect a nursing home patient to show self-care in bathing if the nursing home's policy forbids unattended bathing, or independence in dressing if the staff insists on dressing patients as a matter of expediency.

For a comprehensive examination of functional assessment, the reader is referred to Kane and Kane (1988) and McDowell and Newell (1987).

(continued on p. 588)

The Barthel Index

ACTION	WITH HELP	INDEPENDENT
1. Feeding (if food needs to be cut up = help)	5	10
2. Moving from wheelchair to bed and return (includes sitting up in bed)	5–10	15
3. Personal toilet (wash face, comb hair, shave, clean teeth)	0	5
4. Getting on and off toilet (handling clothes, wipe, flush)	5	10
5. Bathing self	0	5
6. Walking on level surface (or if unable to walk, propel wheelchair)	0*	5*
7. Ascend and descend stairs	5	10
8. Dressing (includes tying shoes, fastening fasteners)	5	10
9. Controlling bowels	5	10
10. Controlling bladder	5	10

A patient scoring 100 BDI is continent, feeds himself, dresses himself, gets up out of bed and chairs, bathes himself, walks at least a block, and can ascend and descend stairs. This does not mean that he is able to live alone: he may not be able to cook, keep house, and meet the public, but he is able to get along without attendant care.

DEFINITION AND DISCUSSION OF SCORING

1. Feeding
   10 = Independent. The patient can feed himself a meal from a tray or table when someone puts the food within his reach. He must put on an assistive device if this is needed, cut up the food, use salt and pepper, spread butter, etc. He must accomplish this in a reasonable time.
   5 = Some help is necessary (with cutting up food, etc., as listed above)

2. Moving from wheelchair to bed and return
   15 = Independent in all phases of this activity. Patient can safely approach the bed in his wheelchair, lock brakes, lift footrests, move safely from bed, lie down, come to a sitting position on the side of the bed, change the position of the wheelchair, if necessary, to transfer back into it safely and return to the wheelchair.
   10 = Either some minimal help is needed in some step of this activity or the patient needs to be reminded or supervised for safety of one or more parts of this activity.
   5 = Patient can come to a sitting position without the help of a second person but needs to be lifted out of bed, or if he transfers with a great deal of help.

3. Doing personal toilet
   5 = Patient can wash hands and face, comb hair, clean teeth, and shave. He may use any kind of razor but he must put in blade or plug in razor without help as well as get it from the drawer or cabinet. Female patients must put on own makeup, if used, but need not braid or style hair.

*Score only if unable to walk.

The Barthel Index (*Continued*)

4. Getting on and off toilet

   10 = Patient is able to get on and off toilet, fasten and unfasten clothes, prevent soiling of clothes, and use toilet paper without help. He may use a wall bar or other stable object for support if needed. If it is necessary to use a bed pan instead of toilet, he must be able to place it on a chair, empty it, and clean it.

   5 = Patient needs help because of imbalance or in handling clothes or in using toilet paper.

5. Bathing self

   5 = Patient may use a bath tub, a shower, or take a complete sponge bath. He must be able to do all the steps involved in whichever method is employed without another person being present.

6. Walking on a level surface

   15 = Patient can walk at least 50 yards without help or supervision. He may wear braces or prostheses and use crutches, canes, or a walkerette but not a rolling walker. He must be able to lock and unlock braces if used, assume the standing position and sit down, get the necessary mechanical aids into position for use, and dispose of them when he sits. (Putting on and taking off braces is scored under Dressing).

6a. Propelling a wheelchair

   5 = If a patient cannot ambulate but can propel a wheelchair independently, he must be able to go around corners, turn around, maneuver the chair to a table, bed, toilet, etc. He must be able to push a chair at least 50 yards. Do not score this item if the patient gets a score for walking.

7. Ascending and descending stairs

   10 = Patient is able to go up and down a flight of stairs safely without help or supervision. He may and should use handrails, canes, or crutches when needed. He must be able to carry canes or crutches as he ascends or descends stair.

   5 = Patient needs help with or supervision of any one of the above items.

8. Dressing and undressing

   10 = Patient is able to put on and remove and fasten all clothing, and tie shoe laces (unless it is necessary to use adaptations for this). This activity includes putting on and removing and fastening corset or braces when these are prescribed. Such special clothing as suspenders, loafer shoes, dresses that open down the front may be used when necessary.

   5 = Patient needs help in putting on and removing or fastening any clothing. He must do at least half the work himself. He must accomplish this in a reasonable time.

   Women need not be scored on use of a brassiere or girdle unless these are prescribed garments.

9. Continence of bowels

   10 = Patient is able to control his bowels and have no accidents. He can use a suppository or take an enema when necessary (as for spinal cord injury patients who have had bowel training).

   5 = Patient needs help in using a suppository or taking an enema or has occasional accidents.

(Continued)

The Barthel Index (*Continued*)

10. Controlling bladder

10 = Patient is able to control his bladder day and night. Spinal cord injury patients who wear an external device and leg bag must put them on independently, clean and empty bag, and stay dry day and night.

5 = Patient has occasional accidents or cannot wait for the bed pan or get to the toilet in time or needs help with an external device.

The total score is not as significant or meaningful as the breakdown into individual items, since these indicate where the deficiencies are.

Any applicant to a chronic hospital who scores 100 BDI should be evaluated carefully before admission to see whether such hospitalization is indicated. Discharged patients with 100 BDI should not require further physical therapy but may benefit from a home visit to see whether any environmental adjustments are indicated.

From Mahoney FI, Barthel DW. Functional evaluation: The Barthel index. Md State Med J 1965; 14(2):61–5; with permission.

Nursing Diagnosis and Management of High-risk Areas in Daily Living

DAILY LIVING WITH VULNERABILITY FOR FALLING

Falls in older persons are not inevitable, but they do occur with sufficient frequency in some groups to warrant consideration as an area of risk in daily living for the elderly.

RISK FACTORS

The risks of falling increase with

Increasing age
The number of chronic diseases present
The number and type of medications being taken
Cognitive impairment
Physical disability

Times of greater risk are those when the elderly person is changing position, i.e., sitting to standing, standing and turning, and walking up stairs.

SIGNS AND SYMPTOMS

Falls contribute to both psychological and physical injury. The older person who sustains little or no injury in a fall may delay or avoid discussing it. This choice may be made to avoid embarrassment or risk of being viewed as less competent in some behavior or activity that has previously been unrestricted or viewed as safe. Providing a safe nonjudgmental climate in which the person can openly discuss falls and accidents is important.

Evidence of falls includes bruises, abrasions, pain, swelling, or fractures. Changes in cognitive function related to pressure from edema or subdural hematoma may also be evidenced.

Psychological damage resulting from falls is more subtle. General comments may express concern about the living situation, indicating that home maintenance is too complicated. Signs of this concern may be evidenced by decreased thoroughness in housekeeping tasks. Fear of living alone may be openly discussed or alluded to.

The once active person may not venture out into the neighborhood and may be observed or report restricting movement within the home. Changes in grooming, dress, and personal appearance may be signals of injury or changing capacity for self-care. Gathering data on eating patterns reveals concerns related to falls in meeting the daily requirements of shopping and food preparation. Information about the availability of support persons—family, friends, and neighbors—is also useful to determine the resources available to the older person.

NURSING DIAGNOSIS

The major nursing diagnoses related to the older person who fall are (1) risk for injury re-

The PGC Instrumental Activities of Daily Living Scale

ACTION	SCORE

A. Ability to use telephone

1. Operates telephone on own initiative—looks up and dials numbers, etc.	1
2. Dials a few well-known numbers	1
3. Answers telephone but does not dial	1
4. Does not use a telephone at all	0

B. Shopping

1. Takes care of all shopping needs independently	1
2. Shops independently for small purchases	0
3. Needs to be accompanied on any shopping trip	0
4. Completely unable to shop	0

C. Food preparation

1. Plans, prepares, and serves adequate meals independently	1
2. Prepares adequate meals if supplied with ingredients	0
3. Heats and serves prepared meals, or prepares meals but does not maintain adequate diet	0
4. Needs to have meals prepared and served	0

D. Housekeeping

1. Maintains house alone or with occasional assistance (e.g., "heavy work-domestic help")	1
2. Performs light daily tasks such as dishwashing, bedmaking	1
3. Performs light daily tasks but cannot maintain acceptable level of cleanliness	1
4. Needs help with all home maintenance tasks	1
5. Does not participate in any housekeeping tasks	0

E. Laundry

1. Does personal laundry completely	1
2. Launders small items—rinses socks, stockings, etc.	1
3. All laundry must be done by others	0

F. Mode of transportation

1. Travels independently on public transportation or drives own car	1
2. Arranges own travel via taxi, but does not otherwise use public transportation	1
3. Travels on public transportation when assisted or accompanied by another	1
4. Travel limited to taxi or automobile with assistance of another	0
5. Does not travel at all	0

(Continued)

The PGC Instrumental Activities of Daily Living Scale (*Continued*)

G.   Responsibility for own medications
1.   Is responsible for taking medication in correct dosages at correct times   1
2.   Takes responsibility if medication is prepared in advance in separate dosages   0
3.   Is not capable of dispensing own medication   0

H.   Ability to handle finances
1.   Manages financial matters independently (budgets, write checks, pays rent, bills, goes to bank), collects and keeps track of income   1
2.   Manages day-to-day purchases, but needs help with banking, major purchases, etc.   1
3.   Incapable of handling money   0

From Lawton MP, Brody EM. Self-maintaining and instrumental activities of daily living. The Gerontologist 1969; 9:177; with permission.

---

lated to falls, (2) environmental structuring to prevent falls and relieve anxiety, (3) impaired mobility causing decreased self-care ability, and (4) decreased self-confidence.

PROGNOSIS

Findings clearly indicate an increased mortality during the first year following a fall. Of elderly patients hospitalized for a fall-related injury, 50% will not survive another year (Nelson and Amin, 1990). Over 75 years old, previous fracture, repeated falls, and institutionalization are factors adversely affecting outcome. Individuals without chronic conditions and those taking few or no medications are at lower risk for falling (Morfitt, 1983).

TREATMENT

Prevention Obviously falls are better prevented than treated. Because quality of life is as important as length of life, limiting activity in the hope that falls will not occur is the least acceptable method of prevention. A more realistic approach is to modify the environment. Although cost may be a limiting factor, many alterations can be implemented that are both acceptable to the older person and minimal in expense. Many environmental modifications are relatively easy to perform and are presented here.

Many falls occur in the *bathroom*. Nonslip bathmats and adhesive-backed nonskid strips easily applied in tub or shower are important

safety measures. Grab bars may be placed at critical locations by tub and toilet to lend support.

Stairwell walls and steps should have contrasting colors. Railings need to be installed on all stairs for support and guidance in indicating position on steps. A piece of fabric, a knob, or some other marker can easily be attached to the rail to indicate the level of the top and bottom steps.

The need for *light* increases with age. Either the number of lights or the intensity of bulbs should be increased in order to keep the environment lighted at a safe level while at the same time avoiding glare. Adequate illumination that does not cause shadows that may be misperceived is extremely important in high hazard areas such as stairs and stair landings. Night lights or lighted switches enable the person who gets up at night to orient himself more easily to the environment and minimize the risk for falling.

Obviously, *obstructions* and obstacles need to be removed wherever possible. Extension and long phone cords can be taped down or covered to minimize the possibility of tripping. Avoid the use of throw rugs. Place furniture out of traffic pathways and adjust to the side of the older person's best vision. Edges of carpeting should be blended into the adjoining floor surface as smoothly as possible. These changes may be more easily discussed than accomplished since most older persons have adjusted to their environment without recognizing hazards and barriers.

Pets may present a unique problem in that, while they offer company and comfort, they are also a potential obstacle. Encourage the individual to use his eyes more actively in scanning the environment. Teaching the technique of turning the head to survey the often-missed periphery of the visual field can help avoid many otherwise overlooked dangers.

Ambulation aids, such as canes, walkers, and crutches, are valuable in providing stability and preventing falls. Those who use canes, crutches, or walkers are less likely to fall. Supportive devices such as braces, knee supports, and elastic (Ace) bandage wraps can offer reassurance that a weak joint is less likely to give out and contribute to a fall. Initial reluctance to use these aids due to feelings of awkwardness or loss of self-esteem may in time turn to increased security and independence when the person becomes comfortable using the device.

Acceptability of Preventive Measures
Since most, if not all, preventive measures for falls will be undertaken in the older person's own living area, it is essential that the person participates in understanding the risks and options. The older person has the primary role in decision-making regarding environmental changes. The nurse's function is to discuss methods for making the environment more fallproof, assist the individual in exploring ideas, and provide feedback. The nurse can also play an active role in identifying community resources when labor or materials are involved and the person's resources are limited. There are often community resources available to the elderly, and the local office on aging can be the initial contact.

Nursing Management of Falls Where falls cannot be prevented, there are certain nursing obligations in terms of management. Nurses need to teach patients at high risk (1) how to protect themselves when they fall, and (2) if injuries occur, how to move across the floor to reach the telephone or furniture. When falls occur it is important that the nurse or family be nonjudgmental. Many falls among the elderly are not preventable. After a fall, support and understanding are essential for the older person.

Older persons who have fallen need to be aware that it is not unusual to feel more effects of the fall on the second or third day than immediately after it. The delayed response of pain and stiffness may range in effect from being uncomfortable to being incapacitated. When nurses know that a fall has occurred, checking back with older person a day or two later to ascertain that he is still managing daily living at an acceptable level is an important action.

At the time of the fall, initiate measures to reduce local pain and swelling (e.g., apply cold to the area, support joints with elastic bandages, and elevate or rest the part). Later, heat to the injured part may bring more comfort, although the initial nursing measure may continue to provide comfort and pain relief for the person.

When risks of falls are great and the person prefers to continue living independently, the nurse can help the individual to set up a "backup situation." Many communities have a program in which volunteers call the older person at a specified time each day. If the person does not answer, someone who lives nearby is notified and checks on the patient. Electronic monitoring devices worn by the older person allow him to alert a monitoring station if the need arises. When alerted, the monitoring station initiates a predetermined protocol, usually notifying a family member or other person. This person has a key or some form of access to the home. Thus, the patient has the security of knowing he will never be left without access to assistance longer than a 24-hour period. With these types of systems, the fear of falling and being unable to get help is a less overwhelming concern.

The reporting of falls of an elderly person is extremely important. With the elderly, fractures may be difficult to see on radiographic film. If pain persists it should be assessed and resolved. Similarly, headaches may indicate skull fractures or head injury, and new or increasing confusion may suggest a subdural hematoma. When the patient relates symptoms that could possibly be related to a fall, the nurse should determine whether a fall has occurred. The nurse may need to serve as an advocate for the older person to ensure that serious attention is given the symptom and that adequate assessment and medical management are undertaken.

EVALUATION

The effectiveness of nursing management and achievement of patient goals can be evaluated using outcome criteria such as the following:

1. Participation of the patient in modifying the home environment for prevention of falls

2. Behavior that assists in the prevention of falls such as increased visual awareness or changes in shoes or clothing
3. Establishment of a daily phone call and alerting systems when indicated
4. Continued activity and mobility in the preferred lifestyle without decreasing physical safety
5. Verbalization of what to do if a fall occurs, symptoms to observe and report, and availability of emergency phone numbers
6. Use of cane, walker, or crutches, if appropriate
7. Maintenance of medication schedules and reporting of effects that may place the individual at risk for falling
8. Adjustment to changes that have been made

DAILY LIVING WITH FRACTURES

Fractures disrupt daily living for the elderly. The consequences include living with the psychophysiologic shock of the trauma and its treatment that create emotional and physical interruption of daily living. Strength and endurance are reduced, temporarily or permanently. Pain, not only in the fracture site, but also in other joints, tends to continue beyond the immediate post-trauma and treatment phase. Immobilization of a part of the body and the associated loss of function and coordination also disrupt particular areas of daily living. As noted in the previous section on falls, self-confidence is also in jeopardy.

RISK FACTORS

Both pathophysiology and patterns of daily living contribute to the risk for fractures. Difficulty in managing daily living effectively following a fracture is a major concern.

Older persons with osteoporosis and vision and balance deficits are at greater jeopardy for falling and sustaining fractures. Individuals who move with an unsteady, halting gait rather than a free-flowing one have greater risk of falling due to lack of stable balance. In the familiar environment of the home, the elderly person may feel less need for vigilance and may become inattentive, either in walking or maintaining a safe environment. The greatest number of fractures occur in the home setting.

Risk factors associated with difficulties in managing daily living following fractures include increasing age, living in housing that does not accommodate to the mobility limita-

tions of the fracture site, and absence of adequate sources of support, such as helpful family, friends, and neighbors as well as a dependable source of primary care. Associated health problems, cognitive deficits, vision deficits, and arthritis also make daily living with a fracture more difficult. Greater risk for dysfunction in daily living is associated with fractures of the hip, vertebra, and with repeated and multiple fractures owing to the extended bed rest required and the longer convalescence.

SIGNS AND SYMPTOMS

Daily living with fractures includes seeking treatment for injury as soon after the fracture as possible. Pain is the predominate symptom of a fracture and is the consequence of edema from the inflammatory response and bleeding compressing the nerves along with muscle spasms. In the elderly, indications of pain may not be as straightforward as in a younger person. Restlessness, apprehension, confusion, and, possibly, denial of pain may be typical pain indicators. The difference in response to pain may be related to usual age-related changes or may be related to the meaning of pain in the life of an elderly person. The apprehension and fear of what the diagnosis and consequent treatment may mean in terms of personal independence and living arrangements may influence an older person to deny or minimize the pain and other symptoms, perhaps subconsciously. Thus, reporting may be delayed and subjective data may understate the degree of discomfort and dysfunction.

Other elderly people may minimize bone and muscle discomforts as the expected consequences of aging. The nurse should be alert for signs of deformity, bruising, and abrasions when a patient complains of bone or joint pain, even when no fall has been reported. Loss of function, including refusal to bear weight, is an important sign and creates a high suspicion of fracture.

Because a fracture is not an anticipated event, there is stress with the sudden change in daily living patterns. As a result of physiologic and psychological stress, the older person, who has not previously been confused, may exhibit signs of disorientation and confusion. Later the patient can develop an overwhelming sense of inadequacy that may manifest itself in apathy, low participation in the rehabilitation regimen, and comments reflecting a concern about how to manage daily living when he is discharged.

Fear about the need to move, even temporarily, to a long-term care facility may be covert or overt.

Evidence that the postfracture older person is managing daily living effectively may be indicated by

Completion of activities of daily living adequately within the constraints of ability

Active involvement of family members or friends during the convalescence and rehabilitation process

Understanding of treatment plan, exercises, and medications as shown by consistency and participation

With fractured wrists, shoulders, and collar bones, clothing may not accommodate the immobilizing devices. Caregivers may see inability to accomplish activities requiring the use of the arm or two hands (e.g., cutting meat, tying shoes, opening cans, changing the bed). With fractures of the vertebra or lower extremities, the activities involved in lifting or walking may not be able to be performed, such as getting groceries, carrying objects, maintaining the cleanliness and orderliness of the home, or caring for a pet.

COMPLICATIONS

Loss of independence, mobility, and self-confidence are the general high-risk complications of fractures in the elderly. Mobility is decreased by loss of joint function, contractures, decreased strength, and decreased endurance, which leads to a loss of independence. Sensory deprivation may be a secondary complication to the loss of mobility and independence as a result of decreased socialization and variation in the environment.

NURSING DIAGNOSIS

Data collected on people who sustain fractures point to several areas for nursing diagnoses. Impaired physical mobility related to altered musculoskeletal function secondary to fracture is a general nursing diagnostic category. The concern about risk for injury related to environmental safety remains a high priority for the individual with a fracture (see the earlier section on environmental factors under Falls). The problems of immobility and areas of daily living affected are determined by the extended pe-

riod of recovery that often accompanies hip and vertebral fractures:

1. Impaired mobility necessitating assistance to meet basic daily care needs
2. Potential relocation to extended care, resulting in loss of control or perceived loss of control for decision-making
3. Pain and anxiety interfering with coping ability
4. Restricted lifestyle R/T immobility and loss of self-confidence

PROGNOSIS

Following fracture, a good predictor for return to previous lifestyle is *having been previously active and involved* so that there is a reason for getting better. The slowness of recovery from illness and trauma in the over-70 age group can lead to frustration and hopelessness. Recognizing small gains and pointing them out to the patient and family become important so that there is continued motivation to improve, rather than give up. Another factor influencing prognosis is the promptness with which rehabilitation exercises are instituted, whether the person is in bed, confined to a chair, or ambulatory. Some form of activity can always be undertaken. Conversely, it is rarely too late to begin a rehabilitative program that will influence prognosis in some manner. Being over 85 years of age carries a higher risk of mortality in hip fractures (Miller, 1990; Kenzora et al, 1984; Lewinnek et al, 1980). Postoperative complications and multiple underlying chronic disorders are associated with a poor prognosis. However, availability of supportive family and friends is strongly associated with a successful return to prefracture status.

NURSING MANAGEMENT

Mobilization Following alignment and fixation, early mobilization is a critical component of nursing management of patients with fractures. Participation of the patient and family in planning for the return to prefracture mobility is vital. The challenge for the nurse and the patient is in finding activities that will help the patient retain and regain strength, flexibility, and endurance that are within present capabilities and are of sufficient interest to maintain consistent progression. Repetitive exercises that are done only to please the nurse and have little value to the patient will soon be discarded. Patient participation is more likely when the person is involved in selecting activities and in devising a meaningful plan of balanced exercise and rest.

Pain   Pain can be distracting, making any task more difficult to achieve. Response to pain varies with individuals. Discomfort is not always manifested in complaints but sometimes in withdrawal and refusal to participate. The cultural influences in assessing the patient's response to pain must be considered. Adequate control of pain and muscle spasm contributes to the person's willingness and ability to move and participate in activities. However, too much medication may make the patient too drowsy to ambulate and exercise. The response to analgesia, including the peak effect time and the duration of relief, is important to consider when planning the administration of drugs in relationship to activities. Analgesics should be given long enough ahead of the proposed activity to be effective during the activity.

Many older people harbor fears related to the use of medication to relieve pain. It is important to listen for cues reflecting how they perceive their pain and the acceptance of pharmacologic therapy as a management approach. Among the fears of older people are the risk of loss of awareness, altered mental status, risk of falls, fear of becoming dependent in terms of medications and self-care, and institutionalization in a long-term care facility. Side effects of analgesics, such as constipation and drowsiness, are very common and bothersome. Repeated explanations and reassurances regarding a drug's actions and potential side effects are needed. The rapport between the patient and the nurse will predict both the accuracy of pain assessment and the effectiveness of management.

Antiembolic Stockings   The use of antiembolic stockings remains controversial. However, for patients immobilized for long periods with hip or vertebral fractures, use can provide circulatory benefits.

EVALUATION

Evaluating the achievement of nursing therapy is based on goals that have been defined for and with the individual person. Factors to consider when evaluating the success of nursing treatment include the following:

1. Identification of realistic short- and long-term goals for convalescence
2. Control and relief of pain in relation to tolerance and activity level
3. Ability to regain use of the fractured part consistent with the desired lifestyle
4. Ambulation with the use of an aid or return to a prefracture level of mobility
5. Employment of safety precautions during transfer and ambulation
6. Involvement in physical and occupational therapy as appropriate

DAILY LIVING WITH OSTEOPOROSIS

Daily living with abnormally low bone mass predisposes the older adult to fracture, the single most important complication of osteoporosis. Osteoporotic fractures are a function of two major phenomena: bone loss and falls or other trauma that cause fractures. To safely and effectively manage daily living with osteoporosis, the older adult needs information and support to slow bone loss and avoid fracture-producing trauma.

RISK FACTORS

Lack of knowledge about factors that lead to bone loss and ways to prevent or retard bone loss increases the risk of osteoporotic fracture. In addition, lack of knowledge about the kinds of trauma that can precipitate fractures and how to prevent them increases an individual's fracture risk. Falls are a major and well-known cause of fracture, but even minor trauma from bending forward, lifting, or twisting the torso can precipitate a vertebral fracture.

SIGNS AND SYMPTOMS

Clues that the older person lacks knowledge or support to slow bone loss and prevent bone trauma are readily apparent through interview and observations. Assess the older person's daily living patterns related to exercise participation, cigarette smoking, diet, and medications. Signs that the individual may have learning needs related to bone loss include lack of weight-bearing exercise, cigarette smoking, inadequate calcium intake, and caffeine or alcohol consumption that exceeds moderation. Medications that can cause bone loss include corticosteroids, L-thyroxine, barbiturates, phenytoin, heparin, aluminum-containing antacids, isoniazid, and methotrexate (Zorowitz et al, 1990).

To evaluate the older person's needs for fracture prevention, assess the individual's environment, behavior, and medication regime for risk factors that could contribute to falls (see Falls, Etiologic Factors). Also observe the older person's body mechanics in a sitting posture and during mobility. The presence of environmental or pharmacologic factors that lead to falls, poor sitting posture, and movements that increase compression forces on vertebrae indicate the older person has learning needs related to fracture prevention.

PROGNOSIS

Prognosis for managing daily living effectively to minimize osteoporosis or live with existing osteoporosis depends on the person's knowledge and motivation to: (1) maintain a lifestyle that promotes retention of bone mass (e.g., weight-bearing exercises at least three times per week, intake of 1500 mg calcium in the diet per day, and avoidance of tobacco and alcohol); (2) minimize stresses on weakened bones (e.g., minimize environmental hazards for falls and avoid activities that stress high-risk bony sites); and (3) adequacy of pain management.

COMPLICATIONS

Inability to maintain an independent lifestyle secondary to fracture can be a major complication of living with osteoporosis. Osteoporotic fractures are a leading cause of hospitalization, nursing home placement, and premature death among older adults.

NURSING DIAGNOSIS

Examples of nursing diagnoses for older adults with osteoporosis include:

Motivation or knowledge deficit about lifestyle and dietary habits that prevent or slow bone loss
Motivation or knowledge deficit about ways to prevent fracture-producing trauma

TREATMENT

The primary objectives for nursing treatments in established osteoporosis are to assist the older adult to slow further bone loss and prevent fractures. Many of the dietary and lifestyle behaviors linked to bone loss are modifiable, provided the older person has sufficient knowledge, support, and motivation to change them. To help slow further bone loss in osteoporosis, offer the older adult information and support to

1. Participate in a planned exercise program, recommended by a physician or physical therapist, at least three times a week. The program should include (Lorig and Fries, 1990): (a) a warm-up routine (10 to 15 minutes of exercise for flexibility and strengthening, especially exercise to strengthen back and stomach muscles), (b) 30 to 60 minutes of moderate weight-bearing exercise like walking, dancing, or bicycling (if this is not realistic, even a modest amount of weight-bearing activity is beneficial), and (c) a cool-down period (5 to 10 minutes of gradual activity reduction and some stretching exercise).
2. Consume adequate calcium in the diet, preferably from low-fat diary food sources (Table 30–5), since calcium from dairy products may be more available to the body than calcium from plant sources and may produce more remodeling and stronger bone than calcium supplements (Solomons, 1986). For older adults with lactose intolerance, lactose-free milk preparations are available, and yogurt is often tolerated by many people who are lactose intolerant. If the older adult cannot get adequate calcium from food sources (i.e., 1500 mg/d for postmenopausal women and 800 mg/d for men), then calcium supplements should be taken with food to increase absorption.
3. Avoid excessive use of caffeine (e.g., coffee, tea, soft drinks, chocolate) and alcohol. Specific guidelines are not available related to caffeine or alcohol consumption and bone loss; however, general guidelines recommend moderation in alcohol consumption (i.e., a daily intake of not more than 24 ounces of regular beer, 10 ounces of wine, or 3 ounces of distilled spirits).
4. Stop smoking cigarettes.
5. Consult with a physician to discuss the risks and benefits of estrogen replacement therapy and, whenever possible, eliminate or reduce drugs that cause bone loss.

To minimize the risk of osteoporotic fracture, advise the older adult to

1. Make the home and surroundings fall-proof (see Daily Living with Vulnerability for Falling, Treatment).
2. Avoid lifting heavy objects or bending forward to pick up objects from the floor.

TABLE 30–5   *Food Sources of Calcium*

Food	Amount	Calcium (mg)
LOW-FAT AND NONFAT DAIRY PRODUCTS		
Nonfat milk	1 cup	300
Low-fat milk (1% fat)	1 cup	300
Low-fat milk (2% fat)	1 cup	295
Nonfat dry milk powder	3 tbsp	280
Nonfat yogurt (plain)	1 cup	450
Low-fat yogurt (plain)	1 cup	415
Low-fat cottage cheese (2% fat)	1 cup	155
Part-skim ricotta cheese	$\frac{1}{2}$ cup	355
Part-skim mozzarella	2 oz	365
OTHER CALCIUM-RICH FOODS		
Almonds	1 cup	75
Broccoli, boiled	1 cup	180
Corn tortilla	1	40
Great northern beans, boiled	1 cup	120
Kale, boiled	1 cup	95
Navy beans, boiled	1 cup	130
Pinto beans, boiled	1 cup	80
Tofu (soybean curd)	$\frac{1}{2}$ cup	130
Canned jack mackeral, bones in	$\frac{1}{2}$ cup	230
Canned salmon, bones in	3 oz	190
Canned sardines, bones in	1 oz	85

Adapted from Lorig K, Fries JF. The arthritis helpbook, 3rd ed. Reading, MA: Addison-Wesley, 1990.

3. Avoid exercises that require forward flexion at the waist (e.g., touching toes, sit-ups).
4. Sit up straight and avoid twisting the torso when getting up from a chair.
5. Get into a car by sitting sideways with both legs outside, then lift both legs and bring them into the car together. Reverse the process to get out of a car.
6. Wear low shoes with cushioned soles and rubber heels to reduce back trauma when walking.
7. Use a cane or walker for poor balance or unsteady gait.
8. Consult with a physician to eliminate, when feasible, drugs that contribute to falls, particularly sedatives, phenothiazines, and antidepressants (see Falls, Etiologic Factors).

EVALUATION

Outcome criteria for the older adult with osteoporosis include the following:

• Participates in a planned exercise program, recommended by a physician or physical therapist, for moderate weight-bearing, flexibility, and muscle strengthening exercises at least three times a week
• Gets adequate calcium in the diet, preferably from low-fat dairy foods (i.e., 1500 mg/d for postmenopausal women and 800 mg/d for men)
• Uses caffeine and alcoholic beverages in moderation
• Does not smoke cigarettes

- Eliminates environmental and pharmacologic risk factors for falls
- Demonstrates body mechanics that minimize compression forces on the vertebrae
- Wears properly fitting, low shoes with cushioned heels and soles for walking
- Uses a cane or walker for loss of balance or unsteady gait

DAILY LIVING WITH ARTHRITIS

Osteoarthritis and rheumatoid arthritis are not inevitably disabling; however, both conditions can impair the older person's capacity for daily living. For example, the pain, movement limitations, fatigue, and depression associated with arthritis, especially rheumatoid arthritis and advanced osteoarthritis, can seriously limit self-care and home maintenance. Fortunately, many resources are available to people with rheumatologic disorders, and nurses can provide valuable support in assisting older adults to effectively manage daily living with arthritis.

RISK FACTORS

The degree of functional impairment from either osteoarthritis or rheumatoid arthritis is largely dependent on the severity of joint involvement. In most cases, osteoarthritis is asymptomatic or relatively mild, and the older person functions with little or no interference in daily activities. Advanced osteoarthritis and rheumatoid arthritis, especially long-standing younger onset disease, are more frequently and severely disabling. Multiple joint involvement and/or severe degeneration of the spine or weight-bearing joints from either type of arthritis increase the risk of functional impairment. Pain, decreased strength, and fatigue increase the risk of disuse and deconditioning that can lead to further functional decline.

Other risk factors for functional impairment in arthritis include age-related physical changes, the presence of other chronic diseases, psychological factors, and environmental barriers (Ettinger, 1990). Age-related physiologic changes such as decreases in muscle mass, strength, balance reflexes, reaction time, sensory input, baroreflexes, and aerobic capacity increase the risk of functional decline in the presence of arthritis. The coexistence of arthritis and one or more chronic diseases (e.g., heart failure, chronic obstructive pulmonary disease,

dementia) significantly increases the risk of functional impairment.

The psychological impact of having a disabling form of arthritis can impair daily living as much as the physical aspects of the disease. Body image changes, stigma, perceived powerlessness, and fear of injury are major psychological stressors that can lead to depression and lack of motivation. Environmental barriers such as physical obstructions or lack of resources (e.g., assistive devices and social support) also diminish the older person's ability to cope with daily living and arthritis.

SIGNS AND SYMPTOMS

Signs and symptoms of ADL and IADL dysfunction are obtained through observation and the older adult or caregiver's report. Ideally, the nurse uses a valid and practical functional assessment tool to assess the older adult's ability to manage daily living with arthritis (see Nursing Assessment of Capacity for Daily Living).

When arthritis impairs IADL status, the older person may report increased difficulty or inability to maintain a clean and comfortable home, go shopping, or prepare meals. Signs of IADL impairment may include disorderly surroundings or a lack of necessary equipment, social support, or environmental adaptations to assist the arthritic person in home management. When arthritis affects ADL status, the older adult may need self-care aids or the assistance of another person to manage personal care. In the absence of adequate resources, the nurse may observe that the older person has consistent problems with mobility, hygiene, or grooming including foot care.

NURSING DIAGNOSIS

Many of the physical, functional, and psychosocial problems the older adult can experience with arthritis are amenable to nursing interventions. The following nursing diagnoses are suggested as guides for planning interventions and outcome criteria for the arthritic older adult:

Pain self-management deficit (acute or chronic)
Potential for disuse syndrome
Impaired physical mobility
Self-care deficit (bathing-hygiene, dressing-grooming, toileting, feeding, or total)

Impaired home maintenance management (mild, moderate, severe, potential, chronic)
Fatigue
Reactive depression (situational)

PROGNOSIS

The functional prognosis for osteoarthritis is quite good, given the number of effective treatments that are available (Mongan, 1990). Unfortunately, the long-term prognosis for rheumatoid arthritis, especially younger onset disease, is usually poor in terms of functional ability, pain, adverse drug reactions, and mortality. Some evidence exists, however, that education and self-management programs can have long-term positive effects on functional ability, pain, and psychological variables in rheumatoid arthritis (Wolfe, 1990).

The functional prognosis for arthritis improves when the older person is motivated to improve, treatment is given early, and multidisciplinary approaches are used appropriately. Functional improvement is unlikely when a person is poorly motivated. Frequently, treating a coexisting depression improves an individual's outlook and motivation for daily activities. Most importantly, it is essential to understand the older person's lifestyle, fears, beliefs, and goals. People are less likely to adhere to treatment recommendations that are inconsistent with their values and preferences for daily living. Early intervention is important to prevent or delay potentially irreversible complications (e.g., contractures, immobility). Finally, functional outcomes can improve through collaborative problem-solving among older adults and caregivers, nurses, physicians, social workers, and physical and occupational therapists.

TREATMENT

The primary objective for nursing treatment in arthritis is to promote the older adult's ability to manage daily living, both functionally and psychosocially. The most effective treatments empower the older adult to be an effective arthritis self-manager (Lorig and Fries, 1990). To effectively manage daily living with arthritis, the older person needs knowledge, resources, and psychosocial coping skills. The following sections describe the basic information and resources that arthritic older adults, or caregivers, need to manage pain, movement, self-care, home maintenance, fatigue, and depression.

Managing Pain Pharmacologic control of pain and inflammation is the cornerstone of medical management for arthritis, but non-pharmacologic techniques can effectively relieve pain and have proven beneficial in clinical trials (Abu-Saad and Tesler, 1986). Pain control techniques can reduce the need for pain medication in mild arthritis or potentiate analgesia when medication is required.

Since anxiety and stress increase pain, many pain management techniques use some form of mental relaxation to reduce anxiety and relax muscles. Techniques include progressive relaxation, guided and vivid imagery, breathing exercises, and distraction (Lubkin, 1990). Readers are referred to McCaffery and Beebe (1989) for specific instructions and indications for using relaxation techniques. Information and training for learning these techniques are also available from the Arthritis Foundation and local arthritis support groups. Relaxation tapes for people with arthritis are also available (see box on p. 599).

The application of heat or cold provides cutaneous stimulation for pain relief. Use ice packs at 10-minute intervals to reduce pain and swelling in acutely inflamed joints. When inflammation subsides, use moist heat from packs, soaks, or baths to reduce spasms and increase joint mobility. Dry heat may also benefit, but use caution when recommending heat treatments to the older adult with coexisting peripheral vascular disease or peripheral neuropathies due to the risk for injury from heat sources.

Other forms of cutaneous stimulation for pain relief are massage, external analgesics, and transcutaneous nerve stimulation (TENS). Recommend massage for sore, tense muscles but caution against massage over joints that are acutely inflamed or infected. Some people benefit from the application of substances containing menthol or methyl salicylate (i.e., oil of wintergreen) especially for nighttime use. The efficacy of TENS is supported by more research than other cutaneous methods of pain control. TENS has proven very effective for bony and neuralgic pain, but less effective for peripheral joint pain (Swezey, 1990). In addition, TENS units are expensive and may be a nuisance for the arthritic person to manipulate if pain relief is only marginal.

Managing Movement When it hurts to move, the natural reaction is to cease activity

Resources for Daily Living with Arthritis

INFORMATION

The Arthritis Foundation
1314 Spring St., NW
Atlanta, GA 20309
(800) 283–7800

List of local chapters, public and professional educational materials, and publications, which include *Bulletin on the Rheumatic Diseases* (free), *Primer on the Rheumatic Diseases, Self-Care for Osteoarthritis and Rheumatoid Arthritis,* and *Self-Care Patient Booklet*

Stanford Arthritis Center Tapes
750 Welch Road, Suite 315
Palo Alto, CA 94304

Relaxation tapes for people with arthritis

Sister Kenny Institute—Abbott-Northwestern Hospital
Research and Education Department
Publications/Audiovisuals Office
2727 Chicago Ave
Minneapolis, MN 55407

Publications and audiovisuals on rehabilitation education, including all aspects of daily living with arthritis

EQUIPMENT

Code: A = Self-care aids and self-help products
B = Mobility and positioning devices
C = Clothing and dressing aids
D = Heat and cold therapy
E = Traction equipment

Alimed Inc.
297 High St
Dedham, MA 02026
(800) 225-2610
A B C

Bruce Medical Supply
411 Waverly Oaks Rd
PO Box 9166
Waltham, MA 92254
(800) 225-8446
(800) 342-8955 (in MA)
A B D

(Continued)

Resources for Daily Living with Arthritis (*Continued*)

FashionAble for Better Living, Inc.
5 Crescent Ave
Rocky Hill, NJ 08533
  A B C D

Graham-Field, Inc.
415 2nd Ave
New Hyde Park, NY 11040
(800) 645-8176
  A B C D E

J.T. Posey Company
5635 Peck
Arcada, CA 91006
(818) 443-3143
  A B C

Medline Industries, Inc.
1200 Town Line Rd
Mundelein, IL 60060
  A B C D

Sammons, Inc.
PO Box 32
Brookfield, IL 60513
(800) 323-5547
  A B C D

Truform Orthotics and Prosthetics
3960 Rosslyn Dr
Cincinnati, OH 45209
(513) 271-4594
  A B D E

and overprotect painful joints. However, disuse soon leads to movement limitations, more pain and stiffness, contractures, and immobility. Individuals with arthritis can minimize or prevent these problems with effective body mechanics and exercise.

Proper body mechanics are simple but sometimes overlooked principles that nurses can teach older adults to decrease joint stress, pain, and fatigue (Table 30–6). Basic principles such as proper body alignment, frequent position changes, and efficient load distribution can prevent unnecessary joint stress and fatigue. Whenever possible, older adults who are overweight should be encouraged to lose weight.

Assistive devices for walking provide stability and decrease load on weight-bearing joints. For unilateral hip or knee involvement, a cane should be used on the unaffected side. When arthritis affects the hips or knees bilaterally, a walker is the appliance of choice. To facilitate good posture and balance, canes and walkers need to be the correct height. As a general rule, there should be 20 to 30 degrees flexion at the elbow when the individual is standing in good posture with a cane or walker.

Several types of splints are useful to relieve pain and maintain joint function. Functional hand splints stabilize joints and protect them from painful motion during daily activities. For

TABLE 30–6 *Body Mechanics for Arthritis: Principles and Applications*

Principle	Application
Proper body alignment minimizes joint and muscle stress	Use efficient sitting posture (i.e., bottom flat on seat, upper back straight, knees slightly higher than hips, feet flat on floor or other surface)
Position changes decrease joint stiffness and prevent contractures	Avoid prolonged sitting; get up and stretch; avoid supporting knees in a flexed position when sitting or lying; lie prone for 30 minutes twice a day
Efficient load distribution decreases joint stress and pain	Use stronger joints or larger surface areas (e.g., elbows, forearms, palms, hips) to manipulate spray cans, doors and drawers, container lids
Excess body weight increases joint stress and pain	Lose excess weight

example, splints that stabilize the wrist or carpometacarpal joint of the thumb can permit rheumatoid arthritis patients to do activities that would otherwise not be possible. If joints are very painful, resting hand splints maintain joints in a functional position and help prevent contractures during rest periods. Occasionally, night splinting is prescribed to reduce the symptoms of carpal tunnel syndrome in rheumatoid arthritis (Swezey, 1990). In any case, the older person or caregiver needs to know that a splint should be worn gradually at first (e.g., 20 minutes every hour) until tolerance for the device increases. Careful inspection of the skin, soft tissue, and joints in areas under and around the splint is very important to avoid skin breakdown.

All joints require exercise to maintain cartilage and optimal function, and arthritic joints are no exception. Studies have shown that arthritis patients who do low-impact aerobic exercise can improve their physical performance without increasing joint pain. Physical and psychological benefits from treadmill exercise programs (Harkom et al, 1985), stationary cycling programs (Nath et al, 1987), and aerobic dance programs (Perlman et al, 1987) for arthritic older adults have been demonstrated.

There are two categories of exercise that can benefit arthritic older adults: recreational and therapeutic. Recreational exercises like swimming and dancing are fun and relaxing and can improve flexibility, strength, and endurance. For older adults with mild and moderate arthritis, regular recreational activity and daily range of motion exercises (Fig. 30–4) are usually adequate to maintain joint flexibility and muscle strength.

Therapeutic exercises are movements prescribed by a physical therapist or physician to treat specific musculoskeletal problems and may include isometric and isotonic strengthening, range of motion, and endurance training. Since multiple joint anomalies can exist in the same individual with arthritis (e.g., pain, swelling, contracture, subluxation), exercise prescription must be carefully done based on individual joint assessment (Swezey, 1990). Frequently, physical therapists teach arthritic patients how to carry out the exercise prescription at home, with little or no special equipment, and periodic reevaluations of the older person's joint status ensure that the regimen is still appropriate.

Exercise recommendations for osteoarthritis and rheumatoid arthritis are summarized in Table 30–7. The nurse's role is to understand exercise recommendations for arthritis, to encourage participation, and to assist individuals who cannot exercise independently to maintain joint flexibility. Collaboration with a physical therapist who can individualize exercise regimes for older adults with arthritis is highly recommended.

Isometric exercise increases muscle strength and is the best type of exercise when joints are actively inflamed. Isometric exercise is performed by contracting a muscle against resistance while keeping the muscle in a fixed position. Maximum contractions held for 6 seconds and repeated 5 to 10 times is a recommended daily regimen to increase muscle strength in ar-

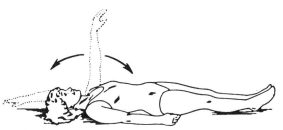

1. Shoulder
Lie on your back. Raise one arm over your head, keeping your elbow straight. Keep your arms close to your ear. Return your arm slowly to your side. Repeat with your other arm.

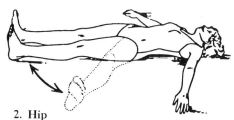

2. Hip
Lie on your back with your legs straight and about six inches apart. Point your toes up. Slide one leg out to the side and return. Try to keep your toes pointing up. Repeat with your other leg.

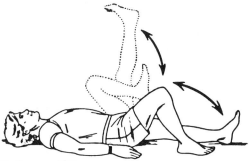

3. Knee and Hip
Lie on your back with one knee bent and the other as straight as possible. Bend the knee of the straight leg and bring it toward the chest. Push the leg into the air and then lower it to the floor. Repeat, using the other leg.

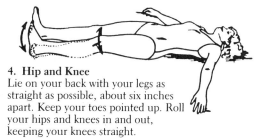

4. Hip and Knee
Lie on your back with your legs as straight as possible, about six inches apart. Keep your toes pointed up. Roll your hips and knees in and out, keeping your knees straight.

7. Knee
Sit in a chair high enough so that you can swing your leg. Keep your thigh on the chair and straighten out your knee. Hold a few seconds. Then bend your knee back as far as possible. Repeat with the other knee.

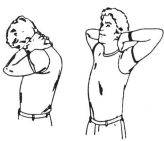

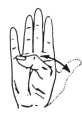

6. Thumb
Open your hand with your fingers straight. Reach your thumb across your palm until it touches the base of the little finger. Stretch your thumb out and repeat.

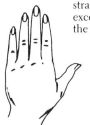

5. Shoulder
a) Place your hands behind your head.
b) Move your elbows back as far as you can. Return to starting position and repeat.

9. Fingers
Open your hand, with fingers straight. Bend all the finger joints except the knuckles. Touch the top of the palm. Open and repeat.

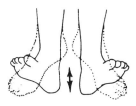

8. Ankle
While sitting a) lift your toes as high as possible. Then, return your toes to the floor and b) lift the heels up as high as possible. Repeat.

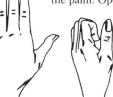

FIGURE 30–4 Active range of motion exercises for arthritis. (From: Arthritis Foundation. Exercise and your arthritis. Atlanta: Arthritis Foundation, 1991; with permission.)

TABLE 30–7 *Exercise Recommendations: Osteoarthritis and Rheumatoid Arthritis*

	OA	RA Inactive	RA Subacute	RA Active
Isometric strengthening	+	+	+	+
Isotonic strengthening*	+	+	±	−
Active range of motion	+	+	+	+
Passive range of motion	−	−	−	−
Endurance training†	+	+	+	−

Abbreviations: OA, osteoarthritis; RA, rheumatoid arthritis.
Symbols: +, recommended; ±, recommended with supervision; −, not recommended.
*Should be low weight, few repetitions, low arc.
†Should be low impact (e.g., walking, bicycling, swimming).
Data from Gerber LH. Exercise and arthritis. Bull Rheum Dis 1990; 39:5.

thritis (Gerber, 1990). Patients should be taught to breathe normally while performing isometric contractions. Because isometric contractions place high demand on cardiac output and can increase blood pressure, medical assessment of the older adult's cardiac status and level of conditioning is recommended before participation in isometric exercise.

Once optimal muscle strength is achieved through isometric exercise, isotonic exercise can be gradually added to increase muscle endurance. The physical therapist can prescribe a program of low resistance, limited repetition weight lifts to increase strength and endurance without accelerating joint damage. Isotonic exercise is contraindicated when joints are acutely inflamed.

Stretching exercise promotes joint flexibility and can lengthen shortened tendons. Active range of motion is recommended for inflammatory and noninflammatory arthritis, but range of motion against resistance should be very limited when joints are actively inflamed. Passive range of motion can also maintain joint range; however, there is some evidence from animal studies that passive range of motion increases inflammation more than active range of motion when joints are already inflamed (Gerber, 1990). Active exercise is preferred over passive movement, whenever possible.

The type and intensity of stretching exercise for arthritis depends on the goal of exercise. Some general guidelines include the following (Swezey, 1990): (1) to maintain joint motion, do two to three simple stretches, held at the maximum achieved range for 3 to 5 seconds; (2) to

increase joint motion, do a more protracted stretch with more repetitions held for 5 to 20 seconds; (3) to overcome soft tissue contractures, repeat stretching exercises as often as hourly, provided the exercise does not cause untoward discomfort; (4) to facilitate joint motion, do the exercises when joints are warm and near midday when joint stiffness is less likely; and (5) to prevent joint injury, reduce the intensity if exercise increases joint pain that does not subside within 2 hours or causes pain and swelling that increase overnight.

Endurance exercises like walking, bicycling, and swimming are recommended when arthritis is nonacute. To be maximally effective, endurance exercise needs to be done for 15 minutes, three to five times a week at 60% of maximum heart rate (Gerber, 1990), but less demanding programs can also benefit low-fit older adults (O'Brien and Vertinsky, 1991). As was emphasized for isometric exercise, medical evaluation of the older person's cardiac status and overall condition must be done before recommending endurance training.

Managing Self-care Numerous self-care aids are available to assist arthritis patients manage bathing, hygiene, dressing, grooming, toileting, and eating (Table 30–8). The nurse's role is to understand how to use and obtain self-care aids and to assist older adults to use them effectively. Collaboration with occupational therapists is recommended for problem solving. Information on obtaining self-care aids is available from the Arthritis Foundation and specialty suppliers.

TABLE 30–8   *Self-care Aids for Activities of Daily Living*

ADLs	Self-care Aids
Bathing and hygiene	Tub and shower benches Grab bars attached to tub or wall Nonskid safety strips or rubber bath mat Built-up handles for faucets Long shower spray hose Long-handled soap sponge or brush Bath mitt Shower caddy for bathing supplies Electric toothbrush and Water-Pik One-handed dental floss holder
Dressing and grooming	Velcro to fasten clothing, shoes Elasticized cuffs, waistbands, shoelaces Low clothing rods in closet Long-handled shoe horn Dressing stick or reacher to pull up pants Large rings, thread, or leather loops on zipper pulls Front-closing bras Buttonhooks Stocking device to pull on socks Long-handled combs and brushes Nailbrushes, nail files, and make-up containers stabilized with suction cups Stand-up mirrors and neck mirrors
Toileting	Toilet safety frame or wall grab bars Elevated toilet seat or commode over the toilet Sanifem, a device that allows a woman to stand while voiding
Eating	Built-up handles on utensils Plate guards Scoop dishes

Adapted from Lorig K, Fries JF. The arthritis helpbook, 3rd ed. Reading, MA: Addison-Wesley, 1990; and Dittmar S. Rehabilitation nursing: process and application. St. Louis: C.V. Mosby, 1989.

Managing Home Maintenance   Self-help products compensate for the functional impairments of arthritis by decreasing joint stress and the work required to perform IADLs (Fig. 30–5).

These products enable the older person to manage daily living tasks like cooking, cleaning, driving a car, and gardening. The nurse's role is to know the principles for using self-help products, the kinds of products that are available, and how to obtain them. Principles for using self-help products and product examples are summarized in Table 30–9. Occupational therapists can provide valuable information about product use and availability, as well as the Arthritis Foundation and specialty suppliers.

Managing Fatigue   Fatigue is commonly associated with rheumatoid arthritis, but fatigue can occur with any type of arthritis. Acute fatigue is a normal warning sign that the body needs physical and/or mental rest. Chronic fatigue, on the other hand, is a prevalent symptom of depression and many other conditions, so fatigue should not be automatically attributed to arthritis until other, potentially reversible, causes of fatigue are ruled out by medical evaluation (e.g., depression, anemia, hypothyroidism).

Assisting the older person to prevent or reduce arthritis-related fatigue is an important aspect of promoting function in daily living. Interventions described previously can reduce fatigue, including mental relaxation techniques, proper body mechanics, exercise, self-care aids, and self-help products. Other fatigue-reducers include activity adaptation and environmental modifications.

Persons with arthritis require a balance between activity and rest to spare joints and prevent fatigue. Recommend scheduled rest periods in the morning and afternoon. Although rest requirements vary among individuals, several short rest periods (e.g., 30 minutes to 2 hours) may be more beneficial than an extended activity break. Excessive rest should be avoided since prolonged inactivity leads to increased stiffness and musculoskeletal complications (e.g., muscle atrophy, contractures, bone loss).

A fatigue diary can be a useful tool for reorganizing schedules based on fatigue patterns (Piper, 1986). Suggest that the individual record activities and fatigue levels on a 24-hour basis for 1 week, then identify sources of fatigue that can be eliminated or rearranged to conserve energy. Finding a balance between activity and rest is the key to reducing fatigue while maintaining functional abilities.

Environmental modifications can also help

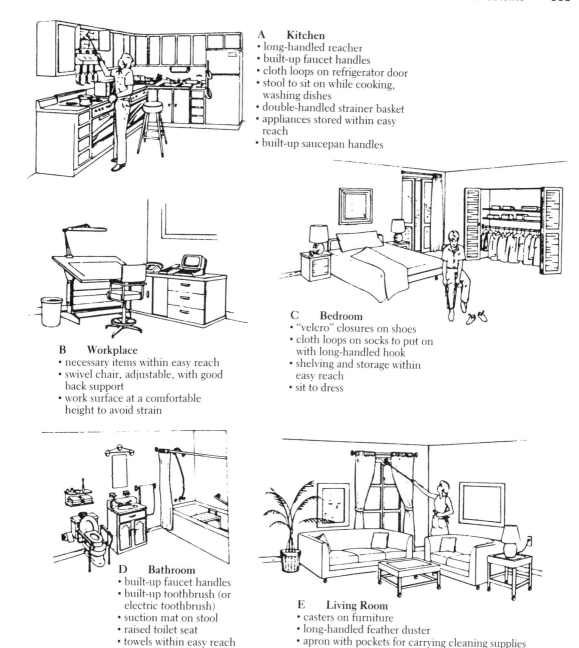

A   Kitchen
- long-handled reacher
- built-up faucet handles
- cloth loops on refrigerator door
- stool to sit on while cooking, washing dishes
- double-handled strainer basket
- appliances stored within easy reach
- built-up saucepan handles

B   Workplace
- necessary items within easy reach
- swivel chair, adjustable, with good back support
- work surface at a comfortable height to avoid strain

C   Bedroom
- "velcro" closures on shoes
- cloth loops on socks to put on with long-handled hook
- shelving and storage within easy reach
- sit to dress

D   Bathroom
- built-up faucet handles
- built-up toothbrush (or electric toothbrush)
- suction mat on stool
- raised toilet seat
- towels within easy reach

E   Living Room
- casters on furniture
- long-handled feather duster
- apron with pockets for carrying cleaning supplies

FIGURE 30–5   Ways to simplify work. (From: Arthritis Foundation. Taking care: Protecting your joints and saving your energy. Atlanta: Arthritis Foundation, 1990; with permission.)

the older person conserve energy and reduce fatigue. Rearranging frequently used items for easy access can minimize the need to bend, stoop, and search. People with arthritis can increase the efficiency of their environment by (1) storing frequently used supplies between eye and hip level, (2) using turntables, stackable storage units, and pull-out racks in cupboards, and (3) using pegboards and hooks to store equipment and tools for easy reach in the kitchen, laundry, and garage (Lorig and Fries, 1990).

TABLE 30–9   *Self-help Products for Home Maintenance: Principles and Product Examples*

Principle	Examples
Products that require less strength to hold and manipulate to decrease joint stress and pain	Lightweight dishes, pots, bowls Enlarged handles for kitchen utensils, writing pens, key holders Enlarged knobs for lamp switches and appliance controls Doorknob extenders and devices to open car doors with the palm Jar openers
Products on wheels minimize the need to lift and carry	Wheeled luggage carriers, trash barrels, shopping carts Utility carts to transport items in the home or at work Furniture on casters
Convenience items to minimize fatigue	Electric food processors, can openers, blenders, garden tools, typewriters, computers Microwave ovens Prepared foods
Products that promote proper body alignment to prevent back strain	Chairs with firm seats, fairly straight backs, right height for efficient sitting posture Long-handled sponges and feather dusters For lumbar arthritis, a firm mattress or bedboard beneath the mattress, lumbar support for driving Back-preserving attachments to operate floor mops, shovels, hoes, rakes

Adapted from Lorig K, Fries JF. The arthritis helpbook, 3rd ed. Reading, MA: Addison-Wesley, 1990.

Managing Depression   Many factors associated with arthritis can predispose to depression, including daily living with chronic pain, fatigue, and functional losses. In addition, body image changes related to deformities, the stigma attached to disability, and lack of resources or social support can all contribute to depression. Major clinical depression requires medical evaluation and treatment, but the nurse can provide important resources and psychological support to older adults with situational depression related to daily living with arthritis.

Providing information, resources, and support that enable the older person to manage daily living with arthritis (i.e., pain, movement, self-care, home-maintenance, and fatigue) can diminish depression by increasing the individual's sense of control. In addition, the older adult who is depressed may need instrumental assistance from the nurse to arrange for assistance in the home, mental health counseling, and other support services from the community. Geriatric social workers familiar with resources in the aging network can be valuable collaborators.

The Arthritis Foundation sponsors local support groups in many communities. Support groups for people with similar conditions can provide an atmosphere of acceptance and understanding, as well as information and opportunities to solve common problems. Arthritis support groups can also help people understand that they are not alone. Seeing and hearing others who are effectively managing daily living with arthritis can inspire hope. A word of caution, however: support groups are not for everyone. The nurse can provide information and encouragement about the benefits of support groups, but the decision to participate rests with the older adult.

EVALUATION

Outcome criteria for daily living with arthritis indicate that the older adult

- Performs functional activities (ADLs and IADLs) at expected optimal levels or
- Verbalizes satisfaction with functional abilities despite limitations

- Demonstrates ability to use self-care aids, self-help products, and mobility devices, as needed
- Verbalizes pain relief and improved function in daily living from selected pain management techniques
- Demonstrates body mechanics that reduce joint stress, pain, and fatigue when sitting, lying, standing, and moving
- Loses weight if overweight (>10% of ideal weight for height, frame, and age) or obese (>20% of ideal weight for height, frame, and age)
- Participates in regular recreational exercise and daily range of motion or
- Participates in a planned exercise program, prescribed by a physician or physical therapist, to maintain or increase muscle strength, joint flexibility, and endurance
- Identifies sources of fatigue in daily living and adjusts schedule to balance activity and rest
- Schedules several short rest periods throughout the day but avoids periods of prolonged inactivity
- Adapts living space so that frequently used supplies are easily accessible
- Verbalizes fatigue reduction and ability to conserve energy
- Expresses feelings related to daily living with a chronic, disabling disease
- Relates psychosocial support from an arthritis support group and/or the nurse relationship or significant others
- Demonstrates ability to obtain community resources, as needed, or has an advocate who can assist in resource management
- Expresses a sense of control in his own ability to manage daily living with arthritis

References and Other Readings

Abu-Saad H, Tesler M. Pain. In Carrieri VK, Lindsey AM, West CM, eds. Pathophysiological phenomena in nursing: human responses to illness. Philadelphia: W.B. Saunders, 1986:235.

Albrich JM, Bosker G. Drug therapy: drug prescribing and systemic detection of adverse drug reactions. In: Bosker G, Schwartz GR, Jones JS, Sequeira M, eds. Geriatric emergency medicine St. Louis: C.V. Mosby, 1990:33.

Barden HS, Mazess RB. Bone densitometry of the appendicular and axial skeleton. Topics in geriatric rehabilitation 1989; 4:1.

Barzel US. Common metabolic disorders of the skeleton in aging. In: Reichal W, ed. Clinical aspects of aging, 3rd ed. Baltimore: Williams & Wilkins, 1989:330.

Barzel US. Estrogen therapy for osteoporosis: is it effective? Hosp Pract 1990; 25:95.

Bauer RL. Assessing osteoporosis. Hosp Pract 1991; 26:23.

Beard K, Walker AM, Perera DR, et al. Nonsteroidal antiinflammatory drugs and hospitalization for gastroesophageal bleeding in the elderly. Arch Intern Med 1987; 147:1621.

Brandt KD. Osteoarthritis. Clin Geriatr Med 1988; 4:279.

Collo MC, Johnson JL, Finch WR, et al. Evaluating arthritis complaints. Nurse Pract 1991; 16:9.

Consensus Development Conference. Prophylaxis and treatment of osteoporosis. Br Med J 1987; 295:914.

Craven R, Bruno PM. Teach the elderly to prevent falls. J Gerontol Nurs 1986; 12:27.

Cummings SR, Browner WS, Grady D, et al. Should prescription of postmenopausal hormone therapy be based on the results of bone densitometry? [editorial]. Ann Intern Med 1990; 113:565.

Cummings SR, Kelsey JL, Nevitt MC, et al. Epidemiology of osteoporosis and osteoporotic fractures. Epidemiol Rev 1985; 7:178.

Custis K. Making sense of bone densitometry. Nursing Times 1990; 86:35.

Dalsky GP, Stocke KS, Eshani AA, et al. Weight bearing exercise training and lumbar bone mineral content in postmenopausal women. Ann Intern Med 1988; 108:824.

Davis MA. Epidemiology of osteoarthritis. Clin Geriatr Med 1988; 4:241.

Dawson-Hughes B, Dallal GE, Kraal EA, et al. A controlled trial of the effect of calcium supplementation on bone density in postmenopausal women. N Engl J Med 1990; 323:878.

Deal CL, Meenan RF, Goldenberg DL, et al. The clinical features of elderly-onset rheumatoid arthritis. Arthritis Rheum 1985; 28:987.

DeGowin RL. The spine and extremities. In: DeGowin & DeGowin's bedside diagnostic examination, 5th ed. New York: Macmillan, 1987:644.

Ettinger WH. Approach to the diagnosis and management of musculoskeletal disease. Clin Geriatr Med 1988; 4:269.

Ettinger WH. Joint and soft tissue disorders. In: Abrams WB, Berkow R, eds. The Merck manual of geriatrics. Rahway, NJ: Merck, Sharp & Dohme, 1990:686.

Fries JF. NSAID gastropathy: the second most deadly rheumatic disease? Epidemiology and risk appraisal. J Rheumatol 1991; 18(suppl 28):6.

Gambrell RD. Estrogen-progestogen replacement and cancer risk. Hosp Pract 1990; 25:81.

Gambrell RD. Estrogen replacement therapy and osteoporosis. Hosp Pract 1991; 26:30.

Gerber LH. Exercise and arthritis. Bull Rheum Dis 1990; 39(6).

Granger CV, Seltzer GB, Fishbein CF. Primary care

of the functionally disabled: assessment and management. Philadelphia: Lippincott, 1987.

Griffin MR, Ray WA, Schaffner W. Nonsteroidal antiinflammatory drug use and death from peptic ulcer in elderly persons. Ann Intern Med 1988; 109:359.

Grisso JA. Exercise. In: Lavizzo-Mourney R, Day SC, Diserens D, Grisso JA, eds. Practicing prevention for the elderly. Philadelphia: Hanley & Belfus, 1989:75.

Grisso JA, Attie M. Prevention of osteoporotic fracture. In: Lavizzo-Mourney R, Day SC, Diserens D, Grisso JA, eds. Practicing prevention for the elderly. Philadelphia: Hanley & Belfus, 1989:107.

Grob D. Prevalent joint diseases in older persons. In: Reichel W, ed. Clinical aspects of aging, 3rd ed. Baltimore: Williams & Wilkins, 1989:314.

Hahn BH. Osteoporosis: diagnosis and mangement. Bull Rheum Dis 1988;38(2).

Hammerman D. The biology of osteoarthritis. N Engl J Med 1989; 320:1322.

Harkom TM, Lampman RM, Banwell BF, et al. Therapeutic value of graded aerobic exercise training in rheumatoid arthritis. Arthritis Rheum 1985; 28:32.

Harris ED. Rheumatoid arthritis: pathophysiology and complications for therapy. N Engl J Med 1990; 322:1277.

Harris WH, Sledge CB. Total hip and total knee replacement. N Engl J Med 1990; 323:725.

Healey LA, Wilske KR. Evaluating combination drug therapy in rheumatoid arthritis [editorial]. J Rheumatol 1991; 18:641.

Hochberg MC. Epidemiology of osteoarthritis: current concepts and new insights. J Rheumatol 1991; 18(suppl 27):4.

Kane RA, Kane RL. Assessing the elderly: a practical guide to measurement. Lexington, MA: D.C. Heath and Company, 1988.

Kane RL, Ouslander JG, Abrass IB. Essentials of clinical geriatrics, 2nd ed. New York: McGraw-Hill, 1989.

Katz S, Ford AB, Moskowitz RW, et al. Studies of illness in the aged: the index of ADL, a standardized measure of biological and psychological function. JAMA 1963; 185:914.

Kenzora J, McCarthy R, Lowell J, et al. Hip fracture mortality: relation to age, treatment, preoperative illness, time of surgery, and complications. Clin Orthop 1984; 186:45.

Kiel DP, Felson DT, Anderson JJ, et al. Hip fracture and the use of estrogens in postmenopausal women: The Framingham study. N Engl J Med 1987; 317:1169.

Kushner I. Does aggressive therapy of rheumatoid arthritis affect outcome? J Rheumatol 1987; 16:1.

Lawton MP, Brody EM. Self-maintaining and instrumental activities of daily living. The Gerontologist 1969; 9:177.

Lewinnek G, Kelsey J, White A, et al. The significance and comparative analysis of the epidemiology of hip fractures. Clin Orthop 1980; 152:35.

Lindsay R. Osteoporosis. Clin Geriatr Med 1988; 4:411.

Lindsay R. Osteoporosis: an updated approach to prevention and management. Geriatrics 1989; 44:45.

Lipsitz LA. The drop attack. J Am Geriatr Soc 1983; 31:617.

Lorig K, Fries JF. The arthritis helpbook, 3rd ed. Reading, MA: Addison-Wesley, 1990.

Lubkin IM. Chronic pain. In: Lubkin IM, ed. Chronic illness: impact and interventions, 2nd ed. Boston: Jones and Bartlett, 1991:111.

Mahoney FI, Barthel DW. Functional evaluation: the Barthel index. Maryland State Medical Journal 1965; 14:61.

Mazanec DJ. Conservative treatment of rheumatic disorders in the elderly. Geriatrics 1991; 46:41.

McCaffery M, Beebe A. Pain: clinical manual for nursing practice. St. Louis: C.V. Mosby, 1989.

McDowell I, Newell C. Measuring health: a guide to rating scales and questionnaires. New York: Oxford University Press, 1987.

Meier D. Disorders of skeletal aging. In: Cassel CK, Riesenberg DE, Sorensen LB, Walsh JR, eds. Geriatric medicine, 2nd ed. New York: Springer-Verlag, 1990:164.

Miller MD. Orthopedic trauma in the elderly. Emerg Med Clin North Am 1990; 8:325.

Mongan E. Arthritis and osteoporosis. In: Kemp B, Brummel-Smith K, Ramsdell JW, ed. Geriatric rehabilitation. Boston: Little, Brown and Company, 1990:91.

Morfitt JM. Falls in old people at home: intrinsic versus environmental factors in causation. Public Health 1983; 97:115.

Mundy GR. New concepts in bone metabolism: clinical implications. Hosp Prac 1991; 26:7.

Murray MD, Brater DC, Tierney WM, et al. Ibuprofen-associated renal impairment in a large general internal medicine practice. Am J Med Sci 1990; 299:222.

Nath A, Webel RR, Kay D, et al. Training effect of aerobic exercise in arthritis patients, abstracted. Clin Res 1987; 35:566A.

Nelson RC, Amin MA. Falls in the elderly. Emerg Med Clin North Am 1990; 2:309.

Nesher G, Moore TL, Zuckner J. Rheumatoid arthritis in the elderly. J Am Geriatr Soc 1991; 39:284.

O'Brien SJ, Vertinsky PA. Unfit survivors: exercise as a resource for aging women. The Gerontologist 1991; 31:347.

Pannush RS, Endo LP. Therapy of musculoskeletal disease. In: Delafuente JC, Stewart RB, eds. Therapeutics in the elderly. Baltimore: Williams & Wilkins, 1988:146.

Perlman SG, Connell K, Alberti J, et al. Synergistic effects of exercise and problem solving education for rheumatoid arthritis patients. Arthritis Rheum 1987; 30:5.

Peyron JG. Is osteoarthritis a preventable disease? J Rheumatol 1991; 18(suppl 27):2.

Piper BF. Fatigue. In: Carrieri VK, Lindsey AM, West CM, eds. Pathophysiological phenomena in nursing: human responses to illness. Philadelphia: W.B. Saunders, 1986:219.

Portenoy RK. Pain. In: Abrams WB, Berkow R, eds. The Merck manual of geriatrics. Rahway, NJ: Merck, Sharp & Dohme, 1990:105.

Pottenger LA. Orthopedic problems. In: Cassel CK, Riesenberg DE, Sorensen LB, Walsh JR, eds. Geriatric medicine, 2nd ed. New York: Springer-Verlag, 1990:212.

Riggs BL. A new option for treating osteoporosis. N Engl J Med 1990; 323:124.

Riggs BL, Hodgson SF, O'Fallon A, et al. Effect of flouride treatment on the fracture rate in postmenopausal women with osteoporosis. N Engl J Med 1990; 322:802.

Riggs BL, Melton LJ. Involutional osteoporosis. N Engl J Med 1986; 314:1676.

Riis B, Thomsen K, Christiansen C. Does calcium supplementation prevent postmenopausal bone loss? A double-blind, controlled clinical study. N Engl J Med 1987; 316:173.

Sculco TP. Orthopedic care in the nursing home patient. In: Katz PR, Calkins E, eds. Principles and practice of nursing home care. New York: Springer, 1989:397.

Senior Medical Review. Arthritic disorders: diagnosis and treatment. 1989; 3:5.

Slemenda CW, Hui SL, Longcope C, et al. Predictors of bone mass in perimenopausal women: a prospective study of clinical data using photon absorptiometry. Ann Intern Med 1990; 112:96.

Smith EL, Reddan W, Smith PE. Physical activity and calcium modalities for bone mineral increase in aged women. Med Sci Sports Exerc 1981; 13:60.

Solomons NW. Calcium intake and availability from the human diet. Clinical Nutrition 1986; 5:167.

Sorensen LB. Rheumatology. In: Cassel CK, Riesenberg DE, Sorensen LB, Walsh JR, eds. Geriatric medicine, 2nd ed. New York: Springer-Verlag, 1990:184.

Sorock GS, Bush TL, Golden AL, et al. Physical activity and fracture risk in a free-living elderly cohort. J Gerontol 1988; 43:M134.

Storm T, Thamsborg G, Steinich T, et al. Effects of intermittent cyclical etidronate therapy on bone mass and fracture rate in women with postmenopausal osteoporosis. N Engl J Med 1990; 322:1265.

Swezey RL. Rheumatoid arthritis: the role of the kinder and gentler therapies. J Rheumatol 1990; 17(suppl 25):8.

Terkeltaub R, Esdaile J, DeCary F, et al. A clinical study of older age rheumatoid arthritis with comparison to a younger onset group. J Rheumatol 1983; 10:419.

Tosteson AN, Rosenthal DI, Melton LJ, et al. Cost effectiveness of screening perimenopausal white women for osteoporosis: bone densitometry and hormone replacement therapy. Ann Intern Med 1990; 113:594.

United States Department of Agriculture (USDA). Continuing survey of food intakes by individuals (CSF II). Washington, DC: USDA Human Nutrition Information Service, 1985.

Vander AJ, Sherman JH, Luciano DS. Human physiology: the mechanisms of body function, 5th ed. New York: McGraw-Hill, 1990.

Watts NB, Harris ST, Genant HK, et al. Intermittent cyclical etidronate treatment of postmenopausal osteoporosis. N Engl J Med 1990; 323:73.

Weins DA. Joint, bone and connective tissue disease in the elderly. In: Bosker G, Schwartz GR, Jones JS, Sequeira M, eds. Geriatric emergency medicine. St. Louis: C.V. Mosby, 1990:453.

Whelton A, Stout RL, Spilman PS, et al. Renal effects of ibuprofen, piroxicam, and sulindac in patients with asymptomatic renal failure. Ann Intern Med 1990; 112:568.

Wilske KR, Healey LA. Remodeling the pyramid—a concept whose time has come [editorial]. J Rheumatol 1989; 16:565.

Wingo PA, Layde PM, Lee NC, et al. The risk of breast cancer in postmenopausal women who have used estrogen replacement therapy. JAMA 1987; 257:209.

Wolfe F. 50 years of antirheumatic therapy: the prognosis of rheumatoid arthritis. J Rheumatol 1990; 17(suppl 22):24.

Woodson GC, Carlson LM. Treating osteoporosis: the etidronate option. Senior Patient 1991; 3:8.

Zeidler H. Epidemiology of NSAID induced gastropathy. J Rheumatol 1991; 18(suppl 28):2.

Zorowitz RA, Luckey M, Meier DE. Metabolic bone disease. In: Abrams WB, Berkow R, eds. Merck manual of geriatrics. Rahway, NJ: Merck, Sharp & Dohme, 1990:710.

31
Renal Failure: Acute and Chronic

NANCY HOFFART

Normal aging includes changes in the kidney and renal function (Chapter 8). However, these changes alone do not predispose the older person to renal failure. Reduced renal function is sufficient for most old people, it is when pathology from another condition occurs that renal failure is likely. Older people are at high risk for both acute and chronic renal failure because they have multiple illnesses and other conditions that predispose them.

Pathophysiology and Medical Management of Acute Renal Failure

Acute renal failure (ARF) is an abrupt cessation of renal function with or without oliguria that can lead to serious complications and death. There are three categories of ARF: prerenal azotemia, intrarenal, and postrenal. Prerenal azotemia is caused by decreased blood flow to the kidneys due to poor systemic perfusion, hypovolemia, altered vascular resistance, or cardiac dysfunction. Intrarenal failure results from injury to the renal tissues because of ischemia or nephrotoxic pigments and drugs. Postrenal failure is caused by interference with flow of the urine from the kidneys, either by obstruction or disruption of the urinary tract.

RISK FACTORS

Renal function deteriorates with age as glomeruli become sclerotic and atrophy. This normal loss of glomerular function does not produce renal failure. Instead, it puts individuals at higher risk if they sustain an insult to the kidney or develop renal involvement associated with another disease. This is generally the scenario when the aged person experiences ARF. Sepsis, intestinal hemorrhage, myocardial infarction, mesenteric ischemia, aortic dissection, dissecting aneurysm, and extensive surgery are conditions that place patients at risk for developing ARF. Additional risk factors for the aged person are multiple myeloma, occlusive disease of the large renal vessels and aorta, and urinary outflow obstruction due to carcinoma. Older persons also are more susceptible to renal damage from aminoglycoside therapy, even when doses are within the normal range (see Chapter 10).

SIGNS AND SYMPTOMS

There are three stages of ARF: oliguric, diuretic, and recovery. Signs and symptoms vary depending on the stage. In the first stage, which lasts 5 to 15 days, the most common symptom is oliguria (urine output < 400 mL/d), although up to 50% of patients who develop ARF are nonoliguric (urine output >800 mL/d). Decreased urine output is accompanied by an increase in serum creatinine and urea nitrogen, fluid volume excess, hyperkalemia, hyperphosphatemia, and metabolic acidosis. Patients with elevated blood urea nitrogen may exhibit symptoms of uremia such as anorexia, nausea, vomiting, pruritis, and changes in affect and mentation.

During the diuretic phase of ARF (which follows the oliguric phase and lasts 1 to 2 weeks) the kidneys show evidence of recovery and begin producing large amounts of unconcentrated urine. Only during the latter part of this stage will the kidneys begin to filter wastes. The last stage of ARF, recovery, lasts several months and is associated with a gradual return of full renal function; signs and symptoms are negligible.

COMPLICATIONS

Fluid and electrolyte disturbances are the most common complications during the oliguric phase of ARF. Patients must be closely monitored to avoid fluid overload and hyperkalemia. Gastrointestinal bleeding and drug toxicity can also occur during this phase. Infectious complications, due to altered immune response and use of invasive treatment procedures, are the most common cause of death in patients with ARF. During the diuretic phase, the patient is at risk for fluid volume deficit and hypokalemia if fluid and electrolyte loss is not monitored and replaced adequately. Complications during recovery are rare.

TREATMENT

Medical treatment is aimed at preventing fluid and metabolic complications. Drug dosages must be altered based on the degree of renal impairment. Dialysis or continuous renal replacement therapy (Price, 1991) is instituted to treat severe volume overload, metabolic disorders, and uremia. During the oliguric and diuretic phases of ARF, patients may be critically ill and cared for in intensive care units.

Nursing care during this time is designed to achieve four goals: maintain fluid and electrolyte balance, prevent drug toxicity, prevent infection, and provide emotional support to the patient and family. As the patient recovers, the focus shifts to include helping the patient re-

turn to normal activity levels (Baer, 1990; Coleman, 1986).

EVALUATION

Treatment of ARF is effective if the patient regains normal renal function. Often, however, this is not the case. Most patients develop ARF as a complication of other serious, life-threatening illnesses. The onset of ARF further compromises their recovery, and death is not uncommon. When a patient with ARF dies, nursing care also should include an assessment of support provided to the patient and family.

Pathophysiology and Medical Management of Chronic Renal Failure

An increasing number of individuals over the age of 70 are being treated for chronic renal failure (CRF). In 1989, 26% of those who began receiving treatment for end-stage renal disease (ESRD) were between 65 and 74 years of age; 15.6% were 75 years of age or older. Between 1988 and 1989 the increase in incidence of treated ESRD for 65- to 74-year-old subjects was 13.2% and for persons 75 and older, the increase was 17.9%; these increases were higher than in all other age groups (USRDS, 1991). The geriatric CRF population presents a challenge for the health care professional because of the multiple dimensions in daily living that are affected by the disease and its treatment.

RISK FACTORS

The cause of CRF in the elderly is frequently another chronic illness. For example, uncontrolled hypertension of short or long duration can damage the glomerular capillaries and in time lead to CRF. Diabetes mellitus, both insulin-dependent and non–insulin-dependent, is a major cause of CRF. The damage is due to vascular changes in the glomerular capillaries. Chronic urinary tract infections or urinary tract obstruction caused by stones or prostatic hypertrophy can cause CRF when treatment of the condition is delayed or inadequate.

Other frequent causes of CRF in the elderly are chronic glomerulonephritis and polycystic kidney disease. Cancer of the kidneys occurs with greater frequency in the aged, but constitutes a small percentage of the number of cases of CRF. Although CRF associated with long-term use of nonsteroidal anti-inflammatory drugs is not currently a large portion of the ESRD population, it is increasing among the elderly.

SIGNS AND SYMPTOMS

Myriad signs and symptoms occur with CRF. They include the following:

Changes in urine output
Edema—peripheral, pulmonary
Fatigue, malaise, sluggishness, weakness
Shortened attention span, inability to pursue cognitive mental tasks, emotional irritability
Anorexia and weight loss; episodes of nausea and vomiting
Insomnia and daytime drowsiness
Memory loss
Vague headaches
Slurred speech, mumbling
Diminished libido and sexual performance
Itching and dry skin
Hypothermia and sensations of coldness
Subtle myoclonus, restlessness, hiccoughs, flapping tremors, muscle jerks, cramps, and tics
Paranoid and compulsive personality changes, anxiety, disorientation, confusion, hallucinations
Unsteady gait, variable paresis
Transiently impaired vision or hearing
Coma, convulsions, death

The severity of symptoms and the person's subjective complaints or ability to tolerate them will depend on how fast renal failure develops. Generally, when it develops over a period of months to years (as occurs with diabetes mellitus, polycystic kidney disease, or chronic glomerulonephritis), the person will experience few symptoms until little renal function remains. With slow progression of the disease, the body is able to adapt to the biochemical changes that occur. On the other hand, when renal failure develops rapidly, such as after removal of cancerous kidneys or due to acute obstructive disease, the person will experience more and more severe symptoms because the body is unable to adapt in a short period.

Symptoms associated with CRF occur because of a buildup of metabolic waste products. The *uremic syndrome* is the term used to iden-

tify the constellation of symptoms caused by the rising level of nitrogenous waste products, although other symptoms contribute to the syndrome. When blood urea nitrogen (BUN) level rises above normal, symptoms appear. (See Chapter 9 for renal laboratory values in the aged.)

Buildup of fluid also contributes to symptoms. As kidneys lose their ability to excrete fluid, peripheral and pulmonary edema develop. As renal function deteriorates, diuretics become ineffective in increasing urine output. If fluid retention persists, congestive heart failure may develop.

Table 31–1 provides laboratory values associated with CRF.

PROGNOSTIC VARIABLES

Morbidity and mortality of the older person will depend primarily on the presence of other organ or system diseases. Individuals who have renal failure in addition to cardiac disease, pulmonary disease, or other major chronic illnesses will have more difficulty withstanding the impact of renal failure and adjusting to the treatment regimen. Psychologic factors also impact on prognosis of the disease. As with any chronic illness, renal failure demands adaptation. If the individual has support and assistance of family and friends, adaptations and adjustments tend to be easier to make.

COMPLICATIONS

Many of the complications experienced by elderly persons with CRF are due to the inability of dialysis to replace all of the functions of the kidney. The most severe medical complications include anemia, renal osteodystrophy, cardiovascular problems, and neuropathy, with less

TABLE 31–1 *Laboratory Values in Chronic Renal Failure*

Blood urea nitrogen greater than 70–80 mg/dL

Serum creatinine greater than 6–8 mg/dL

Creatinine clearance less than 20 mL/min

Serum potassium 3.5–6.0 mEq/L

Serum phosphorus above 5 mg/dL

Serum calcium 8.0–10.5 mg/dL

severe complications being effects on the reproductive and dermatologic systems.

Anemia Anemia is common in people with renal failure. The kidneys are the major site of production of erythropoietin, the hormone that stimulates the bone marrow to produce red blood cells. In CRF erythropoietin production decreases and red blood cell production falls. Alterations in coagulation mechanisms also contribute to the anemia of CRF. Uremia decreases platelet adhesiveness and places the person at higher risk for bleeding. The degree of anemia varies, but hematocrits of 20% to 25% are common. Treatment includes continual assessment and prompt cessation of any bleeding, careful scrutiny to minimize blood sampling during dialysis and at other times, iron supplements when inadequate iron stores are documented, and blood transfusion when the person is unable to tolerate the anemia. Recombinant human erythropoietin recently has become available for treating the anemia of CRF. When the drug is administered parenterally, anemia is corrected, the need for transfusion is decreased, and quality of life is improved (Eschbach et al, 1989). Patients who receive the drug often continue to require iron supplements, and care still must be taken to minimize unnecessary blood loss.

Renal Osteodystrophy Renal osteodystrophy is a second major complication of CRF. This develops very early in the course of renal failure and is initiated by the kidneys' declining ability to excrete excess phosphorus. Because calcium and phosphorus have an inverse relationship, as the serum phosphorus level increases, the serum calcium level decreases. This triggers the beginning of a vicious cycle. Low serum calcium stimulates the parathyroid gland to secrete parathormone, which causes calcium to be resorbed from the bone, eventually resulting in demineralization. This problem is compounded by alterations in vitamin D activity. Kidneys are the site for activation of vitamin D, which is required for the absorption of calcium. As kidney function deteriorates, vitamin D is not activated, leading to a decrease in absorption of dietary calcium from the intestine.

In the early stages, renal osteodystrophy is asymptomatic. In later stages the person may experience bone pain, stress fractures, and deposits of calcium phosphate crystals in soft tissues such as muscle, joints, and blood vessels.

Treatment of renal bone disease often requires a three-step approach. The first goal is to decrease serum phosphorus levels. This is accomplished by administering aluminum hydroxide or calcium carbonate antacids (e.g., Amphojel, Basaljel, Alu-Cap) that bind with phosphorus in the intestine, minimizing its absorption. The second therapeutic measure is administration of calcium supplements if low serum calcium is documented. This aids in maintaining normal serum calcium levels. The final intervention is administration of activated vitamin D or its analogs (e.g., Rocaltrol, calciferol, or dihydrotachysterol) to stimulate calcium absorption. If the combination of these therapies is ineffective and parathormone levels are elevated, a parathyroidectomy may be performed to lower parathormone levels, thus decreasing the demineralization of bones.

Cardiovascular Problems Cardiovascular problems include hypertension, arrhythmias due to electrolyte imbalances, congestive heart failure, myocardial infarction, and pericarditis. These complications are the most frequent cause of death in the aged dialysis population (USRDS, 1991). Hypertension may be caused by fluid and sodium excess or excess of renin production by the diseased kidneys. If the cause is fluid and sodium excess, treatment will include aggressive ultrafiltration during dialysis to remove fluid, plus dietary restriction of both fluid and sodium. When the cause is excess renin production, antihypertensive medications will be required to decrease peripheral vascular resistance, cardiac output, and renin production. Cardiac arrythmias related to potassium and calcium imbalances are treated with dialysis and dietary management. Congestive heart failure develops with fluid overload. The first course of treatment is aggressive fluid removal during dialysis followed by administration of digitalis glycosides (digoxin, digitoxin). Pericarditis is generally an indication of inadequate dialysis, with uremia causing an inflammation of the pericardium. It is treated by increasing the amount of dialysis.

Neuropathy Neuropathy develops because of a buildup of uremic waste products. These affect the central nervous system (CNS) and the peripheral nervous system. Effects on the CNS include headaches, lassitude, memory changes, and decrease in mental function. Both sensory and motor functions of the peripheral nervous system are affected. These changes occur most often in the lower extremities. Many persons experience tingling and restlessness in the extremities and loss of motor strength and grip. Foot drop may develop. Little can be done to lessen neuropathy, although early initiation of dialysis may bring improvement.

Sexuality The reproductive system is affected by renal failure and although reproduction may not be a concern for the 70-year-old individual, the effects of CRF on sexual desire may be. Uremia lessens libido and may cause impotence in men. Anemia may also contribute to loss of energy for sexual activities.

Skin Dermatologic effects of CRF include darkening of the skin and a yellow or sallow tone because of anemia and retention of pigments; dryness due to fluid restrictions; itching related to neuropathy and buildup of waste products; and bruising due to an increased bleeding tendency.

TREATMENT

The elderly person with CRF has four treatment options: conservative management, hemodialysis, peritoneal dialysis, and transplantation. In the past, renal transplantation was rarely offered to individuals over 60 years of age because of poor prognosis due to complications that arise from undergoing major surgery and receiving immunosuppressive medications. Biologic age, however, is not the sole criterion for determining transplant status and in recent years, several authors have reported successful transplantation in persons over 60 years of age (Lundgren et al, 1989; Pirsch et al, 1989; Roza et al, 1989; Schulak et al, 1990). Transplant, however, is the option least likely to be employed for this segment of the ESRD population. In 1989, only 206 transplants were performed in individuals over 65 years of age; this accounted for only 3% of the total number of kidney transplants performed in the United States during that year (USRDS, 1991).

Conservative Treatment The goals of conservative management are preservation of remaining renal function, treatment of any reversible causes of renal failure, relief of symptoms caused by uremia, and education of the individual about renal disease and its treatment. These are achieved through dietary and medication regimens and individualized patient and family instruction.

Conservative management is not a long-term therapy; rather it is the medical treatment instituted when CRF is diagnosed. It is maintained until renal function deteriorates to a point where the person becomes symptomatic. At that point renal replacement therapy (dialysis or transplant) is considered.

The dietary prescription is usually a low protein, low potassium, and low sodium diet coupled with fluid restriction. The medication regimen includes diuretics and aluminum hydroxide or calcium carbonate antacids (phosphate binders). Many persons will require antihypertensive medications, antipruritics, and sodium bicarbonate or Shohl's solution (to treat acidosis). Other important aspects of care include instructing the individual in measures to prevent infection—good hygiene and nutrition.

Hemodialysis and Peritoneal Dialysis These two forms of treatment are both renal replacement therapies and are instituted when the person becomes uremic. Hemodialysis is removal of waste products and excess water by circulation of the blood through an artificial kidney or dialyzer where waste products diffuse into a cleansing fluid and excess water is pulled off by ultrafiltration. Peritoneal dialysis differs in that the cleansing fluid is instilled into the peritoneal cavity and waste products diffuse from the blood circulating through the peritoneal blood supply. Fluid is removed by osmosis. Table 31–2 provides a comparison of hemodialysis and peritoneal dialysis. The selection of treatment depends on a variety of factors.

Transplantation Careful evaluation is necessary to enhance the probability of successful transplantation. This includes an extensive cardiac work-up, evaluation to assess for oncologic processes, either primary or metastatic, and tests to rule out urinary tract obstruction. Elderly patients have been transplanted successfully after cardiac bypass surgery and prostatic resection. Older persons with ESRD generally receive cadaveric transplants because most of their potential living related donors (siblings and parents) are beyond the normal cutoff age for solid organ donation. Thus, the elderly pa-

TABLE 31–2 *Comparison of Hemodialysis and Peritoneal Dialysis*

	Hemodialysis	*Peritoneal Dialysis*
Time required	3–5 hr, 3 times/wk	CAPD: Treatment is continuous but exchanges take $\frac{1}{2}$–1 hr, 3–5 times/d, 7 days/wk CCPD: 7–9 hr, 5–7 times/wk
Dialysis access	Fistula Subclavian catheter	Peritoneal catheter
Location	In-center or home	Home
Advantages	Shorter treatment Efficient removal of metabolic wastes and fluid	Requires no heparinization Few episodes of hypotension or disequilibrium Continuous, therefore more homeostatic
Disadvantages	Requires systemic heparinization Hypotension and disequilibrium occur frequently	High risk of peritonitis Fluid in peritoneum may cause respiratory distress Large protein loss
Contraindications	Marked cardiovascular instability Extreme hypotension Uncontrolled hemorrhage	Open abdominal wounds or stomas Recent bowel surgery Hypercatabolic state Respiratory impairment

Abbreviations: CAPD, continuous ambulatory peritoneal dialysis; CCPD, continuous cycling peritoneal dialysis.

tient who is a candidate for transplant receives dialysis while awaiting a cadaveric organ.

A successful kidney transplant restores normal renal function, but the recipient is at risk of developing organ rejection and complications from long-term immunosuppressive therapy. Corticosteroids, azathioprine, and cyclosporine are the immunosuppressive drugs most commonly used; generally a patient will receive two or more of these drugs.

Treatment Selection The treatment decision is made by the patient, family, and primary care provider. It is critical that everyone involved is knowledgeable about prognosis, complications, cost, and requirements of the options offered. Frequently a patient will change from one treatment to another if problems develop or the current mode is not suitable to the individual.

EVALUATION

In determining effectiveness of the treatment interventions, one must consider the interven-

tion chosen. Evaluating effectiveness of conservative management differs dramatically from evaluating effectiveness of dialysis. In conservative management the success of the treatment will be measured by adequacy of symptom relief, prolongation of renal function, and patient satisfaction with quality of life as renal function deteriorates. In contrast, with either mode of dialysis, one aims at minimizing complications associated with chronic renal failure, keeping laboratory values in the ranges indicated in Table 31–1, and returning the patient to an acceptable quality of life.

Nursing Diagnosis and Management in High-risk Areas of Daily Living with Chronic Renal Failure

CRF and its treatment affect many body systems and carry a high risk of altering normal patterns of daily living for the elderly person. Identifying the difficulties being experienced by the patient and planning nursing interventions to minimize the changes, adapt to the symptoms and the regimen, and finding a satisfying quality of life in the process is challenging. In the geriatric population this becomes a greater challenge because threats to normal lifestyle may be experienced owing to other medical conditions, financial constraints, the home environment, and lack of assistance or support from family, friends, and the community.

DAILY LIVING WITH DIETARY ALTERATIONS

Diet and eating habits are important factors in an individual's lifestyle. Patterns of eating are individualized and encompassed in one's identity. When numerous dietary modifications are prescribed as occurs in CRF, it can become difficult to follow the diet, or even to want to do so. (See the section on low motivation for treatment regimen in Chapter 24, Diabetes.)

The dietary restrictions of conservative management include fluid restriction and a diet that is low in protein, potassium, and sodium. For those on dialysis, dietary modifications include low sodium and potassium intake, vitamin supplements, low phosphorus, fluid restriction, and possible protein supplementation.

RISK FACTORS

Older persons who will experience the greatest difficulty in incorporating the restrictive diet and fluids into their daily living include those who

Are on multiple diets for different conditions
Have low energy (e.g., from anemia) for obtaining and preparing food
Are anorexic or having nausea and vomiting
Are accustomed to ethnic diets that are normally high in sodium
Enjoy the taste of salty foods
Enjoy socializing where food is a central element
Live alone
Eat out often
Have been eating a usual diet that is radically different from that which is prescribed

High-risk times tend to be holidays and family gatherings where requiring different food becomes awkward or difficult.

SIGNS AND SYMPTOMS

Older persons may report distaste for the diet, specific barriers to integrating the diet into their daily living, or anorexia. Primary caregivers or those who prepare food for the person may also report difficulties in meal planning when one person is restricted and others are not.

When an elderly person is not eating according to the prescribed regimen, laboratory values and clinical symptoms serve as indicators of dietary difficulties. Signs and symptoms of fluid overload that may indicate *inability to restrict fluids* include edema, weight gain greater than 2 to 2.5 kg between dialysis treatments, hypertension, shortness of breath, orthopnea, and crackles. An elevated serum potassium level may indicate excess potassium intake, although other conditions such as internal bleeding or tissue damage may also cause it. A diet recall will be required to help confirm the cause of hyperkalemia. If the potassium rises above 6.5 to 7 mEq/L the patient may present with muscle weakness and an irregular heart rate that appears as premature ventricular contractions on electrocardiography and may progress to ventricular tachycardia. In contrast, hyperphosphatemia and hypocalcemia are most often asymptomatic. Instead, monthly serum levels of calcium and phosphorus coupled with annual or semiannual radiographic examinations are needed to assess for problems. Low serum proteins indicate inadequate protein intake. Frequently individuals with CRF lose their appetite for protein. In peritoneal dialysis, protein is lost across the peritoneal membrane and most often results in low serum albumin levels. When serum proteins are low, the body's immune function is impaired and wound healing is delayed.

PROGNOSTIC VARIABLES

The likelihood of difficulty in following the dietary prescription increases with a number of factors. One that is present in many households where more than one elderly person lives is housemates who have opposing dietary prescriptions because they suffer from different medical illnesses. For example, one of the housemates may be on diuretics and be required to follow a high potassium diet. The individual on dialysis will require a low potassium diet. The difficulty of shopping and cooking with opposing meal patterns is more than many persons can handle. In one study, however, dietary compliance was higher for patients who lived with another adult (McKevitt et al, 1986).

Cultural preferences and dietary patterns that have been practiced for a lifetime also make adherence to the diet more difficult. For example, many Asian people will find it difficult to stay on a low sodium diet because of their liberal use of soy sauce and monosodium glutamate in cooking. For patients who are accustomed to eating most meals in a restaurant, it will be more difficult to stay within recommended guidelines. Individuals who have more than one diet to follow due to more than one medical condition face some of the greatest challenges in following their diet. This is best exemplified by the diabetic person who is also on dialysis.

COMPLICATIONS

Complications for the older person who does not understand the diet or does not follow it include malnutrition, signs and symptoms of uremia, the cardiovascular and bone complications identified earlier, and decreased resistance and ability to recover from other pathology.

TREATMENT

Assessment   An initial assessment and determination of the individual's motivation and supports for following the diet will be important. Assess factors such as food preferences, financial resources, cooking facilities and skills, and the meaning of food in the person's life. Once a thorough assessment is completed, make the diagnosis and plan interventions.

Dietary Instruction   Dialysis patients are at risk for malnutrition because of the difficult dietary regimen and poor appetite. Maintaining a nourishing and enjoyable diet within the limitations necessary can best be accomplished through careful dietary instruction of both patient and family and continual reinforcement and encouragement.

First and foremost will be provision of *usable* practical dietary information to the patient and others who may be involved in preparing meals. Make sure they understand how to follow the diet, given their lifestyle and circumstances. This will include negotiating which foods must be omitted, which can be eaten in

moderation, and which are unrestricted. When possible, provide strategies for eating even the most restricted foods on rare occasions, in small amounts. Teaching those who eat in a restaurant how to select restricted foods from a menu or how to deal with pressures to eat when in a social situation can be very helpful. Role playing can be used as a teaching method.

Explore the financial situation and suggest economical foods that provide the necessary nutrients and are acceptable to the person. When it is appropriate refer the person to resources such as Meals on Wheels and senior citizens centers that serve meals. Investigate possible third party payers for special dietary supplements may be necessary and will certainly aid in achieving adherence. Teach the patient some simple strategies for adherence. For example, suggestions that may help the individual control thirst and decrease fluid intake include the following:

Sucking on ice chips, cold sliced fruit, lemon wedges, or hard candy
Using spray mouthwash, sports gum, or rinsing with cold water to relieve dryness
Adding lemon juice to drinking water or water used to make ice cubes
Taking medications with meals
Using small cups and glasses for beverages

EVALUATION

Success in managing the diet effectively in daily living can be monitored in body weight—continual loss or interdialysis gains indicate problems. Diet intake reports and anthropometric measurements provide additional valuable information. Serum levels of phosphorus, calcium, albumin, and potassium are monitored. The older person's report of appetite and satisfaction and success in living with the dietary alterations are important criteria for evaluation.

DAILY LIVING WITH LOW ENERGY

The anemia that accompanies CRF and dialysis contributes to a state of lethargy, easy fatigue, and low energy. Anemia and fatigue are worsened if the person experiences undiagnosed or uncontrolled blood loss. Hematocrits in the low range also contribute to difficulty in sleeping, which further contributes to low energy. Low energy is more common for hemodialysis patients than for peritoneal dialysis patients because anemia is generally less severe with peritoneal dialysis. Patients receiving recombinant human erythropoietin have improved energy levels and are more likely to return to normal levels of activity (Canadian Erythropoietin Study Group, 1989; Evans et al, 1989).

RISK FACTORS

Low energy will be more of a problem for individuals with responsibilities for home maintenance, food preparation, and care of others. Factors in the physical environment also will affect the ability to adapt to low levels of energy. These include numerous stairs in the home and hills or inclines on the way to places the individual may visit. Use of public transportation that is inconvenient and difficult to access (e.g., boarding buses) can cause problems. From a social or recreational standpoint, if the individual has been involved in physical activities it may be harder to have to adjust to the constraints of low energy.

Because all individuals have a time of day during which they are likely to be active and also have different biologic rhythms, the high-risk times will vary from person to person. Some may find they tire quickly in the evening, others in the morning. Often, dialysis patients experience fatigue before treatment because fluid excess may cause respiratory difficulties. Most will be tired immediately following treatment because of rapid changes in body chemistries and fluid removal.

SIGNS AND SYMPTOMS

The older person may complain of fatigue (needing increased sleep and rest), inability to sleep, and depression at the inability to participate in desired activities. Another complaint is increased sensitivity to heat and cold. Often grooming and appearance deteriorate. There may be failure to keep appointments for health care and other activities. Some patients lose interest in eating. Frequently there is depression due to unhappiness with the state of inactivity and a feeling of powerlessness over the situation.

PROGNOSTIC VARIABLES

Low energy will be harder to adapt to if the person has other physical limitations such as muscle weakness, arthritis, cardiac disease or angina, or requires a cane or walker to ambulate.

A sedentary life before onset may predict continued inactivity, but it also may be less stressful to the person. Climate and weather also contribute to both inactivity and frustration with low energy. Extremes of cold and snow in the winter and the heat and humidity of warmer climates may cause undue fatigue.

Managing daily living with fatigue tends to be contingent on daily living requirements, the presence of personal support systems in the home, convenient environment and transportation, and easy access to facilities and services.

COMPLICATIONS

Frustration with inactivity can contribute to depression and a downward spiral in initiative and self-care. Inactivity itself contributes to declines in strength and predisposition to falls, with resultant bruises and fractures. If falls occur near the time of a dialysis treatment, excessive bleeding may result due to anticoagulation. Healing is slow because of poor nutrition; infections may develop. It is not uncommon for the older person to become increasingly socially isolated.

TREATMENT

The first step in providing nursing care for the person with low energy is to assess for and treat blood loss and to increase the hematocrit. Assess for signs of blood loss such as occult blood in the stools, frequent nosebleeds, and bleeding associated with anticoagulation. Also assess whether an iron supplement is needed and make appropriate suggestion to the physician. Observe for other conditions that could contribute to low energy such as stress, lack of sleep, or shortness of breath related to pulmonary edema.

When the physiologic problems have been investigated and treatment initiated, assess environmental and social considerations. Help the person determine which activities should receive high priority and which times of day are higher energy times. Then help to plan a schedule to use energy most efficiently. This may mean eliminating activities that the individual does not enjoy but has done merely out of habit. It may mean doing a favorite activity at a different time of day. In addition to rearranging activities the person is encouraged to pace them, allowing a short rest period as often as necessary or at the *first* sign of fatigue. If the person also is responsible for the care of others, help assess the feasibility of continuing this activity. Are there others who could assume or assist in this task? For all activities assess external resources for support. Are there grocery stores that accept telephone orders and deliver? Does the person belong to a church or social group that provides transportation for medical appointments? Does the public transportation system have special services for the elderly? External resources such as these can relieve many of the constraints imposed by low energy.

EVALUATION

Criteria for evaluating adaptation to low energy will include assessment of the level of activity. The person should be able to participate in activities that bring enjoyment, in addition to performing the normal required activities of daily living. Patient satisfaction with the activity level will indicate successful adaptation and adjustment. Another important determinant of success is mobility without injury.

DAILY LIVING WITH MEDICATION TAKING

The patient with CRF is required to take many medications because of the inability of dialysis to replace normal kidney functions. This is compounded in older persons because they may be taking medications for other medical problems. Medication handling by the body is altered with both age and renal failure (see Chapter 10, Medications).

RISK FACTORS

The elderly person may find it difficult to follow the medication regimen because of forgetfulness, complexity of the regimen, lack of a usable system for ensuring correct medication taking, and intolerable side effects of drugs.

High-risk times for elderly patients are those when

Medications are changed frequently
New medications are added to the regimen
Stressful situations are occurring in the person's life

SIGNS AND SYMPTOMS

Manifestations of difficulty in incorporating medication taking effectively into daily living include the following:

Complaints about having to take "too many medications"
Questions regarding medications
Not having prescriptions refilled with expected frequency
Persistence of symptoms of the condition for which the medication was prescribed
Failure to report significant side effects promptly

PROGNOSTIC VARIABLES

Forgetfulness or a variable schedule of activities alerts the nurse to potential for failure in following the medication regimen. The greater the number of medications taken and the more varied the schedule for administration, the greater the chance for error. A lack of understanding of the importance of the medications or a failure to value medications also may preclude following the regimen.

COMPLICATIONS

If the patient takes medications less frequently or in smaller doses than prescribed there will be inadequate resolution of the problems for which they were prescribed. In contrast, if the medications are being taken in greater doses or frequency than prescribed there may be drug overdose, toxicity, or interactions. Overcompliance—taking the drug despite the appearance of adverse side effects and failing to report the signs and symptoms to the health care provider—can result in unnecessary and dangerous risks to health.

TREATMENT

Assisting the geriatric patient to follow the medication regimen requires careful instruction, reinforcement of instruction, and development of aids or reminders to make the task easier. Do not overload the person with too much information. Begin instruction with the essential information, for example, when to take each drug. If the label reads, "Take 1 tablet with each meal and at bedtime," assess how many meals the person eats and when they eat. It may be necessary, if the drug is to be taken four times each day and the person eats only two times, to alter the wording of the prescription. Other essential information is the name of the drug, a simple explanation of its purpose (no more than one sentence initially), and any problems or reactions to observe for (limit to major items to which the individual is susceptible). Give general instructions that apply to the taking of any medications, including reporting to the nurse or physician any side effects. It is important the individual understand that all old medications and medication bottles must be discarded.

Careful monitoring for side effects, interactions, and complications of medications is a major nursing role. The nurse will probably be communicating with the patient on a more frequent basis than other health care professionals and is in the best position to identify problems early. In the elderly person with renal failure, sedative and analgesic medications have a tendency to cause excess sedation and confusion. At the first sign of these symptoms, assure the person that the problem is not related to medication overuse. Periodically question the person about over-the-counter medications that might be self-prescribed. Remind the person not to take over-the-counter drugs or treatments unless he has checked with the nurse or physician. Table 31–3 identifies medications that commonly are prescribed and those that require dosage alteration or are contraindicated

TABLE 31–3 *Medication Usage in Chronic Renal Failure*

Medication	*Rationale*
MEDICATIONS COMMONLY PRESCRIBED FOR DIALYSIS PATIENTS	
Vitamins B and C Folic acid	Replace water-soluble vitamins lost through the dialyzer during dialysis
Aluminum hydroxide or calcium carbonate antacids	Bind with phosphorus in the gastrointestinal tract to maintain normal serum phosphorus levels
Antihypertensive agents	Control hypertension that is nonresponsive to sodium and fluid restriction
MEDICATIONS CONTRAINDICATED FOR DIALYSIS PATIENTS	
Aspirin	Increases the risk of blood loss and gastrointestinal bleeding in patients who are already at high risk due to platelet dysfunction and gastrointestinal irritability
Magnesium-containing antacids	Magnesium from the antacid is absorbed, serum magnesium levels rise and may lead to toxicity
Tetracyclines	Increase the catabolic rate that results in rise in BUN and uremic symptoms
Acetohexamide Chlorpropamide	May accumulate and cause prolonged hypoglycemia
MEDICATIONS THAT NEED DOSAGE MODIFICATIONS	
Digoxin	Dosage is decreased and/or interval is increased due to risk of drug accumulation and toxicity
Antibiotics	Many require decrease in dose and an increase in the interval due to possible accumulation and toxicity. Some people will require administration of a supplemental dose following dialysis because they are removed as they pass through the dialyzer. Those antibiotics that are sodium or potassium salts must be given with caution for they may lead to hypernatremia or hyperkalemia
Insulin	Dosage generally needs to be reduced since it is partially metabolized by the kidneys
Narcotics, sedatives, and barbiturates	Individuals with CRF frequently show an increased sensitivity to these drugs. It is important to observe for excessive sedation

in uremia. Reference lists covering a broader array of drugs than presented in the table are available (Bennett et al, 1990; Brater, 1985). It behooves the nurse to be particularly astute in administering medications to the person with CRF.

It is beneficial to establish, when possible, one pharmacy or pharmacist to fill the person's prescriptions and to assist in monitoring prescription-filling practices, educating the patient, and observing for drug interactions.

Simple aids can be developed to help the older person remember when and how to take medications. Help the person pick a place to store medications so that they will be seen at times they are to be taken. Small homemade plastic-wrap pouches with individual doses of medications can be stapled to a wall calendar and pulled off. This way the person can set up a whole week's or month's medications at one time. This system is less expensive than some of the trays and medication holders that are available. It may not help the person to remember to take the medications, but if a dosage is missed it will be picked up the next time medications are to be taken. Special instruction for taking medications with small amounts of fluid will be important and will help persons to stay within their fluid restriction. Remind them that any liquid works; it does not have to be water. Taking medications with food, such as applesauce, also may work very well.

EVALUATION

A verbal report by the person on medication taking is a first step in assessing success. Verify the self-report with routine medication checks. Have the patient present all medications and then check refill dates and accuracy and frequency of dosage. Check also for medications no longer prescribed or those that are self-administered. Careful assessment for resolution of problems being treated by the medication is another aspect of evaluation.

DAILY LIVING WITH DEPENDENCE

Dialysis carries with it dependence, both physiologic and psychologic. The patient is dependent on the dialysis machine for life. If treatment is stopped, death occurs in a short period of time. Some individuals are able to accept this physiologic dependence, yet maintain psychologic independence. Others succumb to full dependence in all realms of their life, including dependence on family and friends for all physical, social, and emotional needs.

RISK FACTORS

Risk of dependency increases when the elderly person has comorbid physical problems and low energy, encounters structural barriers, lacks money, transportation, companionship, and is concerned about safety (McKevitt et al, 1986).

High-risk times for increasing dependence include the following:

Periods of acute illness or occurrence of a major complication
Times of increased stress such as a change in living environment or loss of a loved one.

SIGNS AND SYMPTOMS

Dependence is determined or suspected by an unwillingness of the individual to participate in physical care, treatment activities, or decision making related to the treatment. The person may rely on family, friends, and medical staff for assistance with all activities.

It is important to fully assess the situation, because inactivity by the older person may be related to misunderstanding or lack of knowledge about how to participate. In such cases, instruction may facilitate independence.

Psychologic reactions such as depression, anger, despondence, and resignation also are associated with dependency. The person may express feelings of helplessness. Rule out other psychologic or physiologic conditions that may produce the above signs and symptoms.

PROGNOSTIC VARIABLES

If the older person has always been dependent, it will be difficult, if not impossible, to change that pattern. Rather, accept the reality and plan care using the lifelong pattern. An assessment of the family will be important in determining the potential for independence. If the family is one that "does for" the older person, the goal will be to maintain the person's independence and to assist the family in understanding how important it is for the person to be independent in those areas where it is possible. Family members may need help in finding other ways to meet their needs.

COMPLICATIONS

Dependence can progress to deterioration of physical and psychologic well-being and withdrawal from all activities. If the person becomes physically dependent, there will be actual loss of strength and mobility due to inactivity. This may lead to development of other complications such as decubitus ulcers. In extreme cases, psychologic dependence may lead to termination of treatment or suicide.

TREATMENT

Fostering independence begins with the earliest interactions with the older patient. Encourage the patients to do those activities they are capable of. Teach and expect them to learn new self-care activities that may be required in the course of treatment. If the older patient is physically incapable of functioning independently, do not fall prey to assuming a concomitant inability to make decisions regarding the direction of care. Taking away one's decision-making ability can take away the patient's most basic independent function. If depression occurs, help the person to assess the situation for ways to increase involvement in desired activities. Referral for counseling may be warranted. Also rule out drug side effects as depressive agents.

EVALUATION

One can determine the degree of independence by assessing the patient's involvement in decision making and implementation of care, psychologic adaptation, resumption of normal life activities, and general state of happiness.

DAILY LIVING WITH CONSTRAINTS OF THE DIALYSIS REGIMEN

Dialysis is a time-consuming activity that limits one's ability to participate in normal activities such as socializing, travel, and work. The time required for the dialysis procedure includes travel time if the person is dialyzed in a dialysis unit or treatment preparation and cleanup time if the person is on home dialysis. This time, as much as 15 to 45 hours per week, is considerable and leaves fewer hours in which to pursue other activities.

To help the person accommodate to such an infringement, encourage the use of time during the treatment to perform sedentary activities such as reading, crafts, correspondence, and visiting with family and friends. Help the individual to prioritize activities so that valuable time is not spent on things that bring no enjoyment or personal return.

Dialysis can also interfere with the ability to travel. Many people look forward to traveling during retirement and when renal failure develops around this time, the need to begin dialysis may dash all hopes of being able to fulfill those plans. Dialysis is not, however, an absolute contraindication to travel. Most dialysis facilities will accept traveling patients if they make arrangements in advance. Another alternative is the ability to dialyze oneself by going through a home dialysis training program. This opens up more opportunities for travel because many rural or isolated areas do not have dialysis facilities serving the community. There are even companies that plan vacation trips for dialysis patients and provide staff and equipment to perform the treatment while on the trip.

HOME DIALYSIS

Dialysis in the home, performed by the patient with the assistance of a family member or helper, is an excellent form of treatment. It increases the person's independence and minimizes time commitments for travel to a dialysis unit. Many activities can be performed at home that would not be possible during treatment in a facility. With the technical, educational, and emergency support offered through the dialysis unit, treatment is safe and cost effective.

For the older person, home dialysis may be more challenging to institute because the person may find it difficult to assume and learn the responsibilities and procedures due to poor health, lack of confidence in the ability to learn the procedure, or fear of working with technical equipment. However, many older patients and spouses perform home dialysis meticulously. Staff who train the geriatric home dialysis dyad must adopt teaching strategies that encompass adult learning theory and adjust for slower yet more thorough learning. It is important to remember that most older people want to perform something absolutely correctly before they progress to a new learning activity. They strive for mastery.

DAILY LIVING WITH DYING

THE PATIENT PERSPECTIVE

The person with CRF is faced with the inevitability of death if dialysis is stopped (or if it is not initiated). This awareness can be immobilizing. If dialysis is unsatisfactory to the patient, due to poor quality of life or complications, termination of dialysis may be considered.

Frequently a person will ponder this decision alone without talking to family or health care providers. An attentive nurse will discuss this concern when it arises. The patient will have many questions. These might include the following:

Is stopping the treatment interpreted as suicide?
How long does it take to die?
Is it a painful death?

Provide answers, assurance, and acceptance of the patient's concerns.

Legally, termination of dialysis is not considered suicide, but the person's religious or moral beliefs may call it that.
When dialysis is discontinued, death generally occurs within 7 to 10 days.
There is little pain. The person will become lethargic as uremia progresses followed by coma. Death usually occurs from cardiac arrest associated with hyperkalemia.

Fear of death may be more of a concern for the nurse than for the elderly patient (see Chapter 6). The nurse also can provide information and assistance in preparing an advanced directive so that if incapacitated, the patient's preferences for care will be followed.

THE FAMILY PERSPECTIVE

The patient's family also is faced with similar and sometimes more difficult situations. Supportive nursing intervention and a great deal of patience and understanding is required as the family works through feelings and decisions they may have to make. The nurse will need to draw on an understanding of ethics, moral decision making, and death and dying to provide appropriate assistance and support to the individual and family at such a time.

Living with dying, from the family perspective, begins at the time that treatment for CRF begins. The family needs to understand the importance of its role as assistants in the care of the person with CRF. The roles can be minor or major and include things such as food preparation and having to learn about dietary restrictions, providing transportation to and from dialysis or medical appointments, and having the patient move in with them or serving as a home dialysis helper. Whatever the role, it is best that the family members understand its importance and *magnitude* from the beginning. They need to realize that, in time, they may be faced with very difficult decisions.

The situation is most challenging when the elderly person does not tolerate dialysis well and shows a gradual and continual decline in health. This is particularly true if the patient becomes fully dependent or mentally incapacitated and has not prepared an advanced directive. In this situation, all decisions for care and treatment rest with the family. The decision about continuing care often will be an agonizing one. They will be deciding between continuing aggressive treatment with the hopes of improvement or stopping dialysis with the knowledge of certain death. In these cases the family may decide to terminate dialysis. If this is their decision, they will need the same education as described for the patient in the previous section. A prime desire many family members have for their loved ones is that they do not suffer. Reassure them that death due to uremia is not painful.

Nursing care for the patient who terminates treatment will be to provide physical and emotional comfort. Most often all dietary and treatment regimens will be discontinued so that the patient can enjoy the last days without restrictions. Good personal hygiene to cleanse the skin of uremic waste products excreted through perspiration (uremic frost) and to prevent uremic taste and mouth odor will be important. Use of oxygen, elevating the head of the bed, and relief of any constrictions that would exacerbate dyspnea due to fluid overload is advisable. Most important is providing emotional support to the patient and family regarding the acceptance of their decision to stop treatment. Assure them that if they change their mind at the last minute dialysis can be reinstituted.

References and Other Readings

Baer CL. Acute renal failure: recognizing and reversing its deadly course. Nursing 1990; 20:34.

Bennett WM, Aronoff GR, Golpher TA, Morrison G, Singer I, Brater DC. Drug prescribing in renal failure: dosing guidelines for adults, 2nd ed. Philadelphia: American College of Physicians, 1990.

Brater DC. Handbook of drug use, 2nd ed. Lancaster, TX: Improved Therapeutics, 1985.

Canadian Erythropoietin Study Group. The effect of recombinant human erythropoietin upon quality of life and functional capacity of anemic patients on chronic hemodialysis. Kidney Int 1989; 35:195.

Coleman EA. When the kidneys fail. RN 1986; 49:28.

Eschbach JW, Abdulhadi MH, Browne JK, et al. Recombinant human erythropoietin in anemic patients with end-stage renal disease. Ann Intern Med 1989; 111:992.

Evans RW, Rader B, Egrie J, Adamson JW, Eschbach JW. Correction of anemia with recombinant human erythropoietin enhances the quality of life of hemodialysis patients. Kidney Int 1989; 35:246.

Lancaster LE, ed. Core curriculum for nephrology nursing, 2nd ed. Pitman, NJ: American Nephrology Nurses' Association, 1991.

Lundgren G, Persson H, Albrechtsen D, et al. Recipient age—an important factor for the outcome of cadaver renal transplantation in patients treated with cyclosporine. Transplant Proc 1989; 21:1653.

McKevitt PM, Jones JF, Marion RR. The elderly on dialysis: physical and psychosocial functioning. Dialysis and Transplantation 1986; 15:130.

Pirsch JD, Stratta RJ, Armbrust MJ, et al. Cadaveric renal transplantation with cyclosporine in patients more than 60 years of age. Transplantation 1989; 47:259.

Porush JG, Faubert PF. Renal disease in the aged. Boston: Little, Brown, 1991.

Price C. Continuous renal replacement therapy. In: Lancaster LE, ed. Core curriculum for nephrology nursing, 2nd ed. Pitman, NJ: American Nephrology Nurses' Association, 1991.

Richard CJ. Comprehensive nephrology nursing. Boston: Little, Brown, 1986.

Roza AM, Gallagher-Lepak S, Johnson CP, Adams MB. Renal transplantation in patients more than 65 years old. Transplantation 1989; 48:689.

Schulak JA, Mayes JT, Johnston KH, Hricik DE. Kidney transplantation in patients aged sixty years and older. Surgery 1990; 108:726.

Ulrich BT, ed. Nephrology nursing: concepts and strategies. East Norwalk, CT: Appleton & Lange, 1989.

US Renal Data System. USRDS 1991 annual data report. Bethesda, MD: The National Institutes of Health, National Institute of Diabetes and Digestive and Kidney Diseases, 1991.

Zawada ET, Sica DA, eds. Geriatric nephrology and urology. Littleton, MA: PSG Publishing, 1985.

32
Respiratory Problems

SUZANNE C. LAREAU

Pathophysiology and Medical Management of Chronic Obstructive Pulmonary Disease

Chronic respiratory conditions challenge the coping resources of patients and their families, as well as health care providers. Patients must deal with the changes in their health that accompany this progressive disease. Family members must learn to cope with the physical limitations and behavioral changes occurring with the patients. Health care providers must be adept at recognizing the acute and chronic physiologic changes as well as the behavioral changes precipitated by or magnified by the illness. By understanding the interplay among these processes, the nurse is better equipped to establish realistic and therapeutic goals for the patient.

DESCRIPTION

Chronic obstructive pulmonary disease (COPD) is a broad term used to describe patients with chronic bronchitis, asthma, and/or emphysema who have irreversible obstruction to airflow. COPD is probably the most common respiratory problem in the elderly and is the fourth leading cause of death in persons over the age of 65 (National Center of Health Statistics, 1989). COPD is also known by these

names: chronic obstructive lung disease (COLD), chronic airway obstruction (CAO), chronic airflow limitation (CAL), and chronic obstructive airway disease (COAD).

Pure forms of either chronic bronchitis or emphysema may be present but are not as common as combinations of both. Figure 32–1 shows the potential relationship between these conditions. Although this figure does not represent the proportional involvement of these conditions in the general population, it does demonstrate that these conditions can exist alone or in any combination. In this figure, *B* alone represents patients with chronic bronchitis only. Circle *B*, which overlaps with *E*, represents patients with irreversible airway obstruction who have a combination of chronic bronchitis and emphysema.

Where *B* overlaps with both *E* and *A*, this represents patients with irreversible airway obstruction with bronchitis, emphysema, and asthma. Asthma commonly exists on its own but in the elderly is more commonly observed in combination with bronchitis and/or emphysema.

As with most of the chronic lung diseases, tobacco smoke is the major cause for the development of COPD. COPD is therefore one disease that can be prevented. In chronic bronchitis and emphysema, it generally takes 30 years of smoking for patients to become symptomatic for chronic bronchitis or emphysema.

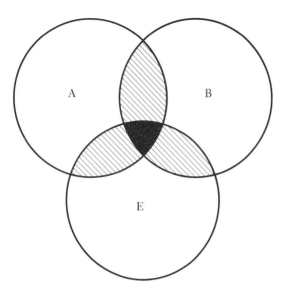

FIGURE 32-1   In chronic obstructive lung disease, several disorders may overlap. A, asthma; B, bronchitis; E, emphysema.

CHRONIC BRONCHITIS

Chronic bronchitis is a condition characterized by chronic or excess production of mucus secretion in the airways. The accumulation of mucus most often manifests itself in patients by a productive cough. The diagnosis of chronic bronchitis is defined as a history of a cough with sputum production occurring on most days for at least 3 months of the year for a minimum of 2 consecutive years. Other disease states producing similar symptoms such as tuberculosis, lung cancer, or cardiac disorders must be ruled out. Anatomically there is hypertrophy and hyperplasia of the mucous glands and a thickening of the bronchial wall. The end result is a reduction in the internal diameter of the airway, creating obstruction to airflow, especially on exhalation.

EMPHYSEMA

Emphysema is defined as an irreversible "condition of the lung characterized by abnormal permanent enlargement of the airspace distal to the terminal bronchiole, accompanied by destruction of their walls, and without obvious fibrosis" (National Heart, Lung, and Blood Institute, 1985). The most common symptom among patients with emphysema is dyspnea on exertion.

Emphysema is a pathologic finding and is a subcategory of other conditions producing respiratory airspace enlargement. Categories of airspace enlargement include simple airspace enlargement and emphysema (Table 32-1). The most common problem of simple airspace enlargement seen in the aged is a condition called the aging lung (formerly called senile emphysema). Approximately half of the population over 70 years of age develop the aging lung (Fishman, 1988). Despite the implied association with aging, it is unknown if age alone is a factor or age combined with environmental factors produce the emphysematous changes (ATS, 1987).

Airspace enlargement of emphysema is subtyped depending on the location of the destruction of the acinus. Panacinar also called panlobular emphysema affects the acinus uniformly. Destruction tends to occur predominantly at the base of the lung. This type of emphysema is observed in patients with the hereditary form of emphysema, alpha$_1$-antiprotease deficiency and can be an incidental finding in the elderly (ATS, 1987).

Centriacinar or proximal acinar emphysema affects primarily the terminal bronchiole and most commonly affects the upper lobes of the lung. There are two forms of this lesion. The first is called centrilobular emphysema and is associated with smoking. The second is coal pneumoconiosis resulting from exposure to coal dust.

Distal acinar or paraseptal emphysema affects the alveolar ducts and sacs, i.e., the distal part of the acinus. The most common condition in which this is seen is in spontaneous pneumothorax of the young adult.

TABLE 32-1   *Respiratory Airspace Enlargement*

1. Simple airspace enlargement
   a. Aging lung (senile emphysema)
   b. Congenital overinflation
2. Emphysema
   a. Panacinar (panlobular)
   b. Centriacinar (proximal acinar)
   c. Distal acinar (paraseptal)

The anatomic changes unique to bronchitis and emphysema are important from a clinical standpoint. Patients with bronchitis produce significant amounts of sputum because of the destruction of the normal mechanisms for airway clearance. These patients experience airway obstruction, hypoxemia, and frequent respiratory infections. Patients with emphysema, on the other hand, produce little sputum. Their airway obstruction is a result of unstable airways due to the loss of alveoli. These patients experience severe dyspnea and are susceptible to respiratory infections. A summary of the differences in symptoms between patients with chronic bronchitis and emphysema are outlined in Table 32–2.

ASTHMA

Asthma is a reversible condition of hyper-responsiveness or irritability of the tracheobronchial tree to stimuli. A principal characteristic of asthma is its paroxysmal nature, i.e., it comes and goes. Symptoms displayed by patients may take the form of wheezing, cough, dyspnea, or chest tightness. Caregivers must be cautious not to depend on wheezing as the major presenting symptom of asthma since any of these symptoms may predominate.

There are many potential causes of asthma. These causes have been categorized as intrinsic and extrinsic. Extrinsic asthma occurs in atopic patients and is precipitated by pollens and exercise. Intrinsic asthma occurs in patients without evidence of atopy and often begins in adult life. Although asthma can be precipitated from a mix of intrinsic and extrinsic causes, the elderly are less likely to experience asthma from allergens. This may be related to a decreased immune response with age. In fact, the diagnosis of asthma in the elderly is difficult because of the overlap of asthma with chronic bronchitis and emphysema, i.e., COPD in this population. Recently, it has been reported that there is a subpopulation of elderly patients with late onset (>65 years) asthma (Braman, et al 1991). It has been postulated that these patients have been misdiagnosed as having COPD. In general, establishing the specific diagnosis of asthma in the elderly is not important unless the diagnosis is critical to the treatment.

EFFECTS OF SMOKING

Tobacco smoke is the prime cause of chronic bronchitis and emphysema, with approximately 20% of smokers developing COPD. Smoking accounts for 90% of the morbidity

---

TABLE 32–2 *Distinguishing Features of Patients with COPD with Predominance of Bronchitis and Emphysema*

	Bronchitis	*Emphysema*
Age of onset	50–60	55–75
Major symptom	Cough	Dyspnea
Sputum	Copious	Scanty
Cough	Present	Occasional
Respiratory infections	Frequent	Occasional
Breath sounds	Crackles	Diminished
Chronic cor pulmonale	Common	Uncommon
Chronic hypoxemia	Severe	Mild to moderate
Chronic hypercapnia	Common	Uncommon
Chest radiography	Normal or fibrosis	Normal or flattened diaphragm with hyperinflation

and mortality from emphysema while environmental factors account for a small percent (US DHHS, 1984). The risk for developing COPD in a 45-year-old man who does not smoke is one chance out of 200 by the age of 60. If this same person were to smoke two packs of cigarettes a day they would have one chance in five (20%) of developing COPD. Their chances decrease to 1 in 15 (7%) if they stop smoking (Higgins et al, 1982).

The normal cleansing mechanism of the airway consists of a sol/gel layer of mucus and ciliary activity that moves mucus up the tracheobronchial tree. Inhaled substances that reach the terminal bronchioles are removed by alveolar macrophages that ingest substances and remove them via either the mucociliary layer or the lymphatics.

Smoking inhibits mucociliary clearance by paralyzing the cilia. Paralysis of cilia results in mucus stasis, which impairs the clearance of bacteria and particulate matter from the airways. Smoking is also believed to increase the release of neutrophil elastase in the lung, which may be the cause of pulmonary emphysema.

Prolonged exposure to smoke results in the permanent loss of cilia, goblet cell hypertrophy, and mucous gland hyperplasia, as seen in chronic bronchitis.

DYNAMICS

NORMAL VENTILATION

The ventilatory volume (ventilation) of a normal resting adult is about 6 L/min. Of this 6 L, approximately 2 L is ventilation that does not participate in respiratory gas exchange, i.e., *dead space ventilation*, leaving a total of 4 L of effective ventilation. The cardiac output (perfusion) of a normal resting adult is about 5 L/min. The ratio of the ventilatory volume (4 L) to the cardiac output (5 L) is called the ventilation-perfusion ratio (V/Q ratio). Nearly 100% of blood flow passes through the pulmonary capillary bed so that the ratio of alveolar ventilation to pulmonary perfusion is normally 4:5 or 0.8. There are enormous variations in the V/Q ratio in different portions of the lung for normal subjects. For example, in the upright position, the base of the lung has both increased ventilation and increased blood flow because of the effects of gravity. Since the increased blood flow is much greater than the airflow, the perfusion is proportionately greater than ventilation and the V/Q ratio is reduced

to about 0.65. Respiratory units at the lung apex have both diminished ventilation and low perfusion, but the perfusion is proportionately lower than the ventilation. The result is an overall V/Q ratio of 3.0.

Although airflow and blood flow relationships are far from ideal even in normal subjects, the lungs have a regulatory mechanism for matching airflow and blood flow at the regional level. For example, a reduction in the local flow of blood such as from a pulmonary embolus is quickly followed by a drop in the carbon dioxide level in the corresponding airway as a result of decreased delivery of carbon dioxide to the alveolus. Respiratory bronchiole and alveolar duct constriction at the site of the embolus follows, so that ventilation is not wasted on an area not receiving blood flow. Additionally, if ventilation is reduced to a small area of lung tissue such as by atelectasis, the resultant decrease in oxygen levels is sensed by the adjacent pulmonary arteriole. Arteriolar spasm occurs with shunting of the blood away from the poorly ventilated lung tissue. In this way lungs function with a minimum of wasted ventilation and blood flow. As long as there is matching of ventilation and perfusion, and the involved area is not too large, arterial blood gases will be normal.

VENTILATION-PERFUSION CHANGES

Because of the differences in lung pathology among patients with COPD, there may be distinctly different changes in ventilation and perfusion. For example, in the patient with primarily emphysematous COPD, destructive changes occur in both alveoli and capillaries. Despite considerable loss of tissue, the patient is generally not hypoxemic. The reason is the equal loss of both alveoli and capillaries, resulting in no mismatching of blood. In contrast, the patient with COPD with primarily bronchitis has a relatively well-preserved capillary bed but ventilation to these areas is impaired. The result is a mismatching of blood where areas of the lung that are poorly ventilated are still being perfused.

INCREASED RESISTANCE TO FLOW

The resistance of airflow is increased in all patients with obstructive lung disease. Depending on the severity of disease, resistance may occur in both the inspiratory and expiratory phases of respiration with resistance greatest on expiration. Overcoming the resistance to airflow in the normal tracheobronchial tree requires about 30% of the total mechanical work of respiration. Resistance to airflow is increased in COPD as a result of any combination of the following: (1) plugging of airways from increased sputum production, (2) mucosal hypertrophy and edema, (3) "floppy" airways due to destruction of the lung parenchyma and loss of structural integrity, and (4) airway narrowing from bronchial smooth muscle contraction due to hyperactivity of the airways.

DIAGNOSIS

The most important of the diagnostic tests used to determine the presence and type of airway obstruction for the patient with COPD are spirometry and diffusion studies. Tests of spirometry evaluate the patient's efficiency in moving air in and out of their lungs and provides some information about the effectiveness of bronchodilators. Tests of diffusion capacity evaluate the effectiveness of gas passing through the alveolar-capillary membrane. The two major categories of lung dysfunction that are evaluated with spirometry are restrictive and obstructive lung diseases (Table 32–3). These tests along with the patient's history allow for the diagnosis of COPD. Tests of lung diffusing capacity evaluate abnormalities in gas exchange across the alveolar-capillary membrane. A reduction in diffusing capacity is seen in emphysema.

SPIROMETRY

There are several measurements taken during spirometry testing. During this test, patients are asked to breathe into a closed circuit tubing

---

TABLE 32–3 *Differences in Spirometry in Patients with Obstructive and Restrictive Lung Disease*

Test	Obstructive	Restrictive
FEV_1 (% predicted)	Reduced	Normal to decreased
FVC (% predicted)	Normal (or reduced)	Reduced
FEV_1/FVC (%)	Reduced	Normal to increased

---

at various lung volumes (Fig. 32–2). Because the lungs are unable to empty completely, measurements of total lung capacity, functional residual capacity, and residual volume must be measured indirectly by other means. The effects of age in spirometry values in normal pulmonary function in men and women are different.

TIDAL VOLUME

The *tidal volume* is the normal amount of air we inhale or exhale when breathing at rest. The tidal volume does not generally change in patients with COPD.

VITAL CAPACITY

The *vital capacity* (VC) is the maximal amount of air expelled after a maximal inhalation. The VC is reduced in patients with restrictive disease due to scarring of lung tissue. It may also be reduced in obstructive lung disease because of air trapping. This latter phenomena occurs because the patient's airways collapse during the exhalation phase and "traps" air in the lungs. So although patients may have a normal amount of air in their lungs, this test is not able to detect the entrapment of air. Tests of diffusion capacity help determine if the restriction is due to air trapping or true restriction of lung tissue.

FORCED VITAL CAPACITY

The *forced vital capacity* (FVC) is the maximum volume of air exhaled after a maximal inhalation. The difference between the VC and the FVC is time. During the FVC, the patient is coached to breathe out as hard and as fast as possible. Figure 32–3 shows a composite of the FVC and how time is integrated into the measurement.

Individuals with normal lungs can exhale about 80% of their VC in 1 second. In patients with airway obstruction, exhalation of air takes longer, with obstruction particularly magnified during the forced expiratory maneuver. For example, if a patient's normal VC is 3000 mL, then they should be able to exhale greater than 2000 mL (80%) within 1 second. This measurement is called the forced expiratory volume in 1 second (FEV_1). The more severe the obstruction, the less the volume of air the patient will be able to exhale within 1 second (Table 32–4,

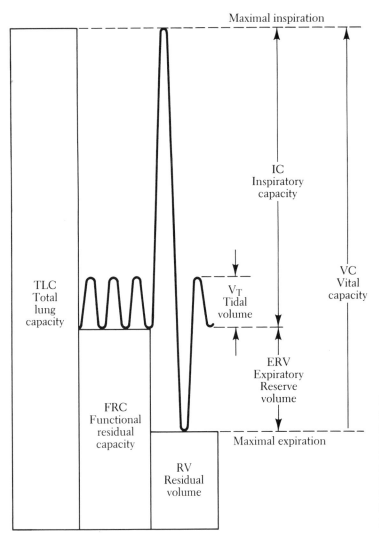

FIGURE 32–2 Lung volumes and capacities measured with spirometry are noted within the dotted lines. Parameters of lung function enclosed in bars must be measured by other techniques. (From Haas A, et al. Pulmonary therapy and rehabilitation. Baltimore: Williams & Wilkins, 1979, p. 48; with permission.)

p. 632). The FEV$_1$ is therefore an important measurement in patients with COPD.

Spirometry is often done with and without the influence of bronchodilators, i.e., before and after bronchodilator studies. Generally, the first test is done after the patient has abstained from bronchodilators for 4 to 6 hours. The test is taken and repeated after the patient has taken an inhaled bronchodilator. Postbronchodilator studies showing improvement (defined as >15% from prebronchodilator values) indicate the patient has reactive airways and emphasizes the value of bronchodilator therapy. The absence of improvement with bronchodilators, however, is not believed to be an indication to alter bronchodilator therapy.

DIFFUSION CAPACITY

The *diffusion capacity* (DLCO) is a test measuring the rate at which carbon monoxide (CO) in the lung combines with hemoglobin in the blood. The results are influenced by: how much surface area in the lung is involved in the transfer of gases between the alveoli and capillaries, the diffusion characteristic of the membrane, and the quantity of hemoglobin available in the vascular bed. During the test, the patient inhales a known quantity of CO and helium mixture. The breath is held for 10 seconds followed by exhalation. The gas diffused is the difference between the amount of mixture initially inhaled and that which was exhaled. Results are expressed as the quantity of CO trans-

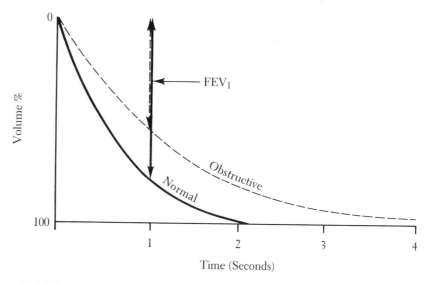

FIGURE 32-3 Spirogram of patient without airway obstruction (normal) compared with patient with obstruction. Reading the lung volume from the lowest (top) value to the highest (bottom) volume, the volume of air exhaled in 1 second is reduced in the obstructed patient. Patients with normal lungs can exhale virtually their entire vital capacity in 2 seconds, whereas those with airway obstruction take longer. (Adapted from Burrows B et al. Respiratory disorders. Chicago: Year Book Medical, 1983, p. 79.)

ferred per minute, per millimeter of mercury, or expressed as the percent of predicted value for that patient.

SIGNS AND SYMPTOMS

The cardinal symptoms of COPD are shortness of breath and cough. Shortness of breath is caused by the increased work of breathing and the cough is due to increased bronchial secretions combined with loss of normal clearance mechanisms. There is a marked decrease in breath sounds owing to decreased movement of air. The expiratory phase of respiration, normally about the same length as inspiration, becomes prolonged. Wheezing may occur because of obstruction to airflow from collapsed airways, excessive mucus, or bronchospasm. The presence of a "barrel chest" with an increased anteroposterior diameter suggests the presence of advanced COPD with resultant hyperinflation. Kyphosis (forward curvature of the thoracic spine) increases anterior chest diameter and should not be confused with the barrel chest of emphysema.

In the advanced state of disease, there may be evidence of weight loss, displacement of the liver lower in the abdomen, hyperpnea and tachycardia with mild exertion, and a low, flat, and relatively immobile diaphragm. Heart sounds may be distant and cyanosis may be present.

IMPACT OF CHRONIC OBSTRUCTIVE PULMONARY DISEASE

The physiologic changes accompanying COPD are often at a physical and psychological cost to the patient. The changes observed in patients with emphysema serve as a good example of this impact. In emphysema, the loss of alveoli results in loss of elastic recoil of the lung. The lungs become hyperinflated, resulting in flattening of the diaphragm from its normal dome shape. This change in shape places the diaphragm in a position that makes it mechanically inefficient. The accessory muscles of ventilation must therefore share a greater than normal role in breathing at rest as well as with exercise. It is important to note three characteristics of accessory muscles. First, the accessory muscles of ventilation are generally inactive during normal, quiet breathing. They become active when high workloads demand

TABLE 32–4   *Spirometric Changes with Airway Obstruction*

Severity of Impairment*	FEV$_1$ (% predicted)	FVC (% predicted)	FEV$_1$/FVC (% predicted)	DL$_{CO}$ (% predicted)
Normal[†]	≥ 80	≥ 80	≥ 75	≥ 80
Mild	60–79	60–79	60–74	60–79
Moderate	41–59	51–59	41–59	41–59
Severe	< 40	< 50	< 40	< 40

*American Thoracic Society (1986).
[†]Figures vary depending on the patient's age, sex, and body size.

their participation. Second, these muscles are not designed to be energy efficient. Therefore, it takes more energy for accessory muscles to carry the burden of breathing than the healthy diaphragm. Third, the major function of these muscles is to mobilize the arms and neck. When they are also called on to play a major role in breathing there is competition for this limited source of energy (Celli et al, 1988). Simple activities requiring motion of the upper arms such as washing hair or reaching overhead may interfere in ventilation in some patients.

DYSPNEA AND COUGH

Chronic dyspnea and chronic cough are the most common problems experienced by patients with COPD. Of the two symptoms, dyspnea is experienced by virtually all patients and has the most impact on the patient, their lifestyle, and family. Dyspnea or shortness of breath in this population is related to the work of breathing and emotion. Dyspnea is experienced when the energy requirements of activities exceed the patient's ability to sustain ventilation to meet these needs. In most individuals without lung disease, dyspnea is a sign that the limit of the physiologic abilities has been approached and is frequently interpreted as being simply out of shape. Dyspnea in these instances is not perceived as frightening and does not result in discontinuing or avoiding the activity. For patients with COPD, however, dyspnea is interpreted much differently. Dyspnea becomes a quickly learned signal to modify behavior and is frequently perceived by the patient to be a sign of impending danger. Few patients continue their activities at the same level once dyspnea begins. Activities that might elicit this discomfort are avoided. Figure 32–4 depicts the progressive limitation in activities induced by dyspnea.

Compounding the avoidance of activities is the effect of dyspnea on anxiety levels. Anxiety and dyspnea are closely linked sensations that can precipitate one another, i.e., anxiety can produce dyspnea and dyspnea can produce anxiety. Dyspnea can therefore be elicited by both physical as well as emotional stimuli. Strategies to deal with dyspnea are discussed later in this chapter.

Cough is another distressing symptom. Cough in patients with COPD is generally stimulated by the presence of secretions and the need for their evacuation. Secretions that are not expectorated can create airway obstruction. For this reason, cough suppressants are not usually given.

Increased secretions are not the sole cause of cough. Patients manifesting asthma can cough from hyperirritability of the airways with little or no sputum production. This irritability can stimulate the cough receptors. Cough in these patients is nonproductive and may be treated with bronchodilators or cough suppressants.

CHANGES IN LIFESTYLE

The disabling effects of COPD usually occur in the fifth to sixth decade of life, a time when most people are planning for retirement. Retirement in and of itself is cause for considerable adjustment, but when retirement is pre-

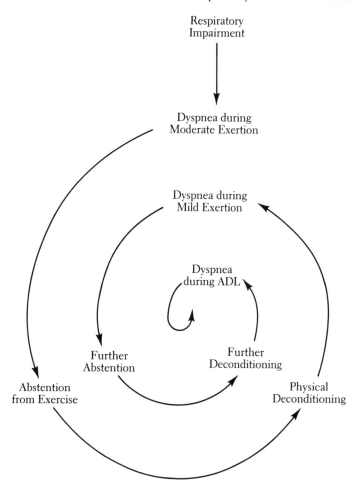

Respiratory
Impairment

Dyspnea during
Moderate Exertion

Dyspnea during
Mild Exertion

Dyspnea
during ADL

Further
Abstention

Further
Deconditioning

Abstention
from Exercise

Physical
Deconditioning

FIGURE 32–4 The cycle imposed by dyspnea on activity levels. (From Haas A, et al. Pulmonary therapy and rehabilitation. Baltimore: Williams & Wilkins, 1979, p. 59; with permission.)

cipitated by disability, the stress can be compounded.

For example, consider the patient with chronic lung disease. COPD develops slowly over 10 to 15 years; however, it is not until the patient has an "event" such as pneumonia, or acute bronchitis, that he begins to understand the long-term nature of the illness. There appears to be a critical point that patients identify as the onset of their COPD. It seems that it is at that point, patients begin to see their future differently. The focus of their life turns from a retirement filled with promise to a retirement feared for its limitations. Unfortunately, this clouded outlook interferes with the patient's ability to objectively differentiate those limitations that are a normal part of aging from those as a result of COPD.

Not surprisingly, patients display signs of depression, anxiety, and loss of self-esteem.

Whether these problems become chronic or not depends largely on a combination of the patient's inner strength and availability of a support system (both professional as well as personal).

ADAPTATION TO CHRONIC ILLNESS

The model of adaptation to chronic illness follows the grieving process described by Engel (1964). This process involves five events:

1. Shock and disbelief
2. Developing awareness
3. Restitution
4. Resolution of the loss
5. Idealization

Adaptation to chronic illness follows a similar pattern:

Disbelief
Developing awareness
Reorganization of relationships with others
Resolution of the loss
Identity change

Patients do not necessarily go through each stage in order. They may skip a stage or be in several stages at one time.

The stage of disbelief begins when the person learns either by diagnosis or change in function that he has a particular condition. This represents a threat to self. The person resorts to denial to protect himself against the impact of it. Behaviors may include a refusal to accept the diagnosis or statements to the fact that something else is causing the symptoms. For example, the person may attribute his shortness of breath to old age or lack of physical condition. The person may avoid medication by refusal or forgetfulness. This is particularly damaging to people with early-to-moderate lung disease, since many continue smoking.

As symptoms progressively worsen, decreasing activity no longer helps. They begin then to become aware of the limitations of their disease and the implications. Many patients struggle with issues of independence. Initially, family members seek to relieve patients of discomfort (usually in the form of dyspnea) by doing things for the patient. Patients, on the other hand, may react to their dependence on others by anger. They may blame those on whom they depend for care, family, friends, a supernatural power, or themselves. When they turn their anger inward, they become depressed. Their fear of the unknown may lead to anxiety about their prognosis. They may become overdependent, withdrawn, or emotionally labile.

In reorganizing relationships with others, the patient must remake contact with his support system, generally the family. The family may go through many of the same stages of adjustment as the patient. These support people may react with fear, resentment, anger, and anxiety. As limitations increase, more responsibility must be assumed, including, sometimes, a return to work because of exhausted finances.

In the stage of resolution, they begin to acknowledge changes in how they see themselves and begins to identify with others who have the same problem. They acknowledge having a loss. Behaviors may include directing derogatory comments toward themselves and over-

emphasizing or preoccupation with dyspnea. They may also seek out others with similar problems by joining support groups for patients with lung disease, e.g., American Lung Association.

Finally, in the stage of identity change the patient feels worthy of respect as a person. He begins to understand the limitations from the pulmonary disease, but the lung condition no longer becomes the entire focus of his life. Behaviors may include acceptance of the illness, and active participation in an exercise program may begin. Plans are made for the future, including vacation plans.

COMPLICATIONS

Persons with COPD are vulnerable to bronchopulmonary infection. These infections contribute to a significant portion of exacerbations. As the disease advances, patients are susceptible to developing hypoxemia, congestive heart failure, upper respiratory infections (and pneumonia), malnutrition, and depression.

Some of the most serious complications of COPD are caused by severe hypoxemia. The chronic presence of arterial oxygen tension below 60 mm Hg may lead to the development of pulmonary hypertension and eventually right-sided heart failure (cor pulmonale). Management of cor pulmonale includes oxygen therapy and diuretics.

In some cases, infection and bronchospasm can lead to respiratory failure and/or severe hypoxemia. Criteria for intubation varies among institutions; however, in general, when respiratory failure causes severe respiratory acidosis (pH < 7.25) intubation and mechanical ventilation may be required. Severe hypoxemia ($PaO_2 < 45$ mm Hg) may also be an indication for intubation if supplemental oxygen does not maintain the patient's oxygen level above 55 mm Hg.

COPD is a progressive disease. The rate of progression varies among individuals depending on environmental exposures, familial history, childhood respiratory illness, and smoking. Smoking plays a significant role in the decline of lung function. For example, in persons who have never smoked and have had limited environmental exposure, the decline in FEV_1 from 20 to 70 years of age averages 10 mL/yr. For smokers, this decline is more than twice as much, or 23 mL/yr. In the person who stops smoking at age 50, this decline is reduced to 17 mL/yr (Camilli et al, 1987).

Survival rates for COPD vary. In one study of 200 persons with COPD, 186 subjects survived after 1 year and 35 survived after 6 years. This represented a 50% mortality before 6 years (Burrows and Earle, 1969). It is known that there is a tremendous variability in survival among patients. Some patients with severe disease live much longer than previously predicted.

MEDICAL MANAGEMENT AND ASSOCIATED NURSING CARE

Treatment of COPD aims to (1) recognize and treat the airway obstruction that is reversible, (2) monitor and treat complications, and (3) provide symptomatic relief and support through techniques of pulmonary rehabilitation. Patients are best helped when all elements of care are integrated into a comprehensive program in which the interdisciplinary health care team communicates regularly and in which the patient and their family are involved.

KNOWLEDGE ABOUT THE DISEASE AND TREATMENT

Many patients with COPD are taught to self-manage infections and bronchodilator therapy. In order to achieve this goal, they must be taught the disease process, signs of infection, signs of airway obstruction (versus anxiety), and indications for treatment.

Early recognition and treatment of infection is important since some patients may experience an infection every 2 to 3 months. If patients have been instructed to self-medicate, they must keep track of the use of antibiotics, understand the need to complete a full course, and inform their physician about the frequency of use.

Anxiety can produce dyspnea, which is often associated by the patient with bronchospasm and the need for a bronchodilator. Patient use of bronchodilators should be discussed to determine their use.

DRUG MANAGEMENT

Most persons with COPD will be on a large number of drugs, probably for the rest of their lives. Because of this, drugs should be carefully monitored for interactions. These drugs include bronchodilators, antibiotics, steroids, diuretics, and oxygen. To participate in the drug regimen effectively, patients need to know the following:

The names of the medications

The purpose and side effects of each medication

The importance of regular use of the medication and appropriate spacing of the dosage (i.e., do instructions that read three times a day means every 8 hours or 9–1–5)

How to evaluate over-the-counter drugs used for respiratory problems

The proper method for using inhalers

How to identify and when to treat respiratory infections

What symptoms should be reported to the nurse or physician

BRONCHODILATORS

Bronchodilators cause a response by their action on the alpha and beta receptors of the sympathetic nervous system. Agents that stimulate the alpha (or excitatory) adrenergic receptors cause bronchial vasoconstriction and are useful as bronchial mucosal decongestants.

Stimulation of $beta_1$-receptors primarily affects the heart. It increases the force of contraction (inotropic effect) and the heart rate (chronotropic effect). Stimulation of $beta_2$-receptors primarily affects the smooth muscles of the tracheobronchial tree by relaxing them.

Bronchoconstriction in reactive airway disease is caused by both irritant-induced bronchospasm and reflex parasympathetic action. In persons with an allergic basis for bronchospasm, inhaled antigens react with specific IgE, an immunoglobulin antibody, to produce potent chemical mediators that activate the vagal reflex (Ziment, 1990). Bronchoconstriction can be blocked by anticholinergic drugs such as atropine.

Bronchodilators have many side effects, most commonly heart palpitation, upset stomach, tremors, insomnia, and urinary retention. The medication that is effective for one person may aggravate another; therefore, frequent changing of medication and dose is common. It is important that symptoms probably related to medication be promptly reported. Another medication most likely can be prescribed.

THEOPHYLLINE

Despite its common use, the method of action of theophylline in achieving bronchial muscle relaxation is poorly understood. It was once believed that increases in cyclic 3′, 5′-adenosine monophosphate (cAMP) was pivotal. Now it is believed that the entry of calcium ions into the muscle cell is most important (Ziment, 1990). Virtually all patients with COPD are placed on theophylline, yet only recently have studies been undertaken to determine the overall benefit of theophylline in COPD patients. In addition to producing relaxation of bronchial muscles, theophylline has been reported to increase the contractility of the diaphragm (Aubier et al, 1981) and relieve dyspnea (Mahler et al, 1985).

Theophylline agents are derivatives of the xanthine family. Since caffeine is also from this family, one occasionally hears of the therapeutic benefits of caffeine for pulmonary patients. Many forms of theophylline are available: oral liquid, tablets, and capsules, rectal solutions and suppositories, and intravenous solutions. Anhydrous forms of theophylline (e.g., Quibron, Choledyl) were once the main agents available. This form of theophylline varies in potency and is rapidly metabolized, making therapeutic levels difficult to both achieve and sustain.

Combination drugs contain aminophylline, ephedrine, and barbiturates (e.g., Primetene, Tedral, Marax). Combination drugs are not desirable since increasing the dosage to obtain the benefit of added theophylline also results in increased dosages of barbiturates and ephedrine.

Therapeutic level of theophylline can be monitored by obtaining serum blood levels. In general, a range of 10 to 20 μg/mL of serum is desirable. It is believed that levels below 10 are not therapeutic. Levels above 20 are known to produce toxicity, including seizures and cardiac arrhythmias. Other side effects of theophylline that can occur within or outside the therapeutic range are nausea, vomiting, nervousness, insomnia, headache, transient diuresis, and gastric acid secretion.

Interpretation of theophylline levels must be made with the knowledge of the peak release and trough levels of the various agents. Most forms of theophylline (e.g., Theodur, Slo-Bid) reach peak levels in 4 to 6 hours while trough levels are attained in 12 hours. Longer acting agents (24 hours) such as Uniphyl and Theo-24 (and in some instances Slo-Bid, depending on patient metabolism) reach peak levels in 10 to 12 hours with trough levels in 24 hours.

In addition to the variability among drugs in reaching therapeutic levels, a number of conditions and drugs are also known to alter the metabolism of theophylline. For example, smokers require much higher doses of theophylline to reach therapeutic levels than nonsmokers. Conversely, smoking cessation can cause levels to plummet. Congestive heart failure, hypoxemia, and drugs such as cimetidine and erythromycin can produce toxic levels (Hendeles and Weinberger, 1983). Patients who suddenly complain of nausea or vomiting may be experiencing sudden changes in their levels secondary to congestive heart failure or other known causes.

SYMPATHOMIMETICS

Sympathomimetic bronchodilators categorize both catecholamines (e.g., epinephrine) and noncatecholamine drugs. *Epinephrine* (adrenalin) is a potent bronchodilator with a short half-life. It shrinks mucosa and dilates the smooth muscle of the tracheobronchial tree. Because of its strong stimulus to the heart, its use is limited to the acute setting to treat severe bronchospasm.

Noncatecholamines include drugs that have both beta$_1$ and beta$_2$ effects as well as drugs that have selective beta$_2$ action. The number of drugs within this category are numerous. Selected older and newer drugs are discussed.

Isoproterenol (Isuprel) has been available for a number of years and is available in liquid or aerosolized form for inhalation. It achieves its bronchodilation action by stimulating the beta-receptors more than the alpha receptors. Because beta$_1$- and beta$_2$-receptors are equally affected, cardiac side effects are common. Its rapid onset of action (minutes) makes it a popular bronchodilator; however, its limited duration of action (20 to 120 minutes) and side effects have limited its usefulness.

Isoetharine (Bronkosol) is for inhaled use and possesses a preferential action on beta$_2$-receptors, with purported minimal effect on beta$_1$-receptors. Although side effects are less than with isoproterenol, many patients experience problems nonetheless.

Metaproterenol (Alupent), terbutaline (Brethine), and albuterol (Ventolin, Proventil) are synthetic beta-adrenergic agents. They are more commonly used due to their selective beta₂ activity. These drugs are available in inhaled and tablet forms. Their longer duration of action and lessened cardiac and CNS effects makes them drugs of choice. Evaluation of patients on bronchodilators is an important part of patient care. Although a excellent bronchodilator response may be produced by these drugs, all are capable of causing disturbing side effects, with the elderly being particularly sensitive. The most common effects are tremors, tachycardia, nervousness, palpitations, and arrhythmias. Because there is such a variety of bronchodilators with comparable potency, patients should not be left to deal with side effects unnecessarily.

ATROPINE

At one time, anticholinergic drugs such as atropine were contraindicated in persons with respiratory problems because of the fear of its drying effects on mucus. Atropine, in the form of ipatropium bromide (Atrovent) has been shown to have powerful bronchodilating capabilities in selected patients with COPD. Additionally, side effects are few: dryness of mouth, cough, and eye irritation with contact. The major limiting factors in its use now is the proper evaluation of candidates and proper dosing. All patients with COPD will not benefit from its use. At this time, most clinicians must rely on patient reports of improvement to determine its usefulness. Lastly, patients must take the drug regularly (i.e., not as needed) and in larger doses than once believed.

STEROIDS

Steroids are anti-inflammatory agents used in the acute stages of asthma and in some patients with COPD. Their actions include preventing antigen-antibody reactions by inhibiting antibody formation, inhibition of cellular mechanisms involving bronchoconstriction, and directly increasing the intracellular concentration of cAMP, thereby producing bronchial muscle relaxation.

There is disagreement about the indications for steroids in both the acute and chronic settings. On the one hand, it is not always possible to document improvement in airway obstruction with testing. On the other hand, many patients report increases in activity tolerance beyond what can be achieved with maximal

bronchodilator therapy. Compounding these unknowns are the number of side effects from steroid use, some of which are irreversible. These side effects include increase in appetite, weight gain, fluid retention, bruising of extremities, acne, hyperglycemia, osteoporosis of the spine and hips, gastric and duodenal ulcers, cataracts, and a decreased resistance to infection.

Despite this formidable list, steroids can be an important part of treatment. Nurses must play an active role in evaluating, educating, and guiding patients. Problems encountered by patients generally center on maintaining or decreasing the dosage of steroid as prescribed. Patients are often tempted to wean themselves from the drug to either avoid the side effects or because of the misconception that they may get addicted. Because long-term steroid use can cause adrenal suppression, reduction of steroids must be carefully supervised. When reducing the dosage, the nurse and patients must be alert to signs of adrenal suppression (hypotension, mental changes, etc.) or worsening of breathing.

Although steroids are generally given in tablet form, intravenous and intramuscular forms are given in the acute setting or by inhalation in the chronic setting. Inhaled steroids can be used as a substitute for tablets (when dose requirements are low) or as a supplement to tablets. Common inhaled forms include triamcinolone acetonide (Azmacort), flunisolide (AeroBid), and beclomethasone (Vanceril or Beclovent).

Problems common to inhaled steroids are inappropriate use of inhaler, misunderstanding of dosing, and improper sequencing of medication. Proper use of inhalers is covered later in this chapter. Dosing problems revolve around not comprehending the importance of taking the inhaler daily and as prescribed. The confusion sometimes arises because of the association with inhaled bronchodilators, which are often ordered to be taken as needed. Patients believe this applies to steroid inhalers as well. Inhaled steroids must be taken daily and in the dosage prescribed. Dosing problems occur because of the fear of the high numbers of inhalations required (four inhalations, five times daily is not uncommon).

When patients are also taking inhaled bronchodilators, the bronchodilator should precede the inhalation of steroids. Bronchodilators can maximize the deposition of steroids.

The most common side effects from inhaled

steroids are cough and localized infection in the mouth with *Candida albicans*. Mouth rinses or gargles after inhaler use reduce the incidence of this infection. Occasionally, oral antifungal treatment is required.

ANTIBIOTICS

Early recognition and treatment of upper respiratory infection is important since infections most likely will progress to more serious problems. Current practice is that antibiotic therapy should begin at the first sign of infection (Table 32–5), but it must be kept in mind that not all patients follow the same pattern of symptoms of infection nor do they normally register an elevated temperature.

Some physicians keep patients supplied with antibiotics with instructions to begin treatment whenever they note a change in sputum color.

The airways of patients with COPD are commonly colonized with *Streptococcus pneumoniae*, *Hemophilus influenzae*, and *Branhamella catarrhalis*. When infection occurs it is generally believed to be from a virus. Traditional approaches to treatment are not applied in most COPD patients, unless there is evidence of a bacterial infection (i.e., fever, changes on chest radiography, hypoxemia). Antibiotic treatment generally consists of sulfa agents, ampicillin, tetracycline, or erythromycin for 7 to 10 days. Other more expensive antibiotics that are effective are doxycline, amoxicillin, and cefaclor.

TABLE 32–5   *Signs and Symptoms of Respiratory Infection*

Increased cough

Increased sputum production

Change in sputum color from normal, i.e., clear, white, or yellow to yellow, green, or gray

Change in sputum consistency from thin and watery to thick and tenacious

Change in sputum amount from normal

Increased dyspnea and/or chest tightness

Decreased activity tolerance

Fever or chills may be but often are not present

A common problem in treatment is convincing patients to complete the course despite improvement in symptoms.

COUGH MEDICINE

When cough is due to an acute infection, antibiotics and inhaled bronchodilators are usually effective. Anesthetic mixtures or lozenges may be taken to soothe the throat. Sedatives and codeine-containing agents are avoided in cases of severe infection where respiratory compromise may occur if the cough reflex is abolished. The effectiveness of guaifenesin (Robitussin, Organidin, Humid LA) is controversial. Patients with tenacious mucus in whom increased fluid intake is not effective may benefit from a trial of guaifenesin-containing agents.

Cough due to dryness may be relieved by simply having the patient breathe vaporized water. Dry cough is common in the winter months when dryness from heating systems occur.

OXYGEN

In general, the indication for oxygen is documented hypoxemia where the arterial oxygen tension (PaO_2) is less than 60 mm Hg or in patients with acute respiratory distress from pneumonia, until such time as an arterial blood gas can be drawn. Flow rates of 2 to 4 L/min are generally sufficient to correct the hypoxemia.

Hypoxemia results from the V/Q mismatch and shunting caused by fluid-filled alveoli as well as the increased metabolic demands for oxygen with fever. Tachycardia is an early sign of hypoxemia. The patient may appear restless, confused, or aggressive. The presence of a decreased urinary output may progress to renal shutdown if hypoxia is prolonged. In some patients, hypotension may occur with progression of disease due to a lowered cardiac output. A decrease in cardiac output results from depressed myocardial function and fluid loss secondary to fever.

Arterial blood gases should be obtained to monitor for hypoxemia and/or respiratory failure. Oxygen administration in the presence of elevated CO_2 (hypoventilation) should be done cautiously. Ordinarily, changes in CO_2 stimulates our drive to breathe. In the presence of hypoventilation ($PaCO_2 > 45$ mm Hg) this normal stimulus to breathe may be ignored by the respiratory center. The center must then rely on low oxygen levels to stimulate respiration. If patients under these circumstances receive oxygen and normalize their oxygen levels (seen by a PaO_2 of > 60 mm Hg), they may then have their drive to breathe removed and stop breathing.

When hypoxemia at rest is documented, oxygen is ordered 24 hours a day. One of the results of a major study of oxygen use showed that periodic oxygen use in hypoxemic patients increased their morbidity and mortality (Nocturnal Oxygen Therapy Trial Group, 1980).

CROMOLYN

Cromolyn (Intal) was introduced over 20 years ago as a treatment for asthma. Its mechanism of action was described as stabilizing the mast cell from releasing mediators (histamine, etc.) that cause bronchospasms. There is reason to believe that it also has other beneficial effects. Cromolyn has been reported to benefit those with both allergic and nonallergic asthma (Bernstein, 1985). Because its action is preventative, cromolyn is not indicated for the acute treatment of bronchospasm.

Recent reports indicate that cromolyn may also benefit patients with COPD. Normally a trial period of 2 to 4 months of treatment is required to evaluate its benefits.

Cromolyn is available only in inhaled forms. Side effects include local irritation of the pharynx and trachea, cough, and bronchospasm. When cromolyn use is preceded by a bronchodilator, cough and bronchospasm can sometimes be avoided.

DIGOXIN

The use of digoxin in patients with COPD is controversial. Of the several proposed benefits, the main indications have been either to improve right ventricular function in cor pulmonale or to treat arrhythmias.

It appears that digoxin may be beneficial in the treatment of right-sided heart failure when accompanied by left ventricular impairment (Ziment, 1990). Treatment of atrial fibrillation may be an indication for digoxin; however, most arrhythmias can be successfully treated with calcium channel blockers.

The consequences of pulmonary disease make patients susceptible to digitalis toxicity. Early signs of toxicity include anorexia, nausea, vomiting, and diarrhea.

DIURETICS

Diuretics decrease the volume of extracellular fluid by causing a loss of salt and water through the kidneys, thus preventing or eliminating edema. Their mechanism of action differs depending on the type of drug.

The thiazides accomplish their action through inhibition of sodium reabsorption in the distal convoluted tubule. The thiazides also reduce arterial pressure by reduction of blood volume and reduction of peripheral vascular resistance owing to their direct action on the smooth muscles of the arteriolar walls.

Side effects include hypokalemia and metabolic alkalosis because there is increased exchange of sodium for potassium and hydrogen ions at the distal convoluted tubule; hyperglycemia because of their direct effect on insulin release and because hypokalemia also reduces release of insulin; and hyperuricemia because thiazides interfere with excretion of uric acid by the distal convoluted tubule.

Furosemide (Lasix) is a loop diuretic and acts by interfering with sodium reabsorption by the ascending portion of Henle's loop. The side effects are the same as those of other thiazides but the hyperglycemia may be milder and hypokalemia, metabolic alkalosis, and hyperuricemia may be more severe.

Certain diuretics are potassium-sparing in that they interfere with the exchange of sodium for potassium and hydrogen ions in the distal convoluted tubule. Spironolactone is the drug of choice in hypertension resulting from steroids.

Patients taking diuretics should be instructed to weigh themselves daily and report any sudden changes to the doctor. Diuretics should be taken early in the day to reduce nocturia. They should also be told of possible problems caused by potassium loss. Symptoms to watch for are fatigue and weakness, "a washed-out" feeling. Eating foods high in potassium may be sufficient to prevent deficiency. Some examples are canned salmon, baked potatoes, frozen lima beans, dried prunes, raisins, bananas, and oranges.

Occasionally potassium supplements such as potassium chloride may be ordered. They should be diluted before ingestion, usually with fruit juice or water. Giving them after meals may minimize gastric irritation. They taste bad and it is difficult to disguise the taste.

ALPHA₁-ANTITRYPSIN REPLACEMENT

A small number of patients with emphysema have developed the disease due to a congenital deficiency of alpha₁-antitrypsin. A deficiency of alpha₁-antitrypsin allows for the uncontrolled action of proteolytic enzymes that digest and destroy the acinar portion of the lung unit. Alpha₁-proteinase inhibitor (Prolastin) has recently been developed to replace the missing inhibitor. This drug may prevent further destruction of lung tissue (Cutter Biological, 1988). Unfortunately inhibitor replacement cannot repair lung tissue that has already been lost. Additionally, because of its specificity for alpha₁-antitrypsin, Prolastin therapy is unlikely to benefit patients with emphysema caused solely from smoking.

Alpha₁-proteinase inhibitor is administered intravenously, once weekly in doses of 60 mg/kg at a rate of 0.08 mL/kg/min. Reported side effects have been negligible but include delayed fever (resolving spontaneously), lightheadedness, dizziness, and mild, transient leukocytosis. Prolastin is purified from fresh human plasma and therefore poses a potential risk for transmitting hepatitis. All patients receiving Prolastin should be immunized against hepatitis B.

The long-term benefits of Prolastin are yet to be determined.

NARCOTICS, SEDATIVES, TRANQUILIZERS, AND ANTIDEPRESSANTS

Most narcotics, sedatives, tranquilizers and antidepressants have respiratory depressant effects, their use has historically been avoided in pulmonary patients. The benefit of many of these drugs has been observed and the high incidence of respiratory failure with these drugs has failed to be documented. On the other hand, in view of the frequent reports and documentation of anxiety and depression in patients, it is reasonable to treat these conditions with counseling and medications. Newer sedatives and tranquilizers with short half-lives (alprazolam, buspirone, triazolam) have made treatment safer. Antidepressants have been shown to alleviate depression and anxiety and

increase the functional levels of COPD patients (McDonald et al, 1990).

Pneumonia

Pneumonia is the fourth leading cause of death among the elderly. Bacteria or viral pneumonias are lung infections for which the elderly, especially those with COPD, are at risk. Bacterial pneumonias occur most frequently among the elderly. Gram-positive diplococcus *Streptococcus pneumoniae* is the cause of bacterial pneumonia in 50% to 90% of community-acquired pneumonias (Donowitz and Mandell, 1985).

Pneumonia can be caused by other organisms but these occur less frequently. Other organisms that can cause pneumonia are gram-negative bacteria (e.g., *Escherichia coli, Klebsiella,* enterobacter), viruses (influenza, herpes), fungi, or mycobacteria (tuberculosis).

Compared with the general population, the elderly and nursing home residents who develop pneumonia are more likely to have *Staphylococcus aureus* or gram-negative bacteria as pathogens. Because pneumococcal pneumonia is the most common pathogen, it will be discussed in detail.

ETIOLOGIC FACTORS

S pneumoniae is a normal inhabitant of the nasal and oral pharynx. Contamination of the lung may occur from aspiration. Whether or not pneumonia develops depends on the interaction between the number and virulence of the bacteria and host defenses.

HIGH RISK

The elderly are particularly vulnerable to pneumonia. A number of common disorders increase the risk of bacterial pneumonia: COPD, congestive heart failure, influenza, alcoholism, corticosteroid therapy, malnutrition, and pulmonary neoplasm.

Upper respiratory infections increase the risk of pneumonia. About 60% to 75% of those who acquire pneumococcal pneumonia have had a preceding upper respiratory infection. Aspiration of infected material into the lower respiratory tract probably begins the infectious process. Viral respiratory infections damage normal lung defenses, making them vulnerable to bacterial invasion.

Aspiration in the elderly is common, occurring secondary to impaired swallowing or reduced cough reflex. Patients are particularly prone to aspiration during sleep and oral or tube feedings. Care during feedings and elevation of the head of the bed can reduce the incidence of aspiration.

DYNAMICS AND SIGNS AND SYMPTOMS

A younger person with pneumococcal pneumonia and some older adults exhibit the classic syndrome of pneumonia. The onset is sudden, with shaking chill, fever, pleuritic chest pain, and cough productive of purulent and/or blood-tinged sputum. In the elderly, signs and symptoms may be more subtle. Lethargy, weakness, anorexia, or confusion may be apparent.

FEVER AND SHIVERING

Fever can rise to 102°F to 106°F (39°C to 41.5°C) usually peaking in late afternoon or evening. Normal temperature of people over 70 is 97°F, so even a temperature of 99°F can be fever in older people (Stengel, 1980). Tachycardia, increased blood pressure, rapid shallow respiration, increased use of accessory muscles of respiration, or shivering may occur.

Chills from fever occur from both the effects of pyrogens as well as vasoconstriction. The energy required to generate heat by shivering is great in terms of caloric expenditure and oxygen use. Proportionately, there is little subsequent heat production for the amount of energy expended (Holtzclaw, 1990). Treatment of fever with ice packs may worsen the shivering, causing the core body temperature to elevate even higher (Holtzclaw, 1990). Furthermore, dehydration (a common problem in the elderly) may alter the thermoregulatory center and interfere with the control of fever.

Control of shivering is best attained through drug therapy. Reduction of environmental factors that aggravate shivering should be instituted, e.g., not exposing patients during bathing, maintaining temperature of the room, warming intravenous infusions, and heating linens.

CYANOSIS

Cyanosis of the lips and nail beds may be seen in patients but are *unreliable signs*. Its appearance may be masked by skin color and anemia.

PHYSICAL SIGNS

Initially, crackles are present on auscultation. Later as the lungs fill with fluid, signs of consolidation may be present. These include dullness to percussion, increased tactile fremitus (vibration felt with the hand on the chest during talking), bronchial breath sounds, whispered pectoriloquy (distinct transmission of whispered sounds), and egophony (long *e* sound transmitted as *ay*). There may be decrease in motion of the chest wall on the affected side.

LEUKOCYTOSIS

The white blood count (WBC) may reach 15,000 to 30,000, usually reaching its peak by the third day. Polymorphonuclear leukocytes make up an abnormal 70% to 90% of the leukocytes. Leukocytosis in the elderly, however, may not occur in 20% of patients (Gleckman, 1985). A normal or low WBC may indicate a fulminating infection with bacteremia. Blood cultures may demonstrate bacteremia in 25% of patients with pneumococcal pneumonia (Frame, 1982). Three blood cultures should be obtained, even in afebrile patients because the incidence of bacteremia is high (15% to 25%).

RADIOGRAPHIC FINDINGS

The radiologic pattern is nonspecific (Nilderman and Fein, 1986). Radiographs may or may not show signs of consolidation.

DIFFERENTIAL DIAGNOSIS

It is extremely important that the diagnosis of pneumonia be made early and treatment initiated because organisms double rapidly and can become overwhelming in just a few hours. Drugs sensitive to the organism must be instituted quickly.

Before starting antibiotics, sputum should be collected for Gram stain, culture, and sensitivity. The nurse plays a crucial role in sputum collections since an inadequate specimen may result in a delay in treatment. Sputum must be from the lower respiratory tract, not saliva.

Sputum from the lungs is generally thick, yellow, green, or pink-tinged. Saliva is generally thin, clear, or frothy. Since many elderly are dehydrated and weakened in their ability to cough, specimens may be difficult to obtain. If patients are unable to raise sputum but have a good cough, sputum induction with hypertonic saline is indicated. Patients who are unable to cough effectively may require suctioning, using a mucus trap for collection. Sputum specimens should be processed immediately to avoid overgrowth with contaminants.

COMPLICATIONS

Pulmonary complications include atelectasis, resulting from bronchial obstruction; delayed resolution beyond the normal 2 to 3 weeks; abscess that causes persistent fever and production of large amounts of purulent sputum; and pulmonary embolus. Empyema is a rare complication.

Pleural effusion occurs in 5% of patients with pneumococcal pneumonia. Rarely does it require aspiration since it resorbs spontaneously.

HERPES SIMPLEX

Herpetic blisters about the mouth are common.

PLEURISY

Inflammation of the pleura results in pleurisy. Pleurisy is characterized by sharp, stabbing pain, accentuated by inspiratory movement. Pain results in splinting of the affected side and rapid, shallow respirations. If the diaphragmatic pleura is involved, pain is referred to the shoulder.

GASTROINTESTINAL SYMPTOMS

Ileus may occur. Ileus is thought to be the result of low oxygen saturation of the blood supplying the bowel. The resulting abdominal distention often adds to the already increased work of breathing.

PROGNOSIS

With prompt and adequate therapy, most patients recover uneventfully. Older persons, however, need to anticipate a longer period of convalescence and a slower return of energy, often a major source of frustration. COPD and cardiac disease may slow the recovery rate even more and can increase the risk of complications. Bacteremia is associated with a 20% to 30% mortality.

MEDICAL MANAGEMENT AND ASSOCIATED NURSING CARE

BED REST

The older person with pneumococcal pneumonia should be hospitalized. Bed rest is required to decrease the body's demand for oxygen. This can be an added danger to someone who is already experiencing airway obstruction. The patient must be reminded to breathe deeply and cough. An incentive spirometer may be helpful in encouraging deep breathing when used every 1 to 2 hours. Frequent position change must also be encouraged, and a footboard should be provided so leg exercises can be practiced at regular intervals.

ANTIMICROBIAL THERAPY

Uncomplicated *S pneumoniae* pneumonia is treated with penicillin in the form of (1) penicillin G procaine, 300,000 U intramuscularly every 8 hours, (2) aqueous crystalline penicillin G, 400,000 U intravenously every 4 hours, or (3) penicillin V, 250 mg by mouth every 6 hours. For persons with penicillin allergy, erythromycin, cephalosporins, clindamycin, or trimethoprim/sulfamethoxazole are effective.

HYDRATION AND AIRWAY MANAGEMENT

Maintaining adequate hydration is important for the regulation of body temperature, electrolyte balance, and facilitating clearance of secretions from the airways. As mucus production increases and fills the airways, water is absorbed, making mucus thick and expectoration difficult and causing airway obstruction. If this process occurs in enough airways, the patient will be unable to meet his need for oxygen. The patient must be kept well hydrated to keep mucus thin and easy to expectorate. Forcing fluids of up to 2000 to 3000 mL daily orally or intravenously can control dehydration. The patient's intake and output must be closely monitored to ensure adequate intake as well as providing information about the patient's renal status. An aerosol unit may be helpful in managing secretions.

Coughing is important to airway clearance. The presence of coarse crackles indicates sputum accumulation in the lung and calls for aggressive measures to get the patient to cough. If unable to cough due to a decrease in responsiveness or inability to cooperate, suctioning may be necessary.

The use of postural drainage (percussion and vibration) is controversial. It appears that if patients raise more than an ounce or two of sputum, drainage may be beneficial. In the elderly, however, if this procedure is used, care must be taken to observe the patient during the procedure to ensure the patient can adequately handle any secretions that become mobilized. Postural drainage may be contraindicated in patients with some cardiac diseases.

OXYGEN

The administration of oxygen is frequently indicated in patients with pneumonia because they have hypoxemia. This is discussed in the section on COPD.

VITAL SIGNS

Because tachycardia and hypotension are signs of cardiac stress, pulse and blood pressure should be monitored frequently. Elevated temperature causes an increase in the basal metabolic rate. This increases the need for calories and protein. Weight loss will occur if adequate calories are not provided and consumed. An increased metabolic rate also causes water and sodium loss by means of diaphoresis. An adequate fluid intake and output must be maintained. An output of 1000 mL/d is considered adequate.

Frequent gown and linen changes may be necessary because of diaphoresis. Some physicians treat the headache that may accompany fever with codeine rather than aspirin, since the diaphoresis that follows administration of aspirin may be more uncomfortable than the headache. Temperature, pulse, and respiration should decrease within 12 to 36 hours after initiation of penicillin, but may not reach normal levels for 4 days or more. Roentgenography will show evidence of clearing more gradually.

PLEURITIC PAIN

Codeine may be given for pleuritic pain unless cough suppression is of concern. An intercostal nerve block or interpleural analgesia may offer relief.

PREVENTING RECURRENCE

Patients with secretions should be instructed in the importance of good bronchial hygiene.

Since 1977 a vaccine effective against 14 types of *S pneumoniae* has been available. Currently a pneumococcal vaccine effective against 23 types is available.

Although two randomized controlled trials among older adults have not shown differences in respiratory disease with vaccinations, blood studies suggest 60% to 80% effectiveness among older people who are vaccinated. Pneumococcal vaccine should be given to adults over the age of 65 and to adults at risk with chronic illnesses such as COPD. One-time vaccination is required. Persons who received the 14-valent vaccine should *not* be given the 23-valent vaccine because adverse reactions with revaccination outweigh the slight advantage of broader coverage.

Flu Shots All persons over the age of 65 are advised to be immunized yearly against influenza. Those with cardiovascular or pulmonary disease or any chronic disease are particularly vulnerable to the flu. There are two major types of influenza type A, which tends to drift and shift among different strains, and type B, which is fairly stable. A single intramuscular injection is required in adults annually. Since strains change yearly, revaccination is required with vaccine specific to the strains known to cause illness for the coming year.

Vaccination should not be administered to people with allergies to eggs.

Many older persons are reluctant to have flu vaccinations. Some report having developed side effects of a cold following injections and therefore have difficulty understanding how the vaccine can prevent illness. With the availability of purer vaccines, side effects are less likely. Less than a third will develop localized erythema and rarely are flu-like symptoms displayed, i.e., fever, malaise, and myalgias.

Vaccination in the early fall is important in order to be maximally protected. If an outbreak of influenza A is recognized and the necessary 2 to 3 weeks protection cannot be obtained, the antiviral agent amantadine can be administered. Amantadine is given 200 mg taken orally, on a daily basis until the epidemic has passed, or for 2 weeks following vaccination. It has been shown to be 70% to 90% effective in young adults. Its effectiveness among the elderly and other high-risk groups is not known.

EVALUATION

When antibiotics are effective, the older patient usually begins to feel better in 2 to 3 days after treatment. Chest radiographs are taken frequently during therapy to check for resolution of the infection. Consolidation may take 10 weeks to resolve on radiography.

Because it will take longer to recover fully than the older person may like, it becomes important for the nurse to be aware of the patient's response to activities and demands of daily living to assess how they are pacing themselves. With time the patient should return to the premorbid state.

Tuberculosis

Tuberculosis is included in this chapter because there presently is a resurgence of the disease in the United States. New cases have increased 10 percent nationwide (Richman, 1992), and many are drug resistant. There are several reasons for this resurgence. People over 75 may have had a primary lesion when they were young and this can be activated by chronic illness and poor nutrition in old age. As the person ages, cell-mediated immunity due to normal aging decreases, increasing the risk for reactivation. Some medications given for chronic conditions, particularly steroids, can cause reactivation of healed lesions. In addition, 25% to 30% of all newly diagnosed cases of tuberculosis are found in people over 65 (Yoshikawa, 1992).

Tuberculosis is a systemic disease, and health care providers should always think of this as a possible diagnosis in someone with a low-grade fever, unexplained weight loss, cough, and/or weakness. These symptoms may happen in normal aging, but patients who present with these symptoms should be checked by skin test and/or chest radiography to rule out tuberculosis.

Tuberculosis is endemic in many foreign countries, especially Southeast Asia. Many people from these countries have immigrated to the United States with untreated or healed disease, placing them at higher risk for infection or reinfection. Patients with acquired immunodeficiency syndrome have a high incidence of tuberculosis and although most of them are young, they may be cared for in nursing homes, increasing the risk to older patients sharing the facility.

The Core Curriculum on Tuberculosis (CDC, 1991) is available free and nursing facilities should have copies. The Centers for Disease Control also have a video tape on Mantoux testing, also free from local health departments. Local health departments have nurses available for lectures and consultation on tuberculosis, and these nurses should be used to review the pathology and treatment of the disease. Another source of information is the American Lung Association, addresses of local chapters are found in the telephone book.

Nursing and Management in Daily Living

DAILY LIVING WITH CHRONIC PULMONARY DISEASE

As with many chronic conditions in the elderly, chronic lung disease often results in a gradual decline in activities. The adaptations and compromises made by patients, however, are not always in their best interest. Decreasing activity levels have direct negative effects on the efficiency of extracting oxygen from the muscles, sleep habits, social support system, and the patient's overall sense of well-being.

RISK FACTORS

Patients with lung disease can be negatively affected by a number of factors. These include:

Living in areas with poor air quality
Cold weather
Exposure to second-hand smoke
Colds or flu
Housing that requires climbing a significant number of stairs
Having to alter a formerly active lifestyle due to activities that exceed their oxygen capabilities or require positions that compromise muscles of respiration

SIGNS AND SYMPTOMS

There are many signs that indicate that individuals are not managing daily living effectively or that their quality of life is not satisfying. Many of these represent symptoms of depression common among both elderly persons and patients with COPD. The patient or others may report that the patient is becoming increasingly sedentary and withdrawing from activities, eating less, or complaining of lack of sleep. Patients may report that they avoid social activities because of fear of infection or anxiety when among others. Some are of the mistaken belief that they will breathe better by moving from one region of the country to another. It is not uncommon to hear patients or their spouse report that the patient sleeps little during the day and/or sleeps upright in a lounge chair at night. This behavior may represent attempts to relieve symptoms of heart failure; however, it is more commonly associated with unexpressed fears of going to sleep and never waking up again.

PROGNOSTIC VARIABLES

A major factor in successfully living with chronic pulmonary disease is working cooperatively with one's caregiver, be they spouse, relative, or friend. Because chronic illness is stressful, behavioral problems frequently emerge. Premorbid personality characteristics become magnified under the stress. Often, the object of negative behaviors is the caregiver. Support systems for both the patient and caregiver are important in keeping the family unit solidified. Counseling by persons aware of the behavioral needs and dynamics of pulmonary patients can be very effective.

COMPLICATIONS

Preoccupation with breathing may result in the older person isolating or alienating himself from others. Fear of dyspnea and/or oxygen deprivation may lead to anxiety and hyperventilation. Sleep deprivation may further aggravate low energy levels.

TREATMENT

Oxygen Therapy When oxygen is ordered, it is important that patients have realistic expectations of its use and understand its application.

The nurse should assess the patient's:

Attitude toward oxygen
Resources for payment
Knowledge of the equipment
Knowledge about the indications for use

Oxygen therapy once meant a life of seclusion, with the person being homebound. Present day systems for delivering oxygen are available that make mobility possible, including travel with oxygen.

The three major types of systems for oxygen delivery are tanks or cylinders of compressed gas, liquid oxygen reservoirs, and oxygen concentrators. The choice of system depends on the cost to third-party payers, cost to the patient, patient mobility, and environment in which the patient lives.

Tanks or cylinders serve as a reservoir for 100% oxygen in the gaseous state, stored under compressed conditions. In most instances, oxygen in cylinders are the cheapest form of oxygen (cost varying among companies) but may be limiting for the patient who is mobile. Since the majority of patients are on continuous oxygen, the length of time a cylinder will last is important (Table 32–6). Cylinders come in several sizes and length of available oxygen will vary. The large cylinders are generally H or K cylinders. For patients requiring oxygen at 2 L/min, an H cylinder will last approximately 55 hours, a K cylinder, longer. Naturally, as flow requirements increase, the tank will last proportionately less time. Smaller tanks, usually in the form of E cylinders, can be made portable with the use of a cart. At 2 L/min, an E cylinder will last 5 hours.

Because of the dangers of the cylinder cracking when it falls, all cylinders must be secured to a stationary source. A tank that cracks on impact will become airborn like a missile due to the high compression of gas within. Patients who may have small children around must take particular care to see that all cylinders are secured.

Another area of hazard, common to all systems of oxygen, is the increased flammability of materials in the presence of oxygen, described under the section on **Safeguards.**

Liquid systems for oxygen apply the principle of oxygen in a liquid state (when brought to low temperatures), as opposed to the gaseous state. Liquid oxygen is stored in an insulated reservoir at −300°F. The liquid vaporizes, converting oxygen to a gaseous state. As this process occurs, the oxygen must either be used by the patient or vented into the atmosphere, because the container does not have the ability to store large quantities of oxygen in gaseous form.

The major advantage of liquid oxygen is its portability. Patients who are ambulatory bene-

TABLE 32–6 *Length of Oxygen Administration with H and E Cylinders*

Liters per Minute	Type of Cylinder H (hr)	E (hr)
1	110	10
2	55	5
3	36.5	3.5
4	27.5	2.5
6	18	1.5
8	13.5	1

fit the most from this source of oxygen delivery since the devices are designed for portability. Full units weigh from 6 to 10 lbs, depending on the type. Since oxygen must be used on a continuous basis in order to avoid waste, this device is not indicated for those who use oxygen less than 24 hours per day, e.g., nighttime use. Potential hazards of liquid oxygen are from frostbite or burns if the skin comes in contact with unprotected areas on the reservoir. The oxygen that is vented from the system is not sufficient to make liquid oxygen a significant hazard.

Concentrators are electrically powered devices that entrain room air, filter out nitrogen and water vapor through a molecular sieve, and collect only the oxygen particles. The result is a concentration of oxygen of 80% to 95%. The concentration diminishes as the flow rate requirements increase; however, a built-in sensor attempts to compensate for the reduced concentration by automatically adjusting (increasing) the flow rate.

In most cases, this less pure form of oxygen is sufficient in patients requiring low flow rates (1 to 3 L/min). However, because of the variability in concentration of oxygen, all patients on concentrators should have their oxygen levels checked on the device they will be using to ensure equivalent amounts of oxygen are being received.

Advantages of the concentrator are their low maintenance, i.e., there is no need to refill reservoirs. The disadvantages include reliance on electricity and therefore need for a backup system (usually an E cylinder) in the event of power failure, lack of portability, inaccuracies at high flow rates, and cost of electricity not covered by third-party reimbursement. Patients on concentrators often use long oxygen tubing for mobility in the home. The tubing can become a physical hazard to the patient or others in the home.

Closely related to the oxygen concentrator is the oxygen *enricher*. This system, like the concentrator, filters out nitrogen but not the water vapor. The collected oxygen is therefore humidified, but the concentration of oxygen is reduced in half (about 40%). Because of the low concentration of oxygen, it is difficult to ensure adequate oxygen levels in the patient.

Oxygen-conserving Devices Newer modalities of delivering oxygen have been developed in the past decade to maximize the oxygen being delivered. Generally, these devices result in an overall cost savings or increase the convenience of taking oxygen.

The major changes include changes in catheter design, delivery through a tracheostomy-like opening, and devices to deliver oxygen only during inhalation. The most significant change in catheter design came with the introduction of the Oxymizer (Chad Therapeutics Inc, Woodland Hills, CA). The *Oxymizer* is a nasal cannula with larger than normal tubing (fitting under the nose) that houses a bladder. This bladder serves as a collection reservoir for oxygen during the exhalation phase of breathing. On inspiration, the reservoir empties and provides a bolus of oxygen, as well as normal flow to the patient. The result is that some patients are able to reduce the required flow rates approximately in half (testing and documentation of oxygen levels during use are required). By reducing flow rates, some patients are able to use smaller receptacles for oxygen or get longer use out of current devices.

The *pulse oxygenator* (e.g., Companion 5, Puritan Bennett Corp., Lenexa, KS) is a device sensitive to the inhalation phase of the patient. This device injects a bolus on inhalation, thereby reducing wasted oxygen on exhalation. This device can reduce oxygen use in half in some patients. Problems may occur with the sensitivity of the device with changes in respiratory patterns, e.g., increase in respiratory rate and depth with exercise.

Transtracheal oxygen is a method of oxygen delivery through a small-bore tubing inserted directly into the trachea. Specially designed catheters are available Since little oxygen is wasted (because it bypasses the upper airway) increased amounts of oxygen are delivered. Flow rates can be reduced to half of what is required with conventional nasal cannulas. This device has been accepted by patients for its aesthetic appearance (it can be camouflaged easily) and for the reduced oxygen requirements.

Ambulation and Travel with Oxygen In most instances, patients who are independently mobile benefit from the liquid system of oxygen because of its portable design. Limitations on reimbursement, however, may dictate the use of cylinders for mobility.

Travel for patients on oxygen should not be discouraged. Many oxygen companies have offices throughout the country and the availability of oxygen can be assured. Travel by plane, train, and water have been enhanced in some instances by an increased awareness of patient needs. Since carriers vary in their restrictions, travelers with oxygen should call to determine their requirements. Just as "shopping around" for the least expensive oxygen company can be cost-saving, so can shopping for a carrier.

Safeguards Although some precautions are necessary, patients should not be made to fear oxygen. Oxygen supports combustion; therefore, any materials (cannulas, clothing, bed linens, etc.) will burn faster in the presence of oxygen. Patients should not work near an open flame or smoke. Smoking is the greatest single fire hazard for patients receiving oxygen (West and Primeau, 1983). Patients receiving oxygen should not smoke.

Evaluation of Oxygen Therapy Patients receiving oxygen should be reevaluated to establish their current oxygen levels under the following circumstances:

When changes in flow rates are made
When the patient's condition changes (e.g., pneumonia, congestive heart failure)
Routinely, at least every year

BREATHING TECHNIQUES

Breathing techniques are taught to control the rate and depth of respiration. The simplest technique, pursed-lip breathing, is often self-taught. Breathing out through pursed lips reminds patients to slow the exhalation phase of breathing. It increases airway pressure and reduces air trapping in patients with COPD. Since this can control dyspnea, there can be a reduction in anxiety associated with its use.

Controlled breathing during activities can reduce dyspnea in patients. In patients with COPD, exhalation is the longest phase of the breathing sequence because of obstruction to airflow. Consequently, activities should be done during exhalation. For example, activities requiring bending or pushing should be preceded by inhalation and the activity performed during exhalation through pursed lips. There is some question about which activities should be performed on inhalation. Some advocate inhalation during activities that require bringing air into the lungs, such as pulling or reaching. Others suggest that any activity requiring effort be performed on the exhalation phase of breathing.

Probably the most important point of breathing with activities is that patients be aware of their pattern. A common problem patients encounter is breathholding with activities. Breathholding can produce dyspnea in and of itself. Patients unconsciously hold their breath when performing strenuous activities such as tying shoes and picking up objects. Emphasis should be placed on the rhythmicity of breathing with energy efficient maneuvers. A general rule of thumb is to have patients take twice as long for exhalation as they do for inhalation. Patients should be taught to perform strenuous activities on exhalation, and not hold their breath. For example, when opening a heavy door, inhale first, then exhale when pushing or pulling the door open.

Abdominal or diaphragmatic breathing was once proposed as a means of "switching" patients from a breathing pattern that consisted of a paradoxical pattern of chest out and stomach in on inhalation, to chest out and stomach out on inhalation. The latter is referred to as diaphragmatic breathing. The belief was that breathing exercises could revert the flattened diaphragm to its dome shape by pushing abdominal contents (through the contraction of abdominal muscles) up against the diaphragm on exhalation. The diaphragm, however, is flattened in patients with emphysema for a number of reasons, but primarily from overinflation of the lungs secondary to the loss of elastic recoil. Since a flattened diaphragm is a normal consequence of irreversible overinflation, breathing exercises alter the shape of the diaphragm temporarily at best.

Abdominal or diaphragmatic breathing exercises may, however, have the beneficial effect of assisting the patient to control the rate and depth of breathing in the acute phase. This can be particularly beneficial during acute dyspnea or anxiety. Diaphragmatic breathing is taught by instructing the patient to place one hand on the chest, and one on the abdomen. The chest wall and abdomen should expand on inhalation. On exhalation the abdominal muscles should contract and press up against the abdominal contents.

STAIR CLIMBING

Stair climbing is an activity that may seem overwhelming to a patient with chronic lung disease, but it can be accomplished by applying breathing techniques and energy-conserving methods. The pattern recommended is to ascend one or two steps on inhalation and two to four steps on exhalation, while breathing through pursed lips. If exhalation is extremely prolonged, climb three steps on inhalation and six on exhalation. Patients who are severely dyspneic may only be able to inhale at rest and take one step on exhalation. The important point is for patients to pace themselves within the limitations of their breathing capacity.

DAILY LIVING WITH MANAGING SECRETIONS

Lung secretions present a variety of challenges in daily living. Very often these problems are managed by the nurse and the patient with minimal input from the physician.

Some of the problems and tasks are associated with removal of lung secretions, maintaining adequate hydration, and social and physical problems associated with coughing, raising, and disposal of sputum.

Retention of lung secretions leads quickly to problems in breathing and infection. On the other hand, coughing and raising sputum are socially unacceptable behaviors. It is sometimes difficult for patients to maintain airway hygiene and still be an acceptable part of a social group.

RISK FACTORS

Accumulation of secretions normally stimulates the cough reflex and secretions are expec-

torated. When the amount and character of the sputum changes or the patient's cough reflex is diminished, the patient is at risk for retention of secretions.

Secretions usually increase in amount due to infection, and high levels of moisture such as a tracheostomy mist may actually induce and increase the secretions. The character of sputum may, on the other hand, change to thick, tenacious sputum. This may be due to dehydration, infection, or an asthmatic episode. Rehydration, antibiotics, or bronchodilators are usually necessary. A reduction in the cough reflex and/or reduction in the normal mucociliary clearance system may occur for a number of reasons: medications such as cough suppressants, sedatives, anesthesia, or hypnotics may alter the cough reflex, as well as generalized weakness or smoking.

SIGNS AND SYMPTOMS

Prevention of secretion problems is the first line of defense against infection. Risk factors that are present should be corrected. The elderly person should be particularly observed for cough effectiveness. Coarse crackles on auscultation frequently indicate the presence of secretions, which can be expectorated. When patients are requested to cough and their attempts are feeble, it is generally a sign of weakness in generating a good cough. Coach the patient to inhale deeply and exhale slowly but as completely as possible until they believe they no longer can push any air out of their lungs. At the end of exhalation, have the patient generate a small cough or huff. This technique may help "milk" the secretions up the airway.

PROGNOSIS

Any factors that inhibit cough, expectoration of sputum, or adequate fluid intake place the patient at risk for improper management of secretions.

COMPLICATIONS

Complications of excess secretions in the lungs include

Risk of lung infection
Hypoxemia from airway obstruction
Impaired sleep due to wakefulness from expectorating secretions

MEDICATIONS

There are a number of medications available to assist with expectorations. Included are mucolytic agents such as guaifenesin agents, solutions of potassium iodide, and acetylcysteine (Mucomyst). There is some controversy in the value of expectorants but most clinicians agree that if the patient does not respond to other techniques, expectorants are worth trying. In general, expectorants should not be taken daily for chronic use. There is empirical evidence that long-term chronic use decreases the effectiveness of the drug.

MANAGEMENT OF HYDRATION

Problems with hydration result from the increased water loss secondary to increased respiratory rate and poor intake of fluids by the elderly. Maintaining adequate hydration is the key to keeping secretions thin enough to be expectorated and may be difficult to achieve in patients in nursing homes. A desired fluid intake is about 3000 mL/d. Nursing responsibilities include the following:

1. Assessing the usual pattern of fluid intake, types of fluids, amounts, and time of consumption
2. Ensuring the patient understands the importance of fluid intake and the relationship between thin secretions and ease of expectoration
3. Working with the patient to develop an acceptable schedule for fluid intake
4. Having the patient keep a diary of intake, in order to identify problems and discuss solutions

For the patient with uncompromised cardiac or renal function, drinking this volume of fluid is necessary to achieve loose secretions. In some instances, a cardiac condition may exist that is so severe that fluid restriction is necessary. Unlike cardiac patients, however, congestive heart failure in pulmonary patients, even in the presence of visible pedal edema, does not warrant fluid restrictions, if the patient is on a diuretic.

The scheduling of fluid intake can be laborious for some patients. The nurse should assess the patient's current drinking habits (a patient diary is often beneficial). Patients may find that filling a 3 quart container with water, daily, helps guide them in understanding the expectations for what constitutes 3000 mL of fluids.

There may be additional sources of fluids that the patient may not realize, such as milk, coffee, tea, juices, and clear soups. Patients are often of the mistaken belief the milk will "make sputum." There is no evidence that this is true.

Increased humidification in the home can reduce the loss of fluids by mouth. When secretions are particularly tenacious, the added moisture from a vaporizer or steam from a shower can be helpful. The mechanism of its usefulness is not clear. It is unlikely that these are sources of hydration, but they may reduce water loss from the airways as well as potentially stimulate the production of secretions.

Urine color is a good indicator of hydration. Too little fluid intake may result in dark urine, and adequate intake may be reflected in a pale urine color.

AIRWAY MANAGEMENT

Impairment of the normal mucociliary clearance mechanism, excess production of secretions, and bronchial inflammation in chronic bronchitis can cause a decrease in airway diameter. In emphysema, loss of elastic support of alveoli and bronchi result in airway collapse and obstruction during cough. Generally during a cough, airways collapse at the level of the trachea. With chronic airway obstruction, premature collapse of airway occurs further down the bronchial tree, trapping secretions lower in the airway.

Teaching effective cough can be an important measure in the care of patients with COPD. Patients should be instructed to cough in the upright position. Instruct the patient to inhale deeply, then during a slow exhalation, cough briefly at successively smaller lung volumes without taking breaths between coughs. The patient should cough at least four times during a single exhalation. This technique is intended to delay the premature collapse of airways. An alternate technique, described previously, involves exhaling maximally, followed by a cough at the very end of exhalation.

BREATHING EQUIPMENT

Equipment Bronchodilators (and other agents) may be given by aerosolization or nebulization over a period of 10 minutes or in a bolus form (metered dose). A number of devices are available for delivering medication or for augmenting the metered-dose delivery (spacing devices).

Nebulized medication breaks up or reduces

the particle of medication to a size small enough to be inhaled deep into the small airways. Particles must be 2 μm or less. Next, the patient must breathe in such a way as to encourage the deep deposition of the medication. Limitations of nebulizers are that much of the nebulized medication becomes wasted because of the large particles produced and difficulty capturing the entire dosage of medication delivered by the device.

The simplest and most portable of the devices is the metered-dose inhaler (MDI) discussed later in this section. A compressor-driven nebulizer device is the other commonly used vehicle for nebulization. This nebulizer operates on electricity and is also available on AC/DC current for use in the automobile. Indications for the power-driven nebulizer are patients who either have difficulty coordinating the hand, mouth, and breathing movements required with the MDI or who are unable to take a deep enough breath with an end-inspiratory pause (seen in patients with acute asthma or very severe obstruction with air trapping).

With the compressor nebulizer, medication is delivered over a period of 5 to 10 minutes (depending on the capabilities of the device). The belief is that the longer period of nebulization (as opposed to the MDI) provides a greater opportunity for the medication to be deposited in the lungs.

Recent studies comparing the MDI with the compressor nebulizer indicate that most patients, even when hospitalized, can obtain as much benefit from a properly administered MDI as they can with the power-driven nebulizer.

Metered-dose Inhaler   Bronchodilators, steroids, Cromolyn, and Atrovent are available in MDI form. Two techniques for inhalation have been proposed: the open and closed mouth methods. Most patients benefit from the open mouth method described in Table 32–7. Areas in which most patients fail are in exhaling just to end-tidal volume, inhaling slowly and deeply, and holding the breath at the end of inhalation.

Studies have shown that of the medication delivered by MDI only 15% reaches the lungs, even when using the proper technique. Proper use of the inhaler is therefore essential.

Spacer Devices   Spacer devices, like the open mouth technique, puts distance between the medication being aerosolized and the mouth.

TABLE 32–7 *Instructions for Metered-dose Inhaler Using the Open Mouth Technique*

1. Shake the container several times
2. Hold the inhaler with mouthpiece parallel to the mouth, about two fingers from the mouth
3. Breathe out normally (not hard) to the end of a normal exhalation (i.e., end tidal volume)
4. Open mouth wide, at the beginning of a *slow* inhalation, depress inhalator, administer *one* spray of the medication
5. Continue to inhale, slowly and deeply
6. Try to hold breath for 5–8 seconds
7. Exhale normally
8. Repeat second inhalation after waiting about 30 seconds

The spacer reduces the amount of direct impaction of the bolus of medication onto the palate or tongue, which ultimately gets swallowed and does not enter the lung. Additionally, the spacer serves as a reservoir to hold the medication in suspension to allow time for the large particles to fall out and smaller particles to remain suspended and inhaled.

The spacing device, such as the Inspirease or Aerochamber, can augment delivery of any of the inhaled medications. Azmacort, however, comes with its own built-in spacer and therefore does not require a spacer. Patients who experience coordination problems may benefit from the spacer since the timing of opening the mouth with activation of the MDI is not crucial. Spacers are also useful in patients who complain of the taste of the medication, since the spacer reduces impaction of large particles in the oropharynx. Atrovent can cause temporary visual impairment if nebulized into the eyes. Spacer devices can reduce this side effect.

Written Instructions   All patients should receive instructions on the use of the device and cleaning instructions. Instructions with the MDI, however, are usually outdated in their description of technique.

Patients who use saline may want to make it for use in certain circumstances. Table 32–8 gives instructions on this.

TABLE 32–8 *Instructions for Making Normal Saline*

Normal saline is used as to dilute for broncho-dilators and other agents. Some bronchodilators and cromolyn compounds come in unit dose packaging with saline added. If the patient wishes to make his own normal saline solution, the following recipe should be used:

1. Place an uncovered, clean quart jar and its lid in a clean saucepan, completely covering with water
2. Cover the saucepan and boil for 10 minutes
3. In another clean saucepan, place $\frac{1}{2}$ teaspoon of *uniodized* table salt in a pint of tap water
4. Cover the pan and boil for 10 minutes
5. Turn off the heat and allow both pans to cool with covers on
6. Pour salt solution into the sterile jar
7. Seal the jar tightly and store in the refrigerator

Homemade saline solution will remain sterile for a week if the jar is tightly sealed and stored under refrigeration

---

Evaluation Patients with either the MDI or nebulizer would be able to (1) explain the purpose of the medication, (2) explain the delivery system, (3) demonstrate appropriate use of the device, and (4) demonstrate proper cleaning of the equipment.

DAILY LIVING WITH SLEEP PROBLEMS

Sleep disturbances in the elderly person are the most frequent reason for psychiatric hospitalization (Mei-Tal and Meyers, 1985). Many elderly persons complain of not being able to sleep as long as they would like. Persons with COPD, most of whom are elderly, have in addition, problems with sleep secondary to both physiologic and psychologic alterations.

Sleep problems in elderly persons are common because consolidated sleep becomes more fractured with age (Webb, 1989). Since most people expect that a "good night's sleep" consists of no awakenings, the elderly may become troubled by the change in their normal sleep pattern. Patients need to be aware that a disruption in sleep will occur.

Despite the disruption in sleep, elderly peo-ple may in fact have a greater total sleep time with age. Some elderly people experience significant changes or extremes of sleep (too little or too much) (Kripke et al, 1979). Of those at these extremes, a greater percentage of elderly sleep longer with age (> 10 hours), while a smaller percentage may in fact reduce sleep time to less than 5 hours. Naps tend to increase with age but only about 10% of the elderly nap chronically.

Medications may disrupt one's normal sleep pattern directly or indirectly. For example, stimulants such as caffeine can promote wakefulness while diuretics may cause the individual to awaken to urinate. In pulmonary patients, theophylline may be too stimulating to some patients. Secretions can also be a problem, since secretions move and pool by gravity during recumbent positions. Patients may no sooner get to sleep before awakening to expectorate or cough. Pulmonary patients also may experience orthopnea at night secondary to congestive heart failure. Hypoxemia also may occur at night in patients with COPD. In general, one can anticipate that oxygen levels will be lower with sleep than during the day.

Situational events may have such a distressing effect on the patient that they are unable to fall asleep. For example, watching a disturbing TV program or hearing of disturbing incidences in the person's life may cause insomnia. Not infrequently, pulmonary patients have a fear of falling asleep believing they will not awaken again. There is no evidence that pulmonary patients have a high incidence of death during sleep.

Sleep disturbances among elderly people are therefore associated with a number of natural life events. Some recommendations for encouraging sleep are listed in Table 32–9. Sleep medications may be indicated for insomnia, but on a periodic basis only. Chronic use of sleep medications alter the patients concept of sleep and can ultimately result in complaints of insomnia despite sleep medications. Additionally, sleep medications should have a short half-life, since a build-up of the medication may occur if not excreted within 8 to 10 hours.

DAILY LIVING WITH NUTRITIONAL DEFICITS

Malnutrition occurs in elderly persons and frequently in patients with severe emphysema. The mechanism of this deficit in emphysema is unknown, but may be related to the increased

---

TABLE 32–9   *Techniques to Enhance Sleep*

---

1. Use the bed for sleep only, avoid its use for watching TV, eating, and obsessing about sleep

2. Omit alcohol and caffeine before bedtime

3. Avoid frequent napping

4. Awaken at the same time each day

5. Engage in daily exercise, but not before bedtime

---

energy requirements by the respiratory muscles or impaired gastrointestinal function.

RISK FACTORS

Elderly people are prone to nutritional problems because of changes in their eating habits. Patients with emphysema increase the risk of malnutrition as their disease progresses.

Elderly persons may experience subtle yet important changes in their lifestyle that result in poor eating habits. Since they may decrease their activity levels, their requirements for food are lessened. By reducing the size of the meal they prepare, they may fail to eat a balanced meal.

Medications may be a cause of altered appetite. Drugs such as theophylline and beta$_2$-blockers can cause nausea. Antibiotics, prednisone, and theophylline may cause an upset stomach.

A reduction in income or inability to obtain transportation to purchase groceries may affect the patient's eating habits. Finally, patients living alone may not take the time to address their nutritional needs properly.

SIGNS AND SYMPTOMS

Loss of appetite appears related to malnutrition but may also occur from depression. In view of the high incidence of depression among the elderly, a loss of appetite is probably common.

Changes in eating habits can also be anticipated in patients who are dyspneic or fatigued. Patients with a decrease in their sensation of taste (from zinc deficiencies or medication) will also have difficulty in maintaining an interest in food. Finally, food preferences may dictate a patient's eating habits. These preferences may not be met in an institutional setting.

Patients who therefore are depressed, dyspneic, or fatigued should be assessed for nutritional deficits. Signs of nutritional deficiencies include weight loss, decrease in activity levels, muscle wasting, lackluster hair, edema, and hepatomegaly.

PROGNOSTIC VARIABLES

Once nutritional deficits among the elderly are recognized, the challenge of altering behavior becomes a goal. It is unclear, however, how improvements in nutrition alter the course of life in the elderly. In patients with COPD, however, malnutrition is a poor prognostic indicator and difficult to reverse.

Attempts at nutritional repletion are hampered by the pulmonary patient's difficulty consuming large quantities of food due to the dyspnea that is created. Eating and the process of digestion increase the work of breathing and may produce hypoxemia. The use of oxygen while eating may be helpful. Repletion has been successful with slow infusion of nutrients by tube feeding. Weight gain and reversal of malnutrition, however, are temporary, returning to previous levels once the feedings are stopped.

COMPLICATIONS

The consequences of malnutrition are alterations in the drive to breathe, changes in lung structure, decrease in the defense mechanisms of the lung, and a decrease in respiratory strength.

Alterations in lung structure may result in airspace enlargement and decrease in elasticity of the lung. The defense mechanisms of the lung that are altered may result in a decrease in surfactant production and an alteration in the immunologic response. The decreased strength of respiratory muscles may contribute to the increase in dyspnea and can result in respiratory failure.

A reduction in oxygen levels can occur during and up to 2 hours after meals. The mechanism for this response is not clear.

TREATMENT

A variety of techniques may be used to encourage the patient's interest in nourishment, stimulate the appetite, and increase caloric intake (Table 32–10).

TABLE 32–10 *Techniques for Improving Oral Intake*

1. Determine the time of day that the patient is usually hungry and serve the biggest meal at that time

2. Obtain patient's favorite food

3. Make snacks readily available

4. Consume snack 1 to 2 hours before bedtime

5. Mix favorite ice cream with beverages such as juices or carbonated drinks

6. Provide hard candy to suck on or chew gum before meals to stimulate taste buds

7. Consume a glass of wine, 30 minutes before meals

8. Provide oral hygiene

Adapted from Openbrier DR, Covey M. Ineffective breathing pattern related to malnutrition. Nurs Clin North Am 1987; 22:225.

Nutritional counseling should begin by assessing the patient's current eating habits, including the kind and quality of the food he or she eats. Patient diaries are useful in identifying patterns of food preferences, including noting empty calorie foods. Patients should be counseled about the need to include foods from the four basic food groups.

In the case of malnutrition, efforts should be made to increase the consumption of foods that are balanced in carbohydrates and protein. Recently, commercially available high protein liquid supplements have been developed and proposed as a means of treating the nutritional problems of pulmonary patients. There is no evidence that these supplements have any advantage over less costly high calorie drinks available at the grocery store. In fact required amounts of protein, carbohydrate, and fat are not known (Wilson et al, 1985) (see Chapter 12).

Significant oxygen desaturation may occur with meals. An oximeter is a noninvasive method of determining the patient's saturation of oxygen and can be easily performed at the bedside and in the home. Documented desaturation with meals is an indication for oxygen supplementation with meals.

EVALUATION

Once the cycle of poor eating habits has been overcome, patients should begin to show signs of interest in food. Weight gain may be an indication of improved nutritional status, along with signs of increased muscle strength (improved cough, increased ambulation).

DAILY LIVING AS SPOUSE OR COMPANION TO THE PERSON WITH CHRONIC OBSTRUCTIVE PULMONARY DISEASE

With COPD, as with any chronic illness, problems in daily living touch those who share the patient's home and life. COPD is an invisible (though not a silent) disease. It presents the risks of being difficult to understand and therefore difficult to accommodate. At the same time, the coughing and sputum management, the medication regimen, and the difficulties in breathing in both waking and sleeping hours are ever-present reminders of the patient's status.

DEMANDS OF DAILY LIVING

Patients' fears of being left alone in the home affect the spouse (or companion) in a number of ways. The spouse may feel limited in where he can go and for how long. Patient anxiety can influence what friends are allowed into the home. The overall restriction in activities for the caregiver can become a serious problem. On the one hand, the patient may develop manipulative behaviors to keep the spouse ever-present, on the other hand, the spouse may become angry with the patient and guilty because he is unsure whether or not the patient's demands are legitimate.

Role changes often occur. Depending on previous roles, the husband may have to cook and clean, or the wife may have to do yardwork.

Respite care is an important alternative for both the patient and caregiver. Despite resistance by the patient, the concept of "time-out" is important for the caregiver to reenergize. Respite programs are frequently available in the community or hospital setting. They may take the form of a 2-hour break or short-term hospitalization in a facility.

As the patient's condition worsens, hospice may be required to deal with the patient dying from complications of COPD.

SEXUALITY

Inability to become sexually aroused or meet the sexual needs of the spouse or companion may occur. Many patients are resigned to the loss of previous levels of sexual involvement while those close to them may feel quite differently.

Patients with severe COPD are limited in their functional levels due to the physiologic limitations in breathing. Medications may also interfere with their sexual performance, e.g., diuretics may alter sexual arousal. Positional changes can be explored with the patient to reduce the breathing requirements on the patient. Oxygen may be ordered to assist the patient in having sex.

The importance of touching and talking should be emphasized as an important mode of communicating sexually. This is an area in which the patient is not limited.

DECISIONS IN TREATMENT AND TERMINAL CARE

The patient and the spouse need to be involved in decisions about the aggressiveness of treatment as the disease becomes more severe or terminal. This includes decisions regarding hospitalization, use of intensive care facilities, tracheostomies, and other life-saving maneuvers. Both the patient and the spouse need support during terminal stages of the illness. Symptoms or situations in which the physician should be called, what to do when someone dies, and/or how to know the patient is dead should be discussed. The nurse can be a supportive person in opening these discussions and helping couples or families relate effectively to each other in the midst of these ongoing stresses.

RISK FACTORS

Couples with prior difficulties in their relationship will truly test the relationship in a chronic care setting. Patients with COPD may be required to reduce the amount of assistance they have previously provided in house maintenance activities and increase the amount of attention surrounding pulmonary care activities. It sometimes appears that patients find it easier to give up activities than struggle to maintain independence. If the spouse or companion has a need to be protective, the relationship may

not suffer immediately. Eventually, however, the caregivers will find themselves hopelessly restricted, i.e., providing for the patient at the expense of his own needs.

Supportive counseling can be useful in any of these situations. The nurse can play an important role as both a listener and a person to clarify the issues.

Frequent hospitalizations absorb a great deal of money and may affect the family's savings. Patients may need assistance with decisions about insurance coverage, Medicare, and Medicaid.

SIGNS AND SYMPTOMS

Observing a couple together can indicate how they are communicating and if changes in communication are occurring. If they visited the physician's office together, but now no longer do this, or if the spouse does not come into the room to hear the discussion of issues with the physician, there could be a problem. Complaints or nit-picking at whatever is said by spouse about the other spouse is a clue that all is not well between the couple. It may be an indicator that the caretaker or spouse is tired, worried, or not understanding what is happening, or it may be a bid for attention from someone instead of having to give all of the time.

The nurse may observe patients developing a lack of interest in themselves evidenced by changes in grooming, deterioration in physical condition, increases in infections and even hospitalization—all of which may indicate interpersonal problems.

COMPLICATIONS

The relationship can be severed by separation or divorce, leaving the patient without this needed support. Physical and emotional health may deteriorate. Lack of compliance with medical regimen can lead to infection and hospitalizations, increased cough, lack of sleep, increased difficulty breathing, not wanting to get up, and giving up usual activities.

PROGNOSIS

The prognosis for managing daily living effectively as the spouse of the older patient with COPD is associated with the following:

Strength and stability of the relationship to the patient

Spouse's levels of physical and emotional strength and endurance

Capacity and desire to understand the pathology and its treatment

Ability to get adequate sleep and rest on a regular basis

Opportunities for genuine respite periods when needed

Availability of effective support from persons among the health professionals giving care to the patient and from family or friends

MANAGEMENT

Maintaining the integrity of the spouse or companion in the family can be important to the well-being of the patient. In some instances the needs of the caregiver may supersede those of the patient.

Relationships The nurse should be alert to subtle clues of changes in the relationship between the patient and their spouse or caregiver, especially in communication and body language. In a private time with the spouse, high-risk areas in daily living can be discussed, e.g., personal goals, worries and fears, depression, feeling neglected, sleep patterns and fatigue level, periods of respite, personal health status, sexuality, thoughts regarding loss of the spouse, and consideration of separations or divorce. Sensitivity is needed in order to permit spouses to share information they desire to share, without invading areas where they prefer to retain privacy.

Talking with the couple together may provide different kinds of information. One may address their strategies in managing daily living with the restrictions of the disease and its treatment, their successes and problems, and their goals and satisfactions. It is important to gather data and acknowledge the successes and strengths in the situation as well as to diagnose areas where the couple could benefit from help.

Where serious problems in the relationship exist or threaten to develop, professional counseling from a pastor, social worker, or psychiatrist may be desirable. The idea can be introduced to the individuals and referrals made if they wish.

Household and Living Environment A review of the household and living environment

should be done. Important areas for consideration include sleeping arrangements, how the patient could have quiet and privacy at times and yet be able to summon help, how the location of equipment and location of the bathroom can be used to make the treatments efficient and less energy consuming. Installation of an intercom or bell system to awaken the spouse or call for assistance can be reassuring to all in the household.

Managing Daily Living in the Terminal Phase of Illness

When the patient becomes terminally ill, many areas of management should be discussed, preferably before the patient is exceedingly ill. It is far better to discuss issues of life support and future hospitalizations when the patient is not feeling pressured to make a decision. Some patients, when approached about their desire for resuscitation measures, misinterpret the request to mean they are about to face imminent death. Timing of the discussion is important.

The wishes of the patient and family regarding termination of care or life support measures needs to be made explicit so that their wishes can be honored. In support of this decision, the patient may have a durable power of attorney for health care or living will (see Chapter 5).

If the patient has decided against future hospitalization, the spouse needs to be informed about others who can augment care in the home. A variety of resources are available. The office nurse, visiting nurse services, local hospice program, or hospital social worker can provide information. Hospice programs can be an important source of support, care, and information to the spouse, companion, and patient.

Home management of the terminally ill patient with COPD may include administration of narcotics to relieve dyspnea.

EVALUATION

Effective management of daily living with chronic and terminal aspects of COPD can be evaluated in terms of the following:

Maintenance of the health and stamina of the spouse

Continuing openness of the spouse in discussing the difficult and positive aspects of daily living and the strategies that are being used

Maintenance of a relationship between spouse and patient that satisfies them both even though there will be the normal disagreement and strains that accompany life-threatening illness

Expressions of the feeling of effective support from health care providers

Expressions of satisfaction with the approach to death and dying even as grieving is occurring

References and Other Readings

American Thoracic Society. Evaluation of impairment/disability secondary to respiratory disease. Am Rev Respir Dis 1987; 133:1205.

Aubier M, De Troyer A, Sampson M, et al. Aminohylline improves diaphragmatic contractility. N Engl J Med 1981; 305:249.

Bernstein IL. Comolyn sodium. Chest 1985; 87s: 68s.

Braman SS, Kaemmerlen JT, Davis SM. Asthma in the elderly. A comparison between patients with recently acquired and long-standing disease. Am Rev Respir Dis 1991; 143:336.

Burrows B, Earle RH. Course and prognosis of chronic obstructive lung disease: a prospective study of 200 patients. N Engl J Med 1969; 280:397.

Camilli AE, Burrows B, Knudson RJ, et al. Longitudinal changes in forced expiratory volume in one second in adults. Effects of smoking and smoking cessation. Am Rev Resp Dis 1987; 135:794.

Celli B, Criner G, Rassulo J. Ventilatory muscle recruitment during unsupported arm exercise in normal subjects. J Appl Physiol 1988;64: 1936.

Centers for Disease Control, Atlanta, GA. Tuberculin skin testing (video).

Core Curriculum on Tuberculosis USDHHS PHS. Centers for Disease Control, Atlanta, GA, 2nd ed. April 1991, 00-5763.

Donowitz GR, Mandell GL. Acute pneumonia. In: Mandell GL, et al, eds. Principles and practice of infectious diseases, 2nd ed. New York: John Wiley, 1985.

Engle GL. Grief and grieving. Am J Nurs 1964; 64:93.

Fishman AP. Pulmonary diseases and disorders, 2nd ed. New York: McGraw-Hill, 1988.

Frame PT. Acute infectious pneumonia in the adult. Basics of Respiratory Disease 1982; 10:1.

Gleckman RA. Community-acquired pneumonia in the geriatric patient. Hosp Pract 1985; 20:57.

Hendeles L, Weinberger M. Theophylline, a "state of the art" review. Pharmacotherapy 1983; 3:2.

Higgins MW, Keller JB, Becker M, et al. An index of risk for obstructive airways disease. Am Rev Respir Dis 1982; 125:144.

Holtzclaw BJ. Shivering. A nursing problem. Nurs Clin North Am 1990; 25:977.

Kripke DF, Simons RN, Garfinkel L, Hammond EC. Short and long sleep and sleeping pills. Arch Gen Psychiatry 1979; 38:103.

Mahler DA, Matthay RA, Snyder PE, et al. Sustained-release theophylline reduces dyspnea in nonreversible obstructive airway disease. Am Rev Respir Dis 1985; 132:22.

McDonald G, Borson S, Gayle T, et al. Alleviation of depression (and anxiety) in COPD improves function but not dyspnea. Am Rev Respir Dis 1990; 141:A508.

Mei-Tal V, Meyers BS. Major psychiatric illnesses in the elderly: empirical study on an inpatient psychogeriatric unit. Part I: diagnostic complexities. Int Psych Med 1985; 15:91.

Merck manual of geriatrics. Rahway, NJ: Merck, Sharpe, & Dohme Research Laboratories, 1990: 441.

National Center for Health Statistics Advanced Report of Final Mortality Statistics 1987. Monthly Vital Statistics Report, vol 38, no. 5, supplement. Hyattesville, MD: Public Health Service, 1989.

National Heart, Lung, and Blood Institute, Division of Lung Diseases Workshop Report. The definition of emphysema. Am Rev Respir Dis 1985; 132:182.

Niederman MS, Fein AM. Pneumonia in the elderly. Geriatr Clin North Am 1986; 2:241.

Nocturnal Oxygen Therapy Trial Group: Continuous or nocturnal oxygen therapy in hypoxemic chronic obstructive lung disease. Ann Intern Med 1980; 93:391.

Official Statement of the American Thoracic Society, Standards for the Diagnosis and Care of Patients with Chronic Obstructive Pulmonary Disease (COPD) and Asthma. Am Rev Respir Dis 1987; 136:225.

Openbrier DR, Covey M. Ineffective breathing pattern related to malnutrition. Nurs Clin North Am 1987; 22:225.

Prolastin Alpha$_1$-Proteinase Inhibitor (Human). Product Monograph. Miles Inc., Cutter Biological, November 1988.

Richman L. A looming public health nightmare. In: Lungs at work. New York: American Lung Association, 1992.

Screening for tuberculosis and tuberculosis infection in high-risk populations and the use of preventive therapy in tuberculosis infection in the U.S. USDHHS, PHS, CDC, Center for Prevention Services, Division of TB Control, Atlanta, GA, May 18, 1990, vol 39, no. RR–8.

Stengel G. Oral temperature in the elderly. Unpublished master's thesis. Seattle: University of Washington Library, 1980.

The health consequences of smoking: a report of the Surgeon General. Chronic obstructive lung disease. US Department of Health and Human Services. Washington, DC: US Government Printing Office, 1984.

Webb WB. Age-related changes in sleep. Clin Geriatr Med 1989; 5:275.

West GA, Primeau P. Nonmedical hazards of long-term oxygen therapy. Respir Care 1983; 28:906.

Wilson DO, Rogers RM, Hoffman RM. Nutrition and chronic lung disease. Am Rev Respir Dis 1985; 132:1347.

Yoshikawa T. Tuberculosis in aging adults. J Am Geriatr Soc 1992; 40:178.

Ziment I. Pharmacologic therapy of obstructive airway disease. Clin Chest Med 1990; 11:461.

33
Common Skin Problems

CONNIE DAVIS

As the outermost tissue layer of the body, the skin provides a protective covering for the inner tissues and organs and is the part of the self that is visible to others. It is a boundary and shield between the body and its environment, assists in the perception of the environment, and performs or initiates many of the adaptations resulting from this perception. The principal functions of the skin are protection, heat regulation, sensation, and body image. Age-related changes in the skin disrupt these functions to varying degrees and in turn create problems in daily living. The normal changes in the skin occurring with aging are discussed in Chapter 8.

Pathophysiology and Medical Management

Skin disorders are relatively common in the elderly, with an estimated 66% of those over 70 having one skin condition and one third of those experiencing two or more (Balin, 1990). The following are factors that influence the development, presentation, and course of skin diseases in the elderly:

1. Normal aging changes
   Atrophy of the reticular endothelial system
   Decreased sebum excretion
   Changes in responsiveness of nerve endings to sensory stimuli
   Alterations in peripheral vascular circulation and fragile blood vessel walls
   Inelasticity of skin, thinner dermis, and decreased attachment between epidermis and dermis
   Increased renewal time due to decreased turnover in stratum corneum (Balin, 1990)
2. Personal factors
   Nutritional status
   Lifelong history of exposure to sunlight, wind, temperature extremes, humidity, radiation, drugs, or occupational hazards
   Emotional responses to life situations
   Chronic diseases
3. Photodamage
   Increased anomalies in elastic fibers
   Thickened walls of venules
   Hyperplasia of sebaceous glands
   Further decreases in the number of immune cells
   Uneven skin pigmentation (Balin, 1990)

In this chapter common skin problems of the elderly are classified by pathologic process: alterations in cell growth, infections, hypersensitive responses, vascular disturbances, and results of trauma (pressure sores, surgical incisions, or accidental wounds). Basic lesion terminology appears in Table 33–1.

TABLE 33–1 *Skin Lesion Terminology*

	Lesion	Characteristics	Examples
PRIMARY SKIN LESIONS			
Flat	Macules	Nonpalpable localized areas of color change. Various shapes. May be associated with scaling	Drug eruptions; petechiae; areas of melanin deposition
Elevated—solid and localized	Papules	Lesions of approximately 0.5 cm in diameter or less. Top and borders of various shapes. Color—lighter, darker, or same as skin	Pedunculated (neurofibromas); round or irregular (senile angiomas); flat-topped (psoriasis); pointed (insect bites)
	Nodules	Lesions ranging in size from about 0.5 to 1 cm in diameter. Extend deeper into skin than papules. Palpation: when lesion is below the dermis the skin slides over it, whereas a dermal lesion moves with the skin	Erythema nodosum; gouty tophi
	Tumors	Lesions larger than 1 cm	Basal cell carcinoma
	Wheals	Irregular; circumscribed area of edema; color varies from pale to red	Insect bites; hives
Fluid-filled elevations	Vesicles	An accumulation of serous fluid within or below the epidermis depending on the site of cell damage. Diameter less than 1 cm	Blisters; second-degree burns
	Bullae	Serous fluid accumulations greater than 1 cm	Bullous pemphigoid
	Pustules	Vesicles or bullae filled with pus. The translucent skin overlying the lesion reveals the color of the contents (e.g., yellow, green, milky)	Infected pimples
SECONDARY SKIN LESIONS			
	Crusts	Formed from materials that seep out of the skin and dry; may be pus, blood, or serum	Impetigo
	Scales	Accumulations of thin plates of dried, cornified epithelium	Psoriasis; exfoliative dermatitis
	Lichenification	Thickening of skin layers, often as a result of repeated rubbing. Normal skin furrows are accentuated.	Atopic dermatitis
	Erosion	Removal of the upper epidermal layer, resulting in a moist surface that does not bleed or scar	Rupture of a blister or vesicle from allergic reaction
	Ulcer	Removal of skin to a depth below the basal cell layer with healing by scar tissue	Stasis ulcer; pressure ulceration
	Scar	Replacement of normal tissue with fibrous tissue	Keloid (hypertrophied scar)
	Atrophy	Decrease in size and number of cells, resulting in thinning and loss of normal skin furrows	

Data from Bates B. A guide to physical examination and history taking, 5th ed. Philadelphia: J. B. Lippincott, 1991.

ALTERATIONS IN CELL GROWTH

Alterations in cell growth may be classified as benign, premalignant, or malignant.

BENIGN EPIDERMAL TUMORS

Benign epidermal tumors include skin tags, corns, calluses, seborrheic keratosis, and kerato-acanthoma. These are common, unsightly, hyperkeratotic lesions that can be treated for cosmetic reasons.

Etiologic Factors Keratoses, or abnormal growth of keratinizing cells of the epidermis, occur as a result of pressure, often pressure on skin that is sandwiched between a bony structure and a shoe surface. The etiology of skin tags is unknown.

Manifestations *Skin tags* are small (pinhead to pea size), soft, pedunculated protrusions of normal-colored skin. *Seborrheic keratosis* (e.g., seborrheic wart, basal cell papilloma) are slightly raised, yellowish or tan 1-cm, "stuck-on" plaques that are sharply circumscribed and covered with a greasy scale. As the lesion ages, it thickens and becomes more brown or brownish black and may have a granular appearance as a result of follicular plugging (DeWitt, 1990). *Hard corns* are found usually on toes. *Calluses*, which are circumscribed thickenings of the horny layer of the skin, occur on the plantar surface of the foot.

Treatment Skin tags and seborrheic keratoses may be removed from troublesome areas for cosmetic reasons using excision, curettage, electrodissection, or application of liquid nitrogen or carbon dioxide (DeWitt, 1990). Treatment of corns include trimming the thickened portion with a surgical knife blade, stretching shoes, and applying pads to relieve pressure. Molded orthoses are used to relieve pressure on calluses. Surgery for malformations can eliminate the cause of calluses or corns. Shoes with fairly rigid soles allow walking with minimal pressure under metatarsal heads.

PREMALIGNANT CONDITIONS

Actinic (solar) and *radiation keratoses* are important keratolytic lesions since they may lead to basal or squamous cell carcinoma. *Leukoplakia* occurs as spots or patches on the mucosal or mucocutaneous tissues such as lips, buccal mucosa, and vulva.

Etiologic Factors Premalignant conditions have been linked to cell damage, including mechanical irritation, radiation exposure, or chronic irritation from tobacco or other substances.

High Risk At high risk are persons experiencing occupational or lifestyle exposure.

Manifestations *Keratoses* are slightly elevated, light brown-black, scaly papules on exposed body surfaces. The surface may be flat, round, or verrucous (wart-like). The scale is adherent and returns each time it is removed. The chronicity of the lesion and its enlargement, induration, and ulceration are significant factors in consideration of the need for dermatologist referral. *Leukoplakia* are discrete, persistent, white plaques that may be either smooth or warty and may fissure or ulcerate. Usually they are free of induration or inflammation unless they transform to squamous cell carcinoma.

Prevention Prevention of keratoses involves wearing protective clothing and use of sunscreen with adequate sun protection factor. Blacks seldom develop solar keratoses because of the pigment and horny protective layer of their skin. Leukoplakia is prevented by avoiding tissue-irritating habits.

Treatment Refer to a dermatologist. A variety of methods are used to remove lesions: surgical excision, cauterization, cryosurgery with liquid nitrogen, and topical application of a 1% to 5% concentration of 5-fluorouracil in propylene glycol. Specimens are examined by a pathologist for diagnostic confirmation. Results usually are curative, especially if the source of irritation is eliminated.

MALIGNANT CONDITIONS

Malignant conditions include basal cell carcinoma, squamous cell carcinoma, and malignant melanoma (Table 33–2).

INFECTIOUS CONDITIONS

Infectious conditions that are relatively common in the elderly are herpes zoster (viral), can-

TABLE 33–2 *Malignant Conditions*

Basal Cell	*Squamous Cell*	*Malignant Melanoma*
HIGH RISK		
Persons with fair skin and chronic sun exposure	Often at site of previous skin lesions such as sunburns, radiation, chronic ulcers, chemical burns, scars or sinus tracts	Occurs in exposed areas of skin
DYNAMICS		
Arises from basal cell. Grows slowly, extends into surrounding tissue. Rarely metastasizes	Arises from squamous cell, grows quicker than basal cell, may metastasize early, especially in lip, tongue, or external genitalia	Invades and metastasizes. Often arises from melanocytes found in moles
MANIFESTATIONS		
Papular with semitranslucent pearly appearance, center can ulcerate into a persistent open sore. May be pigmented, small blood vessels may be visible at border. Crusting can occur 6 months to 1 year. May extend to bone	Single hard conical nodule, invades and destroys surrounding skin. Leaves indurated area with indistinct and elevated border. Attaches to underlying tissues, may become fixed and firm, metastasize to regional lymph nodes	Irregular border, varied colors of blue, red. Irregular uneven surfaces
PREVENTION		
Avoid sun exposure	Avoid sun exposure	
TREATMENT		
Surgical excision, curettage, cryotherapy, electrodissection, radiation, chemotherapy, Moh's micrographic surgery in advanced, recurrent, or clinically ill-defined tumors or in areas where cosmetic considerations or preservation of function is tantamount	Early recognition, surgical excision, curettage, electrodissection, irradiation or chemosurgery	Wide and deep surgical excision, systematic chemotherapy or regional perfusion may be required due to early metastasis

didiasis (yeast [in the fungal family]), and scabies (infestation). Skin infections in the elderly may indicate underlying systemic disorders such as diabetes, lymphoma, or anemia.

The systemic manifestations associated with infectious processes (elevated temperature, increased perspiration, increased heart rate, and elevated neutrophilic count) are not as pronounced in the elderly as in younger persons; therefore, detection of these processes requires close scrutiny of all indicants.

HERPES ZOSTER

Etiologic Factors Herpes zoster (shingles) is caused by reactivation of latent varicella virus (Phillips and Gilchrist, 1990). Approximately 20 percent of the population with a history of prior exposure will experience a reactivation in their lifetimes (Liesegang, 1991).

High Risk The elderly who are experiencing trauma, surgery, or stress are prone to reactivation. Persons with Hodgkin's disease and lymphomas and persons receiving immunosuppressive therapy or irradiation are also at high risk.

Dynamics Pathogenesis is through reactivation of a latent viral infection of the dorsal root ganglia with retrograde spread to the skin. Cause of reactivation is unknown; it may occur in situations listed under high risk.

Manifestations It appears as groups of papulovesicular lesions following a unilateral dermatomal pattern down an arm or more frequently around one side of the lower chest from posterior to anterior midline. The lesions become pustular or occasionally hemorrhagic about a week later and a crust develops. Pain of a burning nature with varying duration and often of extreme severity occurs in most persons. The disorder clears in about 3 to 4 weeks but the pain may persist longer if a postherpetic neuralgia is present, in which case the pain may persist for months to years.

Prevention Infections involving the trigeminal, second or third cervical nerves, or eighth nerve can cause lasting sensorineural problems. Early medical treatment may reduce postherpetic neuralgia. Infections involving the eye are serious. Varicella zoster immunoglobulin provides effective protection and is used for immunosuppressed patients (Judelsohn 1972).

Treatment Sedatives allow for sleep, and high doses of analgesics may be necessary to relieve pain. Calamine lotion and menthol camphor are beneficial. Burrow's or other hypertonic solutions three times a day followed by antibacterial soap or topical antibiotic ointments may be palliative and prevent secondary infection. Isolation precautions are not necessary because transmission of the disorder is not by contact.

Acyclovir in oral doses higher than those used to treat herpes simplex are used to decrease severity of rash and pain (McKendrick et al, 1986; Huff et al, 1988). Tagamet, a histamine blocker, has been used to decrease rash symptoms, and prednisone can promote healing and decrease postherpetic complications.

Complications Postherpetic neuralgia is a common complication. Eaglstein and coworkers (1970) indicate that cortisone therapy will prevent postherpetic neuralgia in the elderly. Eye complications occur in 50 percent of those with ophthalmic involvement and include eyelid scarring, corneal disease, vasculitis, uveitis, and secondary glaucoma (Liesegang, 1991). Cervical sympathetic nerve blocks have been found to relieve herpetic pain and speed up resolution of the eruption in eye lesions. Tricyclics are also used to treat the pain of postherpetic neuralgia (Portenoy, 1990). Capsaicin in an ointment can provide relief for postherpetic neuralgia by depleting the nerve endings of substance P, although some users find the tingling sensation of the ointment unpleasant (Westerman et al, 1988).

CANDIDIASIS (MONILIASIS)

Etiologic Factors Candidiasis is a yeast infection.

High Risk Persons with a debilitating disease are at high risk, as are those taking broad-spectrum antibiotics.

Dynamics Candidiasis needs moisture to grow. It establishes colonies in intertriginous areas, especially at the angle of the mouth, under dentures, under the breasts, and around the anus and perineum.

Manifestations It occurs as excoriated, inflamed areas with sections of white plaques (yeast colonies).

Treatment Dry with a heat lamp and/or topical dehydrating medications. Clotrimazole, miconazole, nystatin, or econazole are used to treat yeast infections (DeWitt, 1990).

SCABIES

Etiologic Factors *Sarcoptes scabiei*, the itch mite, is the causative factor.

High Risk At risk are persons in unhygienic conditions or who bathe infrequently.

Dynamics The organism burrows and moves along under the skin.

Manifestations It appears as a dark line under the skin. Itching over the site is a common symptom. Usually it occurs on inner surfaces of thighs and forearms, under breasts, between the fingers, and around the perineum.

Prevention Personal and environmental hygienic practices will aid in preventing scabies.

Treatment After bathing, a cream or lotion containing permethrin lindane or crotamiton is applied over the entire body. Twenty-four hours after treatment, all clothing and bed linen should be laundered, and treatment with crotamiton is repeated. Items that cannot be washed may be sealed in an airtight bag for 2 weeks. Treatment may be repeated as directed in 7 days. All medications are washed off after treatment. Hydrocortisone cream or calamine lotion is applied for itch, after scabicide treatment is completed. Antibiotics may be necessary for secondary infections (Phillips and Gilchrist, 1990). Itching may persist several weeks after successful treatment.

HYPERSENSITIVE RESPONSES

Dermatoses of an immune (hypersensitive) nature occur at any age. The disorders seen in the elderly may be exacerbations of previous conditions, newly acquired, or result from therapy for other pathology. Among the changes that enhance the possibility of or mute the response to contact dermatitis are (1) increased epidermal permeability due to decreased protective oily secretions; (2) sensitizing substances in contact with the skin longer due to slower turnover of stratum corneum; and (3) decreased absorption through the skin due to decreased dermal blood flow.

CONTACT DERMATITIS

Etiologic Factors Concentration of irritating or allergenic substances in skin tissue is antecedent to contact dermatitis. Common irritants are soaps, detergents, and other cleansing agents. Determination of the cause is more difficult in the elderly due to the delayed and decreased immune response (Balin, 1990). Frequent immersions in water predispose to the condition.

Manifestations Itching, burning, and redness may be followed by papules, vesicles, and edema. Scratching may result in infections. Repeated reactions lead to thickening of the skin.

Treatment Protect from further damage by the use of rubber gloves when handling irritants. Avoid contacts with known irritants.

To decrease itching and reduce edema, cool wet dressings, topical steroids, and antihistamines may be prescribed. Ointments are preferred for use in the elderly due to their occlusive property, lower cost, and lower incidence of allergic reactions. Creams are preferred for intertriginous areas and lotions or solutions for the scalp (Parisier, 1991). Systemic antibiotics are used if infections occur.

VASCULAR DISTURBANCES

BENIGN VASCULAR TUMORS

Vascular disturbances in the elderly range from benign vascular tumors, venous lakes, and purpura that require little or no treatment, to stasis ulcerations that can cause serious disability and require prolonged treatment.

STASIS DERMATITIS/ULCERATIONS

Etiologic Factors Ischemia of lower extremities is the cause of arterial ulcers; venous ulcers result from prolonged venous hypertension (Richelson, 1990).

Dynamics Single or multiple variables are present such as valvular incompetence, chronic venous insufficiency, venous stasis, atherosclerosis, and age changes in the cutaneous vascular supply. The compromised tissue is poorly oxygenated and end products of metabolism accumulate. Healing is slow. Secondary infection is a potential complication. The underlying pathology often is not curable; therefore, the condition becomes chronic (Richelson, 1990).

Manifestations This condition is manifested in erythema, vesicular lesions, edema, hyperpigmentation, and thin, dry skin. With chronicity there is thickened epidermis, indurated scaly papules or plaques, and accentuated skin markings (lichenification). A brownish discoloration produced by hemosiderin is secondary to petechial hemorrhages. Ulcerations may follow from trauma to the area. Itching is severe and scratching may cause breaks in the skin.

Treatment Bed rest with limited mobility is recommended. Elevation of the foot of the bed and sitting with the legs elevated as much as possible helps to drain the veins and minimize edema. This is contraindicated if the ulcer accompanies arterial insufficiency.

Agents used in the care of an ulcer include damp dressings of normal saline. Topical steroids decrease inflammation. Sometimes oral antibiotics are necessary depending on the results of laboratory studies for organisms and sensitivity. When an ulcer is clean, a zinc paste boot (Unnas boot) provides an occlusive medicated bandage for 7 to 10 days. This allows for reepithelialization and healing without the trauma of frequent dressings. Mobility is possible with a boot. Cleanliness is necessary to prevent infection.

With arterial insufficiency, Buerger's exercises may promote circulation. A sequential compression device may be used to assist return of fluid to circulation (Richelson, 1990). Vascular surgery may be necessary to attain adequate blood flow.

Duration of treatment is prolonged, sometimes months. Hospitalization is not necessary if adequate support is available at home.

TRAUMA

Trauma in the elderly results from pressure over bony prominences, surgical wounds, or accidental injury.

PRESSURE ULCERS

A pressure ulcer is defined as a localized area of trauma resulting from a lack of blood supply to the involved tissue (Broadwell and Jackson, 1982). The danger of this condition is high in elderly people with mobility restrictions and protein deficiencies (Ek et al, 1991). Pressure of sufficient extent and duration to interfere with adequate blood flow and hence with tissue nutrition and oxygen will result in necrosis. The extent and duration of pressure necessary to result in tissue damage are not consistent from one person to another.

Etiologic Factors   Primary etiologic factors include pressure, shearing force, friction, and moisture (Levine et al, 1989).

PRESSURE   The greatest pressure occurs in that tissue closest to the bone, leading to damage of muscle and subcutaneous tissue before the ulcer is visible at the surface. Duration of the pressure affects the amount of damage.

The longer the sustained pressure the greater the danger of interference with circulation. Mean capillary pressure is 25 mm Hg; therefore, positional pressure readily occludes the microcirculation. High pressure for a short time is safer to skin than low pressure for long periods (Husain, 1953). Pressure varies with position. Pressure on ischial tuberosities is greater when sitting in a chair with the feet supported than when the feet hang free. The latter situation distributes the weight along the posterior thighs, and thus does not focus pressure on one site. Pressure on the sacral area varies directly with the extent of the elevation of the head of the bed (Lindan et al, 1965). Persons in semi- or high Fowler's position for cardiovascular respiratory problems are at increased risk for postural pressure lesions. The extent of pressure varies with body build (Lindan et al, 1965). Weight-bearing pressure is concentrated over the bony prominences of thin persons, whereas the tissues of an obese person disperse the weight over a larger surface. However, the blood supply to the subcutaneous tissue of an obese person is impaired because blood vessels are not proportionately increased and overall tissue nutrition and oxygenation may be marginal. Additionally, the interstitial area for transport of nutrients is greater in an obese person than one of normal height–weight relationships.

SHEARING FORCES   Shearing occurs when layers of tissue are slid along horizontal planes, changing their normal anatomic relation to each other. Shearing forces on sacral tissues vary directly with increasing elevation of the head of the bed (Goth, 1942). With head elevation, the outer skin tissues adhere to the bed linen but gravity pull displaces the underlying subcutaneous tissue downward. This uneven tissue shift distorts the blood vessels within the tissues, causing angulation and interference with circulation. As noted previously, maintenance of a semisitting position increases susceptibility to sacral tissue trauma.

FRICTION   Friction is created when two surfaces move across each other, such as a patient being dragged across the sheets. This removes the stratum corneum and hastens ulceration.

MOISTURE   Moisture from incontinency, wound exudate, or perspiration contributes to skin maceration and irritation. Overweight individuals are further at risk due to moisture trapped in skin folds.

Risk Factors Weiler et al (1990) studied 373 elderly nursing home residents to determine risk factors for pressure sore development. Odds of having a pressure sore were 31 times higher when signs of malnutrition were present and 24 times higher when infection was present. Ek et al (1991) also studied factors affecting development and healing of pressure sores in the elderly and found protein malnutrition to be a major factor. Conditions such as psychiatric diagnoses (excluding senile dementia of the Alzheimer's type) had nearly threefold increased risk for pressure sore existence. Hip fracture or hypertension increased risk twofold over those patients without these diagnoses. Other factors increasing the odds of pressure sore presence by two to four times included lower scores on mental status examination and incontinence. Risk assessment tools such as the Norton scale (Norton et al, 1975) and the Braden scale (Bergstrom et al, 1987) are currently being tested and used. Table 33–3 lists risk factors for pressure sore development.

Manifestations Manifestations of tissue trauma include

1. Redness that persists for longer than 20 minutes after pressure release
2. Positive blanching test—slow capillary filling following digital pressure
3. Persistent redness or dusky redness
4. Softened (mushy) and/or hardened (indurated) area under site
5. Blister or break in continuity of skin (Pajk, 1990).

Treatment of Wounds Wound healing occurs in the following phases: inflammatory (defensive or reactive), proliferative (generative, fibroblastic or connective tissue phase), and maturation or remodeling (Cooper, 1990). The inflammatory phase takes place 0 to 4 days after injury and is characterized by hemostasis and removal of debris and bacteria. Granulation tissue composed of ground substance, collagen, blood vessels, macrophages, and fibroblasts then forms in the base of the wound, giving it a red, raw, shiny appearance (Bryant, 1987). Epithelial cells replicate at the edges from healthy tissue with newly formed blood vessels (Hess and Miller, 1990). Necrotic or

TABLE 33–3 *Risk Factors for the Development of Pressure Ulcers*

Altered mental status	Infection
	Jaundice
Anemia	Malnutrition
Chronic illness	Obesity
Circulatory deficiencies	Paralysis/decreased sensation
Diabetes mellitus	Pruritis
Diaphoresis	Underweight
Edema	Unrelieved pressure
Fever	Weakness and debilitation
Immobility	
Incontinence	Xerosis

dead tissue inhibits this growth period, which takes between 4 and 24 days. Fibroblasts follow and form a scar that attains approximately 80% of the tensile strength of the surrounding tissue (Cooper, 1990). Remodeling of the scar occurs over several months and up to 2 years. Growth factors such as platelet-derived growth factor, epidermal growth factor, and angiogenic growth factor have been identified that contribute to wound healing (Jackson and Rovee, 1988).

Aging leads to a slowing of healing mechanisms. Inflammatory response, cell migration, proliferation, and maturation slow, as well as epithelialization and wound contraction (Jones and Millman, 1990).

Promoting wound healing includes creating an optimal environment for healing to occur and actively stimulating the healing process (Jackson and Rovee, 1988). Wound healing is promoted by energy conservation, adequate sleep, and thermoregulation. Attention should be paid to correction of systemic perfusion problems such as overhydration or underhydration (Jones and Millman, 1990). Local perfusion to the wound is compromised in the elderly due to changes in peripheral vascular resistance, decreased number of capillaries in skin, and decreased functioning of the immune system. Maintenance of adequate oxygenation is critical in the inflammatory and proliferative phases. Nutritional status is crucial throughout (Cooper, 1990).

DRESSINGS   The knowledge that epithelialization is delayed in a dry environment has drastically changed wound care (Jackson and Rovee, 1988). A variety of wound care products address this issue, e.g., transparent, hydrocolloid and calcium alginate dressings. Occlusive hydrocolloid dressings are applied to noninfected wounds and left in place for up to 7 days. More frequent dressing changes are associated with a decreased healing rate (Myers et al, 1988). The liquefied gel formed by hydrocolloid dressings causes alarm for some practitioners because it resembles pus (Myers et al, 1988). Transparent dressings are believed to promote autolysis or debridement through the action of leukocytes and macrophages. They are suited to uninfected Stage II or Stage III wounds without copious exudate, sinus tracts, or skin folds. Calcium alginates are nonantigenic dressings that gel in the presence of normal saline or wound fluid. They conform to wound contours and are nonadherent. Some practitioners report leaving alginates in surgical wounds without ill effects (Scherr, 1992). The benefits of moist healing include:

Maintenance of tissue hydration and viability
Reduction or elimination of scab formation
Promotion of epithelial migration, proliferation, and differentiation
Decreased time for wound contraction
Decreased inflammation and edema
Reduced pain (Jackson and Rovee, 1988)

Fine, mesh, nonadherent gauze may be used when a dry dressing is desired.

WOUND PACKING   Disinfectants commonly applied to wound packing that have been studied (including hydrogen peroxide, povidone iodine, and sodium hypochlorite) have been shown to damage tissue and/or interfere with healing. Normal saline can be safely used for noninfected wounds. Exudate absorbers such as pastes, gelatinous beads, powders, or calcium alginates (derived from seaweed) absorb drainage, debride, and provide an environment for granulation tissue to form. Wet-to-dry dressing changes have been replaced by a damp-to-moist technique. If the packing is too dry, it can stick to new tissue and cause damage if not soaked well before removal. Packing that is too wet increases bacterial growth and may macerate surrounding healthy tissue (Myers et al, 1988).

Care should be given to securing the dressing. Tape is contraindicated since the thin skin of the elderly may be removed along with the tape. Montgomery straps, skin sealants or barriers, elastic netting, roller gauze, or binders may be used (Hess and Miller, 1990).

SURGICAL WOUNDS

A decreased rate of healing and decreased final wound strength typify primary intention healing in the elderly. Wound dehiscence increases from 1% in patients between the ages of 30 and 39 to 5% in patients over age 70 undergoing abdominal surgery (Balin, 1990). Often the only sign of impending dehiscence is a marked increase in fluid drainage from the wound. Wound care follows the guidelines listed previously.

ACCIDENTAL TRAUMA

The overall increase in accidental trauma in the elderly increases their chance of wounds. Shearing forces, conditions in the environment (such as sharp edges on mechanical aides such as wheelchairs, walkers, or commodes), and factors that lead to falls predispose the elderly to abrasions, lacerations, and bruises. The decreased cohesion between the dermis and epidermis contributes to skin tears so commonly found in the elderly. Treatment of skin tears includes reapproximating the edges if possible and using steri-strips or transparent dressing to hold them in place. The wound care guidelines listed previously can be used for open wounds or skin tears that slough off or cannot be closed.

Nursing Diagnosis and Management of High-risk Areas in Daily Living

Due to the visibility and functional importance of the skin, both age-related changes and the diseases that affect it are intimately involved with daily living in many dimensions. Some of the high-risk areas of daily living are discussed. These include daily living with changed appearance, risks and discomforts of aging skin, dry skin and associated itching, pressure areas, corns, and calluses.

DAILY LIVING WITH CHANGING APPEARANCE

Age-related changes in the skin and hair are among the highly visible evidences of growing old. For some individuals these changes in appearance create problems in daily living associated with self-esteem and body image. Further, cutaneous disorders are aesthetically unappealing and carry the stigma of physical and moral uncleanliness. The person receives messages of rejection from others and inwardly may feel guilty or unworthy.

RISK FACTORS

Probably those at greatest risk are older persons who have been seen as physically attractive or beautiful and those who see their own beauty as the primary basis for interpersonal attractiveness. Those who value remaining young also find living with wrinkles, sagging tissues, and thinning hair a daily difficulty. Risks of decreased self-esteem increase when the older person is a member of family and social groups in which youth and beauty are highly prized or a basis for status, acceptance, and physical closeness.

SIGNS AND SYMPTOMS

Subtle or overt signs that indicate difficulty managing daily living include complaints reflecting sadness, depression, or anger related to appearance; or comments alluding to appearance, disbelief when they look in the mirror, and jokes about use of hair coloring products or wigs. Statements may address their lowered self-esteem or confidence in social situations and their relationships with other people.

Activities to alter the situation may include increased purchases of creams and cosmetics and nail and hair products to improve or disguise the changes. One may also learn of decreases in social contacts or reports that others avoid looking at them and touching them.

PROGNOSTIC VARIABLES

Poor prognosis for managing daily living in a satisfying way is associated with placing high value on the bloom of youth and wrinkle-free appearance, not intervening in the natural course of events with cosmetics or surgery if desired, and not associating with family and friends whose esteem and affection are based on beauty or who themselves are afraid of aging. Failing to see other personal attributes in themselves that make them worthy of self-esteem and other's esteem is also a factor in a poor prognosis for managing changes in appearance in an effective, satisfying way.

TREATMENT

Nurses who relate genuinely and positively to nonappearance traits in the person convey acceptance. Touching, establishing physical contact without conveying distaste, and establishing eye contact are important. Knowledge regarding normal physiologic changes of aging can ease the adjustment to changing appearance. Gaining the older person's perspective can be achieved through careful listening to gather data on what the presenting situation really is from the older person's point of view. The person may be supported and counseled in the use of measures to counteract or disguise age-related changes: cosmetic surgery, hair coloring, wigs, hair transplants, and the effective use of cosmetics and clothing colors and styles that distract from or minimize deficits. The older person may also need help in developing interactional strategies to handle social situations involving appearance, conversation, and behavior and thus gain a greater sense of control. Role playing and rehearsal may also be useful.

EVALUATION

More care with appearance, expressions of greater comfort in social situations, expressions of worth in nonappearance areas, and growing pride in self would be areas of improvement.

DAILY LIVING WITH RISKS AND DISCOMFORTS OF AGING SKIN

Age-related changes in the skin create added risks and discomfort in daily living. This includes *reduced*

Movement of water and chemicals into and out of the skin
Capacity to withstand mechanical trauma
Temperature-regulating capacity
Sensitivity in communicating pain, pressure, touch, temperature, and positional information to the brain (Balin, 1990)

RISK FACTORS

Dryness The normal dryness of aging skin is potentiated by low humidity in the environment, inadequate fluid intake, frequent bathing or washing using soaps or detergents, and the use of alcohol or other defatting solutions on the skin (Fitzpatrick, 1989).

Trauma The thinner, more fragile skin is in greater jeopardy when there is friction, unrelieved pressure for long periods, falls or other accidents, and exposure of the skin to chemicals or bacteria. Aged skin needs protection from photodamage. The muted inflammatory response decreases expression of sunburn even when damage has occurred (Fenske et al, 1989).

Decreased Temperature-regulating Capacity Exposure to extremes of temperature challenges the skin's thermoregulation ability. Diseases that limit the blood supply to the skin further limit response.

Decreased Sensitivity to Stimuli Excessively hot water in the home, exposure to temperature extremes, and insensitivity to pain and pressure put the older person at risk for injuries.

SIGNS AND SYMPTOMS

Presence of bruises, burns, skin abrasions, infections, pressure sores, evidence of dry skin or itching, hypothermia, or hyperthermia would be evidence that daily living is not being managed well.

PROGNOSTIC VARIABLES

The extent of discomfort and the problems in daily living associated with normal skin changes in the older individual vary greatly. The rate and amount of change is quite individual, as is the perception of physical and psychologic discomfort. The presence of other health problems, particularly those that decrease mobility, circulation, and sensory capabilities, obviously place the skin in greater jeopardy and create greater hazards in managing daily living.

TREATMENT

Teaching elderly people methods for minimizing discomfort and coping with skin changes is an important area for nursing intervention.

The following lists suggest actions the nurse may take to prevent and reduce skin-related discomfort.

Minimizing Skin Dryness

1. Restrict the use of soap in bathing to the axillary and genital areas. Use mild soap. Be sure all soap is removed.
2. Use tepid water rather than hot water for bathing.
3. Bathing twice a week is usually sufficient.
4. Apply a nonperfumed emollient to the skin immediately following washing or bathing to prevent loss of the moisture absorbed during these activities. Increase the moisture in the environment by placing room humidifiers or containers of water over heating elements (Fenske et al, 1989).
5. Wear cotton undergarments to minimize skin irritation.
6. Avoid prolonged exposure to wind and sun.
7. Avoid the use of alcohol or alcohol-containing preparations on the skin.
8. Drink 6 to 8 glasses of water per day.
9. Keep water in vases or other containers in rooms or use a room humidifier (Klein, 1988).

Minimizing Skin Absorption of Chemicals and Avoiding Skin Trauma

1. Wear hat, gloves, and long-sleeved garments when out-of-doors to protect from actinic exposure.
2. Wear gloves for dishwashing and other household chores where detergents are used.
3. Rinse hands well with plain water following use of household chemicals if gloves are not worn.
4. Wear gloves and take extra safety precautions when working with sharp equipment such as gardening and hobby tools.
5. Laundering precautions: wash new undergarments before wearing; rinse all clothes well to remove detergents.
6. Pad body surfaces being subjected to mechanical trauma, e.g., the knees when gardening, thimbles when sewing.
7. Avoid contact with extremes of hot and cold water, electric blankets, radiators, and so forth.
8. Avoid tight and constricting clothing such as elastic waistbands and stockings to prevent friction trauma as well as restriction of circulation.

Maintaining Body Temperature

1. Maintain room temperature constant around 65°F (18.5°C) in cold weather.
2. Wear close-knit (not tight) undergarments in the winter to prevent heat loss.
3. Wear hat and gloves in cold weather because heat is lost from head and hands (Besdine, 1990).
4. Wear wool in preference to synthetic fibers; wool provides better insulation.
5. Stocking or bedsocks prevent cold feet during the night.
6. Flannel sheets are warmer than regular sheets as bedclothes.
7. Stay indoors on windy days to avoid the windchill factor, which stresses adaptive mechanisms.
8. Frequent, small meals and warm liquids help to provide heat to the body.
9. Early morning is the period of lowest body metabolic activity; add extra clothes until food and physical movement stimulate the circulation.
10. Body movement stimulates circulation; therefore, alternate physical and sedentary activities (Besdine, 1990).
11. Sedatives and some tranquilizers depress cerebral function and circulation, requiring extra effort to prevent chilling (Besdine, 1990).
12. Wear light, loose but protective clothing in hot weather.
13. Wear a hat to protect against the intense heat on the head in hot weather.
14. Do outdoor work in the early morning and when the area is in the shade. Work for limited periods of time.

Preventing Injury Related to Decreased Sensitivity

1. Check temperature of bath and dishwashing water before immersing parts of the body into it.
2. Cover hot water bottles and ice packs. Remove from contact with skin for a few minutes every 5 to 10 minutes.
3. Observe areas receiving continued pressure resulting in redness or skin breakdown: coccyx, buttocks, heels and toes (from ill-fitting shoes).
4. Walk cautiously on uneven surfaces.
5. Engage in leg movements (to stimulate circulation) before getting up from a sitting position.

Management of Itching

1. Maintain adequate dietary intake of vitamins, especially vitamins A and B and niacin.
2. Avoid dry skin.
3. Use topical antipruritics such as calamine or hydrocortisone cream.
4. Oral medications such as antihistamines (trimeprazine tartrate, hydroxyzine hydrochloride, and diphenhydramine) may decrease itching.
5. Application of pressure over the site may override the itching sensation.
6. Engage in diversional activity.
7. Avoid drafts, which increase the sensation of itch (DeWitt, 1990).

DAILY LIVING WITH PRESSURE AREAS AND POSITIONAL TISSUE TRAUMA

RISK FACTORS

Risk factors in pressure sore development are listed in Table 33–4.

SIGNS AND SYMPTOMS

Several dimensions of daily living, the environment, and the person will yield data on both the risk or presence of pressure lesions.

Data collection should include: information on the presence of immobilizing pathophysiology, areas of bony prominences, weight loss and nutritional status, low serum protein values, urinary continence, and history of circulatory deficits. Observe for presence of emotional depression or apathy. Observe tissues in areas of positional pressure (coccyx, buttocks, scapula areas, feet) (Pajk, 1990).

Patterns of activities in daily living are another source of information. This includes reports or observation of current eating and fluid intake. Data on the nature of activities in a typical day also are important. Where there is risk of foot lesions, observation of gait would be important. In the environment, observation should be made of the surfaces of chairs where most sitting takes place. On the bed observation includes the condition of the bed linen.

PROGNOSTIC VARIABLES

Poor prognosis is associated with declining health and nutritional status, increasing immobility, incontinence, and declining self-care coupled with inadequate primary care.

TABLE 33–4   *Stages of Pressure Sore Development*

Stage I	*Stage II*	*Stage III*	*Stage IV*
Intact epidermis. Hyperemia, induration that blanches when touched. Reversible	Epidermis and dermis open. Distinct edges with inflammation and induration in surrounding tissue. Drainage may be present. Reversible	Ulcer extends to subcutaneous tissue, edges appear rolled and pigmented. Drainage, necrosis, or undermining may be present. May be life-threatening	Extends to muscle or bone. Drainage present. Sinus tracts and wide undermining may be present. Osteomyelitis or septic arthritis of involved bones may be fatal

Adapted from Pajk M. Pressure sores. In: Abrams, Berkow, eds. The Merck manual of geriatrics. Rahway, NJ: Merck & Co, 1990.

TREATMENT

Prevention   The goal of nursing therapy is the prevention of positional tissue trauma. Prevention is based on managing the causative and risk factors. In particular, the activities are designed to prevent prolonged pressure on tissues overlying weight-bearing bony prominences and to avoid shearing forces. Interventions to accomplish this include the following:

A turning schedule that protects the most vulnerable areas, fits with sleeping, eating, visiting, TV, and other ADLs and uses all positions possible before returning to the initial position

Avoidance of the semi-Fowler and high Fowler positions whenever possible to prevent shearing

Half-hourly release of pressure when sitting in a wheelchair

Use of pressure distributing devices such as convoluted foam mattresses and cushions, alternating air pressure mattresses, sheep skin, air-fluidized beds, or gel pads (Braun et al, 1988).

Nutritional status influences susceptibility to pressure lesions. Attention to adequate nutritional and fluid intake will help to keep tissues healthy and resistant to positional trauma.

Moisture in pressure areas from perspiration or incontinence causes softening of the skin and can result in maceration. Keeping the skin dry in pressure areas is important to minimize risk.

Treatment of Pressure Lesions   The nurse plays a critical role in treatment of pressure sores. Choosing or recommending wound care is often the responsibility of the nurse. Knowledge of the healing process, current research and products, physical and financial restraints, and the lifestyle of the individual being treated should all be taken into consideration (Cooper, 1990).

DAILY LIVING WITH CORNS AND CALLUSES

Corns and calluses are benign hyperkeratotic lesions that are often disabling and immobilizing. Foot care to minimize and manage these hyperkeratotic lesions becomes increasingly difficult as aging persons lose the ability to care for their own feet.

RISK FACTORS

With age-related drying of skin and the loss of subcutaneous tissue, the presence of corns and calluses is a growing problem. The lowering of the metatarsal arch with aging increases the risk of calluses on plantar foot surfaces. Arthritic changes in the feet with associated spurs and joint enlargement increase risks. Older persons who still maintain activities involving walking have more risks. Ill-fitting shoes contribute to these lesions.

Age-related losses in flexibility or pathology that reduce the ability to give foot care on a regular basis increase the risk of being further immobilized by corns and calluses. When this is compounded by either the lack of a primary caregiver to manage foot care regularly or the lack of funds to purchase foot care, the risks of reduced ambulation are great.

SIGNS AND SYMPTOMS

The older person may report increasing pain and difficulty in walking as well as the impact this has on activities of daily living. Neighbors or family may report not seeing the person out and about as much or may observe a change in gait.

The nurse may observe a change in gait in clinic visits or in the home setting. Direct observation of the feet will show the presence of the lesions.

TREATMENT

Prevention   Prevention of immobilization or discomfort from corns or calluses involves

Inspection of the feet to determine status
Suggesting or obtaining metatarsal pads to decrease direct pressure of metatarsal bones on the sole of the shoe
Obtaining adequate-fitting shoes—shoes with a deep rounded toe box to permit toes to spread and avoid pressure on tops of toes. Lamb's wool may be used to separate toes and prevent maceration
Assessment of the older person's capacity for self-care of feet and mobilizing of other resources where self-care is not possible
Arranging for regularly scheduled foot care to control the buildup of keratin lesions

Treatment of Corns and Calluses   Soak in water to soften. Rub with emory board after soaking or with very fine sandpaper affixed to a tongue depressor. Calluses and corns usually respond to the use of keratolytic agents that aid in softening and removal of the material. The central core may be removed with liquid nitrogen by the physician. Devices such as metatarsal pads will help to avoid direct pressure and prevent recurrence. Place a small pad with a center cut-out over corns to relieve pressure. If the core is not removed, a new layer of skin forms unless pressure is relieved. Attention to the fit of shoes will also assist in preventing further trauma. Visual disturbances and diminished joint mobility may prohibit self foot care. Family members may need to be instructed.

DAILY LIVING WITH INGROWN TOENAILS

HIGH RISK

At high risk are persons with mobility problems and toenails that curve in at the margins.

DYNAMICS

Nails become thickened, adherent to skin, and turn inward, pressing into the skin.

PREVENTION

Soak feet in water to soften nails. Slide orange stick around under nail to loosen skin adherence. Cut nails regularly—use clippers, keeping nail corners above skin line, and cut straight across. Teach a family member if the person is unable to do self-care.

TREATMENT

Following the above treatment, place a wisp of cotton or lamb's wool gently under the edge of the nail if it can be changed daily.

References and Other Readings

Alvarez O, et al. The effect of occlusive dressings on collagen synthesis and re-epithelialization in superficial wounds. J Surg Res 1983; 35:142.
Balin AK. Aging of human skin. In: Hazzard et al, eds. Principles of geriatric medicine. New York: McGraw-Hill, 1990.
Bates B. A guide to physical examination and history taking, 5th ed. Philadelphia: JB Lippincott, 1991.
Bergstrom N, et al. The Braden scale for predicting pressure sore risk. Nurs Res 1987; 36:205.
Besdine RW. Hyperthermia and accidental hypothermia. In: Abrams, Berkow, eds. The Merck manual of geriatrics. Rahway, NJ: Merck & Co, 1990:35.
Braun JL, Silvetti AN, Xakellis GL. Decubitus ulcers: what really works. Patient Care 1988; 22:22.
Broadwell DC, Jackson BS, eds. Principles of ostomy care. St. Louis: CV Mosby, 1982.
Bryant R. Wound repair: a review. J Enterostom Ther 1987; 14:262.
Cooper DM. Optimizing wound healing: a practice

within nursing's domain. Nurs Clin North Am 1990; 25:165.

DeWitt S. Nursing assessment of skin and dermatologic lesions. Nurs Clin North Am 1990; 25: 235.

Eaglstein WH, et al. The effects of early corticosteroid therapy on the skin eruption and pain of herpes zoster. JAMA 1970; 211:1681.

Ek AC, Unosson M, Larsson J et al. The development and healing of pressure sores related to the nutritional state. Clin Nutr 1991; 10:245.

Fenske NA, Grayson LD, Newcomer VD. Common problems of aging skin. Patient Care 1989; 23:225.

Fitzpatrick JE. Common inflammatory skin diseases of the elderly. Geriatrics 1989; 44:40.

Goth KE. Clinical observations and experimental studies of pathogenesis of decubitus ulcers. Acta Chir Scand 1942; 87(suppl 76):198.

Hess CT, Miller P. The management of open wounds: acute and chronic. Ostomy/Wound Management 1990; 31:58.

Huff JC, et al. Therapy of herpes zoster with oral acyclovir. Am J Med 1988; 85(suppl 2A):84.

Husain T. An experimental study of some pressure effects on tissues with reference to the bedsore problem. J Pathol Bacteriol 1953; 66:347.

Jackson DS, Rovee DT. Current concepts in wound healing: research and theory. J Enterostom Ther 1988; 15:133.

Jones P, Millman A. Wound healing and the aged patient. Nurs Clin North Am 1990; 25:263.

Judelsohn RG. Prevention and control of varicella-zoster infections. J Infect Dis 1972; 125:82.

Kennedy JA. Skin problems of blacks. JAMA 1976; 236:301.

Klein L. Maintenance of healthy skin. J Enterostom Ther 1988; 15:227.

Levine JM, Simpson M, McDonald RJ. Pressure sores: a plan for primary care prevention. Geriatrics 1989; 44:75.

Liesegang TI. Ophthalmic herpes zoster: Diagnosis and antiviral treatment. Geriatrics 1991; 46:64.

Lindan O, et al. Pressure distribution in the surface of the human body. Arch Phys Med Rehabil 1965; 46:378.

McKendrick MW, McGill JI, White JE, Wood MJ. Oral acyclovir in acute herpes zoster. Br Med J 1986; 293:1529.

Myers RB, et al. Report of a multicenter clinical trial on the performance characteristics of two occlusive hydrocolloid dressings in the treatment of noninfected, partial-thickness wounds. J Enterostom Ther 1988; 15:158.

Norton D, et al. An investigation of geriatric nursing problems in hospitals. Edinburgh: Churchill-Livingstone, 1975.

Pajk M. Pressure sores. In Abrams, Berkow, eds. The Merck manual of geriatrics, Rahway, NJ: Merck & Co, 1990.

Parisier DM. Topical steroids: a guide for use in the elderly patient. Geriatrics 1991; 46:51.

Phillips TJ, Gilchrist BA. Skin changes and disorders. In: Abrams, Berkow, eds. The Merck manual of geriatrics. Rahway, NJ: Merck & Co, 1990:1025.

Portenoy RK. Pain. In: Abrams, Berkow, eds. The Merck manual of geriatrics. Rahway, NJ: Merck & Co, 1990:105.

Richelson CN. Leg ulcers. J Enterostom Ther 1990; 17:217.

Scherr GH. Alginates and alginate fibers in clinical practice. Wounds 1992; 4:74.

Weiler P, et al. Pressure sores in nursing home patients. Aging 1990; 2:267.

Westerman R, et al. Effects of topical capsan on normal skin and affected dermatones in herpes zoster. Clin Exp Neur 1988; 29:71.

34
Vision Problems

SUSAN A. MORGAN

Age-related changes in vision are one of the few guarantees for those who live longer. Many persons experience visual changes beginning as early as the late 30s to the early 40s. Changes in vision become more pronounced with increasing age. Along with normal age-related changes the elderly are at increased risk for developing disorders and diseases of the eyes such as cataracts, macular degeneration, glaucoma, diabetic retinopathy (see Chapter 24), optic nerve atrophy, night blindness, and dry eyes. The first four visual pathologies mentioned above account for over 75% of severe visual impairment among elderly Americans (Genesky and Zarit, 1986).

When these pathologic changes occur with other age-related problems, the balance between requirements and resources for daily living may become increasingly precarious. The ability to see is linked closely with the way in which people manage their daily lives. Any loss of vision has a significant impact on independence and preferred lifestyle:

- Medication use becomes hazardous when labels are difficult to read and all the bottles and pills look alike.
- Nutritional intake is altered as difficulties arise with cooking and shopping. Labels on cans cannot be read or the amount of seasoning determined. Burns while cooking become an increased risk.

- Falls and injuries increase with failure to observe objects in the environment or notice surface changes.

One should also be concerned about the emotional health of the person whose vision is failing. These people may experience

- Altered self-image due to loss of independence
- Boredom when the usual forms of diversion—reading, watching television, writing letters, doing crafts, gardening—are lost
- Isolation from the inability to get out caused by the inability to drive, by the difficulty of reading street and bus signs, or the embarrassment (or fear) of looking clumsy or awkward to others

These are only a few of the areas of difficulty an older person may experience with failing vision. The concerns suggest that nursing expertise can be a useful support system to help older people modify their lifestyle and learn new coping skills in order to maintain quality of life.

Normal Changes in the Aging Eye and Resulting Functional Changes

Like all other body systems, the eye is subject to the effects of time. Throughout life, struc-

673

tural and functional changes occur gradually in the eye. Since the pathologic conditions that affect vision in the elderly are closely related to these changes, normal aging of the eye is reviewed followed by specific pathology.

LIDS

Increasing eyelid laxity with aging can result in entropion (inversion of the lids) or ectropion (eversion of the lids). Ectropic lids can pull the lacrimal gland opening away from the scleral surface and cause watery eyes. Entropic lids typically cause corneal conjunctival irritation and watery eyes due to the inward turning of the lower lids and lashes. The elderly may experience decreased temporal and superior visual fields when the upper lid is abnormally low (ptosis). The etiology of blepharotosis can be neuropenic, myogenic, inflammatory, mechanical, or spurious (pseudoptosis).

CORNEA

The cornea tends to cloud with age, losing its luster and transparency. The epithelium develops minor irregularities and corneal fibers thicken as a part of the general decrease in water content that occurs with aging. A white, gray, or yellowish ring may develop around the corneas. This ring, called an *arcus senilis*, represents peripheral corneal degeneration, but does not affect vision. Corneal changes with age do cause increased light scatter and an overall flattening.

IRIS AND PUPIL

Changes in the iris caused by sclerosis result in a narrowed pupillary diameter and a slowed pupillary response. These changes result in an increased need for light, and slowed response to light and dark. Therefore, the pupils of older people normally are small and somewhat constricted.

The narrowed pupil affects the amount of light the older person needs for effective vision. Additionally, reduced retinal illumination, increased light scatter, crystalline lens discoloration and opacification, and uncorrected myopia contribute to changed visual capacity. In many cases the older individual may need to increase the wattage of light bulbs and carry a small flashlight for greater ease in seeing in the dark.

The slowed pupillary response presents several coping difficulties, primarily involving the amount of time needed to adjust to light changes. Entering a darkened room or building results in a period of time when it is difficult to distinguish objects or people. Alternatively, moving out of doors into bright daylight or having a light suddenly turned on in a darkened room causes a glare that is equally blinding. In either case, hazards are posed for older persons if they try to adjust to the environment quickly. Night lights, canes, an unhurried pace, and a helpful arm promote safety and aid adjustment at these times.

Because of these changes in the iris and the resulting nyctalopia (night blindness), night driving can become a problem. The inability to accommodate quickly to oncoming headlights, particularly with the glare of wet streets, plus the subsequent blackness after a car has passed, causes many older individuals to give up night driving completely. This has the effect of changing social lifestyles; and unless alternative transportation can be arranged, elderly persons are captives in their own environments.

LENS

The changes in the lens have the greatest impact on vision and are associated with major coping problems. The lens is formed like an onion with the oldest tissue in the middle and the youngest at the periphery. As cellular growth slows with age, the lens comes to have a larger proportion of old to new tissue. Its center gradually yellows and becomes less flexible, making it difficult for the ciliary muscle to change the shape of the lens. A slowed and less complete accommodation for near vision results that is called presbyopia. A more profound effect of aging is the development of cataracts, wherein changes in the protein structure of the lens cause it to become opalescent—a normal though pathologic result of aging. Additionally, the epithelium atrophies, water clefts form in the cortex, lens fibers fragment, and crystals such as calcium and cholesterol deposit on the lens.

CILIARY MUSCLE

Over time, the atrophied ciliary muscle becomes stiff and less functional. This, along with the decreased compliance of the lens, contribute to the loss of accommodation. Because the eye brings visual images to focus on the retina by changing the shape and thus refractive power of the lens, near vision requires the greatest amount of work by the ciliary muscle. Therefore, as the muscle loses its ability to contract, near vision is compromised. Starting usually in their 40s, people who have never worn corrective lenses before will need to wear reading glasses, and others may add bifocals or trifocals to existing corrections.

VITREOUS

With age the gelatinous vitreous shrinks and the collagen material of which it is composed tends to become semisolid. Fibrillar aggregates cause shadows to be projected on the retina and result in *floaters* or vitreous opacities appearing in the field of vision. To some degree these opacities are normal, but they may be symptomatic of pathology such as uveitis, retinal hemorrhage, or retinal detachment. Therefore, any sudden change in the kind or amount of floaters warrants a complete fundoscopic examination.

The extent to which normal floaters bother people is highly variable. A recreational sharpshooter or seamstress will complain of them much more than someone who plays bridge or cooks as a hobby.

RETINA AND MACULA

Except for the macula, the retina shows the fewest changes associated with age. The aging retina becomes thinner due to loss of neural cells but only when vascular changes interrupt the blood supply or changes occur in the pigment is its function compromised.

In contrast, the macula is highly vulnerable to age-related sclerotic changes. Since its function is associated with detailed vision, even a very small change will be readily noted by the patient as either visual distortion or loss of acuity. Most often such changes are associated with macular degeneration.

Pathophysiology and Medical Management

CATARACTS

The term *cataract* refers to any clouding or opacity of the lens. Cataracts are a normal consequence of aging and occur to some degree in all people over the age of 70. Diabetes and hypoparathyroidism increase the risk of cataracts as do some drugs such as ophthalmic drop preparations of steroids and anticholinesterase drugs. Other causes of cataracts include radiation, trauma, infrared light, electric shock, anterior uveitis, heterochromic iritis, thromboangiitis obliterans, and congenital anomalies. Recently, radar in communications and microwave ovens have demonstrated a role in cataract formation (Boyd-Monk and Steinmetz, 1987). Cataracts are a bilateral disorder in aging; however, cataract development usually occurs asymmetrically.

Types of Cataracts Cataracts vary in terms of location and density. The opacity may be diffuse or scattered. It may be located centrally or peripherally. The location will determine the nature of difficulties individuals experience and the type of compensatory behavior in which they engage.

WEDGE-SHAPED OR CENTRAL CATARACTS

If the cataract is located in the central area of the lens, vision will be better in dim light when the pupil is dilated. In bright light the pupil constricts and the person may become almost totally blind. Therefore, people with central cataracts habitually read in dim light and keep room lights at a minimum level. Behavior to deal with sudden exposure to bright light or manage in brightly lit areas becomes important to enhance safety and maintain activity.

NUCLEAR OR SCATTERED CATARACTS

Scattered cataracts produce an effect of multiple mirrors in the eye. As the light refracts differently off each opacity, people with this type of cataract complain predominantly of glare. They read better with an eye shade and often wear a broad-brimmed hat outdoors. Habitually they use their hands to shield their eyes from glare or wear tinted or dark glasses.

SUBSCAPULAR OR PERIPHERAL CATARACTS

Opacities located in the periphery of the lens usually do not cause coping problems until they grow into the pupil area. Often they are discovered only in the doctor's office when the pupil is widely dilated. Occasionally a spike will invade the central portion of the pupil and cause a splitting or doubling of images.

Signs and Symptoms The earliest symptoms of cataract are caused by a swelling of the lens before the formation of any visible opacity. This swelling artificially increases the power of the lens and for some people causes a temporary improvement in near vision, commonly referred to as "second sight." Some people experience a need for frequent prescription changes during this time because the swelling changes refractive error. This early stage of cataract development is highly variable; it may be either so short or so long as to go unnoticed.

Almost all cataract patients complain of progressive, painless decrease in vision as well as reduced near vision, altered color perception, eye fatigue, headaches, increased light sensitivity, blurred or multiple vision, and image distortion in which straight lines appear wavy (Morse et al, 1987). It is not unusual for some people to become irritable as they work harder to see through their developing cataracts.

Diagnosis Diagnosis of cataracts is confirmed by direct visualization of the lens opacity and the inability to visualize details of the fundus. Being informed of this diagnosis can be traumatic to some patients, especially if they equate having cataracts to blindness. Accurate information, appropriate to each patient's presenting situation, needs to be provided at a time when the person is able to hear and assimilate the information provided.

Prognosis Older persons need to know that most cataracts grow very slowly over many years. Even with the most dense cataract the person will still be able to discern light, some color, and shadow movements. Surgery is indicated when glasses can no longer improve vision and normal activities such as reading or driving are being compromised. Surgery will improve vision 90% to 95% if other eye pathology does not coexist.

Treatment The treatment for cataracts is surgical removal. The exact method of removal varies depending on the patient, the ophthalmologist, and to some extent the area of the country. The objective in each case is the same: to remove the opaque natural lens and restore vision by using a removable contact lens, intraocular lens implant, or glasses.

Most ophthalmologists are performing cataract surgery on medically stable patients on an outpatient basis. Usually one eye is operated on at a time and local anesthesia is preferred to eliminate the risk of postoperative vomiting with its associated rise of intraocular pressure, as well as its general compromising effect on the respiratory tract.

An *intracapsular extraction* is the traditional method of cataract removal. It involves making an incision halfway around the cornea and extracting the lens in its capsule through a widely dilated pupil. An *extracapsular cataract extraction* differs only in that the posterior capsule of the lens is not removed. In either case, a partial iridectomy is done to ensure that secondary glaucoma does not occur should the vitreous humor move forward and block the flow of the aqueous humor from the eye. The corneal incision is closed with nylon sutures that usually do not need to be removed.

Increasingly cataract surgery involves the insertion of an intraocular lens following a cataract extraction. In 1982, 70% of the cataract surgeries performed in the United States were associated with an intraocular lens implant (Stark et al, 1983). The implant is either inserted into the anterior or posterior chamber or is affixed to the iris. The advantages of the intraocular lens are that the person can see quite well immediately following surgery. It eliminates the discomfort and distortion of cataract glasses; and unlike removable contact lenses, which can be difficult for the elderly to manipulate, it requires no care.

AGE-RELATED MACULAR DEGENERATION

Age-related macular degeneration (AMD) is a condition in which the macula no longer functions well due to deterioration of the central area of the retina. It is the leading cause of new cases of legal blindness in the United States in persons over age 65 and is thought to be present in about 11% of the elderly aged 65 to 74 and 28% of those aged 75 to 85. The cause is thought to be related to a decreased blood supply to the sensitive nerve endings in this region, an accumulation of waste products, and tissue atrophy. Certain systemic diseases, genetic inheritance, and nutritional factors have been implicated as well (Eifrig and Simons, 1983). In some cases abnormal blood vessel growth under the retina damages the macula. Both eyes almost always are affected.

People afflicted with AMD complain that their central vision is either so dark or so distorted that they no longer can see. Usually the condition worsens gradually and, in advanced cases, is as though a hole had been punched in the center of the visual field. Usually the best corrected vision these people can achieve is 20/200 and, therefore, they are classified as legally blind.

AMD responds poorly to medical treatment. Although many forms of treatment have been tried, none has been found effective. The argon laser has been tried with one form of the disease that afflicts about 10% of those diagnosed. The laser photocoagulation treatment obliterates the abnormal new blood vessels, thereby preventing hemorrhages and scar tissue from forming in the sensitive macular area. Persons with this form of AMD need to seek treatment early, because the condition remains in its treatable form for only a few weeks.

Lacking central vision, people with AMD no longer can read, watch television, drive a car, play cards, do handwork, or recognize faces. By scanning to use peripheral vision, they are able to get around, cook, clean, garden, and, in general, manage much of their daily routines. These people need a great deal of reassurance and to be told that they will never become totally blind from macular degeneration. By using peripheral vision they should be able to care for themselves and function with a relative degree of independence.

GLAUCOMA

There are two types of glaucoma: open angle and angle closure. The first is the more common form and is an insidious chronic condition. The second, often characterized by an acute condition, requires surgery if blindness is to be avoided. Glaucoma also can occur secondary to infection, injury, swollen cataracts, and tumors.

The incidence of glaucoma increases from ages 40 to 70, affecting about 2% of the population over 40. Therefore, all eye examinations and physicals on persons over age 40 should routinely include tonometry readings to check for glaucoma. Where there is a family history of the disease, members should be checked annually. Glaucoma occurs in African-Americans four to five times more frequently than in Caucasians.

CHRONIC OPEN ANGLE GLAUCOMA (PRIMARY)

Chronic open angle glaucoma (COAG) results from an obstruction to the normal flow of aqueous humor from the eye caused by changes in the trabecular meshwork of the canal of Schlemm. The resultant backup of fluid increases the intraocular pressure, gradually damaging the optic nerve and causing a progressive loss of visual field. COAG has genetic associations with diabetes.

Signs and Symptoms COAG commonly is diagnosed during a routine eye examination when the eye pressure is found to be above normal or changes are seen in the optic nerve. Because the symptoms are nonexistent or vague, few people are ever aware that they have anything wrong with their eyes. Unrecognized symptoms may include halos and colored rings around lights, nonspecific eye problems, occasional browache, and slow, progressive loss of peripheral vision.

Diagnostic signs include increased intraocular pressure, shallow anterior chamber angle, visual field defect, and pathologic cupping of the optic disk.

Only after the disease has damaged the optic nerve will the patient become aware of blind areas in his visual field.

Treatment The treatment of glaucoma is aimed at maintaining eye pressure within normal limits either by decreasing the production of fluid or aiding its outflow. This is done by using medication. The type, strength, and frequency of medication are selected on the basis of tonometry readings, peripheral field examinations, and changes seen in the optic disk. Frequently prescribed drugs are shown in Table 34–1.

If visual field loss and pressure cannot be controlled with medication or the medication regimen significantly disrupts the patient's lifestyle, surgery may be proposed. Noninvasive laser trabeculoplasty or surgical trabeculectomy may be considered in order to establish an alternative pathway for the aqueous humor to drain from the eye. Patients need to understand that these alternatives may or may not alleviate the need for drops and that there will be no improvement on vision already lost. Fur-

TABLE 34–1   *Drugs Prescribed for Treatment of Chronic Glaucoma*

Drug	Strength	Action
Ophthalmologic solution		
Timolol	0.25%–0.5%	Beta-adrenergic blocker—decreases aqueous production
Pilocarpine	1%, 2%, 4%	Parasympathomimetic—enlarges the drainage channels, increasing the outflow and reducing intraocular pressure
Epinephrine	1%–2%	Sympathomimetic—constricts blood vessels, decreasing aqueous production
Phospholine iodine	0.06%–0.125%	Anticholinesterase agent—inhibits action of cholinesterase, increasing the concentration of acetylcholine. Action similar to a parasympathomimetic
Diamox (tablets)	125–250 mg	Carbonic anhydrase inhibitor—inhibits aqueous production and promotes diuresis

ther, although these alternatives may substantially lower intraocular pressure, they do not decrease the need for medical follow-up to ensure that the pressure continues to remain normal and drainage continues.

ACUTE ANGLE CLOSURE GLAUCOMA (PRIMARY)

Angle closure glaucoma is the less common form of the disease. It is characterized by acute attacks that may cause permanent loss of vision unless treated promptly. This type of glaucoma is characterized by a sudden increase in intraocular pressure caused by the complete closure of the drain angle.

Signs and Symptoms   Symptoms of angle closure glaucoma relate to the rapid increase in intraocular pressure. These include intense eye pain, secondary nausea and vomiting, injected watery-appearing eye, blurred smoky vision, and red and green halos around lights. Diagnostic signs are high intraocular pressure, mid-dilated and nonreactive pupil, corneal edema, congested episcleral and conjunctival vessels, shallow anterior chamber, and a gonioscopically verified angle closure. If it is untreated, blindness can occur within 24 to 36 hours.

Medical Treatment   The immediate treatment of angle closure glaucoma is to use an intravenous push injection of 500 mg of Diamox (acetazolamide) and then apply miotic drops every 10 to 15 minutes to constrict the iris and pull it away from the drain angle. Mannitol is

given to diurese the patient and to slow the production of aqueous fluid. Narcotics are given for pain. Surgery is almost always performed immediately following an acute attack or if the pressure cannot be relieved. The usual surgical procedure consists of bilateral peripheral iridectomies since the disease almost always involves both eyes. The argon laser is used for the iridectomy, and the procedure can be done on an outpatient basis.

Because angle closure glaucoma poses such a severe visual risk, any patient with a history of critically narrowed angles or prodromal attacks should be examined thoroughly. Prophylactic surgery may be recommended.

DRY EYES

Just as age effects the secretion of other glands, lacrimal secretions also may decrease over time. For some individuals this results in a chronic condition referred to as "dry eye." While never a cause of blindness, it can be the source of great discomfort. Hormonal changes are presumed to play a part in these changes because the condition is more frequently seen in postmenopausal women. Some systemic disorders and certain drugs can contribute to keratitis.

Symptoms that become more marked toward the end of the day include a mild-to-severe sensation of having a foreign body in the eye, photophobia, a tendency to close the eyes, and a desire to rub them frequently. Since mild infections usually are present secondary to these symptoms, the patient also may complain of itching and burning. When examined with a microscope the surface of the cornea appears to have been superficially stippled with a pin, a condition referred to as punctate keratitis.

Unfortunately there is no cure for dry eyes. Treatment is directed toward managing causative drugs, eliminating the secondary infections, and providing artificial lubrication for the eye itself. During the day artificial tears can be used; at night a greasy ointment such as Lacri-Lube provides relief. This condition can be so uncomfortable that it is often difficult for patients to accept that the doctor can do little to help them even though they have a good visual prognosis.

Nursing Diagnosis and Management of High-risk Areas in Daily Living

All people who survive to the seventh decade and beyond will experience age-related changes in vision. Additionally, some of these people will experience pathology. Each of these changes will alter vision in some way and thus affect the myriad vision-related aspects of daily living. Alterations in vision associated both with aging and with most types of pathology tend to be gradual, and rarely do persons become totally blind. They may retain some central vision as with glaucoma, or some peripheral vision as with age-related macular degeneration, or they may see shapes and shadows as with cataracts. Given the gradualness of the change, the fact that some degree of vision is usually retained, plus the somewhat slower, often less demanding, pace of life in these decades, most older persons adapt well to these changes and continue to manage their daily living independently. Some people will experience difficulties and are well served by perceptive, appropriate nursing care.

Nurses can and should "fine tune" their assessment abilities, including use of the direct opthalmoscope (Boyd-Monk, 1991). In addition to funduscopic assessments, nurses, practitioners, and clinical nurse specialists can assess eye structures, visual fields, accommodation, central vision, extraocular movements, lacrimal functioning, visual acuity, color discrimination, visual-spatial ability, light sensitivity and dark adaptation, reaction to glare, and adaptive devices. When abnormalities are found, the nurse refers the patient for definitive medical diagnosis and treatment.

DAILY LIVING WITH ALTERED VISION

When vision becomes limited, for whatever reason, individuals must learn new styles of coping with the activities and demands of daily living. Memory and the other senses of hearing and touch become increasingly important to maintain independence. Routine tasks become increasingly more difficult and fatiguing, and usual sources of diversion are less possible. Where age limits agility, the increased fear of falling keeps some people from venturing into unknown areas, because stairs and curbs create new hazards. Even a change in the texture of floor surface, from carpeting to linoleum, can create uncertainty and one can observe visually impaired persons testing with the sole of their shoes to determine changes in level.

RISK FACTORS

Those who tend to experience the greatest difficulty in adjusting to altered vision include the following:

Persons who have never been able to accept any impediments to their lives
Persons with other deficits and pathology (e.g., arthritis, balance problems, past stroke)
Absence of family, neighbors, or community services to assist with activities where vision limits capabilities
Persons with deficits in memory
Persons whose primary activities and diversions are vision related and who refuse to alter the form of the diversion in order to continue it (e.g., sewing, knitting, crocheting with larger size thread or yarn, reading large-print books)

SIGNS AND SYMPTOMS

Evidence that older persons are not managing well with their altered vision may be in the form of either subjective or objective data. They may report the following:

Fatigue in carrying out routine activities of daily living because of the extra strain of diminished vision
A feeling of isolation from other people

Concern about being accurate when taking medication

Reluctance to venture into unfamiliar areas or request assistance from others

Dismay about having to "impose on other people so much"

Frustration with their inability to continue vision-oriented activities in their customary way

Boredom because their days have become "terribly long"

The clinician or family member may observe the following:

Food spots on clothing that once was immaculate, mismatched stockings, odd combinations of colors in shoes, slacks, and coat

Less skill used in applying makeup, particularly blush, eyeshadow, and eyebrow pencil

Burns, bruises, and abrasions on the extremities

Lack of eye contact, or the person looks just past your ear

Uncertainty in the way the person walks and moves about the room, touching door frames and chairs and feeling out floor surfaces with the foot because of a loss of depth perception

PROGNOSTIC VARIABLES

The ability to manage daily living in an effective and satisfying way when vision is lost or diminished is primarily related to a positive attitude and the ability to adapt to alternative activities. Being able to manage is also affected by having consistent acceptable personal support for crucial activities and events that otherwise would be limited because of visual impairment and by the person's ability to accept help offered in a positive affirmative manner. This last point is particularly important if help is to be offered on a continuing basis.

COMPLICATIONS

Social isolation, trauma, unsafe medication taking, nutritional deficits, and failure to thrive are potential complications of visual loss in the elderly.

TREATMENT

Nursing care to assist the individual with the management of daily living begins with an assessment interview.

How do you spend your day?

What kind of work do you do? (Even if they are retired, older people use the word "work" to describe their daily activities.)

What do you do for pleasure?

What is your living situation like? (environment, pets, etc.)

How much help do you receive from neighbors, family, or friends? How do you feel about accepting help? Asking for it?

How do you manage your food shopping and preparation?

How do you manage transportation? What are the biggest problems you encounter?

Has your social life changed in any way because of changes in your vision?

How do you manage medications?

What aspects of your daily living are of most concern?

On the basis of the diagnoses derived from such an assessment, nursing interventions can be planned that will address specific problem areas. These interventions may address safety issues (*e.g.*, handrails, lighting, small rugs, pets underfoot), memory problems and misplacing unseen items, transportation techniques (timing buses, script for asking help from strangers), social situations (planning, rehearsals), and mobilizing support systems, as well as the behavior, attitude, and psychosocial well-being of the person seeking and learning to accept help.

DAILY LIVING WITH OPEN ANGLE GLAUCOMA AND ITS MEDICAL REGIMEN

Persons with COAG are required to incorporate a consistent schedule of ophthalmic medication into their daily living to keep the intraocular pressure within its normal range and minimize damage to the optic nerve. They also need to maintain a lifestyle that does not increase intraocular pressure. If damage to the optic nerve does occur, they must adjust to living with loss of peripheral vision.

Three fundamental principles serve as a foundation for nursing interventions with the person who has glaucoma:

1. *Once a diagnosis of glaucoma is made, treatment must be continued for the rest of one's life.* Glaucoma, like diabetes, at this time can only be treated; it cannot be cured. Patients may find this difficult to comprehend or believe, particularly when they are experienc-

ing no discomfort. Others, believing modern medicine can cure any condition, may mistrust a health care provider who tells them they must take medication for the rest of their lives.

2. *Eye pressure tends to increase whenever the pupils are dilated or the system is placed under physical or emotional stress.* This has implications for the timing of medications. Because the pupils dilate during sleep, drops always should be taken before retiring and the first thing in the morning. During periods of life change, emotional excitement, or anxiety, patients often need to increase either the strength or frequency of their medication. Patients need to learn to be aware of these times and notify their physician when stressful events occur in their lives.

3. *Drops prescribed to be taken several times during the day should be spaced at regular intervals.* Often older patients complain that they think about taking their drops and then cannot remember if they have. In such instances it is best that the patient take additional medication rather than the possibility of having taken none at all. The same is true if a patient must skip or miss a dose. In this instance patients should be told to take their drops as soon as they remember or are able to do so, and then to return to their regular schedule even though the time interval may be shortened. For older people with memory problems, it is best to link their eye-drop schedule to other routine activities such as lunch, dinner, a television show, or before an afternoon nap.

RISK FACTORS

Most people with glaucoma become very faithful (some compulsively) to their prescribed schedule of eye drops and medications. Those at risk for neglecting their prescribed regimen include people who

Are in the denial stage of accepting the diagnosis because of its "silent" nature
Have poor memories and therefore cannot adhere to a schedule
Are unable to understand the nature of glaucoma and its treatment and thus lack a logical rationale for compliance

The time of highest risk for failure to maintain the medication regimen occurs when glaucoma patients are institutionalized in either an acute or long-term care setting. Nurses frequently do not give priority to glaucoma medications, and patients either cannot or are not permitted to administer these medications for themselves.

SIGNS AND SYMPTOMS

Difficulties in daily living may occur with either changes in vision or failure to incorporate the medication regimen into daily living. The most frequent complaint concerning vision tends to focus on the inability to see in dim light and bumping into things, due to blind areas in the field of vision. Problems with medication compliance are evidenced by increased intraocular pressure as measured by tonometer readings and loss of vision.

PROGNOSTIC VARIABLES

A good prognosis for integrating glaucoma and its treatment into daily living is associated with

Accepting the diagnosis
Having a family history of glaucoma where relatives have experienced loss of vision due to poor compliance
Living a relatively structured lifestyle
Being able to self-administer eye drops
Avoiding admission to a hospital or nursing home with its attendant loss of control over medication

Participating in evening activities may become contingent on family or friends providing transportation.

COMPLICATIONS

The complication for which the glaucoma patient is at highest risk is vision loss related to increased intraocular pressure from either failure to adhere to the medication regimen or uncontrollable stress and tension.

MANAGEMENT

"Night Blindness" (Nyctalopia) Glaucoma patients experience difficulty seeing at night whether or not their pupils are constricted. Night driving can be particularly difficult and hazardous both for the patients and their families, and options should be considered for alternative forms of transportation during the hours of darkness. Other strategies for managing at

night include using night lights, canes, flashlights, and higher wattage light bulbs.

Medication Regimen Management of the medication regimen involves helping older persons think through their daily living pattern and consider the strategies for incorporating the medication regimen into it. When treatment is initiated, patients should be told that the drops may give them a slight headache or "pulling" sensation to their eyes. Since most glaucoma drops constrict the pupil, people with central cataracts may complain of vision loss because the smaller pupil prohibits them from looking around their opacity.

Nurses in any setting need to be aware of the specific effect glaucoma drops may have on their patients' visual status, be alert to predictable problems, and where indicated, institute assistance in helping them manage daily living activities. When working with older glaucoma patients, help them to do the following:

Plan a schedule that fits their given lifestyle.
Explore ways to tie medication times to routinely scheduled activities.
Understand that if a dose is forgotten, it is better to take more medication or have a shorter interval between doses than to go without medication.
Think through and rehearse in their minds social situations during which they may need to take their eye drops, and strategies they will use to manage this comfortably.
Schedule office calls for tonometry readings at different hours of the day since intraocular pressure can vary.

In addition to eye drops, carbonic anhydrase may be prescribed for patients who need longer acting control. Patients for whom this medication is prescribed need to know that it

Should be taken at bedtime to provide coverage during sleep when the pupils dilate and the intraocular pressure is likely to rise
Initially has a diuretic effect and can interrupt sleep unless fluids are restricted late in the day
May cause hypokalemia, especially if taken in addition to other potassium-wasting diuretics
May cause tingling of the fingers and toes, indicating that a potassium supplement may need to be prescribed

Patients with kidney disease, hypertension, and glaucoma often find themselves caught between the different medical managements of these various problems. Frequently it is the alert nurse who, by careful questioning of the patients' general health and lifestyle, discerns potential problems and keeps other health care providers aware of the risks their mutual patients may be experiencing.

Stress and Tension Periods of emotional tension can override the effect of medication and cause intraocular pressure to increase. Nurses, alert to those who may be experiencing stress, should discuss the following with their patients:

The role anxiety and tension play in glaucoma, situations and times in their lives when they are likely to be at risk, and options or strategies for avoiding or managing these times
Strategies for controlling intraocular pressure in the presence of anxiety or tension, e.g., rest, medication, increasing the medication, contacting the physician
The effect caffeine and caffeine-containing substances have on intraocular pressure

Institutionalization Glaucoma patients vary markedly in their ability to adjust to their chronic condition. Most become very faithful in adhering to their schedule and can become acutely distressed if it is altered. Because these patients tend to be rather high-strung individuals, they often experience a great deal of anxiety if any change in living situation results in their losing control of their medication schedule, e.g., nursing homes or some retirement settings where the staff control dispensing of medications. Glaucoma patients have been taught that if they do not comply to the prescribed medication schedule, they risk optic nerve damage and blindness. Having internalized this risk, these patients become fearful when others do not comply to their schedules. This fear is real and nurses should give it the attention and urgency appropriate to its reality. Strategies that may help are to do the following:

Rehearse negotiating with nurses or others in an institutional setting to maintain the medication schedule
Request a physician's order for self-administration

Share their realistic fears of eye damage as a way of influencing staff to adhere to the medication schedule

Drug Interactions Persons with glaucoma need to be alert to the effect other medications may have on their eyes. They should be advised to do the following:

Read the labels of all over-the-counter preparations or check with the pharmacist about effects a drug may have on intraocular pressure.

Avoid all cold medications containing antihistamines.

Avoid all medications containing caffeine, e.g., Anacin, APC, Nodoz.

Tell anyone prescribing or giving medications in an emergency that they have glaucoma.

Wear a Medalert identification tag.

Avoid all stomach medications that contain atropine-like substances.

EVALUATION

Evaluation will concern the older person's comfort with the medication regimen in whatever living situation exists, the management and integration of coexisting medical conditions and treatments, and the management of stress.

DAILY LIVING WITH CATARACT SURGERY

Cataract surgery decisions are based on the person's disability, the potential effect of the surgery, and the risk of adding to the disability. For those elderly who consider cataract surgery, the alterations they experience in their daily living fall into three time periods: the decision-making period, the preoperative planning period, and the postoperative management period.

DECISION-MAKING PERIOD

Numerous factors enter into the decision of whether or not to have cataract surgery. The nurse plays an important role in helping the person understand the surgery and any temporary restrictions it may impose, the time considerations involved, and the nature of the visual outcome. It is important that the nurse explore with older persons their understanding of what they have been told and help them acquire enough knowledge to make informed decisions.

Sometimes the decision to have surgery is made before vision becomes severely limited. Factors that contribute to this decision include the following:

Inability to carry out usual activities comfortably; reading, sewing, watching TV, driving safely

Having surgery done before retiring for insurance purposes

Having paid the year's deductible for Medicare coverage

Ensuring adequate vision to pass a driver's license renewal examination (Older persons often have a difficult time reacquiring a driver's license once it is lost)

Being able to enjoy anticipated travel or holiday plans

Occasionally the nurse will encounter a patient who does not complain despite a large amount of visual loss. This person may be waiting for the doctor to suggest surgery or may be unduly frightened of having eye surgery. Talking with the person about fears and the types of problems he is having will provide the nurse with an understanding of the factors influencing his decision making. When appropriate, the nurse can clear up any misunderstandings about the surgery and its risks. These data can then be incorporated into the doctor's discussion with the patient. The decision to have cataract surgery should be the patient's, not a physician talking the patient into the procedure.

Timing The time frame of surgery should be discussed and arranged to fit comfortably into the person's lifestyle. Many people have surgery during the winter months so that they will be able to work in the garden during the summer. Others want their surgery done in early fall so that they will be able to see well enough by the holiday season to participate in family activities.

Information should be given so that patients can not only schedule surgery to meet their needs but also plan their lives to accommodate any limitations they may experience.

Expectations In addition to the time elements involved, other considerations include the patient's expectations about the experiences he will have in the process of having surgery and the nature of the vision postoperatively. The following areas have been found important:

The types of experiences that friends and acquaintances have reported about cataract surgery and its associated vision changes

The desire to retain binocular vision for work or hobby

The fear of having to function without the assistance of a mate or companion

The expectation the patient has of wearing contacts or glasses or having an intraocular lens implanted

Once surgery is scheduled, a complete physical examination with laboratory tests is required. Ask the patient if he is taking aspirin. If he is, it should be stopped several weeks before surgery to reduce the risk of bleeding postoperatively.

POSTOPERATIVE MANAGEMENT PERIOD

Although there is some variation in the prescribed care for the cataract patient postoperatively, the goals are the same. They are to prevent increased intraocular pressure, stress on the suture line, hemorrhage into the eye, and infection.

In general, the following guidelines apply during the immediate postoperative period:

Return home after the surgery—most procedures are done in outpatient surgery

Patch the operative eye only for the first 24 hours. Wear the eye patch when napping or at night to protect the eye

Avoid bending, stooping, lifting heavy objects, rapid head movements, and coughing

Use pillows to avoid rolling to the operative side.

Insert eye drops and ointments as prescribed

Do not squeeze eyelids together tightly as this puts pressure on the eye

Do not participate in any strenuous activities

Use common sense; only the patient knows when he has had enough

If an intraocular lens is not inserted, vision is limited to shapes and shadows until a corrective lens is prescribed

Report any sudden pain, increase in redness, loss of vision, swelling and/or discharge immediately to a physician

Some restrictions continue and affect daily living during the next several weeks while the corneal incision is healing. The postoperative cataract patient should do the following:

Continue to avoid all bending, stooping, and lifting for 2 weeks

Avoid long car trips and crowds where jostling might occur

Do not take airplane trips for 1 month

Other Resources

American Council for the Blind	(202) 833–1251
American Diabetes Association	(212) 541–4310
American Foundation for the Blind	(212) 620–2000
American Printing House for the Blind	(502) 895–2408
Association for Macular Disease	(212) 605–3719
Bureau of Blind and Visually Handicapped	(202) 245–0918
Center for Independent Living	(212) 674–7580
Council of Citizens with Low Vision	(800) 733–2258
Mainstream	(800) 424–8089
National Association for Visually Handicapped	(212) 889–3141
National Federation for the Blind—Special Interest Groups	(301) 659–9311
National Library Service	(800) 424–8567
National Society to Prevent Blindness	(800) 221–3004
Vision Foundation	(617) 926–4232

- Wash your hands with soap and water.

- Look toward ceiling with *both eyes open*.

- Pull lower lid down – steady your hand on your forehead.

- Put a drop of medicine or small strip of ointment (¼ inch) in the sac behind the lashes of the lower lid.

- The tip of the dropper or ointment tube should not touch the eyeball itself.

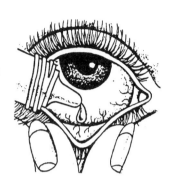

- After instilling the drop do not blink and keep the eyelids closed for 2 minutes.

- Do not give more than one eye medicine at a time – **wait 5 minutes between medicines.**

- When using both ointments and drops, use the ointment *AFTER* the drops.

FIGURE 34–1 Directions for giving eye drops or ointment.

- A mirror will be helpful if you are doing this alone.

Exercise caution in hazardous areas where falls might occur

Avoid coughing, sneezing, vomiting, and Valsalva maneuvers

Swimming and exercise classes should be avoided until authorized by a physician

Medications Eye drops and ointment are a routine component of postoperative therapy. Some patients are fearful they may injure their eye when instilling them. Since most cataract surgery is done on an ambulatory-day surgery basis (Fig. 34–1) teaching patients how and when to instill any ophthalmic medications prescribed should begin in the office preoperatively. Assistive devices for eye medication administration are available for patients who have arthritis, tremors, or other manual dexterity challenges.

Visual Outcome Following Surgery If an intraocular lens has *not* been inserted, vision following surgery is restored by wearing either eyeglasses or a contact lens. These are prescribed several weeks to months following surgery, after the corneal incision has healed and all visual distortion has cleared.

A major drawback to cataract glasses is that they position the corrective lens 14 to 15 mm in front of the natural lens position, causing a 33% magnification of the visual field. Since the brain cannot fuse images of such disparate size, double vision results unless both eyes have been operated or a contact lens is worn on the operative eye. A contact lens more closely approximates the position of the natural lens, reducing the magnification to 8% and allowing binocular vision.

The advent of the intraocular lens has revolutionized cataract surgery by resolving the problem of visual field magnification and the difficulties inherent for older persons in wearing either cataract glasses or contact lenses. Patients who have had an intraocular lens implanted see well without glasses and only need to wear a standard lens to correct any minor unresolved refractive error and to provide reading vision.

Summary

Nurses play an important role in helping older persons with visual impairment adapt and adjust their patterns of daily living to accommodate to their loss of vision. For those whose loss is compounded by other system pathology, this adjustment may be incomplete, involving dependence and institutionalization. However, for the majority of people the adjustment is complete and made gracefully over time as alternate resources are found. The goal is to assist the elderly person to optimal function and optimal lifestyle.

References and Other Readings

Allinson R. Glaucoma. Geriatric Medicine Update and Board Certification Review Course, February 1–5, 1990.

Arentsen J. The dry eye. J Ophthal Nurs Tech 1987; 6:134.

Boyd-Monk H. How to use a direct ophthalmoscope. J Ophthal Nurs Tech 1991; 10:23.

Boyd-Monk H, Steinmetz C. Nursing care of the eye. Norwalk, CT: Appleton & Lange, 1987.

Brenner A. Diagnostic tests and procedures: applying the nursing process. Norwalk, CT: Appleton & Lange, 1987.

Bressler N, Bressler S, Fine S. Age-related macular degeneration. Surv Ophthalmol 1988; 32:375.

Dangel M, Hovener W. Drugs and the aging eye. Geriatrics 1981; 38:133.

Edmonds S. Resources for the visually impaired. J Ophthal Nurs Tech 1990; 9:14.

Eifrig D, Simons K. An overview of common geriatric ophthalmologic disorders. Geriatrics 1983; 38:55.

Engelstein J. Cataract surgery: current options and problems. Orlando, FL: Grune & Stratton, 1984.

Genesky S, Zarit S. In: Rosenbloom A Jr, Morgan M. Vision and aging. New York: Professional Press Books, Fairchild Publications, 1986.

Gerali P, DiVerde M. Glaucoma high risk alert. J Ophthal Nurs Tech 1991; 10:34.

Glaser J. History taking. In: Duane T, ed. Clinical ophthalmology. Hagerstown, MD: Harper & Row, 1984.

Goldstein J. Ocular side effects of systemic drugs. J Ophthal Nurs Tech 1986; 5:103.

Goldstein J. Pharmacology of ophthalmic drugs. Part I. J Ophthal Nurs Tech 1987; 6:146.

Goldstein J. Pharmacology of ophthalmic drugs. Part II. J Ophthal Nurs Tech 1987; 6:193.

Gordon A, Katz N. Reaching out to the older person. J Visual Impair Blind 1987; 81:301.

Jairath N, et al. Effective discharge preparation of elderly cataract day surgery patients. J Ophthal Nurs Tech 1990; 9:157.

Kwitko M, Weinstock F, eds. Geriatric ophthalmology. New York: Grune & Stratton, 1985.

Morse A, Silberman R, Trief E. Aging and visual impairment. J Visual Impair Blind 1987; 81:308.

Parker P. The eyecare group. J Ophthal Nurs Tech 1990; 9:240.

Pavan-Langston P, Dunkel E. Handbook of ocular drug therapy and ocular side effects of systemic drugs. Boston: Little, Brown and Company, 1991.

Resler M, Tumulty G. Glaucoma update. Am Nurs J 1983; 83:752.

Roach V. Diabetic retinopathy. J Ophthal Nurs Tech 1988; 7:166.

Rosenbloom J Jr, Morgan M, eds. Vision and aging. New York: Professional Press Books, Fairchild Publications, 1986.

Roy F. Ocular differential diagnosis, 4th ed. Philadelphia: Lea & Febiger, 1989.

Stark L, Obrecht G, eds. Presbyopia. New York: Professional Press Books, Fairchild Publications, 1987.

Stark W, et al. Trends in cataract surgery and intraocular lenses in the United States. Am J Ophthalmol 1983; 96:304.

Sullivan N. Vision in the elderly. J Gerontol Nurs 1983; 9:228.

Swearinger P. Manual of nursing therapeutics, 2nd ed. St. Louis: C.V. Mosby, 1990.

Todd B. Using eye drops and ointments safely. Geriatr Nurs 1983; 5:53.

Tripathi R, Tripathi, B. Lens morphology, aging and cataract. J Gerontol 1983; 38:258.

Weale R. The eyes of the elderly. Geriatric Med Today 1985; 4:29.

Yannuzzi L, Gitter K, Judson, P. Lasers in ophthalmology. J Ophthal Nurs Tech 1988; 7:199.

Yurick A, et al. The aged person and the nursing process, 3rd ed. Norwalk, CT: Appleton & Lange, 1989.

Index

Page numbers followed by "f" indicate an illustration; those followed by "t" indicate tabular material; drug names are indicated by **boldface** type.

ISBN 0-397-54898-2

90000